Biomedical Engineering and Information Systems:
Technologies, Tools and Applications

Anupam Shukla
Indian Institute of Information Technology and Management Gwalior, India

Ritu Tiwari
Indian Institute of Information Technology and Management Gwalior, India

Medical Information Science REFERENCE

MEDICAL INFORMATION SCIENCE REFERENCE

Hershey · New York

Director of Editorial Content: Kristin Klinger
Director of Book Publications: Julia Mosemann
Acquisitions Editor: Lindsay Johnston
Development Editor: Dave DeRicco
Publishing Assistant: Natalie Pronio
Typesetter: Michael Brehm
Production Editor: Jamie Snavely
Cover Design: Lisa Tosheff
Printed at: Lightning Source

Published in the United States of America by
Medical Information Science Reference (an imprint of IGI Global)
701 E. Chocolate Avenue
Hershey PA 17033
Tel: 717-533-8845
Fax: 717-533-8661
E-mail: cust@igi-global.com
Web site: http://www.igi-global.com

Library of Congress Cataloging-in-Publication Data

Biomedical engineering and information systems : technologies, tools, and applications / Anupam Shukla and Ritu Tiwari, editors.
p. ; cm.
Includes bibliographical references and index.
Summary: "Bridging the disciplines of engineering and medicine, this book informs researchers, clinicians, and practitioners of the latest developments in diagnostic tools, decision support systems, and intelligent devices that impact and redefine research in and delivery of medical services"--Provided by publisher.
ISBN 978-1-61692-004-3 (h/c)
1. Biomedical engineering. 2. Medical informatics. I. Shukla, Anupam, 1965- II. Tiwari, Ritu, 1977-
[DNLM: 1. Biomedical Engineering--methods. 2. Bioengineering--methods. 3. Biotechnology--methods. 4. Information Systems. W 36 B615 2010]
R856.B495 2010
610.28--dc22

2010009790

British Cataloguing in Publication Data
A Cataloguing in Publication record for this book is available from the British Library.

Editorial Advisory Board

List of Reviewers

Table of Contents

Detailed Table of Contents

Microfluidics has shown very good effects in both fundamental and applied research in the field of vascular bioengineering, biotechnology, biomedicine and bio-informatics. In this chapter, we describe the basic principles of microfluidic flow and fabrication techniques as well as explanation of current research and development in the applications of microfluidic devices in diagnostic and prognostic vascular bioengineering. The field is still in its initial stage and has a tremendous reseacrh as it matures to deliver commercially real life products.

In this chapter investigate the effect on charged particles of three possible combinations of alternating and static electromagnetic fields: (i) AC electric field and DC magnetic field (ii) AC magnetic field and DC magnetic field (iii) AC electric field and AC and DC magnetic field.

In this chapter authors try to explain difficulties in biomedical engineering in society and scientific research. Being intrinsically multi- and inter-disciplinary, biomedical engineering lacks precise ethical rules that delineate and delimit professional responsibility, thus blurring the ethical understanding of biomedical engineering. The solution seems to lie in giving due place to human virtues. In the coming days, bioethical issues are expected to be increasingly complicated and dominating the decision-making process owing to the advancements in sciences, and the ever-complicated cases handled by healthcare professionals.

The current work presents a medical watermarking method through contour detection and recovery for the authenticity of bio-medical images, which uses the region growing algorithm and human visual system (HVS). The proposed scheme makes the use of watermarking in biomedical for security purpose.

In this chapter, describe a new idea for measurement of accelerometers and gyroscopes devices in the real life application. They are also explaining the weakness and difficulties of current devices. They proposed some idea to remove problems with the help of fast Fourier transform (FFT).

We present a novel electrical impedance tomography algorithm for reconstruction of layered biological tissues with piecewise continuous plane-stratified profiles. The algorithm is based on the reconstruction scheme for piecewise constant conductivity profiles, which utilizes Legendre expansion in conjunction with improved Prony method.

In this chapter work an attempt is made to develop an intelligent Decision support system (IDSS) using the pathological attributes to predict the fetal delivery to be done normal or by surgical procedure. Soft computing technique namely Artificial Neural Networks (ANN) are used for simulator. The attributes from dataset are used for training & testing of ANN models.

In this chapter we deal with the methods to handle these situations. The continuous research in machine learning and biomedical field has resulted in a large amount of database being created for many diseases, which becomes very difficult to fit as an input to the simulator for training. This increases the dimensionality of the problem and ultimately leads to poor performance. We discuss the method of division of the attributes to reduce the training time and complexity.

In this chapter author's try to give the best model for breast cancer among available models in the world. Now a day's computer systems are widely used in medical diagnosis systems. In biomedical research they are still finding efficient methods, which can deal with all types of data as well as medical images. These modellings tools include, Hidden Markov Model (HMM), Fuzzy Logic (FL) and Artificial Neural Network (ANN) can highlight the important features that play pivotal roles in the classification an aid physicians to diagnose and prognosticate breast cancer.

There is a necessity of efficient and effective techniques, which can clearly separate individual MUAPs from the complex EMG without loss of diagnostic information. This chapter deals with the techniques of decomposition based on statistical pattern recognition, cross-correlation, Kohonen self-organizing map and wavelet transform.

Cryopreservation of sperm has many applications in agriculture, biotechnology, and clinical medicine. The spermatozoon is a very specialized cell that loses the ability of biosynthesis, repair, growth and cell division during the final phase of spermatogenesis. Cryopreservation of sperm generally requires a reduction or arrest of the metabolism of cells, thereby prolonging their life. It is difficult to analyze the beneficial/detrimental effects of a particular compound on sperm cryopreservation. We have briefly discussed the knowledge and limitations of the current semen cryopreservation technology and mainly focused on the development of a simple cryopreservation model using chemically-defined medium and goat cauda-epididymal sperm.

In this chapter, we describe the Computational methods for prediction of recognition helices for C2H2 zinc fingers that bind to specific target DNA sites could provide valuable insights for researchers interested in designing specific zinc finger proteins for biological and biomedical applications. Zinc finger protein-DNA interaction patterns, challenges in engineering the recognition-specificity of zinc finger proteins, the computational methods of prediction of proteins that recognize specific target DNA sequence and their applications in molecular therapeutics.

Preface

This book is basically the result of 20 years of teaching the material to Electronics communication, Information Technology, Computer Science Engineering, Bioinformatics, Biotechnology Engineering and biomedical engineering students. Some of the "students" have also been faculty and post graduate. I am very grateful to them for their patience and tolerance as it progressed from crude notes to its present form.

We describe in chapter 1, Microfluidics is the manipulation and control of fluids in small scale, and has heralded a new age in science as evidenced by the rapid increase in the amount and quality of academic and industrial research output in this area in the recent times. Microfluidics has shown tremendous promise in both fundamental and applied research in the field of vascular bioengineering. In this review, we outline the basic principles of microfluidic flow and fabrication techniques, and describe the recent advances in the applications of microfluidic devices in diagnostic and prognostic vascular bioengineering. The field is still in its infancy and has a great potential for research and development as it matures to deliver commercially viable products. This review, focusing on the current status of microfluidic applications to diagnose and treat blood-related disorders, should be a valuable and opportune addition to the literature of interest to both academia and industry.

We describe in chapter 2, Electromagnetic fields (EMF) are essential to various applications directly involving humans. Fears about the biological effect of exposure to electromagnetic fields drive enormous research into this area. This research generates conflicting results, and consequently, uncertainty regarding possible health effects. This chapter studies a nonlinear Lorenz model describing interactions among charged particles and combined alternating (AC - alternating current) and static (DC - direct current) electromagnetic fields, for various combinations of frequencies, field strengths and relative angle (θ) between the AC and DC magnetic fields. We investigate the effect on charged particles of three possible combinations of alternating and static electromagnetic fields: (i) AC electric field and DC magnetic field (ii) AC magnetic field and DC magnetic field (iii) AC electric field and AC and DC magnetic field. Then the behavior of the particle in these fields with different initial conditions and strong directional effects is observed when the angle between AC and DC magnetic fields is varied. The results show that the cyclotron resonance frequency is affected by charged particles' initial position and initial velocity. Further, we observe strong effects of electric and magnetic fields on a charged particle in a biological cell with initial position and initial velocity.

We describe in chapter 3, Biomedical engineering is an advanced and relatively new field in the healthcare sector. Owing to the very nature of the various professional challenges faced by healthcare professionals, the moral and ethical values seem to have taken the backburner. The factors contributing to it may include a sound knowledge of the healthcare professional on the legally-permissible ethical values, and the desperate situations requiring precise split-moment decision-making. No technological advancement without a human face is worth it, and hence, during the course of the degree, a biomedical engineering student needs to be exposed to various ethical issues through theory, live cases and demonstrations. Being intrinsically multi- and inter-disciplinary, biomedical engineering lacks precise ethical rules that delineate and delimit professional responsibility, thus blurring the ethical understanding of biomedical engineering. The solution seems to lie in giving due place to human virtues. In the coming days, bioethical issues are expected to be increasingly complicated and dominating the decision-making process owing to the advancements in sciences, and the ever-complicated cases handled by healthcare professionals. A global healthcare and ethics-related online open-access portal may serve as a common platform for all the stakeholders in the interest and ethical growth of biomedical engineering in particular and medical sciences in general.

We describe in chapter 4, a medical watermarking method through contour detection and recovery for the authenticity of bio-medical images, which uses the region growing algorithm and human visual system (HVS). The proposed scheme makes the use of neighbourhood region for converting non-specific discontinuous region into specific continuous contour data. This contour as a fragile watermark is embedded in the perceptually insignificant, spatially selected detail coefficients using sub band adaptive threshold scheme along with the EPR as a robust one. Here, a new type of non-oblivious detection method is also proposed. The improvement in performance is supported through experimental results. The reported result shows improvement in visual and statistical invisibility of the hidden data. Moreover, this algorithmic architecture utilizes the existing allocated bandwidth in the data transmission channel in a more efficient manner.

We describe in chapter 5, the use of inertial sensors to measure human movement has recently gained momentum with the advent of low cost micro-electro-mechanical systems (MEMS) technology. These sensors comprise accelerometer and gyroscopes which measure accelerations and angular velocities respectively. This chapter investigates the spectral evaluation of individual sensor errors and looks at the effectiveness of minimizing these errors using static digital filters. The primary focus is on the derivation of foot displacement data from inertial sensor measurements. The importance of foot, in particular toe displacement measurements is evident in the context of tripping and falling which are serious health concerns for the elderly. The Minimum Toe Clearance (MTC) as an important gait variable for falls-risk prediction and assessment, and therefore the measurement variable of interest. A brief sketch of the current devices employing accelerometers and gyroscopes is presented, highlighting the problems and difficulties reported in literature to achieve good precision. These have been mainly due to the presence of sensor errors and the error accumulative process employed in obtaining displacement measurements. The investigation first proceeds to identify the location of these sensor errors in the frequency domain using the Fast Fourier Transform (FFT) on raw inertial sensor data. The frequency content of velocity and displacement measurements obtained from integrating the inertial data using a well known strap-down method is then explored. These investigations revealed that large sensor errors occurred mainly in the low frequency spectrum while white noise exists in all frequency spectra. The efficacy of employing a band-pass filter to remove a large portion of these errors and their effect on the derived displacements is elaborated on. The cross-correlation of the FFT power spectra from a highly accurate optical measurement system and processed sensor data is used as a metric to evaluate the performance of the band-pass filter at several stages of the processing stage. The motivation is that a more fundamental method would require less computational demand and could lead to more efficient implementations in low-power and systems with limited resources, so that portable sensor based motion measurement system would provide a good degree of measurement accuracy.

We describe in chapter 6, Image reconstruction by electrical impedance tomography is, generally, an ill-posed nonlinear inverse problem. Regularization methods are widely used to ensure a stable solution. Herein, we present a novel electrical impedance tomography algorithm for reconstruction of layered biological tissues with piecewise continuous plane-stratified profiles. The algorithm is based on the reconstruction scheme for piecewise constant conductivity profiles, which utilizes Legendre expansion in conjunction with improved Prony method. This reconstruction procedure, which calculates both the locations and the conductivities, repetitively provides inhomogeneous depth discretization, i.e., the depths grid is not equispaced. Incorporation of this specific inhomogeneous grid in the widely used mean least square reconstruction procedure results in a stable and accurate reconstruction, whereas, the commonly selected equispaced depth grid leads to unstable reconstruction. This observation establishes the main result of our investigation, highlighting the impact of physical phenomenon (image theory) on electrical impedance tomography; leading to a physically motivated stabilization of the inverse problem, i.e., an inhomogeneous depth discretization renders an inherent regularization of the mean least square algorithm.

We describe in chapter 7, an intelligent Decision support system (IDSS) using the pathological attributes to predict the fetal delivery to be done normal or by surgical procedure. The pathological tests like Blood Sugar (BR), Blood pressure (BP), Resistivity Index (RI) and systolic / Diastolic (S/P) ratio will be recorded at the time of delivery. All attributes lie within a specific range for normal patient. The database consists of the attributes for cases 2 i.e. normal and surgical delivery. Soft computing technique namely Artificial Neural Networks (ANN) are used for simulator. The attributes from dataset are used for training & testing of ANN models. Three models of ANN are trained using Back-Propagation Algorithm (BPA), Radial Basis Function Network (RBFN), Learning Vector Quantization Network (LVQN) and one hybrid approach is Adaptive Neuro-Fuzzy Inference System (ANFIS). Hence in our present research the ANFIS is the model whom efficiency and result are best .The ANFIS is the best network for mentioned problem. This system will assist doctor to take decision at the critical time of fetal delivery.

We describe in chapter 8, intelligent systems has spread its fruits to the field of biomedical engineering as well; where a series of models are being applied to automatically detect diseases based on some parameters or inputs. The continuous research in this field has resulted in a large amount of database being created for many diseases which becomes very difficult to train. Also the number of attributes is under constant rise. This increases the dimensionality of the problem and ultimately leads to poor performance. In this chapter we deal with the methods to handle these situations. We discuss the mechanism to divide data between different sub-systems. We also discuss the method of division of the attributes to reduce the training time and complexity. The resultant systems are able to train better due to low computational cost and hence give better performance. We validated this with the Breast Cancer database from the UCI Machine Learning repository and found our algorithm optimal.

We describe in chapter 9, Breast cancer is the second most common cancer in the world and is difficult to accurately identify and treat. Diagnostic computational tools can be used effectively, with high degree of accuracy, to determine and distinguish between the two known types of breast cancer namely benign and malignant. These modeling's tools include, Hidden Markov Model (HMM), Fuzzy Logic (FL) and Artificial Neural Network (ANN) can highlight the important features that play pivotal roles in the classification an aid physicians to diagnose and prognosticate breast cancer. Moreover, recent advancement in nanotechnology indicates that with the aid of nanoparticles, nanowires, nanorobots and nanotubes breast cancer can be totally eradicated. The chapter highlights the limitations of the current therapies used in breast cancer and discusses the concept of nanotechnology as a possible future therapy.

We describe in chapter 10, the information extracted from the EMG recordings is of great clinical importance and is used for the diagnosis and treatment of neuromuscular disorders and to study muscle fatigue and neuromuscular control mechanism. Thus there is a necessity of efficient and effective techniques, which can clearly separate individual MUAPs from the complex EMG without loss of diagnostic information. This chapter deals with the techniques of decomposition based on statistical pattern recognition, cross-correlation, Kohonen self-organizing map and wavelet transform.

We describe in chapter 11, In most healthcare systems, this is achieved through exchange of medical information, phone calls and conversations. In an ideal world, this exchange of health information between disparate providers, healthcare systems, laboratories, pharmacies and payers would be achieved electronically and seamlessly. The potential benefits of electronic health exchange are improved patient care, increased efficiency of the healthcare system and decreased costs. The reality is that health information is electronically exchanged only to a limited extent within local communities and regions, much less nationally and internationally. One main challenge has been the inability of health information exchange organizations to develop a solid business case.

We describe in chapter 12, the World Wide Web has made available a large variety of medical information and education resources only dreamed of two decades ago. This review discusses a number of Web-based e-Medical education concepts and resources likely to be of interest to the medical education community as well as a number of other groups. The resources described focus especially on those that are free and those that have an interactive component. The importance of interactivity and its role in the "constructivist" approach to education is emphasized. Problem-based learning in medical education is also discussed. In addition, the importance of "Web 2.0" and related developments is discussed, along with an overview of Web-based medical simulation software that can complement medical education programs.

We describe in chapter 13, despite the importance of medical records, relatively little is known about medical transcription, a process through which voice files are transformed into healthcare documentation. This lack of knowledge is evident in academic research with no previous studies of medical transcriptionists (MTs) or the medical transcription service organizations (MTSOs) in existence despite the central role of the industry in the creation of healthcare documentation. While its general aim is to document the impact of technology on the process of medical transcription, the topic resides in a broader array of issues that include the impact of technology on the workplace, and how assumptions of work drive technological design. The central issue being examined is what is the extent to which technology can replace workers and how design decisions impact practice by either facilitating or impeding it. Given the thing being produced is vital for medical treatment, resolving this question is not only of academic interest, but important to everyone who has a medical record.

We describe in chapter 14, Making the knowledge and expertise of human experts more widely available through computer consultation systems has been recognized as an important tool for improving the access to high quality health care. The software development exploits the potential of human intelligence such as reasoning, making decision, learning (by experiencing) and many others. Artificial intelligence is not a new concept, yet it has been accepted as a new technology in computer science. It has been applied in many areas such as education, business, medical and manufacturing. This chapter explores the potential of artificial intelligence techniques in medical applications.

We describe in chapter 15, Cryopreservation of sperm has many applications in agriculture, biotechnology, and clinical medicine. The spermatozoon is a very specialized cell that loses the ability of biosynthesis, repair, growth and cell division during the final phase of spermatogenesis. Cryopreservation of sperm generally requires a reduction or arrest of the metabolism of cells, thereby prolonging their life. Semen samples of mammalian species are diluted with a suitable diluent [containing a complex extender (e.g., egg-yolk, milk, milk-whey), cryoprotectant (e.g., glycerol)] and processed through different freezing protocol prior to storage in liquid nitrogen (-196C). Despite the use of complex media and cryoprotectants, a substantial portion of the cells die during freezing and thawing (recovery rate do not exceeds more than 50%). As the complex media contain large numbers of undefined biomolecules (proteins, lipids, carbohydrates), it is difficult to analyze the beneficial/detrimental effects of a particular compound on sperm cryopreservation.

We describe in chapter 16, Custom-designed zinc finger proteins attached to various DNA-modifying domains can be used to achieve highly specific genome modification, which has tremendous applications in molecular therapeutics. Analysis of sequence and structure of the zinc finger proteins provides clues for understanding protein-DNA interactions and aid in custom-design of zinc finger proteins with tailor-made specificity. Computational methods for prediction of recognition helices for C2H2 zinc fingers that bind to specific target DNA sites could provide valuable insights for researchers interested in designing specific zinc finger proteins for biological and biomedical applications. In this chapter, we describe the zinc finger protein-DNA interaction patterns, challenges in engineering the recognition-specificity of zinc finger proteins, the computational methods of prediction of proteins that recognize specific target DNA sequence and their applications in molecular therapeutics.

Dr. Anupam Shukla and Dr. Ritu Tiwari
Indian Institute of Information Technology and Management Gwalior, India

Chapter 1
Microfluidic Applications in Vascular Bioengineering

Anand Srinivasan
The University of Texas at San Antonio, USA

José L. López-Ribot
The University of Texas at San Antonio, USA

Anand K. Ramasubramanian
The University of Texas at San Antonio, USA

ABSTRACT

Microfluidics is the manipulation and control of fluids in small scale, and has heralded a new age in science as evidenced by the rapid increase in the amount and quality of academic and industrial research output in this area in the recent times. Microfluidics has shown tremendous promise in both fundamental and applied research in the field of vascular bioengineering. In this review, we outline the basic principles of microfluidic flow and fabrication techniques, and describe the recent advances in the applications of microfluidic devices in diagnostic and prognostic vascular bioengineering. The field is still in its infancy and has a great potential for research and development as it matures to deliver commercially viable products. This review, focusing on the current status of microfluidic applications to diagnose and treat blood-related disorders, should be a valuable and opportune addition to the literature of interest to both academia and industry.

INTRODUCTION

Blood, the vascular tissue, is vital for nutrient transport, immune-surveillance, hemostasis, and wound healing, all of which are critical in order to maintain normal physiology (Lichtman, et al., 2006; Rosenberg & Aird, 1999). Consequently, the pathophysiology of a large number of diseases can be traced to abnormalities in blood flow and function. Hence, assays for composition and function of blood are crucial in both diagnosis and treatment of diseases (Barone & Feuerstein, 1999; Danesh, Collins, Appleby, & Peto, 1998; VanWijk, VanBavel, Sturk, & Nieuwland, 2003).

Blood is a complex tissue comprised of both cellular and acellular components. The cellular components are composed of erythrocytes, leukocytes, and platelets, and the acellular components

DOI: 10.4018/978-1-61692-004-3.ch001

are comprised of lipids, lipoproteins, carbohydrates, and numerous proteins of widely differing structural and functional attributes. Blood-based assays often require isolating and identifying certain specific cell population or molecular entity as a marker for the presence and activity of diseases (Packard & Libby, 2008). For instance, the presence of antibody against varicella indicates the immunization status against chicken pox (Gilden, Cohrs, Mahalingam, & Nagel, 2009); or the presence and number of CD45+ lymphocyte population is a measure of the severity of myeloid leukemia (Countouriotis, Moore, & Sakamoto, 2002). Hence, sample preparation process, which may involve separating one or more components of the blood, is the first and important step for blood assays. Upon extraction of the components of interest, the next step is functional assay or molecular analysis to obtain the requisite clinical or scientific information. This is achieved by identifying specific proteins on cell surface such as cluster of differentiation (CD) markers or identifying free proteins or lipids present in the plasma by using detection systems such as optical or fluorescence read-outs. Thus, the entire process usually takes at least a few hundred microliters to a few tens of milliliters of sample volume. Furthermore, such a process involves separation of cells from plasma, and isolation and retrieval of specific population of cells or proteins for detection and analysis (Gatti, et al., 2009; Kraemer & Maurer, 1998). Unfortunately, these assays suffer from a number of disadvantages: large sample volumes, long assay time period or low throughput, lack of sensitivity, and often a need for a centralized test station. These disadvantages adversely impact diagnosis, treatment and patient recovery thus increasing healthcare costs, morbidity and even mortality rates.

Recent progress in multiplexed, high-throughput screening (HTS) methods, particularly, microfluidics has greatly alleviated these problems, thus making blood-based assays rapid, reliable, informative, and inexpensive (Bange, Halsall, & Heineman, 2005; D'Orazio, 2003; Whitesides, 2006). The greatest advantage of microfluidic technology is miniaturization, which substantially cuts down reagent use, analysis time and assay costs, and minimizes or eliminates labor intensive steps (D'Orazio, 2003). Over the last decade, microfluidic technology has been bolstered by advances on several fronts: transfer of know-how and skills on microfabrication from microelectronic industry, liquid handling and dispensing capability, process control and automation, development of novel materials, and development of better analytical tools for detection (Verpoorte & De Rooij, 2003). As a result, microfluidics is poised to revolutionize the field of wet-lab science in just the same way microelectronics revolutionized the semi-conductor industry about a generation ago. Literature reports indicate that the number of patents issued for microfluidic devices have increased from less than 20 in 1998 to more than 350 in 2004 (Haber, 2006).

Of interest, microfluidics is particularly suited for vascular bioengineering applications because the *in vitro* flow system can be designed to accurately mimic the *in vivo* blood flow patterns or hemodynamics, thus making the microfluidic assays physiologically relevant. Microfluidic systems offer a number of advantages including miniaturization, laminar flow characteristics, large surface area to volume ratio, and decrease in reaction time. Microfluidic applications in vascular bioengineering have seen a leap in past few years as evidenced by the rapid increase in the amount and quality research output in this area. A 'web of science' search on 'microfluidics and blood' show that on an average less than two articles were published every year till 2003, but has risen steadily ever since with nearly 45 articles in 2008 alone.

In this review, we will highlight some of the important advances in microfluidics applications in vascular bioengineering. First, we will discuss the principles that govern flow in microfluidics. Next, we will detail the various fabrication techniques that are employed for the design of microfluidic devices. Finally, we enumerate a number of different applications of the microfluidic devices in vascular research focusing on problems of fundamental interest, and also diagnostic and therapeutic applications.

FLOW IN MICROFLUIDIC DEVICES

Microfluidic devices control and manipulate flow in dimensions of a few tens to a few hundreds of micrometers (Minerick, 2008; Stone, Stroock, & Ajdari, 2004). While we most commonly encounter macroscopic flow such as surface waves or supersonic jets, microscopic flow or flow in microchannels is not visually obvious. However, it is ubiquitous in nature such as water flow in plant sap, flow through gills of a fish, or blood flow in microvessels (Vogel, 1994). Fluid flow in small scale exhibits a number of interesting effects, which can be used creatively for the development of novel devices. 'Small scale' refers to length scales wherein the dimensions of the flow channel are comparable to that of molecular or suspended entities in the fluid. At these length scales, the interfacial and intermolecular interactions become important and the laws of continuum mechanics start to breakdown. For instance, it is well documented that the behavior of molecules at small length scales of the order of a few nanometers, particularly at a phase interface is different from that of the bulk properties (Israelachvili, 2006). In microcirculation through capillaries, the rheology of blood is distinctly different from larger vessels since at small capillary diameters (< 200 μm), the size of the vessel becomes comparable to that of the diameter of blood cells (Popel & Johnson, 2005).

Most microfluidic devices take advantage of the fact that as the length decreases, the surface area ($\sim L^2$) to volume ($\sim L^3$) ratio ($1/L$) increases linearly, thus making interfacial and intermolecular interactions more important. This allows us to utilize surfaces to more effectively impart forces to manipulate and alter bulk fluid flow (Minerick, 2008). Probably the most important quantity in fluid mechanics is Reynolds number, defined as $Re = Lv\rho/\mu$, where L is length, v is velocity, and ρ and μ are density and viscosity of the fluid respectively. Reynolds number represents the ratio of inertial to viscous forces that drive fluid flow (Bird, Stewart, & Lightfoot, 1960). At a Reynolds number below 2000, the flow is laminar, i.e., the fluid moves as parallel sheets with only diffusive (viscous) transport between the layers. On the other hand, at high Reynolds number, the flow is turbulent with considerable, often irreproducible and chaotic mixing. For an incompressible, Newtonian fluid, the fluid flow is governed by Navier-Stokes equation: $\mathrm{Re}\left[u \bullet \nabla u\right] = -\nabla p + \nabla^2 u$, where u is velocity, and p is pressure. Thus, because of the small length scale of microfluidic devices, flow is inherently laminar at low Reynolds number (Re ~0), and the inertial term on the left is negligible compared to the pressure and viscous terms on the right. Such flow, also called creeping flow, is controlled by viscous forces that enable precise manipulation of diffusion and reaction rates.

Another parameter which is particularly important in multiphase flow is "Capillary number" (Shui, Eijkel, & van den Berg, 2007). Capillary number is defined as $Ca = \eta v/g\sigma$, where η is viscosity, v is flow velocity, g is geometrical constant and σ is surface tension. Capillary number is the ratio of viscous to surface tension forces, thus defining the ability of individual drops to remain as drops without coalescing under laminar flow conditions. Though the capillary number does not directly account for dimensions, the increase in surface area to volume ratio in microfluidic chambers can result in an increase in the interfacial area and the interactions between different phases in a multiphase system. Thus, in microfluidic devices, the increase in interfacial area between multiple phases can be exploited for controlling

Table 1. Driving forces typically used in generating flow in microfluidic devices

Driving force	Generator	Reference
Pressure gradient	Syringe pump	(Kline, Runyon, Pothiawala, & Ismagilov, 2008)
Centrifugal force	Rotation on source axis	(Cho, et al., 2007)
Surface tension	Capillary action	(Martinez, Phillips, Butte, & Whitesides, 2007)
Magnetic force	External magnetic field	(Yang, Lien, Huang, Lei, & Lee, 2008)
Electric field	Dielectrophoresis	(Kulp, Vaher, & Kaljurand, 2005)

reaction rates, interfacial transport, mixing, and separation processes.

In addition, because of the ability to apply larger surface forces, flow through microfluidic channels can be accomplished in a number of ways which may not be possible in macroscopic flow. The commonly used driving forces for blood-based assays are listed in Table 1.

A number of other force fields have been reported in other systems elsewhere (Stone, et al., 2004). The pressure driven flow is typically generated using a syringe pump (Kline, et al., 2008) or gravity flow, and the centrifugal force driven flow is generated by rotation (Cho, et al., 2007) with respect to the source reservoir as axis. Flow can also be generated in microfluidic systems using an external magnetic field (Yang, et al., 2008) or electric field (Kulp, et al., 2005), and are needed at much lower strength than in macroscopic systems. The electric field driven flow is generated because of electro-kinetic force, which arises when the fluid in contact with the wall gets polarized because of the adsorption of ions from the fluid on to the wall of the channel. This polarization becomes particularly important in small channels and can be utilized to manipulate fluid flow in microsystems.

FABRICATION OF MICROFLUIDIC DEVICES

The idea of lithography was culled from the notion of Alois Senefelder dating back to the 18th century, and it literally means "writing on stone". Over the recent years, lithographic techniques have been adapted to create Lab-On-Chip (LOC) devices that enable miniaturization, integration and automation of biochemical assays ideal for high-throughput analysis of biological samples (Abdelgawad, et al., 2008; Weibel, DiLuzio, & Whitesides, 2007). The basic principle of lithography is creating patterns of interest on metallic or polymeric substrates by etching or deposition, and can be achieved in a number of different ways, such as photolithography, soft lithography, electron-beam lithography, magnetic lithography, and paper-based lithography. Of these, photolithography and soft lithography have been exploited for a variety of biomedical applications because of the processing advantages and versatility. Paper-based lithography is becoming increasingly popular because of ease-of-use and low cost. Since a majority of microfluidic applications involve structures a few tens to hundreds of nanometers, a Class 10,000 or less clean-room facility is desirable in order to prevent obvious hindrance from air-borne contaminants.

Photolithography

Photolithography has been extensively used in the fabrication of semiconductors to construct Integrated Circuits, and Micro Electro Mechanical Systems (MEMS). Microfluidics chips by photolithography are fabricated in a fashion similar to that of semiconductor chips, and the process is outlined in Figure 1. (A). First a polymeric photoresist such as SU-8, is layered on top of a silicon wafer, followed by a mask which has the one-dimensional topography of the negative of the desired pattern(Becker & Gärtner, 2008). The mask-photoresist-wafer is exposed to UV light, which results in a pattern on the wafer (Figure 1. [A]). The duration of UV treatment determines the geometry of the microstructure. After removal of the mask, the photoresist is washed off by chemical treatment to produce the 'master'. Finally, the fabricated silicon masters are sealed to glass to create microfluidic channels. These silicon-based chips are robust and have been used for a number of biomedical applications (Becker & Gärtner, 2008; R. Huang, et al., 2008). Photolithography can generate microstructures as small as 100 nm (Xia & Whitesides, 1998). Despite the durability of devices made using silicon wafers and glass, photolithography has a few disadvantages including the inability to pattern non-planar three dimensional structures and in fabricating flow control units such as pumps and valves. These limitations that arise due to the rigidity of the silicon and glass substrates have forced photolithography to make way for soft lithography (Quake & Scherer, 2000).

Soft Lithography

Soft lithography or "Smart lithography" is expedient in using a soft material (elastomer) which is flexible, inert for biological samples, cheaper than silica and easy to concoct (Whitesides, 2006). Poly(dimethylsiloxane) or PDMS is most commonly used since it is a cheap, rubber-like elastomer with good optical transparency and biocompatibility. In order to create patterns of interest, a mold that has the inverse topography of the desired pattern is fabricated using photolithography (Figure 1. [B]). The 'Replica molding' process involves casting the PDMS elastomer base for the mold with a suitable curing agent. The elastomer now has the inverse topography of the mold. After curing, the PDMS elastomer is peeled off the mold and stuck to a flat glass substrate, both of which have previously been activated by oxygen plasma treatment. This results in irreversible covalent bonding through a condensation reaction resulting in a Si-O-Si bond. Thus it is possible to have channel operation with pumps at a pressure of about 350 kPa without any leakage or failure (Xia & Whitesides, 1998). The softness and ease of fabrication of PDMS have been particularly advantageous in the construction of microfluidic devices with channels of varying cross-section, valves, pumps and mixers (Unger, Chou, Thorsen, Scherer, & Quake, 2000). Valves are fabricated with crossed channel architecture with a thin layer of polymer sheet in between two perpendicular channels so that when pressure is applied to the upper (control) channel, it shuts the flow in the lower (main flow) channel (Figure 1. [C]). The response time of devices actuated in this fashion is ~1 ms, and the applied pressure is ~100 kPa so that a 100 μm by 100 μm area gives actuation force ~1 mN (Unger, et al., 2000). Pumps are constructed in a similar fashion with the top control channel actuating many fluid channels beneath, all of which discharge into a common manifold. The top control channel is opened and closed at high frequencies (10 kHz or more) thrusting the liquid forward. Mixers are constructed as circular channels wherein the liquid is trapped by closing the inlet and outlet (on either side in Figure 1. [D]), and opening and closing air valves cyclically to mix the trapped liquid. Such devices have found applications in several fields (Chou, Spence, Scherer, & Quake, 1999; Effenhauser, Bruin, Paulus, & Ehrat, 1997; Fu, Spence, Scherer, Arnold, & Quake, 1999). Soft lithography can print microstructures of lateral dimensions as small as 30-100 nm. A variety of polymers, sol-gel, colloidal materials, and biological macromolecules can be patterned directly by this technique.

Paper-Based Microfluidics

Paper-based microfluidic devices are constructed from patterned paper (Figure 1. [E, F]). Test paper strips are covalently conjugated with detection

Figure 1. Schematic of microfabrication techniques. (A) Photolithography: The mask-photoresist-wafer is exposed UV to create the desired pattern on the wafer. The photoresist is washed off, and the wafer is sealed with a glass substrate to generate microfluidic channels; (B) Soft lithography: Casting a microchannel with an optically transparent biocompatible elastomer on a suitable mold and sealed with a glass substrate; (C) Microvalves: Valves are fabricated with crossed channel architecture separated by a thin polymer sheet. The flow through the bottom channel is controlled by air flow in the top channel, which deflects the polymer sheet; (D) Micromixers: Fluid trapped in the central circular loop is mixed by propelling fluid flow at high frequencies through pneumatically controlled air flow; (E) Paper-based microfluidics (2D): Fluid flow driven by capillary effect is exploited for particulate detection of the sample by colorimetric or fluorimetric detection; (F) Paper-based microfluidics (3D): Alternating stacks of paper and tape are arranged such that capillary-driven flow generates streams of fluids cross each other without mixing (adapted from (A.W. Martinez, et al., 2008))

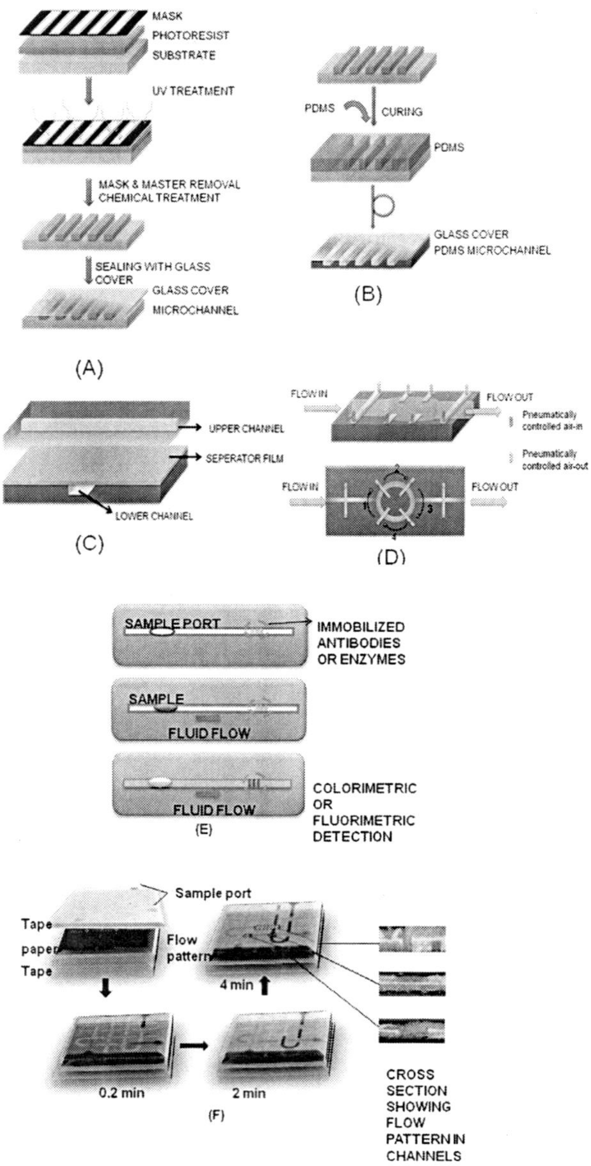

antibodies or enzymes that bind to the protein of interest (Martinez, et al., 2007; A. W. Martinez, et al., 2008). The sample is dropped on the strip, and is allowed to wet the strip by capillary action. If the protein is present in the sample, it can bind to the antibody or can be hydrolyzed by the enzyme immobilized on the strip. This results in a fluorimetric or a colorimetric signal, which can be quantified with a detector or a reader. This idea can be extended to multiple microchannels which are separated by hydrophobic coating that are carved out on a single strip of paper. Such systems can be used for multiplexed assays. Paper-based devices offer numerous advantages including inexpensive substrate, capillary action for conducting samples that precludes any need for external pumps, ease of construction, and contamination-free operation. Paper-based systems have found a number of applications in recent years including chromatographic separation, on-chip glucose and protein assay (Martinez, et al., 2007). Recently paper-based microfluidics were also used for 3D microfluidic bioassays, wherein paper and double-sided adhesive tape were patterned and stacked in 3D such that fluid flows within and between layers of paper (Martinez, Phillips, & Whitesides, 2008). This arrangement results in distribution of samples into thousands of arrays of detection zones. Such multiplexed paper-based devices are truly high-throughput and are advantageous for diagnosis in low-resource settings.

MICROFLUIDIC APPLICATIONS

Fundamental Understanding of Blood Physiology

Cardiovascular diseases, including heart attack and stroke, are the leading cause of morbidity and mortality in the western world (Koch, et al., 2009). Formation of blood clots or thromboses in blood vessels result in heart attack and stroke. Central to thrombosis is platelet activation and aggregation which is initiated in response to agonists such as ADP or collagen or a reactive surface such as those containing tissue factor (Ishii-Watabe, Uchida, Mizuguchi, & Hayakawa, 2000). Hence accurate assessment of platelet function in response to the agonists is very important for the discovery and development of new therapeutic strategies to combat cardiovascular diseases.

In order to understand platelet aggregation and thrombus formation, *in vivo* animal models have remained a holy grail (Furie & Furie, 2005). However, *in vitro* models that mimic human physiology, such as parallel plate flow chambers have been particularly attractive to tease-out the mechanisms underlying coagulation and bleeding disorders, such as the interaction of platelets with thrombogenic surfaces (R. A. Kumar, et al., 2003; Turner, Moake, & McIntire, 2001). Typically, such flow chambers require more volume of blood, which may be easy to obtain from humans or large animals but is rather difficult from small lab animals like rat or mice. A variety of experiments are only possible with small lab animals, such as with genetically engineered organisms, and often an *in vitro* flow model utilizing only small volumes of blood sample can be very helpful for understanding disease pathophysiology.

A microfluidic flow chamber is particularly advantageous for using small volumes of reagents (Neeves, et al., 2008; Sarvepalli, Schmidtke, & Nollert, 2009). The wall shear stress (τ_W) experienced by cells in flow is given by $\tau_W = \dfrac{6Q\mu}{b^2h}$, where Q is volumetric flow rate, μ is viscosity, and b and h are width and height of the channel respectively. Thus, as the channel dimensions decrease, the flow rate needed to obtain similar wall shear stresses decreases. Sarvepalli *et al.* demonstrate that a 50 μm deep PDMS channel can comfortably be used in place of the conventional flow chambers. These channels, as shown in Figure 2. (A), can be used to study platelet adhesion to thrombogenic (collagen) and non-thrombogenic (albumin) surfaces. Along similar

Figure 2. Microfluidics for studying blood physiology. (A) A microfluidic flow channel demonstrating the differential adhesion of platelets to collagen and not to albumin; (B) Fluorescently-labeled reagents and sample are loaded onto separate wells on the top of a Y channel and allowed to mix as they flow through the channel. The presence of molecules of interest is detected when they bind to the fluorescent reagent downstream (adapted from (Koch, et al., 2009)); (C) The threshold patch size of tissue factor on a surface needed for initiating the clotting process can be detected by microfluidics (taken from (Kastrup, et al., 2007))

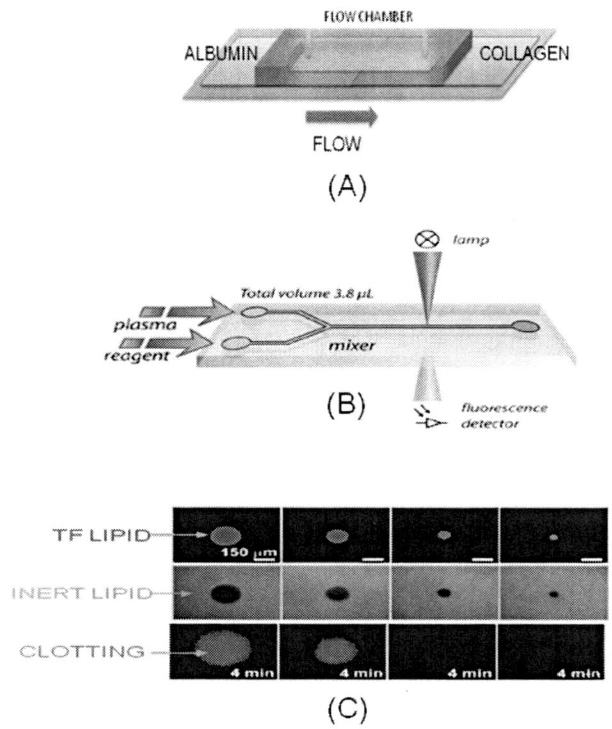

lines, a multiplexed high throughput model was developed by Gutierrez *et al* in which the shear-dependent adhesion of platelets obtained from wild-type and integrin β_3-deficient mice on collagen and fibrinogen coated surfaces were studied simultaneously over a range of shear stress using less than 100 µl blood (Gutierrez, et al., 2008). Kantak *et al.* have developed another multiplexed microchannel model to simultaneously study shear activation of platelets on a number of surfaces assembled layer-by-layer in parallel microchannels (Kantak, Gale, Lvov, & Jones, 2003). In addition to platelet adhesion studies, other cell adhesion studies have also been performed in microfluidic chambers recently including dynamic adhesion of infected erythrocytes to different substrata (Antia, Herricks, & Rathod, 2007), and adhesion of neutrophil to endothelial monolayers (Schaff, et al., 2007). An *ex vivo* autoperfusion model to study blood cell adhesion can be constructed by connecting the microfluidic chip to the artery of an anesthetized rat thereby preventing animal sacrifice (Hafezi-Moghadam, Thomas, & Cornelssen, 2004).

Lab-on-chip devices can also be used for rapid and inexpensive diagnostic tests for clotting factors in plasma. Qualitative and quantitative assessment of clotting factors is critical for evaluating coagulation disorders. Thrombin generation test (TGT) is one of the diagnostic tests used currently to measure coagulation disorder but is very complex, expensive, time consuming and laborious, which can be improved using a microfluidic device (Hemker, et al., 2003). Koch *et al* have devised a microfluidic chamber wherein the sample and reagents can be loaded onto separate wells on the top of a Y channel, and are allowed to mix as they flow through the channel (Figure 2. [B]) (Koch, et al., 2009). The reagents are labeled fluorescently, and hence can be detected by a fluorescence detector. This system reduced the usage of sample volume by more than 30-fold compared to conventional TGT. A microfluidic channel fabricated with soft lithography was used to monitor the agonist-induced platelet activation as measured by ratiometric determination of induced calcium flux in fluor-loaded human platelets (Tran, et al., 2005). This microfluidic assay can screen as many as 900 compounds per hour, with a sensitivity of 5-20 platelets, which is impossible to realize in a conventional assay.

In addition, the transport of activators and inhibitors in a flowing stream of blood can influence the blood clotting process by altering the local concentration of these species (Diamond, 2001; Lo & Diamond, 2004). Microfluidic systems can precisely control the diffusion and reaction length and time scales so that the kinetics of blood clotting can be measured accurately which may not be possible in macroscale studies. Ismagilov and co-workers describe a number of experimental systems and arrive at insightful conclusions on coagulation kinetics (Kastrup, et al., 2008; Kastrup, Shen, Runyon, & Ismagilov, 2007; Runyon, Johnson-Kerner, & Ismagilov, 2004; Runyon, Johnson-Kerner, Kastrup, Van Ha, & Ismagilov, 2007). An interesting example is the identification of a threshold patch size that is necessary for the initiation of coagulation cascade. It was found that the initiation of clotting of platelet rich plasma on to tissue factor embedded in phospholipid patches requires at least a patch diameter $\geq 165\mu m$, suggesting that protein clustering and avidity can be critical in initiating a positive feedback loop (Figure 2. [C]). An extension of this work focused on local bacterial threshold response needed to initiate coagulation since wound healing and coagulation often accompanies microbial infection in blood (Kastrup, et al., 2008). The authors use bacterial surface patterning (a few hundred micrometers in size), and bacteria encapsulated in gel microdroplets containing magnetic particles in a microfluidic channel to study the threshold number of bacteria needed for the coagulation of whole blood. The authors conclude that this threshold bacterial patch size varies with the bacterial strain. Hence this method can be useful in screening strains that can cause clotting during bacterial sepsis, which is important in immunocompromised and immunosuppressed patients.

CELL SEPARATION

The isolation and analysis of cellular components of blood is important for several diagnostic and therapeutic applications. This has been a daunting task because of the number of different cell populations, and the large variation in their concentration. In addition, the isolation has to be pure, free of contaminating cells and gentle without causing any damage. For instance, accurate diagnosis of immune diseases requires isolation of lymphocytes expressing a particular antigen from a large population of blood cells. Microfluidics-based separation techniques have exploited the differences in the physicochemical and biological properties of the blood cells. The heterogeneity in their magnetic, electrical, rheological, physical, and biochemical attributes help the cells differentially segregate under an externally imposed field. These fields are sufficient to segregate the cells in order to obtain a highly pure population and hence no additional labeling or modification steps are required. In addition, because of the large surface area to volume ratio of microfluidic devices, sufficiently large fields can be created over small distances thus enabling

Table 2. Cellular composition of human blood and their mechanical properties (Lichtman, et al., 2006)

Type	Cell Number (/μL)	Mean Volume (Fl)	Elastic Modulus (Dyn/cm²)
Erythrocytes	4100–5900	88	400000 (Dulinska, et al., 2006)
Platelets	172000–450000	6.6	1700 (Schmid-Schonbein, Sung, Tozeren, Skalak, & Chien, 1981)
Leukocytes	4400–11300	525-4200	410 (Haga, Beaudoin, & Strony, 1998)
Neutrophils	900–10800		
Lymphocytes	100–3600		
Monocytes	140–620		
Eosinophils	20–790		

efficient separation. In this section, we will discuss some of the important microfluidic devices that are used for the separation of blood cells.

Separations Based on Biomechanical Properties

Blood consists of ~45% cells including erythrocytes, leukocytes, and platelets, in plasma. As shown in Table 2, these cells have vastly different biomechanical properties and the particulate suspension nature of blood results in unique flow properties in microcirculation (Lichtman, et al., 2006).

Erythrocytes, because of their biconcave discoid shape and greater deformability tend to flow in the center of the blood vessels by forming reversible aggregates ('rouleaux'), thus leaving a plasma-rich zone closer the wall. Such segregation leads to two important outcomes: (i) leukocyte margination, which increases the concentration of leukocytes closer to the vessel wall, and (ii) plasma skimming, which is the uneven distribution of cells and plasma at nonsymmetrical bifurcations (Wootton & Ku, 1999).

Biomimetic devices that simulate these physiological processes have been used for the efficient separation of plasma from cells (Cokelet, Soave, Pugh, & Rathbun, 1993; Shevkoplyas, Gifford, Yoshida, & Bitensky, 2003; Shevkoplyas, Yoshida, Munn, & Bitensky, 2005). In one of the early studies in this direction, Cokelet *et al.*, used lithography to generate microvascular networks on a silicon substrate. Channels, which are ~20 μm diameters were etched on glass, and electrofused to each other to form bifurcations and channels. The channels faithfully mimicked flow in the microvasculature, and this study formed the basis for a number of novel microfluidic blood cell isolation devices (Russon, Sethu, Irimia, Mindrinos, & Calvano, 2008; Shevkoplyas, et al., 2003). Shevkoplyas used a network of rectangular microchannels of ~70 μm width to enhance leukocyte margination progressively from erythrocyte depleted channels, thus resulting in more than 30-fold enhancement in leukocyte population after a single flow-through of 7 mm (Figure 3. [A]). These devices have also been used as a point-of-care diagnostic for separating and analyzing leukocyte samples from patients with inflamed tissues following burn injury or trauma (Russon, et al., 2008; Sethu, et al., 2006). Again, using similar principles and engineering of single channels for uneven particle distribution, it is possible to obtain more than 90% erythrocyte separation efficiency at a relatively high flow rate of 5 ml/min (Jaggi, Sandoz, & Effenhauser, 2007). These designs were based on simulating fluid-particle-wall interactions using computational fluid dynamics (CFD) wherein the equations of conservation of mass and momentum are solved to predict the streamlines of cells in a flow field. It is possible to obtain even higher separation efficiencies (>97% leukocytes) using 'streamline-engineered' bifurcation channels wherein particles beyond a critical particle radius are swept along a straight line, and those with smaller radii are diverted into side channels that are perpendicular to the main channel (S. Zheng, Liu, & Tai, 2008).

The separation efficiency obtained by variations in channel dimensions and bifurcations can be enhanced by incorporating a higher level of sophistication using microstructures inside the channel. The microstructures alter the streamlines of fluid flow, influence the residence time of the cells in the channel, thus amplifying the subtle differences in the physical properties of the cells to obtain very high separation efficiencies. Some of the microstructures that are used in fluid flow include weirs, posts, walls, and sieves. The geometry and positioning of the structures within the microchannel can be designed for optimal cell separation by modeling flow profiles and particle trajectories using CFD simulations (Panaro, Lou, Fortina, Kricka, & Wilding, 2005; S. Zheng, et al., 2008). Both experimental and theoretical studies (Yuen, et al., 2001) have shown that use of microsieves can result in an efficient separation than that obtained using an unobstructed channel. An improvement to this 'dead-end filtration' is a cross-flow filtration design proposed by (Chen, Cui, Liu, & Li, 2008) and (Davis, et al., 2006), which utilizes a micropost array parallel to the flow direction that separates the RBC and WBC from plasma, which are collected in three separate channels.

Separations Based on Biochemical Properties

Constitutive and induced changes in receptor expression levels on target cells can be utilized effectively for the isolation of these cells for a number of biomedical and clinical applications. For instance, the target cells could be circulating tumor cells (Adams, et al., 2208; Murthy, Sin, Tompkins, & Toner, 2004; Nagrath, et al., 2007) or hematopoietic stem cells (Narasipura & King, 2009). The isolation and characterization of circulating tumor cells (CTC) can serve as an indicator for the clinical management of several cancer-related diseases, since these cells are known to be produced during the early stages of tumorigenesis and metastasis. The isolation of hematopoietic stem cells (HSPC) is vital for the restoration of hematopoietic function and survival of cancer patients.

The differences in biochemical properties between cell types can be used selectively for very efficient isolation of cell populations of interest using microfluidic channels. The fundamental idea is the differential capture of cells based on the qualitative and quantitative variations in receptor expression levels, which results in disparity in the interaction characteristics with ligand coated flow channels. The receptor–ligand molecular interactions pertinent to blood cells are typically non-covalent interactions with a bond strength of nano- to piconewtons, which is sufficient to hold cells to surfaces under flow conditions (shear stress of 1-5 dyn/cm^2) similar to those found in blood vessels (Dammer, et al., 1996; R.A. Kumar, et al., 2003). Thus it is possible to isolate cells from blood by capturing them by the binding of cell surface receptor to their cognate ligand. Revzin *et al* developed a microfabricated system for capturing more than 95% of CD5+ T-lymphocytes from blood samples, by coating the microwells with anti-CD5 antibody (Revzin, Sekine, Sin, Tompkins, & Toner, 2004) (Figure 3.[B]). The authors also adapted this prototype for enumerating the circulating CD4+ T-lymphocyte population, which is an important indicator of HIV status. Another interesting and clinically useful application of microfluidic cell separation was demonstrated recently for the high efficiency isolation of CTC using a microfluidic separation device containing antibody-coated microposts. Since CTC are rare (1 in 10^9 cells) their isolation presents a major challenge, and microfluidic devices are particularly useful for such high efficiency cell sorting (Fu, et al., 1999). High cell capture efficiencies can be achieved by optimizing the cell trajectories in a flow stream, the duration of contact and detachment due to fluid force (i.e., on- and off-rate kinetics), and avidity of receptors on cell surface and ligands on microposts. This device was able to identify CTC in more than 99% of blood samples of patients with breast, prostate or colon cancer, and importantly, does not require sample pre-treatment.

In addition to these diagnostic applications, microfluidic cell separations based on receptor–ligand interactions have shown promise in the development of cell-based therapy. Hematopoietic stem cell enrichment of high purity is important in stem-cell based therapies, and has posed tremendous challenges in separating a very small cell population amongst numerous other cell types. Such efficient separation was accomplished by coating surfaces with molecules that bind selectively to the stem cells. Again, the large surface area to volume ratio of microfluidic channels is valuable in increasing the capture probability of cells on-to ligand-coated walls. Murthy *et al* coated surfaces with anti-CD45+ antibody and were able to isolate a population with more than 95% CD45+ cells, independent of the input cell composition (Murthy, et al., 2004). Recently, King and others have developed an implantable device coated with P-selectin for selective enrichment of CD34+ and CD45+ HSPC (Narasipura, Wojciechowski, Duffy, Liesveld, & King, 2008; Wojciechowski, et al., 2008). Though these single flow-through devices do not produce a highly pure population, their efficiency can be further improved by optimizing the flow rates and cell trajectories and the duration of contact between the cells and ligand-coated surfaces.

Separation Based on Magnetic Properties

Magnetic cell sorting (MACS) commonly refers to the separation of cells based on the attachment of magnetic particles to cells. Paramagnetic beads, about 10-100 nm diameter, are coated with antibodies specific for the cells of interest, and the cells are then sorted by the application of an external magnetic field. Though static MACS is commonly employed, superimposition of a hydrodynamic flow field often results in more efficient separation (Berger, Castelino, Huang, Shah, & Austin, 2001). Microfluidic systems are especially advantageous for MACS because the small length scale of the device greatly enhances the magnetic field strength, and hence obviates the need for a strong magnet. This feature has led to the design of a number of microfluidic devices which separate RBC from other cell types due to the inherent magnetic properties of RBC. RBCs contain hemoglobin, an iron-containing protein with substantial paramagnetic moment in the deoxygenated state. In contrast, other blood cells are diamagnetic. While conventional techniques require a large magnetic field and have proven to be very difficult for the separation of RBCs, the advent of microfluidic technologies have made such separations feasible. In a magnetic gradient field superimposed on a flow field, the net force acting on a particle is a balance of the magnetic and hydrodynamic forces given below respectively:

$$F_{mag} = \chi H \frac{dH}{dx} \frac{4}{3} \pi R^3$$
$$F_{hydro} = 6\pi \mu R v$$
$$F_{mag} = F_{hydro} \Rightarrow v = \frac{2}{9} \frac{\chi H R^2}{\mu} \frac{dH}{dx}$$

where χ is magnetic susceptibility, H is magnetic field strength, R is radius, μ is viscosity, and v is velocity. Thus by adjusting the magnetic field strength it is possible to move and separate particles of different magnetic properties. Berger (Berger, et al., 2001), Qu (Qu, et al., 2008), and Iliescu (Iliescu, Xu, Barbarini, Avram, & Avram, 2009) describe different types of designs in which nano-structured ferromagnetic wires or dots were incorporated to the bottom of the flow chamber. These structures greatly amplify the magnetic field gradient and the RBCs are deflected by the magnetic field. In contrast, other cell types are unresponsive to the magnetic field and move with the hydrodynamic flow. This results in the separation of ~95% of RBC using a relatively low magnetic field of ~0.3 T. Such separation can be seen in Figure 3. (C), where at the end of the wire, the RBCs are deflected upon application of the magnetic field (Qu, et al., 2008). Huang *et al* have used a similar approach for the separation of nucleated RBC from blood as a diagnostic tool for maternal and fetal health conditions in pregnant women (R. Huang, et al., 2008). Two microfluidic separation devices were used sequentially: the first one separated nucleated RBCs and WBCs from non-nucleated RBCs based on size differences, followed by a second separation based on the magnetic properties of RBCs and WBCs. This size-magnetic combination as a separation technique was effective in separating 99.99% of nucleated RBCs, and compares very well with conventional assays. This technology holds a lot of promise for label-free, continuous labeling for diagnostic purposes.

Figure 3. Microfluidics for cell separation. (A) Efficient separation of leukocytes from erythrocytes in a bifurcating channel of unequal diameter (taken from (Shevkoplyas, et al., 2005)); (B) Isolation of cell population based on differential receptor-ligand binding in coated channels (taken from (Revzin, et al., 2004)); (C) Separation of RBCs from other blood cells is possible using a magnetic wire in a flow channel (taken from (Qu, et al., 2008))

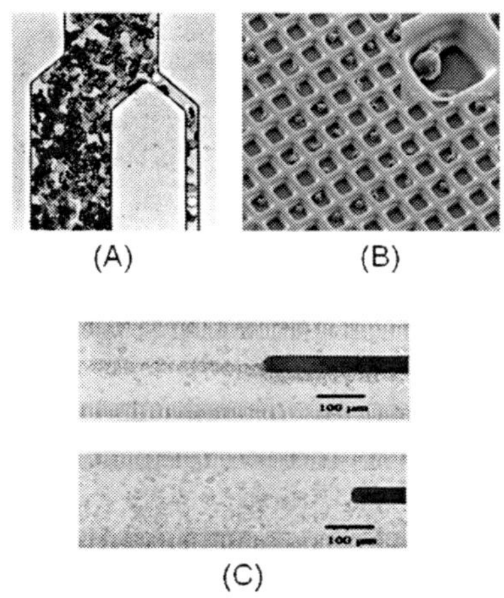

DETECTION OF PATHOGENS

The lab-on-chip technology has miniaturized many important biological assays like PCR (Hashimoto, et al., 2004), DNA analysis and sequencing (Goedecke, et al., 2004), immunoassays (Moorthy, et al., 2004), and intra- and inter-cellular assays (McClain, et al., 2003). These techniques have been used for rapid, reliable and inexpensive detection of microbial pathogens in the blood.

Detection of pathogen in a biological fluid sample is possible with a microfluidic biosensor using fluorescence or label-free detection systems. The pathogens are captured on surfaces through antigen-antibody interactions, and the DNA is extracted for analysis. A microfluidic biosensor for rapid and reliable identification of pathogenic organisms was developed by Zaytseva *et al* (Zaytseva, Goral, Montagna, & Baeumner, 2005). In this biosensor, bacterial cells were first lysed to release a single stranded DNA or RNA ('test probe'), part of which can then bind to their complementary strand attached on to a liposome (Figure 4. [A]). The liposomes carry fluorophore cargo. Another part of the test probe also hybridizes with a complementary capture probe attached to a magnetic bead, which in turn can be captured to an external magnet from a flowing stream. The captured magnet-DNA-liposome is irradiated with a laser, which results in the release of fluorophores from the liposome, which can be detected with an imager. The large surface area of the bead enhances the overall binding affinity by four fold, and the use of liposomes with a large cargo of fluorophores (10^5/liposome) increases the fluorescence intensity by 10 fold. This process takes only 15 min and is capable of continuous sampling in a microfluidic channel. In order to improve the sensitivity of this system to detect low levels of pathogens (as low

Figure 4. Microfluidics for pathogen detection. (A) Target RNA hybridizes to a test probe which is complexed to a fluorphore-loaded liposome, and to a capture probe complexed to a magnetic bead. This hybridization complex can be captured with an external magnet, and detected using laser irradiation (adapted from (Zaytseva, et al., 2005)); (B) Sample containing antigen of interest, and antibody-conjugated magnetic beads were incubated in the incubation chamber, and mixed using the membrane-type micromixer. An on-chip magnet holds the beads in place, while the unbound particles are washed away using the buffer. Next, fluorescent secondary antibodies were allowed to bind the antigen captured on the bead. The pathogen-antibody magnetic bead complexes were subsequently transported into a microfluidic focusing unit by means of the pneumatic controlled pumps and valves, and focused using two neighboring sheath flows. The fluorescent signal from the secondary antibodies on the beads is detected by a PMT module as the sample flows past the detection region. This signal, through a pneumatic controller, activates downstream microvalves, which can turn on or off resulting in the sorting of the target into the collection chambers (taken from (Yang, et al., 2008))

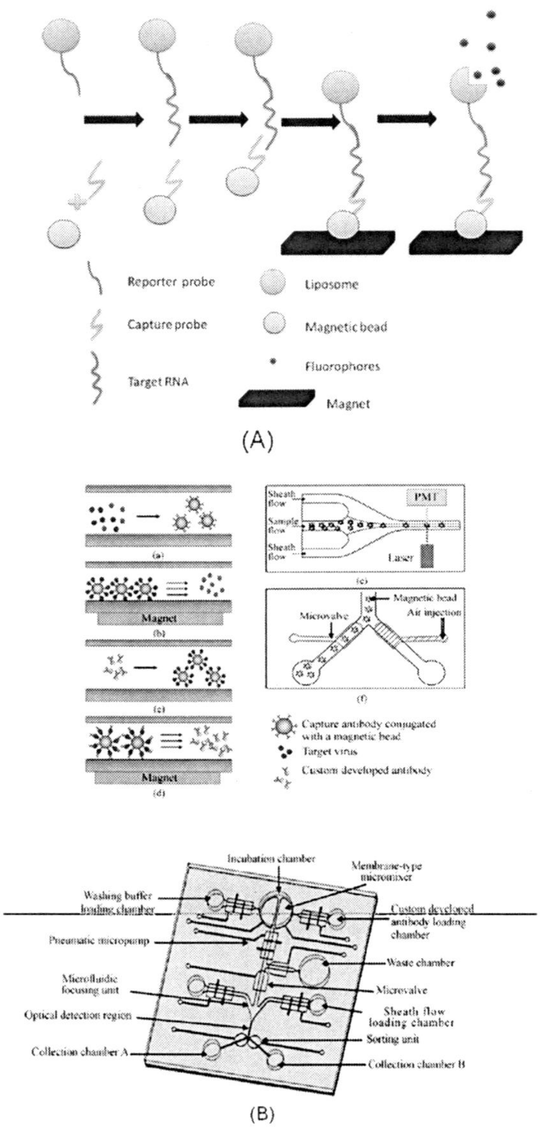

as 2 cfu/μl), Beyor *et al.*, increased the capture efficiency by using a fluidized bed of magnetic beads in the microfluidic channels (Beyor, Seo, Liu, & Mathies, 2008). An automated pneumatic pump produces multiple flutters, which repeatedly drives the sample through the bead bed thus increasing the capture efficiency. After the cells have been loaded, PBS is washed over the beads to remove uncaptured cells. The magnetic field is then switched off so that the bead with the pathogen can be flushed out with buffer and can be used for PCR analysis.

In spite of the rapid and reliable cell counting capabilities of the conventional flow cytometers, factors such as instrument size, large sample volume, laser power consumption and complicated control systems (Huh, Gu, Kamotani, Grotberg, & Takayama, 2005) have made miniaturization of flow cytometers desirable or sometimes even necessary. Lab-on-chip flow cytometers are advantageous over their conventional counterparts by being portable, consuming less analyte volume, cheaper and also reliable (Yang, et al., 2006; Yang, et al., 2008) (Figure 4. [B]). Lab-on-chip flow cytometers can be used for detecting the presence of pathogens in a sample by binding the pathogens to antibody-coated fluorescent beads under flow, and observing the fluorescence intensity. In a microfluidic device for viral detection, 100 μl of sample and 10 μl of anti-pathogen antibody-conjugated magnetic beads (6 μm diameter) were allowed to incubate in the incubation chamber, and mixed using the membrane-type micromixer. An on-chip magnet holds the beads in place, while the unbound particles are washed away using the buffer. Next, 2 μl of custom-made fluorescent secondary antibodies were loaded into the incubation chamber through the reagent-loading chamber and incubated for another 10 min, and the washing step was repeated. The pathogen-antibody magnetic bead complexes were subsequently transported into a microfluidic focusing unit by means of pneumatically controlled pumps and valves, and focused by two neighboring sheath flows. The fluorescent signal from the secondary antibodies on the beads is detected by a PMT module as the sample flows past the detection region. This signal, through a pneumatic controller, activates downstream microvalves, which can turn on or off resulting in the sorting of the target (virus) into the collection chambers.

IMMUNOASSAYS

Identification of antigens and antibody in the sera and other biological fluids is critical for clinical and diagnostic purposes, drug discovery, vaccination, and also for understanding the pathophysiology of immune disorders (Farber, 1999; Nasir & Jolley, 1999; Sundberg, Chow, Nikiforov, & Wada, 2000). These applications often demand the ability to perform multiple parallel reactions using small sample volume because of the limitations in obtaining human blood samples. As a result, microfluidic devices are particularly suited for performing immunoassays in body fluids or biological samples. The large surface-to-volume ratio in microfluidic devices increases the intermolecular interactions compared to macroscale devices. This implies that, in microfluidic devices, the reactions are kinetic-controlled, and not transport-controlled. This has resulted in greatly reducing the assay time from a few hours using conventional techniques to less than a few minutes using microfluidic devices. Conventional immunoassays called ELISA are performed in multiwell plates, where individual wells represent small reactors in which the antigen (antibody) in sera interacts with antibody (antigen) immobilized on the plate or a bead, and the reactions are monitored by fluorescence or optical read-outs. These assays typically take several hours primarily because of the time needed for the molecular entities to diffuse close to each other for a reaction to occur. On the other hand, microfluidic immunoassays are controlled by reaction rate, and enable us to perform multiplexed assays, i.e., multiple reactions under more than one condition.

A clever development in multiplexed assays is plug-based microfluidics. This system essentially simulates the isolated, multi-well environment by utilizing segmented flow microfluidic technology to perform individual assays in "plugs" (Figure 5. [A]). The plugs are aqueous droplets containing sample and analyte surrounded by an inert carrier fluid (such as buffer or gas) (Kline, et al., 2008; Song, Chen, & Ismagilov, 2006; B. Zheng & Ismagilov, 2005; B. Zheng, Tice, & Ismagilov, 2004) and the reaction is monitored by evaluating the change in optical properties of the plug due to the reaction between the test sample and the analyte as they move through the channel. The ability of the plugs to stay as individual drops is determined by Capillary number (*Ca*). The residence time of the plug in the channel corresponds to the reaction or incubation time in the channel. These tests can be easily multiplexed by fabricating microchannels in PDMS, such that each droplet can be used as an individual microreactor or an assay well (Duffy, McDonald, Schueller, & Whitesides, 1998; McDonald, et al., 2000; B. Zheng, Tice, Roach, & Ismagilov, 2004). This is termed as three phase liquid-gas-liquid flow or hybrid approach, since the liquid plugs are separated by gas. The plug-based microfluidics has shown to be successful in high-throughput blood grouping assays using a microfluidic antibody array (Figure 5. [A]). The interaction between antigens on RBC surface and serum antibodies was monitored from RBC agglutination in individual droplets or plugs, that have previously been loaded with antibodies specific for A, B, or D antigens (Kline, et al., 2008). This remarkably reduced the assay duration to 46 s, compared to 45 min when using conventional well-plates. The plug-based system has numerous advantages including decreased evaporation rate (B. Zheng & Ismagilov, 2005), ease of fluid handling (Roach, Song, & Ismagilov, 2005), and minimum analyte dispersion and diffusion issues (Liau, Karnik, Majumdar, & Cate, 2005). This technology has been extended for single cell enzymatic assay (He, et al., 2005), determination of clotting time of blood (Song, Li, Munson, Van Ha, & Ismagilov, 2006), analysis of protein expression (Aharoni, Griffiths, & Tawfik, 2005; P. S. Dittrich, Jahnz, & Schwille, 2005), and cell signaling pathways (El-Ali, Gaudet, Gunther, Sorger, & Jensen, 2005), and DNA fingerprinting (Burns, et al., 1998).

An innovative, fully integrated microfluidic device for rapid, one-step detection of pathogen by ELISA or PCR has been developed recently (Cho, et al., 2007; B. S. Lee, et al., 2009; W. C. Lee, Lien, Lee, & Lei, 2008) (Figure 5. [B]). Cho *et al.*, from Samsung have demonstrated detection of Hepatitis B virus and *E. coli* bacteria in whole blood in a single step, using a circular microfluidic chip, which contains channels and chambers in a circular disc (Cho, et al., 2007). This technique, called "Lab-on-a-CD", has variously been used for cell lysis (J. Kim, et al., 2004), PCR amplification (Lagally, Emrich, & Mathies, 2001), ELISA (Honda, Lindberg, Andersson, Hoffman, & Takei, 2005), and blood alcohol assays (Steigert, et al., 2006). This process is a breakthrough as it takes only 12 min with 100 μl for the entire operation involving plasma separation, mixing with magnetic beads conjugated with antibodies specific for viral or bacterial antigens, washing and DNA extraction, and PCR amplification of the DNA and detection. Further, this process has only one manual step of loading the whole blood into the CD, while the conventional assay takes at least 10 steps. In "lab-on-a-CD", first plasma is separated from cells by centrifugation. Then, plasma is incubated with antibody-coated, magnetic, laser-sensitive microbeads, so as to bind the pathogenic antigen to the beads. Since diffusion is not a limiting factor, even short incubation times can ensure that the antigen binds to beads strongly. The microbeads are then irradiated with a laser, which results in absorption of heat and cell lysis, and the DNA from the pathogen is released. The DNA is then amplified and detected using PCR. This principle lends itself easily to analyze RNA samples, immunoassays, and blood

Figure 5. Microfluidics for immunoassays. (A) Plug-based microfluidics. Fluorescently labeled analytes and samples, when injected into a steady stream of gas flowing through a microfluidic channel, forms nanoreactor plugs. ABO and D blood typing of samples with antibody array (multiple plugs loaded with different antibodies) leading to optical detection of RBC aggregation in the plugs (adapted from (Kline, et al., 2008)); (B) A 'lab-on-CD' analyzer along with the microfluidic disc design showing the detailed layout of channels, chambers and valves (taken from (Cho, et al., 2007; B. S. Lee, et al., 2009))

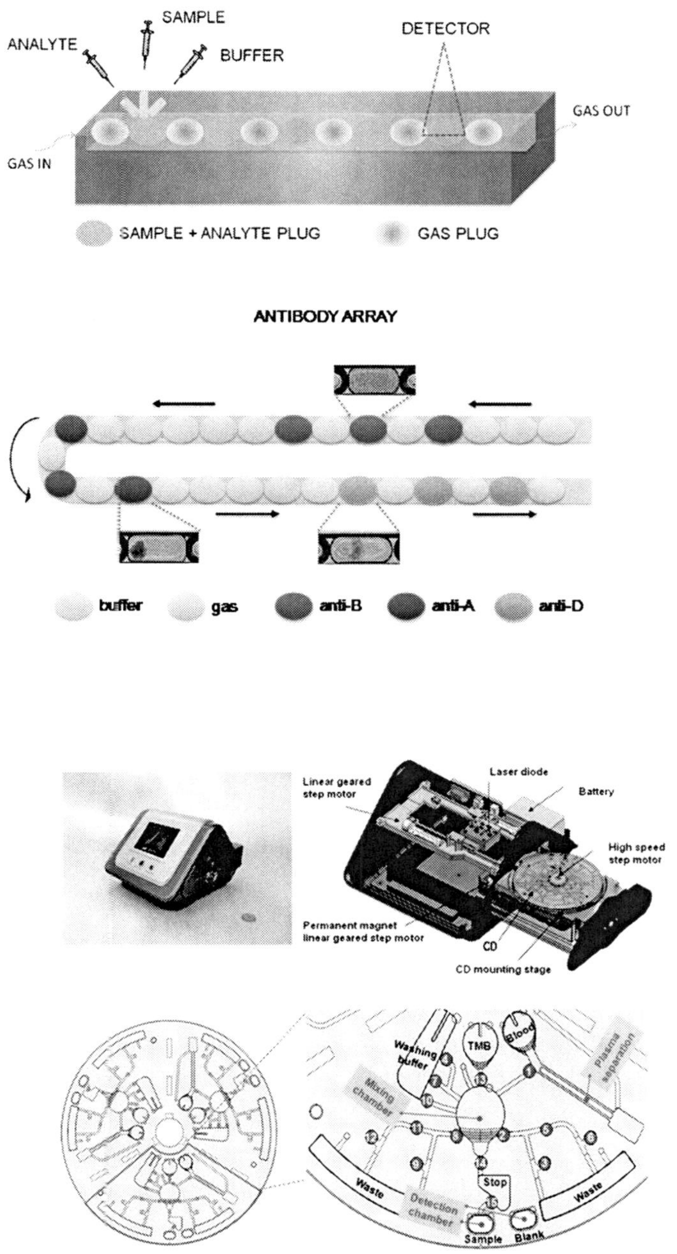

(B)

chemistry analysis. The device uses centrifugal forces to move fluid through the channels, and laser-operated microvalves for precise control of fluid transfer between different chambers. In comparison to the conventional ELISA, the operation time was reduced from over 2 hours to less than 30 min while maintaining similar detection limits.

DRUG DISCOVERY

The discovery and development of new drugs is an expensive, arduous and very long process. Recent estimates place the cost at a whopping \$1.7b and nearly 13 years of development (Sollano, Kirsch, Bala, Chambers, & Harpole, 2008). Furthermore, despite the increasing R&D costs, the number of new chemical entities (NCE) has remained constant over the 10-year period (1996-2006). Thus, the chasm between promise on the lab bench and delivery to the market is widening. Recent advances in high-throughput screening (HTS) technologies using microfluidic devices have shown tremendous potential in narrowing this gap (Kumar & Clark, 2006).

Many important factors that influence the rates of chemically induced or enzyme-catalyzed reactions, like temperature, heat and mass transfer and concentration distribution can be efficiently controlled in a microfluidic device. These advantages make many multiple reaction steps and on-chip analysis to be performed in a very short span of time, usually within few minutes, thereby screening large libraries of probable drugs in short time (P.S. Dittrich & Manz, 2006). Furthermore, microfluidic chips are very well suited for combinatorial synthesis of drugs *in situ*. As shown in Figure 6, by using interconnected networks of channels with valves and pumps, different reactants can be mixed together, thus enabling multiplexed drug screening (Adamson, Mustafi, Zhang, Zheng, & Ismagilov, 2006; P.S. Dittrich & Manz, 2006).

Microfluidics offers numerous advantages in all three phases of drug testing namely, sampling, processing and analysis (Kang, Chung, Lang, & Khademhosseini, 2008), which have been used, in a rather limited way, for the development of new drugs for clotting disorders. For instance, Tsuchiya has developed a microneedle system for minimially invasive blood extraction and *in situ* processing to separate plasma proteins from other cells (Tsuchiya, Nakanishi, Uetsuji, & Nakamachi, 2005). The proteins can then be tested for assessing the affinity of drug candidates that block their function, thus reducing clotting. Diamond and colleagues (Neeves, et al., 2008), and Sarvepalli *et al* (Sarvepalli, et al., 2009) describe a microfluidic system for testing a large number of thrombotic and thrombolytic drug candidates particularly from mice, where the current technology is limited because of the amount of blood that could be drawn from these animals. Microfluidic chips can also be connected to animal models through venous catheters so that previously administered drug compounds (Kralj, Sahoo, & Jensen, 2007) can easily be obtained and analyzed without involving any loss in separation and organic-solvent based extraction. A number of good reviews have been published on the use of microfluidic devices for drug discovery and development, which could provide perspectives for exploring the use of these devices for the discovery of new drugs in blood-related disorders (P.S. Dittrich & Manz, 2006; Jahnisch, Hessel, Lowe, & Baerns, 2004; Kang, et al., 2008). For instance, enzymatic assays (Rondelez, et al., 2005) could be suitably adapted for studying the efficacy of anti-coagulants, microbead-based screening assays for peptide-binding drugs (Nolan & Sklar, 1998), enumeration and cell sorting such as epitope-tagged β_2-adrenergic receptors associated with cardiovascular diseases (B. Huang, et al., 2007), label-free photonic biosensors for receptor-ligand binding (Maerkl & Quake, 2007), and toxicity and bioavailability studies of different organs using

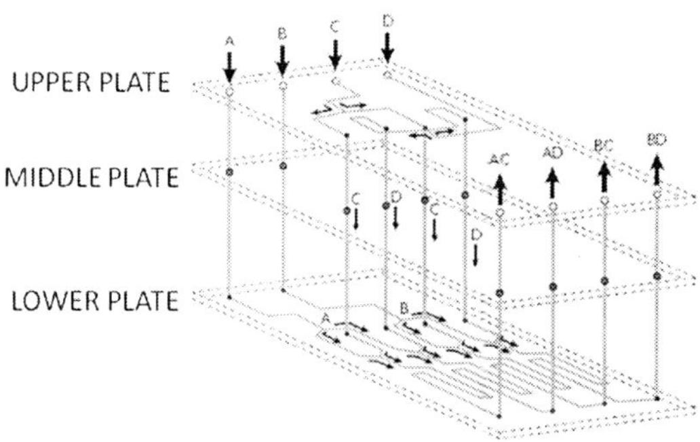

Figure 6. Microfluidics for drug discovery. Schematic of a microfluidic system for combinatorial syntheses in a three-dimensional microchip (P.S. Dittrich & Manz, 2006)

microfluidic channels as surrogate blood vessels (Sin, et al., 2004). See Figure 6.

OUTLOOK

Microfluidics offers a plethora of opportunities for both basic and applied research in vascular bioengineering. A number of these opportunities arise from not only from the need to better understand disease pathophysiology, but also to develop cost-effective and reliable devices for rapid diagnosis, and the discovery of novel therapeutics. Successful development of microfluidic devices requires a better understanding of fluid mechanics, and associated physical and chemical phenomena in small scales, which is currently not well understood. Computational and experimental fluid dynamics can help in visualizing flow of complex fluids such as blood with suspended cells and dissolved proteins in different configuration, geometry, and topography. This will aid in achieving high-value applications through novel approaches for driving flow, interactions between various cells and surfaces, and chemical reactions.

Another important and active research area is new fabrication techniques and materials which will scale microfluidics down to nanofluidics. Various modifications to conventional lithographic techniques such as edge lithography and embossing can create devices with a spatial resolution of 1-10 nm. Alternate to the conventional top-down techniques are bottom-up approaches of building larger structures from smaller units such as self-assembled monolayers which can faithfully replicate repeating structures with sub nanometer resolution. Examples of these approaches include design and construction of devices using DNA and protein as structural and functional subunits. It is conceivable that we could obtain cues from naturally occurring ion and protein channels to construct novel devices for precise flow regulation. Biological molecules can also be exploited for the development of 'self-driven' motors for driving pumps and valves used in microfluidic devices (T. Kim, et al., 2009). These biological nanomotors utilize ATP as an energy source and have better energy efficiency than conventional motors. Though the force generated by a single motor such as kinesin is only a few piconewtons, the atomic precision of these motors allows us to integrate multiple units to produce the torque necessary to drive microfluidic flows. Though the biomimetic and nanoscale engineered devices are still in the early stages of development, they hold interesting challenges and great promise for commercial applications.

An important application of microfluidics is diagnosis, and hence better detection and analysis techniques will be invaluable. It is often desired to rapidly detect as low as picomolar quantities of a molecular entity in small sample volumes, particularly in 'point-of-care' settings. Such requirements demand highly sensitive, label-free detection reagents such as quantum dots (QD), which are nanocrystals of photoluminiscent particles such as CdS (Medintz, Uyeda, Goldman, & Mattoussi, 2005). Integrating quantum dots with high precision optical detection techniques such as Surface Plasmon Resonance can provide attractive biomarker tools for the early detection of cancer or fungal infection, which has not been possible before (Homola, 2008).

We have outlined here some of the important applications of microfluidic technologies in vascular bioengineering. While this review is in no way meant to be exhaustive in the rapidly expanding field of microfluidics, we hope it has given the reader an appreciation that there is indeed, as a wise man once said, 'plenty of room at the bottom' (Feynman, 1960). The application of microfluidics to study and treat vascular diseases are still in its infancy: some of the tools already exist and need meaningful collaborations between materials scientists and physicians to refine these tools, while some others need innovative ways of building tools and translating research from the 'bench-to-bedside-to-community'. Nevertheless, the small scale manipulation of blood is ultimately of paramount importance and fraught with interesting and rewarding challenges that should keep researchers busy and excited for several years to come.

REFERENCES

Abdelgawad, M., Watson, M. W. L., Young, E. W. K., Mudrik, J. M., Ungrin, M. D., & Wheeler, A. R. (2008). Soft lithography: masters on demand. *Lab on a Chip*, *8*(8), 1379–1385. doi:10.1039/b804050h

Adams, A. A., Okagbare, P. I., Feng, J., Hupert, M. L., Patterson, D., & Gottert, J.. (2208). Highly efficient circulating tumor cell isolation from whole blood and label-free enumeration using polymer-based microfluidics with an integrated conductivity sensor. *Journal of the American Chemical Society*, *130*, 8633–8641. doi:10.1021/ja8015022

Adamson, D. N., Mustafi, D., Zhang, J. X. J., Zheng, B., & Ismagilov, R. F. (2006). Production of arrays of chemically distinct nanolitre plugs via repeated splitting in microfluidic devices. *Lab on a Chip*, *6*(9), 1178–1186. doi:10.1039/b604993a

Aharoni, A., Griffiths, A. D., & Tawfik, D. S. (2005). High-throughput screens and selections of enzyme-encoding genes. *Current Opinion in Chemical Biology*, *9*(2), 210–216. doi:10.1016/j.cbpa.2005.02.002

Antia, M., Herricks, T., & Rathod, P. K. (2007). Microfluidic modeling of cell-cell interactions in malaria pathogenesis. *PLoS Pathogens*, *3*(7), e99. doi:10.1371/journal.ppat.0030099

Bange, A., Halsall, H. B., & Heineman, W. R. (2005). Microfluidic immunosensor systems. [Review]. *Biosensors & Bioelectronics*, *20*(12), 2488–2503. doi:10.1016/j.bios.2004.10.016

Barone, F. C., & Feuerstein, G. Z. (1999). Inflammatory mediators and stroke: New opportunities for novel therapeutics. [Review]. *Journal of Cerebral Blood Flow and Metabolism*, *19*(8), 819–834. doi:10.1097/00004647-199908000-00001

Becker, H., & Gärtner, C. (2008). Polymer microfabrication technologies for microfluidic systems. *Analytical and Bioanalytical Chemistry*, *390*(1), 89–111. doi:10.1007/s00216-007-1692-2

Berger, M., Castelino, J., Huang, R., Shah, M., & Austin, R. H. (2001). Design of a microfabricated magnetic cell separator. *Electrophoresis*, *22*(18), 3883–3892. doi:10.1002/1522-2683(200110)22:18<3883::AID-ELPS3883>3.0.CO;2-4

Beyor, N., Seo, T. S., Liu, P., & Mathies, R. A. (2008). Immunomagnetic bead-based cell concentration microdevice for dilute pathogen detection. *Biomedical Microdevices*, *10*(6), 909–917. doi:10.1007/s10544-008-9206-3

Bird, R. B., Stewart, W. E., & Lightfoot, E. N. (1960). *Transport Phenomena*. New York: John Wiley and Sons.

Burns, M. A., Johnson, B. N., Brahmasandra, S. N., Handique, K., Webster, J. R., & Krishnan, M. (1998). An integrated nanoliter DNA analysis device. *Science*, *282*(5388), 484–487. doi:10.1126/science.282.5388.484

Chen, X., Cui, D. F., Liu, C. C., & Li, H. (2008). Microfluidic chip for blood cell separation and collection based on crossflow filtration. *Sensors and Actuators. B, Chemical*, *13*, 216–221. doi:10.1016/j.snb.2007.07.126

Cho, Y. K., Lee, J. G., Park, J. M., Lee, B. S., Lee, Y., & Ko, C. (2007). One-step pathogen specific DNA extraction from whole blood on a centrifugal microfluidic device. *Lab on a Chip*, *7*(5), 565–573. doi:10.1039/b616115d

Chou, H. P., Spence, C., Scherer, A., & Quake, S. (1999). A microfabricated device for sizing and sorting DNA molecules. *Proceedings of the National Academy of Sciences of the United States of America*, *96*(1), 11–13. doi:10.1073/pnas.96.1.11

Cokelet, G. R., Soave, R., Pugh, G., & Rathbun, L. (1993). Fabrication of in vitro microvascular blood flow systems by photolithography. *Microvascular Research*, *46*, 394–400. doi:10.1006/mvre.1993.1062

Countouriotis, A., Moore, T. B., & Sakamoto, K. M. (2002). Cell surface antigen and molecular targeting in the treatment of hematologic malignancies. [Review]. *Stem Cells (Dayton, Ohio)*, *20*(3), 215–229. doi:10.1634/stemcells.20-3-215

D'Orazio, P. (2003). Biosensors in clinical chemistry. [Review]. *Clinica Chimica Acta*, *334*(1-2), 41–69. doi:10.1016/S0009-8981(03)00241-9

Dammer, U., Hegner, M., Ansemetti, D., Wagner, P., Dreier, M., & Huber, W. (1996). Specific antigen/antibody interactions measured by force microscopy. *Biophysical Journal*, *70*, 2437–2441. doi:10.1016/S0006-3495(96)79814-4

Danesh, J., Collins, R., Appleby, P., & Peto, R. (1998). Association of fibrinogen, C-reactive protein, albumin, or leukocyte count with coronary heart disease - Meta-analyses of prospective studies. [Review]. *Jama-Journal of the American Medical Association*, *279*(18), 1477–1482. doi:10.1001/jama.279.18.1477

Davis, J. A., Inglis, D. W., Morton, K. J., Lawrence, D. A., Huang, L. R., & Chou, S. Y. (2006). Deterministic hydrodynamics: Taking blood apart. *Proceedings of the National Academy of Sciences of the United States of America*, *103*(40), 14779–14784. doi:10.1073/pnas.0605967103

Diamond, S. L. (2001). Reaction complexity of flowing human blood. [News Item]. *Biophysical Journal*, *80*(3), 1031–1032. doi:10.1016/S0006-3495(01)76083-3

Dittrich, P. S., Jahnz, M., & Schwille, P. (2005). A new embedded process for compartmentalized cell-free protein expression and on-line detection in microfluidic devices. *ChemBioChem*, *6*(5), 811–814. doi:10.1002/cbic.200400321

Dittrich, P. S., & Manz, A. (2006). Lab-on-a-chip: microfluidics in drug discovery. *Nature Drug Discov.*, *5*, 210–218. doi:10.1038/nrd1985

Duffy, D. C., McDonald, J. C., Schueller, O. J. A., & Whitesides, G. M. (1998). Rapid prototyping of microfluidic systems in poly(dimethylsiloxane). *Analytical Chemistry*, *70*(23), 4974–4984. doi:10.1021/ac980656z

Dulinska, I., Targosz, M., Strojny, W., Lekka, M., Czuba, P., & Balwierz, W. (2006). Stiffness of normal and pathological erythrocytes studied by means of atomic force microscopy. *Journal of Biochemical and Biophysical Methods*, *66*(1-3), 1–11. doi:10.1016/j.jbbm.2005.11.003

Effenhauser, C. S., Bruin, G. J. M., Paulus, A., & Ehrat, M. (1997). Integrated capillary electrophoresis on flexible silicone microdevices: Analysis of DNA restriction fragments and detection of single DNA molecules on microchips. *Analytical Chemistry*, *69*(17), 3451–3457. doi:10.1021/ac9703919

El-Ali, J., Gaudet, S., Gunther, A., Sorger, P. K., & Jensen, K. F. (2005). Cell stimulus and lysis in a microfluidic device with segmented gas-liquid flow. *Analytical Chemistry*, *77*(11), 3629–3636. doi:10.1021/ac050008x

Farber, G. K. (1999). New approaches to rational drug design. *Pharmacology & Therapeutics*, *84*, 327–332. doi:10.1016/S0163-7258(99)00039-X

Feynman, R. P. (1960). There's plenty of room at the bottom. *Engineering and Science*, 22–36.

Fu, A. Y., Spence, C., Scherer, A., Arnold, F. H., & Quake, S. R. (1999). A microfabricated fluorescence-activated cell sorter. *Nature Biotechnology*, *17*, 1109–1111. doi:10.1038/15095

Furie, B., & Furie, B. C. (2005). Thrombus formation in vivo. *The Journal of Clinical Investigation*, *115*, 3355–3362. doi:10.1172/JCI26987

Gatti, R., Antonelli, G., Prearo, M., Spinella, P., Cappellin, E., & De Palo, E. F. (2009). Cortisol assays and diagnostic laboratory procedures in human biological fluids. [Review]. *Clinical Biochemistry*, *42*(12), 1205–1217. doi:10.1016/j.clinbiochem.2009.04.011

Gilden, D., Cohrs, R. J., Mahalingam, R., & Nagel, M. A. (2009). Varicella zoster virus vasculopathies: diverse clinical manifestations, laboratory features, pathogenesis, and treatment. [Review]. *The Lancet Neurology*, *8*(8), 731–740. doi:10.1016/S1474-4422(09)70134-6

Goedecke, N., McKenna, B., El-Difrawy, S., Carey, L., Matsudaira, P., & Ehrlich, D. (2004). A high-performance multilane microdevice system designed for the DNA forensics laboratory. *Electrophoresis*, *25*(10-11), 1678–1686. doi:10.1002/elps.200305897

Gutierrez, E., Petrich, B. G., Shattil, S. J., Ginsberg, M. H., Groisman, A., & Kasirer-Friede, A. (2008). Microfluidic devices for studies on shear-dependent platelet adhesion. *Lab on a Chip*, *8*(9), 1486–1495. doi:10.1039/b804795b

Haber, C. (2006). Microfluidics in commerical applications: an industry perspective. *Lab on a Chip*, *6*, 1118–1121. doi:10.1039/b610250f

Hafezi-Moghadam, A., Thomas, K. L., & Cornelssen, C. (2004). A novel mouse-driven ex vivo flow chamber for the study of leukocyte and platelet function. *American Journal of Physiology. Cell Physiology*, *286*, C876–C892. doi:10.1152/ajpcell.00500.2003

Haga, J. H., & Beaudoin, A. J. W., J.G., & Strony, J. (1998). Quantification of the passive mechanical properties of the resting platelet. *Annals of Biomedical Engineering*, *26*, 268–277. doi:10.1114/1.118

Hashimoto, M., Chen, P. C., Mitchell, M. W., Nikitopoulos, D. E., Soper, S. A., & Murphy, M. C. (2004). Rapid PCR in a continuous flow device. *Lab on a Chip*, *4*(6), 638–645. doi:10.1039/b406860b

He, M. Y., Edgar, J. S., Jeffries, G. D. M., Lorenz, R. M., Shelby, J. P., & Chiu, D. T. (2005). Selective encapsulation of single cells and subcellular organelles into picoliter- and femtoliter-volume droplets. *Analytical Chemistry*, *77*(6), 1539–1544. doi:10.1021/ac0480850

Hemker, H. C., Giesen, P., Al Dieri, R., Regnault, V., de Smedt, E., & Wagenvoord, R. (2003). Calibrated automated thrombin generation measurement in clotting plasma. *Pathophysiology of Haemostasis and Thrombosis*, *33*, 4–15. doi:10.1159/000071636

Homola, J. (2008). Surface plasmon resonance sensors for detection of chemical and biological species. *Chemical Reviews*, *108*, 462–493. doi:10.1021/cr068107d

Honda, N., Lindberg, U., Andersson, P., Hoffman, S., & Takei, H. (2005). Simultaneous multiple immunoassays in a compact disc-shaped microfluidic device based on centrifugal force. *Clinical Chemistry*, *51*(10), 1955–1961. doi:10.1373/clinchem.2005.053348

Huang, B., Wu, H., Bhaya, D., Grossman, A., Granier, S., & Kobilka, B. K. (2007). Counting low-copy number proteins in a single cell. *Science*, *315*(5808), 81–84. doi:10.1126/science.1133992

Huang, R., Barber, T. A., Schmidt, M. A., Tompkins, R. G., Toner, M., & Bianchi, D. W. (2008). A microfluidics approach for the isolation of nucleated red blood cells (NRBCs) from the peripheral blood of pregnant women. *Prenatal Diagnosis*, *28*(10), 892–899. doi:10.1002/pd.2079

Huh, D., Gu, W., Kamotani, Y., Grotberg, J. B., & Takayama, S. (2005) Microfluidics for flow cytometric analysis of cells and particles. *Physiological Measurement*, *26*(3), R73–R98. doi:10.1088/0967-3334/26/3/R02

Iliescu, C., Xu, G., Barbarini, E., Avram, M., & Avram, A. (2009). Microfluidic device for continuous magnetophoretic separation of white blood cells. *Microsystem Technologies*, *15*, 1157–1162. doi:10.1007/s00542-008-0718-9

Ishii-Watabe, A., Uchida, E., Mizuguchi, H., & Hayakawa, T. (2000). On the mechanism of plasmin-induced platelet aggregation: implications of the dual role of granule ADP. *Biochemical Pharmacology*, *59*, 1345–1355. doi:10.1016/S0006-2952(00)00279-3

Israelachvili, J. (2006). *Intermolecular and surface forces*. New York: Academic Press.

Jaggi, R. D., Sandoz, R., & Effenhauser, C. S. (2007). Microfluidic depletion of red blood cells from whole blood in high-aspect-ratio microchannels. *Microfluid. Nanofluid.*, *3*, 47–53. doi:10.1007/s10404-006-0104-9

Jahnisch, K., Hessel, V., Lowe, H., & Baerns, M. (2004). Chemistry in microstructured reactors. *Angewandte Chemie International Edition*, *43*, 406–446. doi:10.1002/anie.200300577

Kang, L., Chung, B. G., Lang, R., & Khademhosseini, A. (2008). Microfluidics for drug discovery and development: From target selection to product lifecycle management. *Drug Discovery Today*, *13*(1), 1–13. doi:10.1016/j.drudis.2007.10.003

Kantak, A. S., Gale, B. K., Lvov, Y., & Jones, S. A. (2003). Platelet function analyzer: shear activation of platelets in microchannels. *Biomedical Microdevices*, *5*(3), 207–215. doi:10.1023/A:1025708225412

Kastrup, C. J., Boedicker, J. Q., Pomerantsev, A. P., Moayeri, M., Bian, Y., & Pompano, R. R. (2008). Spatial localization of bacteria controls coagulation of human blood by 'quorum acting'. [Article]. *Nature Chemical Biology*, *4*(12), 742–750. doi:10.1038/nchembio.124

Kastrup, C. J., Shen, F., Runyon, M. K., & Ismagilov, R. F. (2007). Characterization of the threshold response of initiation of blood clotting to stimulus patch size. [Article]. *Biophysical Journal*, *93*(8), 2969–2977. doi:10.1529/biophysj.107.109009

Kim, J., Jang, S. H., Jia, G. Y., Zoval, J. V., Da Silva, N. A., & Madou, M. J. (2004). Cell lysis on a microfluidic CD (compact disc). *Lab on a Chip*, *4*(5), 516–522. doi:10.1039/b401106f

Kim, T., Cheng, L.-J., Kao, M.-T., Hasselbrink, E. F., Guo, L. J., & Meyhofer, E. (2009). Biomolecular motor-driven molecular sorter. *Lab on a Chip*, *9*, 1282–1285. doi:10.1039/b900753a

Kline, T. R., Runyon, M. K., Pothiawala, M., & Ismagilov, R. F. (2008). ABO, D blood typing and subtyping using plug-based microfluidics. *Analytical Chemistry*, *80*(16), 6190–6197. doi:10.1021/ac800485q

Koch, K., van Berkel, S. S., van de Wal, M. M. E. B., Nieuwland, P. J., van Hest, J. C. M., & Rutjes, F. P. J. T. (2009). Thrombin generation test in microfluidic systems. *Journal of Applied Physics*, *105*, 102012–102017. doi:10.1063/1.3116634

Kraemer, T., & Maurer, H. H. (1998). Determination of amphetamine, methamphetamine and amphetamine-derived designer drugs or medicaments in blood and urine. [Review]. *Journal of Chromatography. B, Analytical Technologies in the Biomedical and Life Sciences*, *713*(1), 163–187. doi:10.1016/S0378-4347(97)00515-X

Kralj, J. G., Sahoo, H. R., & Jensen, K. F. (2007). Integrated continuous microfluidic liquid-liquid extraction. *Lab on a Chip*, *7*(2), 256–263. doi:10.1039/b610888a

Kulp, M., Vaher, M., & Kaljurand, M. (2005). Miniaturization of sampling for chemical reaction monitoring by capillary electrophoresis. [Article]. *Journal of Chromatography. A*, *1100*(1), 126–129. doi:10.1016/j.chroma.2005.11.018

Kumar, R. A., & Clark, D. S. (2006). High-throughput screening of biocatalytic activity: application in drug discovery. *Current Opinion in Chemical Biology*, *10*(2), 162–168. doi:10.1016/j.cbpa.2006.02.033

Kumar, R. A., Dong, J.-f., Thaggard, J., Cruz, M. A., Lopez, J. A., & McIntire, L. V. (2003). Kinetics of GPIbα-vWF-A1 tether bond under flow: effect of GPIbα mutations on the association and dissociation rates. *Biophysical Journal*, *85*, 4099–4109. doi:10.1016/S0006-3495(03)74822-X

Kumar, R. A., Dong, J. F., Thaggard, J. A., Cruz, M. A., Lopez, J. A., & McIntire, L. V. (2003). Kinetics of GPIb alpha-vWF-A1 tether bond under flow: Effect of GPIb alpha mutations on the association and dissociation rates. [Article]. *Biophysical Journal*, *85*(6), 4099–4109. doi:10.1016/S0006-3495(03)74822-X

Lagally, E. T., Emrich, C. A., & Mathies, R. A. (2001). Fully integrated PCR-capillary electrophoresis microsystem for DNA analysis. *Lab on a Chip*, *1*(2), 102–107. doi:10.1039/b109031n

Lee, B. S., Lee, J. N., Park, J. M., Lee, J. G., Kim, S., & Cho, Y. K. (2009). A fully automated immunoassay from whole blood on a disc. *Lab on a Chip*, *9*(11), 1548–1555. doi:10.1039/b820321k

Lee, W. C., Lien, K. Y., Lee, G. B., & Lei, H. Y. (2008). An integrated microfluidic system using magnetic beads for virus detection. *Diagnostic Microbiology and Infectious Disease*, *60*(1), 51–58.

Liau, A., Karnik, R., Majumdar, A., & Cate, J. H. D. (2005). Mixing crowded biological solutions in milliseconds. *Analytical Chemistry*, *77*(23), 7618–7625. doi:10.1021/ac050827h

Lichtman, M. A., Beutler, E., Kipps, T. J., Seligsohn, U., Kaushanksy, K., & Prchal, J. T. (2006). *William's Hematology*. New York: McGraw-Hill.

Lo, K., & Diamond, S. L. (2004). Blood coagulation kinetics: high throughput method for real-time reaction monitoring. [Article]. *Thrombosis and Haemostasis*, *92*(4), 874–882.

Maerkl, S. J., & Quake, S. R. (2007). A systems approach to measuring the binding energy landscapes to transcription factors. *Science*, *315*(5809), 233–237. doi:10.1126/science.1131007

Martinez, A. W., Phillips, S. T., Butte, M. J., & Whitesides, G. M. (2007). Patterned paper as a platform for inexpensive, low-volume, portable bioassays. *Angewandte Chemie International Edition*, *46*, 1318–1320. doi:10.1002/anie.200603817

Martinez, A. W., Phillips, S. T., Carrilho, E., Thomas, S. W., Sindi, H., & Whitesides, G. M. (2008). Simple telemedicine for developing regions: Camera phones and paper-based microfluidic devices for real-time, off-site diagnosis. *Analytical Chemistry*, *80*(10), 3699–3707. doi:10.1021/ac800112r

Martinez, A. W., Phillips, S. T., & Whitesides, G. M. (2008). Three-dimensional microfluidic devices fabricated in layered paper and tape. *Proceedings of the National Academy of Sciences of the United States of America*, *105*, 19606–19611. doi:10.1073/pnas.0810903105

McClain, M. A., Culbertson, C. T., Jacobson, S. C., Allbritton, N. L., Sims, C. E., & Ramsey, J. M. (2003). Microfluidic devices for the high-throughput chemical analysis of cells. *Analytical Chemistry*, *75*(21), 5646–5655. doi:10.1021/ac0346510

McDonald, J. C., Duffy, D. C., Anderson, J. R., Chiu, D. T., Wu, H. K., & Schueller, O. J. A. (2000). Fabrication of microfluidic systems in poly(dimethylsiloxane). *Electrophoresis*, *21*(1), 27–40. doi:10.1002/(SICI)1522-2683(20000101)21:1<27::AID-ELPS27>3.0.CO;2-C

Medintz, I. L., Uyeda, H. T., Goldman, E. R., & Mattoussi, H. (2005). Quantum dot bioconjugates for imaging, labeling, and sensing. *Nature Materials*, *4*, 435–446. doi:10.1038/nmat1390

Minerick, A. R. (2008). The rapidly growing field of micro and nanotechnology to measure living cells. *A.I. Ch.E.J.*, *54*(9), 2230–2237.

Moorthy, J., Mensing, G. A., Kim, D., Mohanty, S., Eddington, D. T., & Tepp, W. H. (2004). Microfluidic tectonics platform: A colorimetric, disposable botulinum toxin enzyme-linked immunosorbent assay system. *Electrophoresis*, *25*(10-11), 1705–1713. doi:10.1002/elps.200405888

Murthy, S. K., Sin, A., Tompkins, R. G., & Toner, M. (2004). Effect of flow and surface conditions on human lymphocyte isolation using microfluidic chambers. *Langmuir*, *20*, 11649–11655. doi:10.1021/la048047b

Nagrath, S., Sequist, L. V., Maheswaran, S., Bell, D. W., Irimia, D., & Ulkus, L. (2007). Isolation of rate circulating tumor cells in cancer patients by microchip technology. *Nature*, *450*, 1235–1239. doi:10.1038/nature06385

Narasipura, S. D., & King, M. R. (2009). P-selectin-coated microtube for the purification of CD45+ hematopoietic cells directly from human peripheral blood. *Blood Cells, Molecules & Diseases*, *42*(2), 136–139. doi:10.1016/j.bcmd.2008.12.002

Narasipura, S. D., Wojciechowski, J. C., Duffy, B. M., Liesveld, L. J., & King, M. R. (2008). Purification of CD45+ hematopoietic cells directly from human bone marrow using a flow-based P-selectin-coated microtube. *American Journal of Hematology*, *83*(8), 627–629. doi:10.1002/ajh.21204

Nasir, M. S., & Jolley, M. E. (1999). Fluorescence polarization: An analytical tool for immunoassay and drug discovery. *Combinatorial Chemistry & High Throughput Screening*, *2*, 177–190.

Neeves, K. B., Maloney, S. F., Fong, K. P., Schmaier, A. A., Kahn, M. L., & Brass, L. F. (2008). Microfluidic focal thrombosis model for measuring murine platelet deposition and stability: PAR4 signaling enhances shear-resistance of platelet aggregates. [Article]. *Journal of Thrombosis and Haemostasis*, *6*(12), 2193–2201. doi:10.1111/j.1538-7836.2008.03188.x

Nolan, J. P., & Sklar, L. A. (1998). The emergence of flow cytometry for sensitive, real-time measurements of molecular interactions. *Nature Biotechnology*, *16*, 633–638. doi:10.1038/nbt0798-633

Packard, R. R. S., & Libby, P. (2008). Inflammation in atherosclerosis: From vascular biology to biomarker discovery and risk prediction. [Review]. *Clinical Chemistry*, *54*(1), 24–38. doi:10.1373/clinchem.2007.097360

Panaro, N. J., Lou, X. J., Fortina, P., Kricka, L. J., & Wilding, P. (2005). Micropillar array chip for integrated white blood cell isolation and PCR. *Biomolecular Engineering*, *21*, 157–162.

Popel, A. S., & Johnson, P. C. (2005). Microcirculation and hemorheology. *Annual Review of Fluid Mechanics*, *37*, 43–69. doi:10.1146/annurev.fluid.37.042604.133933

Qu, B.-Y., Wu, Z.-Y., Fang, F., Bai, Z.-M., Yang, D.-Z., & Xu, S.-K. (2008). A glass microfluidic chip for continuous blood cell sorting by a magnetic gradient without labeling. *Analytical and Bioanalytical Chemistry*, *392*, 1317–1324. doi:10.1007/s00216-008-2382-4

Quake, S. R., & Scherer, A. (2000). From micro to nanofabrication with soft materials. *Science*, *290*(5496), 1536–1540. doi:10.1126/science.290.5496.1536

Revzin, A., Sekine, K., Sin, A., Tompkins, R. G., & Toner, M. (2004). Development of a microfabricated cytometry platform for characterization and sorting of individual leukocytes. *Lab on a Chip*, *5*, 30–37. doi:10.1039/b405557h

Roach, L. S., Song, H., & Ismagilov, R. F. (2005). Controlling nonspecific protein adsorption in a plug-based microfluidic system by controlling interfacial chemistry using fluorous-phase surfactants. *Analytical Chemistry*, *77*(3), 785–796. doi:10.1021/ac049061w

Rondelez, Y., Tresset, G., Tabata, K. V., Arata, H., Fujita, H., & Takeuchi, S. (2005). Microfabricated arrays of femtoliter chambers allow single molecule enzymology. *Nature Biotechnology*, *23*, 361–365. doi:10.1038/nbt1072

Rosenberg, R. D., & Aird, W. C. (1999). Vascular-bed - Specific hemostasis and hypercoagulable states. [Review]. *The New England Journal of Medicine*, *340*(20), 1555–1564. doi:10.1056/NEJM199905203402007

Runyon, M. K., Johnson-Kerner, B. L., & Ismagilov, R. F. (2004). Minimal functional model of hemostasis in a biomimetic microfluidic system. [Article]. *Angewandte Chemie International Edition*, *43*(12), 1531–1536. doi:10.1002/anie.200353428

Runyon, M. K., Johnson-Kerner, B. L., Kastrup, C. J., Van Ha, T. G., & Ismagilov, R. F. (2007). Propagation of blood clotting in the complex biochemical network of hemostasis is described by a simple mechanism. [Article]. *Journal of the American Chemical Society*, *129*(22), 7014–7015. doi:10.1021/ja072602p

Russon, A., Sethu, P., Irimia, D., Mindrinos, M. N., & Calvano, S. E. (2008). Microfluidic leukocyte isolation for gene expression analysis in critically ill hospitalized patients. *Clinical Chemistry*, *54*(5), 891–900. doi:10.1373/clinchem.2007.099150

Sarvepalli, D. P., Schmidtke, D. W., & Nollert, M. U. (2009). Design considerations for a microfluidic device to quantify the platelet adhesion to collagen at physiological shear rates. *Annals of Biomedical Engineering*, *37*(7), 1331–1341. doi:10.1007/s10439-009-9708-z

Schaff, U. Y., Xing, M. M., Lin, K. K., Pan, N., Jeon, N. L., & Simon, S. I. (2007). Vascular mimetics based on microfluidics for imaging the leukocyte - endothelial inflammatory response. *Lab on a Chip*, *7*(4), 448–456. doi:10.1039/b617915k

Schmid-Schonbein, G. W., Sung, K.-L. P., Tozeren, H., Skalak, R., & Chien, S. (1981). Passive mechanical properties of human leukocytes. *Biophysical Journal*, *36*, 243–256. doi:10.1016/S0006-3495(81)84726-1

Sethu, P., Moldawer, L. L., Mindrinos, M. N., Scrumpia, P. O., Tannahill, C. L., & Wilhelmy, J. (2006). Microfluidic isolation of leukocytes from whole blood for phenotype and gene expression analysis. *Analytical Chemistry*, *78*, 5453–5461. doi:10.1021/ac060140c

Shevkoplyas, S. S., Gifford, S. C., Yoshida, T., & Bitensky, M. W. (2003). Prototype of an in vitro model of the microcirculation. *Microvascular Research*, *65*, 132–136. doi:10.1016/S0026-2862(02)00034-1

Shevkoplyas, S. S., Yoshida, T., Munn, L. L., & Bitensky, M. W. (2005). Biomimetic autoseparation of leukocytes from whole blood in a microfluidic device. *Analytical Chemistry*, *77*, 933–937. doi:10.1021/ac049037i

Shui, L., Eijkel, J. C. T., & van den Berg, A. (2007). Multiphase flow in microfluidic systems - Control and applications of droplets and interfaces. *Advances in Colloid and Interface Science*, *133*, 35–49. doi:10.1016/j.cis.2007.03.001

Sin, A., Chin, K. C., Jamil, M. F., Kostov, Y., Rao, G., & Shuler, M. L. (2004). The design and fabrication of three-chamber microscale cell culture analog device with integrated dissolved oxygen sensors. *Biotechnology Progress*, *20*(1), 338–345. doi:10.1021/bp034077d

Sollano, J. A., Kirsch, J. M., Bala, M. V., Chambers, M. G., & Harpole, L. H. (2008). The economics of drug discovery and the ultimate valuation of pharmacotherapies in the marketplace. *Clinical Pharmacology and Therapeutics*, *84*(2), 263–266. doi:10.1038/clpt.2008.117

Song, H., Chen, D. L., & Ismagilov, R. F. (2006). Reactions in droplets in microfluidic channels. *Angewandte Chemie International Edition*, *45*, 7336–7356. doi:10.1002/anie.200601554

Song, H., Li, H. W., Munson, M. S., Van Ha, T. G., & Ismagilov, R. F. (2006). On-chip titration of an anticoagulant argatroban and determination of the clotting time within whole blood or plasma using a plug-based microfluidic system. *Analytical Chemistry*, *78*(14), 4839–4849. doi:10.1021/ac0601718

Steigert, J., Grumann, M., Brenner, T., Riegger, L., Harter, J., & Zengerle, R. (2006). Fully integrated whole blood testing by real-time absorption measurement on a centrifugal platform. *Lab on a Chip*, *6*(8), 1040–1044. doi:10.1039/b607051p

Stone, H. A., Stroock, A. D., & Ajdari, A. (2004). Engineering flows in small devices: Microfluidics toward a lab-on-a-chip. *Annual Review of Fluid Mechanics*, *36*, 381–411. doi:10.1146/annurev.fluid.36.050802.122124

Sundberg, S. A., Chow, A., Nikiforov, A., & Wada, H. G. (2000). Microchip-based systems for target validation and HTS. *Drug Discovery Today*, *5*, S92–S103. doi:10.1016/S1359-6446(00)80100-2

Tran, L., Farinas, J., Ruslim-Litrus, L., Conley, P. B., Muir, C., & Munnelly, K. (2005). Agonist-induced calcium response in single human platelets assayed in a microfluidic device. *Analytical Biochemistry*, *341*, 361–368. doi:10.1016/j.ab.2005.02.024

Tsuchiya, K., Nakanishi, N., Uetsuji, Y., & Nakamachi, E. (2005). Development of blood extraction system for health monitoring system. *Biomedical Microdevices*, *7*(4), 347–353. doi:10.1007/s10544-005-6077-8

Turner, N. A., Moake, J. L., & McIntire, L. V. (2001). Blockade of adenosine diphosphate receptors P2Y(12) and P2Y(1) is required to inhibit platelet aggregation in whole blood under flow. [Article]. *Blood*, *98*(12), 3340–3345. doi:10.1182/blood.V98.12.3340

Unger, M. A., Chou, H. P., Thorsen, T., Scherer, A., & Quake, S. R. (2000). Monolithic microfabricated valves and pumps by multilayer soft lithography. *Science*, *288*(5463), 113–116. doi:10.1126/science.288.5463.113

VanWijk, M. J., VanBavel, E., Sturk, A., & Nieuwland, R. (2003). Microparticles in cardiovascular diseases. [Review]. *Cardiovascular Research*, *59*(2), 277–287. doi:10.1016/S0008-6363(03)00367-5

Verpoorte, E., & De Rooij, N. F. (2003). Microfluidics meets MEMS. [Review]. *Proceedings of the IEEE*, *91*(6), 930–953. doi:10.1109/JPROC.2003.813570

Vogel, S. (1994). *Life in moving fluids* (2nd ed.). Princeton, NJ: Princeton University Press.

Weibel, D. B., DiLuzio, W. R., & Whitesides, G. M. (2007). Microfabrication meets microbiology. *Nature Reviews Microbiology*, *5*(3), 209–218. doi:10.1038/nrmicro1616

Whitesides, G. M. (2006). The origins and the future of microfluidics. *Nature*, *442*, 368–373. doi:10.1038/nature05058

Wojciechowski, J. C., Narasipura, S. D., Charles, N., Mickelsen, D., Rana, K., & Blair, M. L. (2008). Capture and enrichment of CD34-positive haematopoietic stem and progenitor cells from blood circulation using P-selectin in an implantable device. *British Journal of Haematology*, *140*(6), 673–681. doi:10.1111/j.1365-2141.2007.06967.x

Wootton, D. M., & Ku, D. N. (1999). Fluid mechanics of vascular systems, diseases, and thrombosis. [Review]. *Annual Review of Biomedical Engineering*, *1*, 299–329. doi:10.1146/annurev.bioeng.1.1.299

Xia, Y., & Whitesides, G. M. (1998). Soft lithography. *Angewandte Chemie International Edition*, *37*, 550–575. doi:10.1002/(SICI)1521-3773(19980316)37:5<550::AID-ANIE550>3.0.CO;2-G

Yang, S. Y., Hsiung, S. K., Hung, Y. C., Chang, C. M., Liao, T. L., & Lee, G. B. (2006). A cell counting/sorting system incorporated with a microfabricated flow cytometer chip. *Measurement Science & Technology*, *17*(7), 2001–2009. doi:10.1088/0957-0233/17/7/045

Yang, S. Y., Lien, K. Y., Huang, K. J., Lei, H. Y., & Lee, G. B. (2008). Micro flow cytometry utilizing a magnetic bead-based immunoassay for rapid virus detection. *Biosensors & Bioelectronics*, *24*(4), 855–862. doi:10.1016/j.bios.2008.07.019

Yuen, P. K., Kricka, L. J., Fortina, P., Panaro, N. J., Sakazume, T., & Wilding, P. (2001). Microchip module for blood sample preparation and nucleic acid amplification reactions. *Genome Research*, *11*(3), 405–412. doi:10.1101/gr.155301

Zaytseva, N. V., Goral, V. N., Montagna, R. A., & Baeumner, A. J. (2005). Development of a microfluidic biosensor module for pathogen detection. *Lab on a Chip*, *5*(8), 805–811. doi:10.1039/b503856a

Zheng, B., & Ismagilov, R. F. (2005). A microfluidic approach for screening submicroliter volumes against multiple reagents by using preformed arrays of nanoliter plugs in a three-phase liquid/liquid/gas flow. *Angewandte Chemie International Edition*, *44*(17), 2520–2523. doi:10.1002/anie.200462857

Zheng, B., Tice, J. D., & Ismagilov, R. F. (2004). Formation of arrayed droplets of soft lithography and two-phase fluid flow, and application in protein crystallization. *Advanced Materials (Deerfield Beach, Fla.)*, *16*(15), 1365–1368. doi:10.1002/adma.200400590

Zheng, B., Tice, J. D., Roach, L. S., & Ismagilov, R. F. (2004). A droplet-based, composite PDMS/glass capillary microfluidic system for evaluating protein crystallization conditions by microbatch and vapor-diffusion methods with on-chip X-ray diffraction. *Angewandte Chemie International Edition*, *43*(19), 2508–2511. doi:10.1002/anie.200453974

Zheng, S., Liu, J.-Q., & Tai, Y.-C. (2008). Streamline-based microfluidic devices for erythrocytes and leukocytes separation. *Journal of Microelectromechanical Systems*, *17*(4), 1029–1038. doi:10.1109/JMEMS.2008.924274

KEYTERMS AND DEFINITIONS

Antibody: An antibody is a type of protein produced by the body's immune system when the immune system detects harmful substances, called antigens. Antibodies are important in resistance against disease, in allergy, and in blood transfusions, and can be utilized in laboratory tests for the detection of antigens.

Antigen: A substance that when introduced into the body stimulates the production of an antibody. Antigens include toxins, bacteria, foreign blood cells, and the cells of transplanted organs.

Blood Typing: The process of identifying an individual's blood group by serologic testing of a sample of blood involving classification of blood by inherited antigens associated with erythrocytes (red blood cells). Without identification of these factors, blood transfusion from an incompatible donor may result in destruction of red cells or coagulation.

Combinatorial Synthesis: A process which allows for the simultaneous generation and rapid testing for a desired property, of large numbers of chemically related compounds. For example any of the compound from set **A** = $\{A_1, A_2, \ldots\}$ can be combined with set **B** = $\{B_1, B_2, \ldots.\}$ to produce **AB** = $\{A_1B_1, A_1B_2, \ldots.\}$

ELISA: Enzyme Linked Immunosorbent Assay is a sensitive immunoassay that uses an enzyme linked to an antibody or antigen as a marker for the detection of a specific protein, especially an antigen or antibody. It is often used as a diagnostic test to determine exposure to a particular infectious agent, such as the AIDS virus, by identifying antibodies present in a blood sample.

Epitope: A localized region on the surface of an antigen that is capable of eliciting an immune response and of combining with a specific antibody to counter that response.

Ex Vivo: Technique where part of the organism is placed in an external environment, without minimum alteration to the natural conditions.

In Vitro: The technique of performing a given procedure in an external environment, i.e., outside of a living organism, such as in a "test tube" or Petri dish.

In Vivo: Any experimental procedure performed within a living organism.

Ligand: A charged or uncharged molecule or a protein that can chemically bind to another molecule or a protein (called receptor) to from a complex. The Ligand-Receptor complex triggers a cascade of cellular response.

Mutant: A genetic variation in a normal organism that exhibits genotypic (sometimes even phenotypic) variations, such that the resultant is different from the wild type of the same kind.

PCR: The polymerase chain reaction (PCR) is a laboratory technique for "amplifying" a specific DNA sequence. PCR is extremely efficient and sensitive; it can make millions or billions of copies of any specific sequence of DNA, even when the sequence is in a complex mixture.

Receptor: A molecular structure (usually a protein) or site on the surface or interior of a cell that binds with a ligand including hormones, antigens, drugs, or neurotransmitters, to produce some effect in the cell.

Wild Type: The *typical* form (phenotype) of an organism, strain, protein, gene, or characteristic as it occurs in nature.

Chapter 2
Analysis of Biological Effect of AC-DC Electromagnetic Fields using the Lorenz Model

Malka N. Halgamuge
The University of Melbourne, Australia

Chathurika D. Abeyrathne
The University of Melbourne, Australia

Priyan Mendis
The University of Melbourne, Australia

ABSTRACT

Electromagnetic fields (EMF) are essential to various applications directly involving humans. Fears about the biological effect of exposure to electromagnetic fields drive enormous research into this area. This research generates conflicting results, and consequently, uncertainty regarding possible health effects. This chapter studies a nonlinear Lorenz model describing interactions among charged particles and combined alternating (AC: alternating current) and static (DC: direct current) electromagnetic fields, for various combinations of frequencies, field strengths and relative angle (θ) between the AC and DC magnetic fields. We investigate the effect on charged particles of three possible combinations of alternating and static electromagnetic fields: (i) AC electric field and DC magnetic field (ii) AC magnetic field and DC magnetic field (iii) AC electric field and AC and DC magnetic field. Then the behavior of the particle in these fields with different initial conditions and strong directional effects is observed when the angle between AC and DC magnetic fields is varied. The results show that the cyclotron resonance frequency is affected by charged particles' initial position and initial velocity. Further, we observe strong effects of electric and magnetic fields on a charged particle in a biological cell with initial position and initial velocity.

DOI: 10.4018/978-1-61692-004-3.ch002

INTRODUCTION

Electromagnetic radiation can be either ionizing (ultraviolet, X-ray and gamma rays) or non-ionizing radiation (microwave, radio waves, infrared, visible light and near ultraviolet), according to the frequency or wavelength of the radiation. Generally, either excitation or ionization can take place when radiation is absorbed by tissue. Ionization arises once radiation transports adequate energy to eliminate an electron from an atom or molecule. Excitation arises when radiation excites the motion of the atoms or molecules, or when it excites an electron from an engaged orbital into a higher-energy orbital. Electromagnetic radiation which does not hold enough energy to ionize atoms or molecules is called non-ionizing radiation.

Amplitude modulated radiofrequency fields were used in early experimental work. The amplitude modulation has been recognised as a significant factor in generating biological effects. Hence, later on electric and magnetic fields were used in experiments. Theoretical models that clarify the interaction between low frequency magnetic fields and biological tissue are crucial. Several experiments indicate an enhancement of the biological effect of certain resonance frequencies (Liboff, 1987; Liboff, Rozek, Sherman, McLeod, & Smith, 1987; McLeod, Smith, Cooksey, & Liboff, 1987; Smith, McLeod, Liboff, & Cooksey, 1987). The resonance frequencies may possibly be linked to the magnitude of the local geomagnetic field (Blackman, Benane, Rabinowitz, House, & Joines, 1985; Blackman, Kinney, House, & Joines, 1989). Further, amplitude windows were found, suggesting that stronger magnetic fields do not constantly involve rigorous biological consequence (Blackman et al., 1989).

In this chapter, we analyze the biological effects of non-ionizing radiation, in particular the behavior of charged particles exposed to alternating and static electromagnetic fields in a biological cell. Investigating the biological effects of electromagnetic fields covers a broad range of disciplines: basic biology, fundamental physics and biophysics, fundamental chemistry, biochemistry and electrical engineering (Barnes, 2006). According to the AC electric and magnetic signal, the model can be linear or non-linear. Both linear and non-linear models are considered in our analysis. A previous study (Thompson et al., 1995) of a nonlinear Lorenz model describing interaction between charged particles and combined AC and DC magnetic fields investigated the different combinations of field strengths, frequencies and relative angles between AC and DC magnetic fields in a vacuum. In this chapter, we investigate the effects on charged particles in a biological cell due to three possible combinations of alternating and static electromagnetic fields. The intention of this analysis is to clarify some of the basic characteristics in terms of the simplest possible model, which includes at least the crucial elements of the interaction of charged particles exposed to all combinations of AC and DC electromagnetic fields. See Figure 1.

ELECTRIC & MAGNETIC FIELDS

Electric and magnetic fields are interrelated. Electric fields are formed by voltage and measured in volts per meter (V/m) or newton per coulomb (N/C). Magnetic fields are induced by alternating current and measured using the derived quantity magnetic flux density (B) in webers per square meter (Wb/m^2), tesla (T) or gauss (G) where 1 μT = 10 mG. Magnetic fields only present when the appliance is turned on while electric fields can exist without any current flow (Habash, 2004). Electric fields proceed on static and moving ions, while magnetic fields only act on moving ions. Magnetic fields penetrate biological bodies without attenuation, even though electric fields are usually highly filtered from the cell interior. The speed and direction of the ion's motion are affected by electric force, as electric force is in the direction of the electric field. However, magnetic

Figure 1. Coordinate system: DC magnetic field B_0, AC electric field E and AC magnetic field B_{1z}. Here, DC magnetic field, B_0, is in the vertical y – z plane and a uniform AC electric field, E, is in x direction perpendicular to the y – z plane and AC magnetic field B_{1z} is in z direction perpendicular to the y – z plane

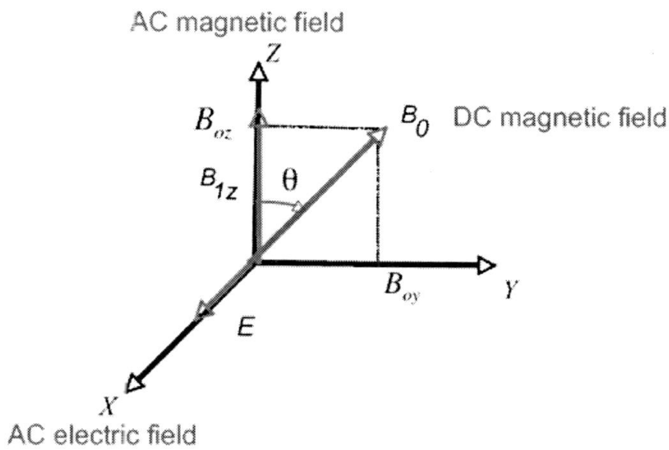

force on moving ions with velocity *v* is always perpendicular to *v*. Therefore, magnetic force cannot change its speed, although it changes the direction of the ion (Popp, 1994). Further, electromagnetic field strength decreases rapidly when we move away from the sources.

Direct current fields are steady with respect to the direction, strength and rate of flow. Alternating current fields change their direction, strength and rate of flow regularly with time. AC current does not flow gradually in a single direction; it changes direction *P* times per second or *P* cycles per second: it's so called "Hertz" (Hz). The electromagnetic spectrum covers the frequency range of 3 kHz to 300 GHz (ICNIRP). These fields can be classified according to the frequency range: extremely low frequency (ELF) fields and very low frequency (VLF) fields. ELF fields are defined as those having frequencies up to 3 kHz and VLF fields cover the frequency range 3 - 30 kHz. Because of the quasi-static nature of electromagnetic fields at these frequencies, electric and magnetic fields act independently of one another and are measured separately (Habash 2004).

The general public is today exposed to various sources of static and alternating electromagnetic fields; both manmade and naturally created fields. The electromagnetic fields are produced artificially with frequencies up to 300 GHz. Examples of natural static electric fields are thunderstorms and electricity; the earth's magnetic field (0.035 - 0.07 mT) is an example of a natural static magnetic field (Noble, 2005). Man-made static magnetic fields which are generated with DC current can be 1000 times stronger than the earth's natural magnetic field. Magnetic Resonance Imaging (MRI) uses magnetic fields 300,000 times stronger than the earth's. Any residential or occupational site is subject to coincident exposure from many electromagnetic sources, external and internal to the site itself. Some examples of manmade electromagnetic field sources are given in Table 1.

BIOLOGY

Superficial tissues, cells and nerves can be influenced by electromagnetic fields. Similarly specialized cells collectively execute certain particular functions. The total of these cells is called tissue and there are many types of tissues all over the living being. Tissues contain cells, neurons and

Table 1. Sources of manmade electromagnetic fields

	Sources of Electromagnetic Fields
External	High voltage power lines, transformers, underground cables, substations, transportation system (trains, trams & electric and hybrid cars), cellular antennas, cell towers, Wi-Fi hot spots, WiMAX, broadcast towers (AM, FM, television), RFID.
Internal-Workplace	Computers, printers, scanners, photocopiers, fax machines, fluorescent lights, heaters, telephone switching systems, security systems, Personal Digital Assistances (PDAs), cellular and codeless phones, wireless networks.
Internal-Residential	Internal wiring, meters, electrical main panels, sub-panels, grounding systems, hairdryers, electric shavers, electric blankets, TV, radio, video players, stereo systems, lighting, air conditioners, electric heaters, refrigerators, electric ovens, electric cookers, toasters, coffee machines, microwave ovens, washing machines and dryers, sewing machines, vacuum cleaners and other household appliances, cellular and codeless phones.

extracellular materials. Superficial tissue is fatty and lying under the skin, is the nearest part of the body to the surroundings. Thus, environmental changes are mostly sensed initially by the tissues and conducted by them. There are several types of animal tissues: muscle tissue, connective tissue, nervous tissue and epithelial tissue, which have different functions. The muscles, organs and other soft structures of the body are bounded by a band of fibrous connective tissue (Mader, 2008).

The cell is the smallest element of living organisms. Human organisms are multicellular, with approximately 10^{14} cells each with a typical size of 10 μm. Living cells are naturally active and dynamic, and some cells, such as nerve and muscle cells are excitable. A cell membrane, also called plasma membrane, covers each of these cells. The cell membrane protects the cell, separating the cell substance from its outside environment. The membrane mainly consists of a lipid bi-layer, but it also contains several protein molecules in the lipid, many of which penetrate all the way through the membrane. The fat soluble substances, such as carbon dioxide and oxygen, can penetrate the lipid layer easily. On the other hand it is not permeable to water soluble substances, such as ions, urea and glucose. However, free ions, such as K^+, Na^+, Cl^- and Ca^{++} on both sides of every cell membrane, can move across in different concentrations. These ions control the cell volume, help the signaling process and create a strong electric field between both sides of the cell membrane (Panagopoulos, Messini, Karabarbounis, Philippetis, & Margaritis, 2000). That is, the membrane can be affected by the difference in ion concentration on the two sides of the membrane. The ions from a high concentration area move to a low concentration area. This potential difference depends on the polarity of ions. The protein ion channels are classified according to gating types such as voltage gated, mechanically gated and ligand gated channels, and the opening and closing of channels are based on these mechanisms. Each channel is specific for only one type of ion and hence there are particular ion channels for calcium ions, sodium ions, chloride ions, and potassium ions. The membrane potential governs the transition of the voltage gated channels between a closed and open state through an open channel protein gate, the ions can enter or exit the cell.

A nerve is a cordlike, enclosed, collection of peripheral axons, which are long and slender projections of neurons. Nerves are only found in the peripheral nervous system. Nerves are categorized into groups based on their function, the direction that signals are conducted and where they connect to the central nervous system. Nerves sense the internal and external surroundings. A synchronized motion of K^+ and Na^+ ions across the nerve cell membrane is called a nerve signal. Information is communicated by the nerves in the form of electrochemical impulses which are extremely fast. This information is changed from electrical to chemical and then back to electrical. Nerves

Figure 2. The structure of a neurcn, neuron cell and neuron cell membrane. The free ions displace due to external electromagnetic fields and change the potential difference across the membrane which may influence the opening and closing of ion-protein channels. A synchronized motion of ions across the nerve cell membrane is called a nerve signal. These nerve impulses allow neurons to understand the surroundings

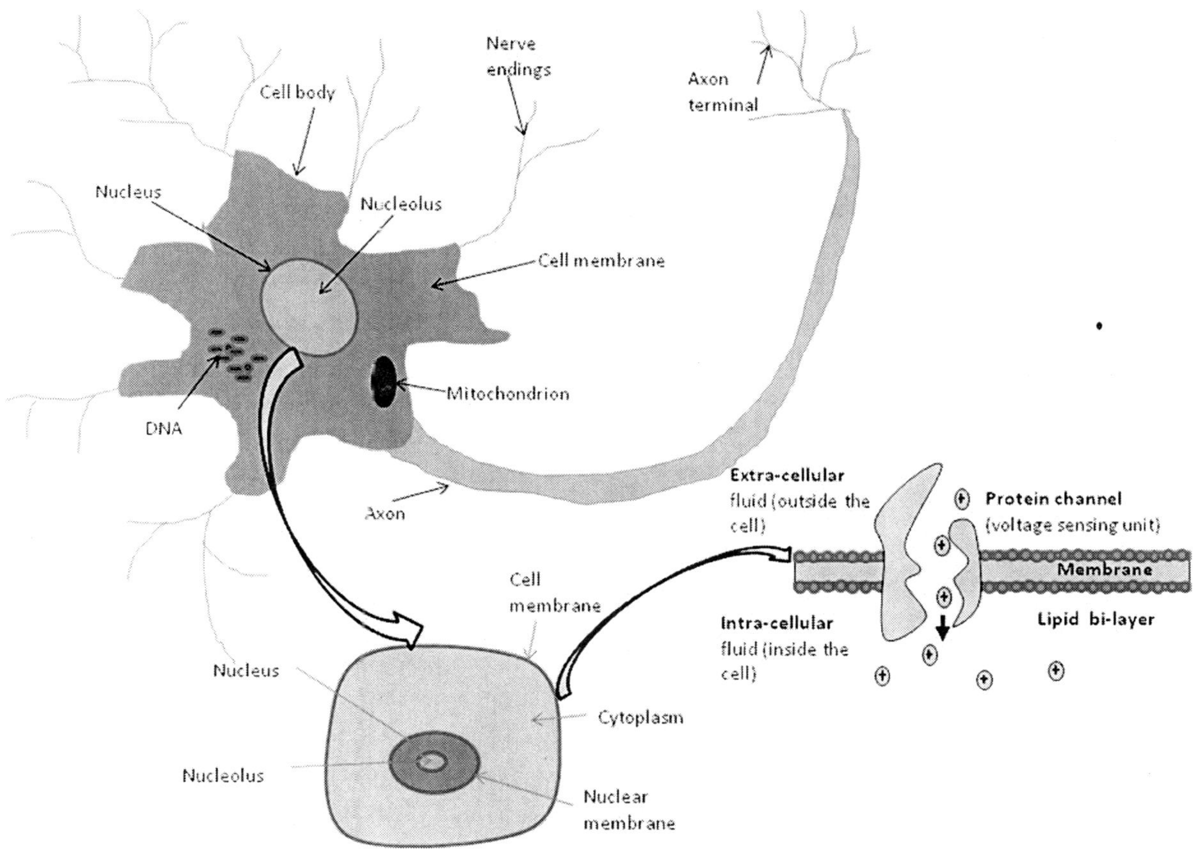

provide a common pathway for these impulses. These signals move from one area of the membrane to another along the axon to the nerve cell. The electrochemical signals are carried by the nerves in different areas of the nervous system, such as between the brain and the tissues. All the essential components of the cell, such as nucleus and mitochondria are in the cell body. The neuron dies if the cell body dies. Cell bodies are grouped together in clusters. The small, branch-like nerve endings of the cells are called dendrites, which create connections to other cells. This allows the neuron to understand the surroundings by communicating with other cells. Nerve endings can be found on one or both ends of the cell (Guyton & Hall, 2006). Figure 2 explains the structure of the neuron cell membrane, neuron cell and neuron.

BIOLOGICAL EFFECTS OF ELECTROMAGNETIC FIELDS

The acceptable exposure level to extremely low frequency magnetic fields is still controversial in terms of magnetic field strength. Realistically, magnetic fields are impossible to shield. They penetrate deeply into the cells and tissues and of and exposed person. On the other hand, electric fields can be shielded successfully and our body is not electrically homogeneous. It is crucial to understand the association between electric and magnetic fields outside and inside biological systems, which significantly varies with frequency and strength. Electric fields are significantly reduced by several orders of magnitude inside biological tissues from their values in air, external to the tissues. In magnetic fields, induced fields are same as external fields (Habash, 2004).

In the past half-decade, substantial work has been done to verify the effects of electromagnetic fields on biological systems over the whole frequency spectrum. Quite a lot of research effort has considered the connection between electric and magnetic field from the biological effects of high-voltage power lines (Bier, 2006; Cooper, Garny, & Kohl, 2003; Valjus, 1996). Recently interest changed from the strong electric field of high power voltage lines to reasonably weak magnetic fields produced by electrical appliances and distribution lines. Until the 1980s, the research on extremely low frequency fields related principally to electric fields, however, later this expanded into ELF magnetic fields (Durney, Rushforth, & Anderson, 1988). There are electric and magnetic fields more or less everywhere we go that utilize 50 or 60 Hz of electric power. Hence, extremely low frequency (ELF, 0 - 300 Hz) fields are very important from a public health point of view. Despite the fact that the interaction of electromagnetic fields with biological systems has been investigated, there are biophysical mechanisms which can explain many of the observed biological effects of low frequency magnetic fields (Habash, 2004). Since the use of mobile communications is exploding, with 25% of the earth's population owing a mobile phone, we should consider the relevance of theoretical models that relate the interaction between low frequency magnetic fields and biological matter to radiofrequency electromagnetic fields.

We can measure the external quantities of electric and magnetic fields, and internal quantities can be measured as current density and specific absorption rate (SAR). The SAR measures the energy absorption rate by the body that can be manifested as heat (Durney, Massoudi, & Iskander, 1986). Skin penetration depth is inversely proportional to the frequency of the field, and hence the higher the frequency, the shallower the skin depth. For example, for 10 GHz frequency skin penetration is about 0.4 cm. The International Committee of Non-Ionizing Radiation Protection (ICNIRP) has introduced exposure limit values for electromagnetic fields. Exposure above 100 kHz can lead to considerable absorption of energy, and hence, temperature increases. According to ICNIRP limits (ICNIRP Guidelines), to avoid affecting the nervous system, basic exposure limits have given according to frequency range. Signals between 0 - 100 kHz limits are provided on current density. When the signal is between 100 kHz - 10 GHz, limits are provided on both current density and SAR to prevent high, localized tissue heating. Finally, if the signal is between 10 - 300 GHz limits are provided on power density to prevent excessive heating in tissue.

1. *Low Frequency Electromagnetic Fields (LF EMF)* - Frequency is between 30 - 300 kHz and wavelength is 1 - 10 km. This is in the low frequency range, and is therefore considered a non-thermal electromagnetic field. The induced current carries electric currents in the body and leads to nerve excitation. Hence, the limiting factor for LF EMF is current density (A/m^2).
2. *High Frequency Electromagnetic Fields (HF EMF)* - Frequency is between 3 - 30 MHz and wavelength is 10 - 100 m. This is in the microwave range, considered a thermal electromagnetic field. This leads to very high penetration depth; hence, body heating (by setting water dipoles into rotation) occurs. Thus, limiting factor for LF EMF is SAR (W/kg).

3. *Very High Frequency Electromagnetic Fields (VHF EMF)* - Frequency is between 30 - 300 MHz and wavelength is 1 - 10 m. This is in the infrared, visible light range (higher than microwave range). This leads to very low penetration depth, causing skin burns due to body heating. Hence, the limiting factor for VHF EMF is power density (W/m^2). According to the World Health Organization (WHO), induced electric fields are more than one million times weaker than the external field.

In cellular dynamics, electrical activity of excitable cells has beenn extensively studied (Panagopoulos, Karabarbounis, & Margaritis, 2002; Panagopoulos et al., 2000). Dielectric data for body tissue and the underlying mechanisms of interaction at the cellular, sub-cellular and molecular levels are vital to study. The position of the biological system with respect to the field, availability of an electric or magnetic component or both, amplitude and gradient of the field, frequency spectrum and timing are some essential parameters for the biological effects of electromagnetic fields. The principal role of the interaction between electromagnetic fields in a biological system depends on the cell membrane (Adair, 1991; Eichwald & Walleczek, 1998; Magnussen, 1999). The cellular studies have rigorously addressed the biophysical mechanisms of the interaction of weak electromagnetic fields on biological tissues. The electromagnetic bio-effects of relatively weak signals can be produced with a time-varying electric field, *E(t),* which is induced from an applied time-varying magnetic field, *B(t)* (Pilla 2006). The possibility for the channel to be open will be influenced from an external field, and thus the current of ions into the cell. An AC electric field will apply oscillating force on the free ions on the outside of the cell and in channel protein. When the amplitude of the ions' force vibration exceeds some threshold value, the oscillating ions will give a false signal to the channel protein voltage sensor for opening or closing the channel. This external field sets up a periodic force on each free ion that can pass across plasma membrane. Due to this force, the ion is displaced a certain distance from its initial position (Panagopoulos et al., 2000). Panagopoulos et al. (Panagopoulos et al., 2000; 2002) have shown that this vibration of electric charge is able to irregularly gate electro-sensitive channels on the plasma membrane, and thus cause interference the cell's electrochemical balance and function. Authors developed a mathematical model by considering AC electric and magnetic fields' influence on cells (Panagopoulos et al., 2000). However, this phase needs to be considered in detail to identify with the complicated details of electromagnetic interactions in cell plasma membranes in the presence of noise.

The ions formed under the influence of ionizing radiation in the tissue cells are highly reactive and can break DNA strands, thus causing many alterations. There is a probability to form various cancerous growths because they move in the tissue to the blood stream and then over the whole body. As a result of cancerous tissue growth, normal tissues slowly undergo nutritive death. Low frequency electric fields arise from electric charges and external electric fields induce charges on the body's surface. Because of the conducting nature of the tissues, the external electromagnetic fields can induce electromagnetic fields in the tissues. Thus, the body's surface charge produces a current density inside the body. Low frequency magnetic fields arise from the motion of electric charges and are strongest close to the device. This results from an induced electric field and the circulation of electric currents according to Faraday's law. The magnitude of induced field and the current density is proportional to the loop radius. Hence, the strongest electric fields are induced when the loop dimensions are greatest. At very high frequencies, since all energy is immersed in a small region, the heating of the skin is significant.

At extremely low frequencies the internal field is extremely small; however, the wavelength is large for low frequencies, so the radiation of energy can penetrate through the body extensively. Strong low frequency fields are capable of inducing electric currents which lead to nerve excitation. This stimulated membrane of a nerve fiber causes slight leakage of ions through protein ion channels in the membrane to its interior. The membrane potential is changed by these ions, which in turn causes more channels to open, thus changing potential. These potential changes in turn cause the electrical current to flow along both inside and outside the fiber and further increase potential changes. Until the nerve signal goes to the end of the fiber this process continues. These membrane potentials change the cells' functions (Guyton & Hall, 2006).

A number of experiments indicate an enhancement of the biological effects investigated for certain resonance frequencies (Liboff, 1987; Liboff et al., 1987; McLeod et al., 1987; Smith et al., 1987). Some theoretical models are considered below, with particular emphasis on the ability to modify the function of proteins in the cell membrane. Previous work (Litovitz, 1991) has showen a hypothesis, that there should be steady oscillating electromagnetic fields for a certain period of time (approximately 1 s) to obtain a biological effect. This permits us to differentiate between external fields and thermal noise fields, even if they might be lesser than the noise fields (Habash, 2004).

RESONANCE AND ITS APPLICATION

A cyclotron is a particle accelerator which accelerates charged particles using high frequency alternating voltage. Cyclotron resonance frequency is a distinctive function of charge to mass ratio ($\psi\ q/m$) and intensity of magnetic field $\omega_c = (\psi\ q/m)B$. When the external field is tuned to the cyclotron frequency of the ion or to its harmonics, the effect accomplishes its maximum. Further, cyclotron resonance can occur when AC electric fields are tuned to the cyclotron frequency of the specific ion.

The Ion Cyclotron Resonance (ICR) Model

The Ion Cyclotron Resonance (ICR) model is one of the first models that described the event of resonance frequencies' correlation to the magnitude of the geomagnetic field. The ICR model was formulated by Liboff (McLeod & Liboff, 1986), is reporting the movement of ions in a magnetic field. This model considers an ion moving in a static magnetic field B and a time varying electric field E which is the basis of the ion's acceleration. Cyclotron resonance means that an AC electric field is tuned to the *cyclotron frequency* of the specific ion. This occurs when the AC electric field is perpendicular to the DC magnetic field in the absence of an AC magnetic field, or when an AC magnetic field is parallel to the DC magnetic field. The ICR model explains the incident of resonance frequencies, but, does not indicate how the response might vary with different AC flux densities.

Ion Parametric Resonance (IPR) Model

The IPR model depends on the frequency of the AC magnetic field, the flux densities of the AC and DC magnetic fields, and charge to mass ratio of the target ions. Since the basic signal to noise issues might not be resolved in the ICR model, the primary form of the IPR model was proposed by Lednev (Lednev, 1991) and later by Blanchard et al. (Blanchard & Blackman, 1994; Blanchard, Blackman, & House, 1995). This considers the oscillation (in a given direction) of an ion bound to a protein (Calmodulin), in a time-varying magnetic field. The model was disproved but then defended by Adair (Adair, 1992, 1998) and Engström extended this model over a number of studies (Engstrom, 1996, 1997; Engstrom &

Bowman, 2004). According to the IPR model, at cyclotron resonance, bio-effect reaches maximum when $B_{AC}/B_{DC} = 1.84$, where it follows the Bessel function as $J_1(B_{AC}/B_{DC})$, for parallel AC and DC magnetic fields. Blanchard and Blackman have experimentally and else, theoretically demonstrated a different functional motif of biological effects' dependency. According to them bio-effects follow the Bessel function as $J_1(2B_{AC}/B_{DC})$ and the maximum effect is at $B_{AC}/B_{DC} = 0.9$ (Blanchard & Blackman, 1994). Later, Koch (Koch, Sommarin, Persson, Salford, & Eberhardt, 2003) supported this model using experimental demonstrations.

Lednev (Lednev, 1991) and others (Binhi, 2000; Blackman, Blanchard, Benane, & House, 1994; Blanchard & Blackman, 1994; Engstrom, 1996; Liboff, 1985; Liboff, 1987; Liboff, Williams, Strong, & Wistar, 1984; Blackman, Blanchard, Benane, & House, 1995; Blackman, Blanchard, Benane, House, & Elder, 1998; Muehsam & Pilla, 1994; Chiabrera, 1992; Coulton, 2000; Hendee et al., 1996; Shuvalova, Ostrovskaya, Sosunov, & Lednev, 1991; Chiabrera, 1989) formulated an IPR quantum method which modeled an ion, bound in a trap, as a charged oscillator, characterized by several vibrational energy levels, to recover thermal noise problems in the ICR model (Pilla, 2006). This is based on the Zeeman Effect, where existence of a static magnetic field might split the energy level of the bound ion into two sublevels. The Larmor frequency, which is half of the cyclotron frequency, is the difference between these two energy levels (Pilla, 2006).

Application of Resonance

Cyclotrons can be used to cure cancers. Magnetic Resonance Imaging (MRI) is a good example. The resonance condition in IPR occurs in MRI, except with static magnetic fields. The main dissimilarity between IPR and MRI is that in IPR, the AC and DC magnetic fields are parallel to each other, while they are perpendicular to each other in MRI (Halgamuge, Persson, Salford, Mendis, and Eberhardt, 2009).

A recent example of using resonance is the *Wireless Power System*, transferring electrical energy through magnetic field without wires. Devices can be charged without wires as the electromagnetic waves are transmitted through air. This uses low frequency electromagnetic waves to transmit longer distances, and possibly somewhat high frequency waves in shorter distances. Here, both transmitter and receiver should use the same resonant frequency. If the communication distance is less than one wavelength, it is called a near field; if higher, it is called far field. To keep a pure magnetic field, the distance should be less than one wavelength. WiTricity (http://www.witricity.com/index.html) found that this technology is safe as the power is transferred through the magnetic field, not through the electric far field.

Electron cyclotron resonance is also used for efficient plasma generation. Some of the activities dependent on electron cyclotron resonance technology are semiconductor manufacturing (DRAM memories), particle accelerators, and painting plastic bumpers for cars. The nuclear magnetic resonance is used to determine the structure of chemical compounds, for data acquisition in the petroleum industry, and for process control in oil refineries and magnetometers.

ANALYSIS OF LORENZ MODEL

If a particle of charge q moving with a velocity v experiences a force F, independent of v, then this region is to be distinguished by an electric field. However, if the charged particle experiences a force which depends on v, then this region is to be distinguished by a magnetic field. The force, F, is given by $F = qv \times \mathrm{B}$, where B is the magnetic flux density (Rao, 2004). In other terms, magnetic force is proportional to the magnitude of v and orthogonal to v and B. The force due to electric field, E is proportional to it and is given by $F = qE$.

In physics, force will apply on a particle due to an electric and/or magnetic field. External fields deploy a periodic force on each free ion which can pass across plasma membrane (Thompson et al., 1995; McLeod et al., 1987). Due to this force, the ion is displaced distance r from its original position. Three forces are considered which influence each particle's movement: (i) An alternating force due to an external electric or magnetic fields: (ii) A damping force proportional to the velocity of the ion, since the ion moves in a viscous medium (iii) A restoration force due to a slight distortion of ion equilibrium. This force is proportional to the displacement of the ion. The particle, because of the above forces, will be accelerated and displaced. The force F on a particle due to E electric field and B magnetic field, in the vicinity of a cell's plasma membrane is given by, $F = mdv/dt + m\upsilon v + m\omega_3^2 r = \psi q(E + v \times B)$, where υ is the drag coefficient, ψ is the particle valence, q is the electric charge of the particle of mass m, v denotes the velocity of the particle at time t and ω_3 is the self-oscillating frequency.

The drag coefficient illustrates the drag or resistance of a particle in a moving fluid. This depends on the particle's size and shape as well as the fluid viscosity. The nature of drag coefficient depends on the flow of the liquid. In the Laminar flow of liquid, where viscous forces are leading, the drag coefficient has the dimensions of s^{-1}, even though for turbulent flow fluids the drag coefficient is dimensionless. Usually, in the body, the blood flow is laminar. However, under conditions of high flow (e.g.: in the ascending aorta and stenotic heart valves), laminar flow can be disrupted and become turbulent. The resonant behavior vanishes with the increasing drag. The bound lifetime is inversely proportional to viscosity. Long bound times on the order of 1 s in calcium - calmodulin requires $\upsilon \approx 1\ s^{-1}$. The drag coefficient for shorter bound lifetimes, such as 1 ms, require values on the order of $\upsilon = (10^2 - 10^3)$ s^{-1}. The bound lifetime for free ions in a medium with a viscosity equal to that of bulk water, $\upsilon = 10^{13}\ s^{-1}$, will be in the order of 10^{-12} s. For a given value of viscosity, lower values for the oscillator frequency ω_3 result in weaker binding and thus lower bound lifetimes (Muehsam & Pilla, 1996). Since the self-oscillating frequency of free ions is so small it can be considered a constant $\omega_3 = const./\omega$. The self-oscillating frequency depends on the bound life time. When ω_3 is small, the ion's movement due to restoration force is negligible (Panagopoulos et al., 2000).

The static magnetic field, B_0 is in the y–z plane of the alternating electric field, E is in x direction of the alternating magnetic field and B is in z direction as shown in Figure 1. We choose E and B arbitrarily to be at 90^0, such that alternating $E = (E_x, 0, 0)$, static $B_o = (0, B_{oy}, B_{oz})$, and alternating $B = (0, 0, B_{1z})$.

The Non-Linear and Linear Equations of Motion

The aim of this section is to observe nonlinearity and linearity in the motion of charged particles. In the effect on a charged particle of combined AC - DC electromagnetic fields, mainly considering initial position and speed to cyclotron resonance forms a background to this work (Halgamuge, Abeyrathne, Mendis, 2009).

AC Electric Field and DC Magnetic Field

In this case, combined AC electric and DC magnetic field is considered. Here E varies sinusoidal with time, as $E(t) = E_1 \sin ky \cos kx \sin \omega t$, where E_1 is the electric field intensity, $k = \omega/c\sqrt{2}$, angular frequency $\omega = 2\pi f$, f frequency, and c is speed of light. The force due to alternating electric field and static magnetic field considering a nonlinear model is given by replacing ky by y, kx by x and ωt by t. The displacement in x, y and z directions are given by the forces in these directions:

$$x'' + \hat{\upsilon}x' + \omega_3^2 x = \beta_1 \sin y \cos x \sin t + \omega_{oz} y' - \omega_{oy} z',$$

$$y'' + \hat{\upsilon}y' + \omega_3^2 y = -\omega_{oz} x',$$

$$z'' + \hat{\upsilon}z' + \omega_3^2 z = \omega_{oy} x'. \tag{1}$$

Considering dimensionless quantities, where $\hat{\upsilon} = v/f$, $\omega_{oy} = \psi\, q\, B_{oy} /m\, \omega$, $\omega_{oz} = \psi\, q\, B_{oz} /m\, \omega$, $\beta_1 = \psi\, qE_1/m\, \beta_0$ and $\beta_0 = \psi\, qE_0/m$. Here $\omega_{oy} = \omega_o \sin\theta$ and $\omega_{oz} = \omega_o \cos\theta$ characterize the dimensionless cyclotron resonance frequencies, which depend on the static magnetic fields in *y* and *z* directions, respectively.

Thus, the linear model for alternating electric and static magnetic fields, replacing *sin y* by *y* and *cos x* by 1 is given by the forces in *x*, *y* and *z* directions:

$$x'' + \hat{\upsilon}x' + \omega_3^2 x = \beta_1 y \sin t + \omega_{oz} y' - \omega_{oy} z',,$$

$$y'' + \hat{\upsilon}y' + \omega_3^2 y = -\omega_{oz} x',$$

$$z'' + \hat{\upsilon}z' + \omega_3^2 z = \omega_{oy} x'. \tag{2}$$

The electric field exerts a force only in *x* direction since the electric field is in that direction. The resultant displacement can be obtained by the vector summation of the displacements in all three directions. In these fields, the particle must displace in the electric field's direction, which is perpendicular to the static magnetic field.

AC Magnetic Field and DC Magnetic Field

The influence of AC magnetic field and DC magnetic field on particles motion is examined. Here *B* varies sinusoidal with time, as $E(t) = B_1 \cos kx \cos ky \cos \omega t$ where B_1 is the magnetic field intensity. The non-linear model is given by considering the displacement in *x*, *y* and *z* directions due to the forces on the particle:

$$x'' + \hat{\upsilon}x' + \omega_3^2 x = \left(\omega_{oz} + \omega_1 \cos x \cos y \cos t\right) y' - \omega_{oy} z',$$

$$y'' + \hat{\upsilon}y' + \omega_3^2 y = -\left(\omega_{oz} + \omega_1 \cos x \cos y \cos t\right) x',$$

$$z'' + \hat{\upsilon}z' + \omega_3^2 z = \omega_{oy} x', \tag{3}$$

where $\omega_1 = \psi q\, B_1 / m\omega$. This dimensionless parameter gives the angular frequency due to the strength of the AC magnetic field.

The linear model is given by taking $\cos x = \cos y = 1$, and the forces in *x*, *y* and *z* directions are:

$$x'' + \hat{\upsilon}x' + \omega_3^2 x = \left(\omega_{oz} + \omega_1 \cos t\right) y' - \omega_{oy} z',$$

$$y'' + \hat{\upsilon}y' + \omega_3^2 y = -\left(\omega_{oz} + \omega_1 \cos t\right) x',$$

$$z'' + \hat{\upsilon}z' + \omega_3^2 z = \omega_{oy} x'. \tag{4}$$

The alternating magnetic field influences the particle's motion in *x* and *y* directions only because this field is in the *z* direction. The particle displaces perpendicular to both alternating and static magnetic fields.

6.1.3 AC Electric Field and AC and DC Magnetic Field

In the presence of alternating fields, the E and B fields are coupled together via Maxwell's equations. Here, $\nabla E = \rho/\varepsilon$, $\nabla B = 0$, $\nabla \times E = -\partial B/\partial t$ and $\nabla \times B = \mu\varepsilon\, \partial E/\partial t + \mu J$, where ρ is the charge density, J is the conductive current density, ε is the permittivity and μ is the permeability of the medium. The spatial dependence of E and B will induce nonlinearities in the Lorenz model. The resultant magnetic field due to static and alternating magnetic fields is $B = B_{oy}\hat{y} + (B_{oz} + B_1)\hat{z}$.

Assuming there are no external forces, (i.e. $\rho = 0, J = 0$), $E_{1x}\,\hat{x} + E_{1y}\,\hat{y} = c^2 \int (\partial B_1/\partial x\ \hat{x} + \partial B_1/\partial y\ \hat{y})\, dt$.

The nonlinear model is given by considering the displacement in x, y and z directions due to the forces in these directions:

$$x'' + \hat{\upsilon}x' + \omega_3^2 x = \left(-\omega/2\right)\cos x \sin y \sin t + \left(\omega_{oz} + \omega_1 \cos x \cos y \cos t\right)y' - \omega_{oy}z',$$

$$y'' + \hat{\upsilon}y' + \omega_3^2 y = \left(\omega_1/2\right)\sin x \cos y \sin t - \left(\omega_{oz} + \omega_1 \cos x \cos y \cos t\right)x',$$

$$z'' + \hat{\upsilon}z' + \omega_3^2 z = \omega_{oy}x'. \tag{5}$$

Thus, the linear model is given by considering the forces in x, y and z directions:

$$x'' + \hat{\upsilon}x' + \omega_3^2 x = \left(-\omega_1/2\right)y \sin t + \left(\omega_{oz} + \omega_1 \cos t\right)y' - \omega_{oy}z',$$

$$y'' + \hat{\upsilon}y' + \omega_3^2 y = \left(\omega_1/2\right)x \sin t - \left(\omega_{oz} + \omega_1 \cos t\right)x',$$

$$z'' + \hat{\upsilon}z' + \omega_3^2 z = \omega_{oy}x'. \tag{6}$$

An alternating electric field is induced in both x and y directions by an alternating magnetic field in z direction. Hence, the force of the alternating magnetic field influences the particle motion in x and y directions only.

NUMERICAL RESULTS AND DISCUSSION

The behavior of the particle motion for various combinations of the dimensionless quantities $\omega_{0,}$ ω_1, β and the angle θ between AC and DC magnetic fields, is analyzed in this section. Here zero drag is assumed. The influence of the AC electric field and DC magnetic field on particle displacement in x, y and z directions is shown in Figures 3 and 4. The resonance is observed at $\omega = \omega_{0,}\omega_0/2$ when the initial velocity of particles is zero. The initial velocity influences the particle displacement significantly. When ω_1 is fixed and smaller than ω_0, the only clear effect in both the linear and nonlinear models is cyclotron resonance at $\omega_0 = 1$. Hence, at this point external field frequency ω = cyclotron frequency, ω_c. These two figures show that the maximum particle displacement occurs at zero fields and this is experimentally demonstrated (Binhi, Alipov, & Belyaev, 2001; Lednev et al., 1996). However, in the nonlinear model there are small resonants at other frequencies except at the cyclotron frequency. Thus, the non-linear model does not verify the ICR behavior of charged particles.

The particle displacement varies with angle and ω_0, due to the initial conditions. Hence the angle of maximum displacement varies. Theoretically, for parallel magnetic fields and a perpendicular electric field, the effect maximizes at cyclotron resonance conditions. There is no displacement in z direction if the initial conditions are zero in that direction. If there is an initial condition in z direction, the particle displacement is constant with ω_0, and there is no resonance. However, if either x or y has a initial condition, the particle moves in both directions, whereas for zero initial conditions the displacement is zero in both directions. The existence of an initial velocity and increasing initial conditions increases the particle's displacement. The amplitude and direction of the resonant at $\omega_0 = 1$, vary with the initial conditions. For some initial conditions the resonant does not occur. Moreover, displacement is higher for the AC electric field than the AC magnetic field. However, the existence of an initial velocity makes the displacement similar for all three cases.

The effect of non-linearity on the IPR model can be illustrated in Figures 5 and 6. These figures show the particle's displacement with B_{AC}/B_{DC} for $\theta = 0$, $y(0) = 1$ and $\omega_0 = 1$. Figure 5 shows the particle's motion for the linear model; Figure

Figure 3. Linear model for AC electric and DC magnetic field: The particle displacement with zero drag, $\omega_1 = 0.1$, $\omega_3 = 0.001$, $\theta = 0^0$ and initial positions $x(0) = y(0) = z(0) = 1$

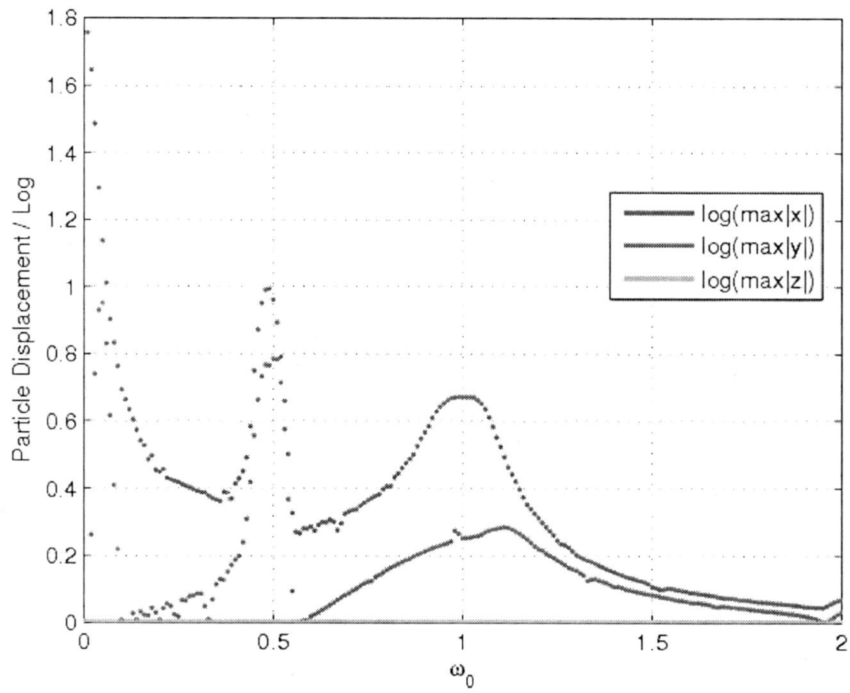

Figure 4. Linear model for AC electric and DC magnetic field: The particle displacement with zero drag, $\omega_1 = 0.1$, $\omega_3 = 0.001$, $\theta = 0^0$, initial positions $x(0) = y(0) = z(0) = 1$ and initial velocities $x'(0) = y'(0) = z'(0) = 1$

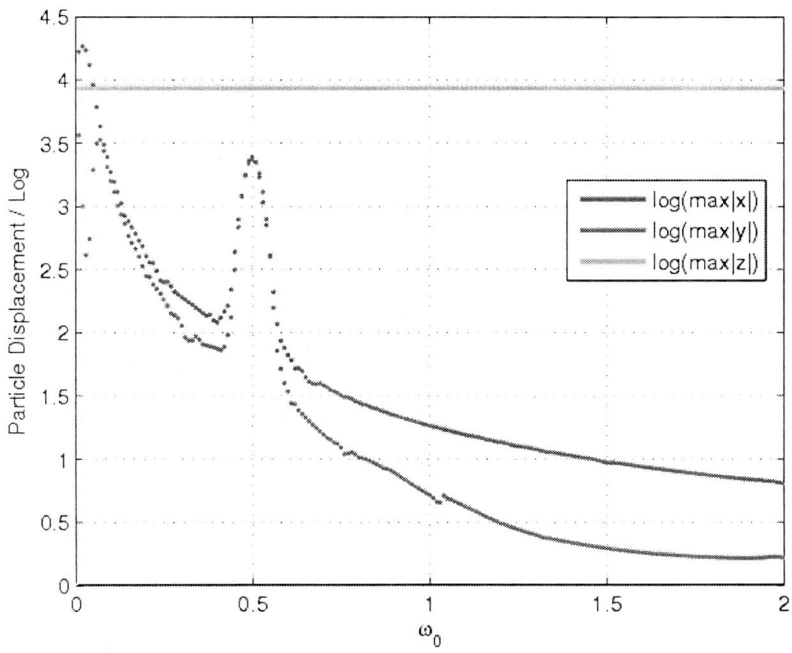

Figure 5. Linear model for AC and DC magnetic field: The particle displacement with zero drag, ω_0 = 1, ω_3 = 0.001, $\theta = 0^0$ and initial positions y(0) =1

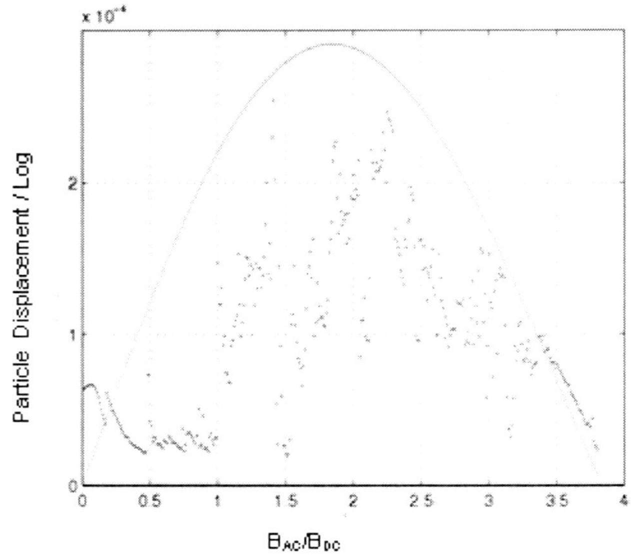

Figure 6. Non-linear model for AC and DC magnetic field: The particle displacement with zero drag, ω_0 =1, ω_3 = 0.001, $\theta = 0^0$ and initial positions y(0) =1

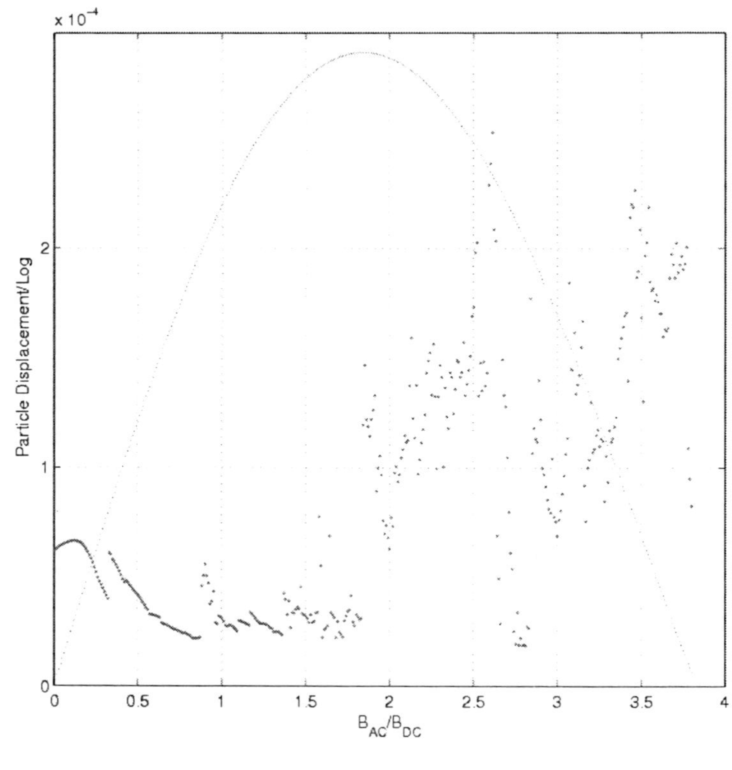

Figure 7. Linear model for AC electric and AC, DC magnetic field: Resonance windows with zero drag, $\omega_3 = 0.001$, $\theta = 0^0$ and initial positions $x(0) = y(0) = z(0) = 1$

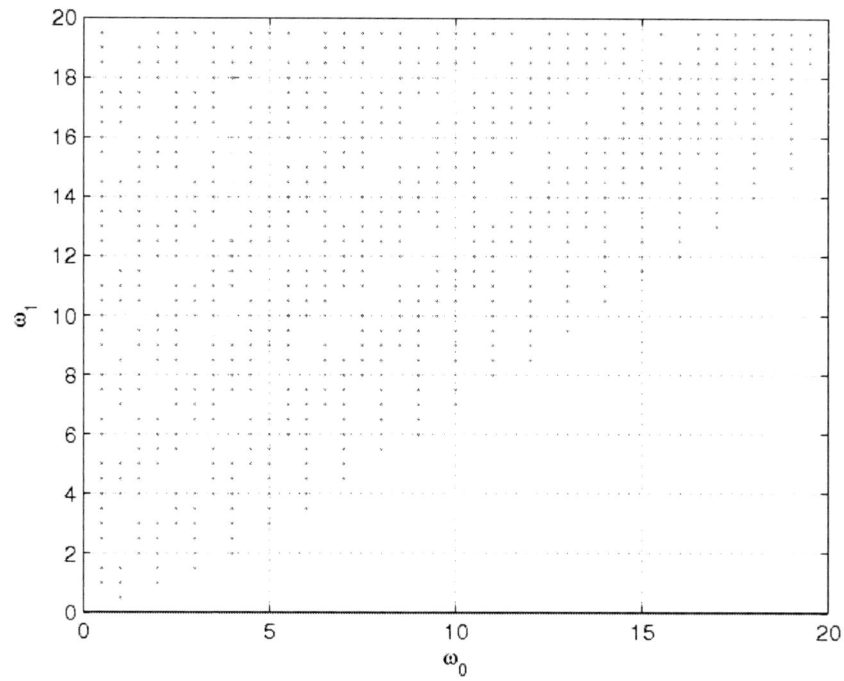

6 shows for the nonlinear model. This model does not follow the Bessel function, while the linear model follows it such that the maximum occurs at $B_{AC}/B_{DC} = 1.84$. We observed the IPR model for an AC electric field and DC magnetic field as well as for AC electric and AC and DC magnetic fields when $\theta = 0$ for both the linear and non-linear models. In neither case does the particle follow the Bessel function. Further, the linear AC, DC magnetic field model only verified Lednev's model, not Blackman and Blanchard's model. More experimental verification is required to clarify this behavior.

Figure 7 shows the resonance windows for the linear model of AC electric and AC, DC magnetic fields when $\theta = 0$. The figure illustrates the dimensionless particle displacement in the x direction when it exceeds 10 in 50 time steps. The windows are regularly spaced, as in Figure 6. Figure 8 illustrates the particle's displacement with a varying angle, θ, and ω_0. The particle shows a resonant behavior at $\omega_0 = 1$. The maximum displacement occurs for $\theta = 90^0$. Further, the particle's motion is altered with the existence of noise. This model becomes physically impossible with increasing initial conditions, integration time and field densities because the particle's displacement becomes higher than the biological cell dimensions.

CONCLUSION

This chapter analyzed in detail the behavior of a charged particle in a biological cell exposed to different combinations of electric and magnetic fields. Our results show that an alternating electric field influences the particle's displacement, and therefore the cell more than does an alternating magnetic field. When alternating and static

Figure 8. Non-linear model for AC electric and DC magnetic field: The particle displacement in x direction with zero drag, $\omega_1 = 0.1$, $\omega_3 = 0.001$, $\theta = 0^0$ and initial positions $x(0) = y(0) = z(0) = 1$

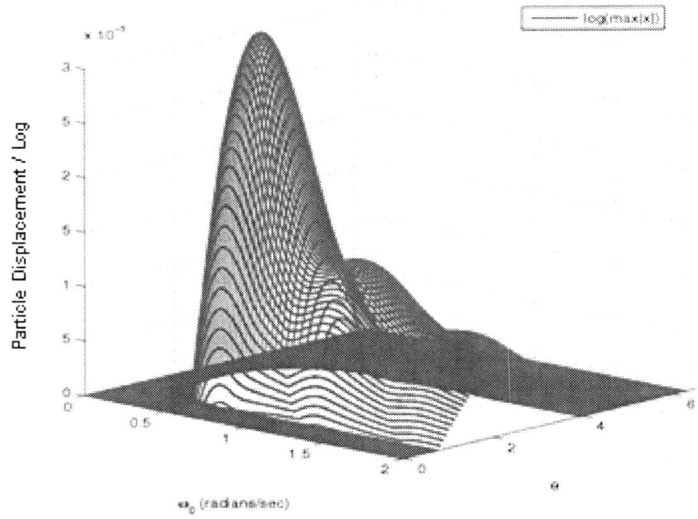

magnetic fields are parallel to each other, and an alternating electric field is perpendicular to the magnetic field, the maximum displacement occurs. The particle's displacement in a biological cell due to electric and magnetic fields is sensitive to initial positions and initial velocities of the particle. This indicates the frequency and angle where maximum displacement occurs can be changed.

FUTURE RESEARCH DIRECTIONS

Complicated and sensitive research procedure needs to be designed to determine the biological effects of a low frequency electromagnetic field. The lack of such sensitivity generates a high possibility of deriving inconsistent results (Habash, 2004). The lack of skills and experience of scientists can be a reason for this inconsistency. Hence, it is necessary to analyze existing results and carry on properly structured and independent research all over the world. This research is highly required to reduce the gap of information.

REFERENCES

Adair, R. K. (1991). Constraints on biological effects of weak extremely-low-frequency electromagnetic-fields. *Physical Review A., 43*(2), 1039–1048. doi:10.1103/PhysRevA.43.1039

Adair, R. K. (1992). Criticism of lednev mechanism for the influence of weak magnetic-fields on biological-systems. *Bioelectromagnetics, 13*(3), 231–235. doi:10.1002/bem.2250130307

Adair, R. K. (1998). A physical analysis of the ion parametric resonance model. *Bioelectromagnetics, 19*(3), 181–191. doi:10.1002/(SICI)1521-186X(1998)19:3<181::AID-BEM6>3.0.CO;2-Y

Barnes, F. S. (2006). *Bioengineering and biophysical aspects of Electromagnetic fields*. Boca Raton, FL: CRC.

Bier, M. (2006). How to evaluate the electric noise in a cell membrane? *Acta Physica Polonica B, 37*(5), 1409.

Binhi, V. N. (2000). Amplitude and frequency dissociation spectra of ion-protein complexes rotating in magnetic fields. *Bioelectromagnetics, 21*(1), 34–45. doi:10.1002/(SICI)1521-186X(200001)21:1<34::AID-BEM6>3.0.CO;2-8

Binhi, V. N., Alipov, Y. D., & Belyaev, Y. I. (2001). Effect of static magnetic field on E. coli cells and individual rotations of ion - protein complexes. *Bioelectromagnetics, 22*, 79–86. doi:10.1002/1521-186X(200102)22:2<79::AID-BEM1009>3.0.CO;2-7

Blackman, C. F., Benane, S. G., Rabinowitz, J. R., House, D. E., & Joines, W. T. (1985). A role for the magnetic-field in the radiation-induced efflux of calcium-ions from brain-tissue invitro. *Bioelectromagnetics, 6*(4), 327–337. doi:10.1002/bem.2250060402

Blackman, C. F., Blanchard, J. P., Benane, S. G., & House, D. E. (1994). Empirical-test of an ion parametric resonance model for magnetic-field interactions with pc-12 cells. *Bioelectromagnetics, 15*(3), 239–260. doi:10.1002/bem.2250150307

Blackman, C. F., Blanchard, J. P., Benane, S. G., & House, D. E. (1995). The ion parametric resonance model predicts magnetic-field parameters that affect nerve-cells. *The FASEB Journal, 9*(7), 547–551.

Blackman, C. F., Blanchard, J. P., Benane, S. G., House, D. E., & Elder, J. A. (1998). Double blind test of magnetic field effects on neurite outgrowth. *Bioelectromagnetics, 19*(4), 204–209. doi:10.1002/(SICI)1521-186X(1998)19:4<204::AID-BEM2>3.0.CO;2-5

Blackman, C. F., Kinney, L. S., House, D. E., & Joines, W. T. (1989). Multiple power-density windows and their possible origin. *Bioelectromagnetics, 10*(2), 115–128. doi:10.1002/bem.2250100202

Blanchard, J. P., & Blackman, C. F. (1994). Clarification and application of an ion parametric resonance model for magnetic-field interactions with biological-systems (1994). *bioelectromagnetics, 15*(5), 493-493.

Blanchard, J. P., & Blackman, C. F. (1994). Clarification and Application of an Ion Parametric Resonance Model for Magnetic Field Interactions with Biological Systems. *Bioelectromagnetics, 15*, 217–238. doi:10.1002/bem.2250150306

Blanchard, J. P., Blackman, C. F., & House, D. E. (1995). Clarification and application of ion parametric resonance model for magnetic-field interactions with biological-systems - reply. *Bioelectromagnetics, 16*(4), 274–275. doi:10.1002/bem.2250160413

Chiabrera, A. B. B., Kaufman J. J., & Pilla A. A. (1989). Interaction Mechanisms of Low Level Electromagnetic Fields in Living Systems. Genoa, Italy: University of Genoa.

Chiabrera, A. (1992). From the Langevin-Lorentz to the Zeeman model of electromagnetic effects on ligand-receptor binding. *Bioelectrochemistry and Bioenergetics, 28*, 355–365. doi:10.1016/0302-4598(92)80025-C

Cooper, P. J., Garny, A., & Kohl, P. (2003). *Cardiac electrophysiology: Theoretical considerations of a potential target for weak electromagnetic field effects*. Oxford, UK: Oxford University Press.

Coulton, LA, B. A., Van Lierop JE, and Walsh MP. (2000). The effect of static magnetic fields on the rate of calcium/calmodulin-dependent phosphorylation of myosin light chain. *Bioelectromagnetics, 21*, 189–196. doi:10.1002/(SICI)1521-186X(200004)21:3<189::AID-BEM6>3.0.CO;2-L

Durney, C. H., Massoudi, H., & Iskander, M. F. (1986). Radiofrequency radiation dosimetry handbook (4 ed.). New York: Wiley.

Durney, C. H., Rushforth, C. K., & Anderson, A. A. (1988). Resonant AC – DC magnetic fields: calculated response. *Bioelectromagnetics*, *9*, 315–336. doi:10.1002/bem.2250090402

Eichwald, C., & Walleczek, J. (1998). Magnetic field perturbations as a tool for controlling enzyme-regulated and oscillatory biochemical reactions. *Biophysical Chemistry*, *74*(3), 209–224. doi:10.1016/S0301-4622(98)00180-X

Engstrom, S. (1996). Dynamic properties of Lednev's parametric resonance mechanism. *Bioelectromagnetics*, *17*(1), 58–70. doi:10.1002/(SICI)1521-186X(1996)17:1<58::AID-BEM8>3.0.CO;2-5

Engstrom, S. (1997). What is the time scale of magnetic field interaction in biological systems? *Bioelectromagnetics*, *18*(3), 244–249. doi:10.1002/(SICI)1521-186X(1997)18:3<244::AID-BEM7>3.0.CO;2-2

Engstrom, S., & Bowman, J. D. (2004). Magnetic resonances of ions in biological systems. *Bioelectromagnetics*, *25*(8), 620–630. doi:10.1002/bem.20028

Guyton, C., & Hall, J. E. (2006). *Textbook of medical physiology*. Philadelphia: Elsevier Inc.

Habash, R. (2004). *Biological Effects of Electromagnetic Fields, Handbook of Engineering Electromagnetic Fields*. Boca Raton, FL: CRC Press.

Halgamuge, M. N., Abeyratne, C. D., & Mendis, P. (2009). *Effect of Cyclotron Resonance Frequencies in Particles Due to AC and DC ElectroMagnetic Fields*. Paper presented at the World Academy of Science, Rome, Italy.

Halgamuge, M. N., Persson, B. R. R., Salford, L. G., Mendis, P., & Eberhardt, J. L. (2009). Comparison between Two Models for Interactions between Electric and Magnetic Fields and Proteins in Cell Membranes. *Environmental Engineering Science*, *26*(10), 1473–1480. doi:10.1089/ees.2009.0014

Hendee, S. P., Faour, F. A., Christensen, D. A., Patrick, B., Durney, C. H., & Blumenthal, D. K. (1996). The effects of weak extremely low frequency magnetic fields on calcium/calmodulin interactions. *Biophysical Journal*, *70*(6), 2915–2923. doi:10.1016/S0006-3495(96)79861-2

Koch, C., Sommarin, M., Persson, B. R. R., Salford, L. G., & Eberhardt, J. L. (2003). Interaction between weak low frequency magnetic fields and cell membranes. *Bioelectromagnetics*, *24*(6), 395–402. doi:10.1002/bem.10136

Lednev, V. V. (1991). Possible mechanism for the influence of weak magnetic-fields on biological-systems. *Bioelectromagnetics*, *12*(2), 71–75. doi:10.1002/bem.2250120202

Lednev, V. V. (1991). Possible mechanism for the influence of weak magnetic fields on biological systems. *Bioelectromagnetics*, *12*, 71–75. doi:10.1002/bem.2250120202

Lednev, V. V., Srebnotskaya, L. K., & L'Yasova, I., Y. N., Rozhdestvenskaya., Z. Y., Klimov, A. A., Belova, N. A., et al. (1996). Magnetic parametric resonance in bio-systems: experimental verification of the predictions of a theory using regenerating planarians Dugesia tigrina as a test system. *Biophysics*, *41*, 825–835.

Liboff, A. (1985). Cyclotron resonance in membrane transport. In *Interactions between Electromagnetic Fields and Cells*. New York: Wiley.

Liboff, A. R. (1987). *S. S., and McLeod BR.* Mechanistic Approaches to Interactions of Electric and Electromagnetic Fields with Living Systems.

Liboff, A. R., Mc, S. S. D., & Leod, B. R. (1987). Mechanistic Approaches to Interactions of Electric and Electromagnetic Fields with Living Systems. *Bioelectrochemistry and Bioenergetics*, *35*(1-2), 71–79.

Liboff, A. R., & McLeod, B. R. (1987). *Mechanistic Approaches to Interactions of Electric and Electromagnetic Fields with Living Systems*. Amsterdam: Springer.

Liboff, A. R., Rozek, R. J., Sherman, M. L., McLeod, B. R., & Smith, S. D. (1987). CA-2+-45 cyclotron-resonance in human-lymphocytes. *Journal of Bioelectricity*, *6*(1), 13–22.

Liboff, A. R., Williams, T., Strong, D. M., & Wistar, R. (1984). Time-varying magnetic-fields - effect on DNA-synthesis. *Science*, *223*(4638), 818–820. doi:10.1126/science.6695183

Litovitz, T. A. K., D.; Mullins, J.M. (1991). Effect of coherence time of the applied magnetic field on ornithine decarboxylase activity. *Biochemical and Biophysical Research Communications*, *178*, 862–865. doi:10.1016/0006-291X(91)90970-I

Mader, S. S. (2008). Human Biology (10 ed.): McGraw Hill Higher Education.

McLeod, B. R., & Liboff, A. R. (1986). Dynamic characteristics of membrane ions in multifield configurations of low-frequency electromagnetic-radiation. *Bioelectromagnetics*, *7*(2), 177–189. doi:10.1002/bem.2250070208

McLeod, B. R., Smith, S. D., Cooksey, K. E., & Liboff, A. R. (1987). Ion-cyclotron resonance frequencies enhance Ca++-dependent motility in diatoms. *Journal of Bioelectricity*, *6*(1), 1–12.

Muehsam, D. J., & Pilla, A. A. (1994). Weak magnetic-field modulation of ion dynamics in a potential well - mechanistic and thermal noise considerations. *Bioelectrochemistry and Bioenergetics*, *35*, 71–79. doi:10.1016/0302-4598(94)87014-4

Noble, D., McKinlay, A., & Repacholi, M. (2005). Effects of static magnetic fields relevant to human health. *Progress in Biophysics and Molecular Biology*, *87*(2-3), 171–372.

Panagopoulos, D. J., Karabarbounis, A., & Margaritis, L. H. (2002). Mechanism for action of electromagnetic fields on cells. *Biochemical and Biophysical Research Communications*, *298*(1), 95–102. doi:10.1016/S0006-291X(02)02393-8

Panagopoulos, D. J., Messini, N., Karabarbounis, A., Philippetis, A. L., & Margaritis, L. H. (2000). A mechanism for action of oscillating electric fields on cells. *Biochemical and Biophysical Research Communications*, *272*(3), 634–640. doi:10.1006/bbrc.2000.2746

Shuvalova, L. A., Ostrovskaya, M. V., Sosunov, Y. A., & Lednev, V. V. (1991). Effect of parametric resonance magnetic-field on the rate of Ca2+-calmodulin dependent myosin phosphorylation. *Doklady Akademii Nauk SSSR*, *317*(1), 227–230.

Smith, S. D., McLeod, B. R., Liboff, A. R., & Cooksey, K. (1987). Calcium cyclotron-resonance and diatom mobility. *Bioelectromagnetics*, *8*(3), 215–227. doi:10.1002/bem.2250080302

Thompson, C. J., Briggs, K. M., Farrell, P., Fleming, A., Hocking, B., & Joyner, K. (1995). Nonlinear dynamics of charged-particles interacting with combined ac-dc electromagnetic-fields. *Physica A*, *220*(3-4), 471–484. doi:10.1016/0378-4371(95)00162-Z

Valjus, J. (1996). Health risks of electric and magnetic fields caused by high-voltage systems in Finland. *Scandinavian Journal of Work, Environment & Health*, *22*(2), 85–93.

ADDITIONAL READING

Adair, R. K. (1998). Extremely low frequency electromagnetic fields do not interact directly with DNA. *Bioelectromagnetics*, *19*(2), 136–137. doi:10.1002/(SICI)1521-186X(1998)19:2<136::AID-BEM14>3.0.CO;2-O

Adair, R. K. (2000). Static and low-frequency magnetic field effects: health risks and therapies. *Reports on Progress in Physics*, *63*(3), 415–454. doi:10.1088/0034-4885/63/3/204

Binhi, V. N. (2000). Rotation of biological systems in magnetic fields: Splitting of spectra of some magnetobiological effects. *Biofizika*, *45*(4), 757–759.

Binhi, V. N., & Blackman, C. F. (2005). Analysis of the structure of magnetic fields that induced inhibition of stimulated neurite outgrowth. *Bioelectromagnetics*, *26*(8), 684–689. doi:10.1002/bem.20180

Binhi, V. N., Chernavskii, D. S., & Rubin, A. B. (2006). The temperature factor and magnetic noise under the conditions of stochastic resonance of magnetosomes. *Biofizika*, *51*(2), 274–277.

Binhi, V. N., & Savin, A. V. (2003). Effects of weak magnetic fields on biological systems: physical aspects. *Physics-Uspekhi*, *46*(3), 259–291. doi:10.1070/PU2003v046n03ABEH001283

Blackman, C. F., Andrews, P. W., Ubeda, A., Wang, X., House, D. E., & Trillo, M. A. (2001). Physiological levels of melatonin enhance gap junction communication in primary cultures of mouse hepatocytes. *Cell Biology and Toxicology*, *17*(1), 1–9. doi:10.1023/A:1010980112946

Blackman, C. F., Benane, S. G., & House, D. E. (1995). Frequency-dependent interference by magnetic fields of nerve growth factor-induced neurite outgrowth in PC-12 cells. *Bioelectromagnetics*, *16*(6), 387–395. doi:10.1002/bem.2250160607

Blackman, C. F., Benane, S. G., House, D. E., & Joines, W. T. (1985). Effects of ELF (1-120 Hz) and modulated (50 Hz) RF fields on the efflux of calcium-ions from brain-tissue invitro. *Bioelectromagnetics*, *6*(1), 1–11. doi:10.1002/bem.2250060102

Coulton, LA, B. A., Van Lierop JE, and Walsh MP. (2000). The effect of static magnetic fields on the rate of calcium/calmodulin-dependent phosphorylation of myosin light chain. *Bioelectromagnetics*, *21*, 189–196. doi:10.1002/(SICI)1521-186X(200004)21:3<189::AID-BEM6>3.0.CO;2-L

Durney, C. H. (1992). Interactions between electromagnetic-fields and biological-systems. *Annals of the New York Academy of Sciences*, *649*, 19–34. doi:10.1111/j.1749-6632.1992.tb49593.x

Durney, C. H., Cutillo, A. G., & Ailion, D. C. (2000). Magnetic resonance behavior of normal and diseased lungs: spherical shell model simulations. *Journal of Applied Physiology*, *88*(4), 1155–1166.

Dutta, S. K., Ghosh, B., & Blackman, C. F. (1989). Radio frequency radiation-induced calcium-ion efflux enhancement from human and other neuroblastoma cells in culture. *Bioelectromagnetics*, *10*(2), 197–202. doi:10.1002/bem.2250100208

Engstrom, S., & Fitzsimmons, R. (1999). Five hypotheses to examine the nature of magnetic field transduction in biological systems. *Bioelectromagnetics*, *20*(7), 423–430. doi:10.1002/(SICI)1521-186X(199910)20:7<423::AID-BEM3>3.0.CO;2-W

Engstrom, S., Markov, M. S., McLean, M. J., Holcomb, R. R., & Markov, J. M. (2002). Effects of non-uniform static magnetic fields on the rate of myosin phosphorylation. *Bioelectromagnetics*, *23*(6), 475–479. doi:10.1002/bem.10035

Grande, D. A., Magee, F. P., Weinstein, A. M., & McLeod, B. R. (1991). The effect of low-energy combined ac and dc magnetic-fields on articular-cartilage metabolism. *Annals of the New York Academy of Sciences*, *635*, 404–407. doi:10.1111/j.1749-6632.1991.tb36510.x

Heden, P., & Pilla, A. A. (2008). Effects of pulsed electromagnetic fields on postoperative pain: A double-blind randomized pilot study in breast augmentation patients. *Aesthetic Plastic Surgery*, *32*(4), 660–666. doi:10.1007/s00266-008-9169-z

Hendee, S. P., Greenwald, R. M., & Crisco, J. J. (1998). Static and dynamic properties of various baseballs. *Journal of Applied Biomechanics*, *14*(4), 390–400.

Jenrow, K. A., Smith, C. H., & Liboff, A. R. (1996). Weak extremely-low-frequency magnetic field-induced regeneration anomalies in the planarian Dugesia tigrina. *Bioelectromagnetics*, *17*(6), 467–474. doi:10.1002/(SICI)1521-186X(1996)17:6<467::AID-BEM6>3.0.CO;2-1

Jenrow, K. A., Zhang, X., Renehan, W. E., & Liboff, A. R. (1998). Weak ELF magnetic field effects on hippocampal rhythmic slow activity. *Experimental Neurology*, *153*(2), 328–334. doi:10.1006/exnr.1998.6902

Lavine, L. S., Shamos, M. H., Liboff, A. R., Lustrin, I., & Rinaldi, R. A. (1972). Electric enhancement of bone healing. *Science*, *175*(4026), 1118. doi:10.1126/science.175.4026.1118

Lednev, V. V. (1995). Clarification and application of ion parametric resonance model for magnetic-field interactions with biological-systems - comment. *Bioelectromagnetics*, *16*(4), 268–269. doi:10.1002/bem.2250160410

Lednev, V. V. (1996). Bioeffects of weak combined, static and alternating magnetic fields. *Biofizika*, *41*(1), 224–232.

Lednev, V. V., Srebnitskaya, L. K., Ilyasova, E. N., Rozhdestvenskaya, Z. E., Klimov, A. A., & Tiras, H. P. (1996). Weak combined magnetic field tuned to the parametric resonance of the nuclear spins of hydrogen atoms increases the proliferation of neoblasts in regenerating planarians Dugesia tigrina. *Doklady Akademii Nauk*, *348*(6), 830–833.

Lednev, V. V., Srebnitskaya, L. K., Khromov, A. S., & Rogdestvenskaya, Z. E. (1994). Weak magnetic-fields affect ca-calmodulin dependent myosin phosphorylation in suspension myofibrils. *Journal of Muscle Research and Cell Motility*, *15*(2), 219–219.

Liboff, A. R. (1974). Electrically mediated growth mechanisms in living systems - introductory-remarks. *Annals of the New York Academy of Sciences, 238*(OCT11), 5-6.

Liboff, A. R. (2002). Comment on "Extremely low frequency magnetic fields can either increase or decrease analgesia in the land snail depending on field and light conditions" by Frank S. Prato, M. Kavaliers, and A.W. Thomas. *Bioelectromagnetics*, *23*(5), 406–407. doi:10.1002/bem.10028

Liboff, A. R. (2009). Electric Polarization and the Viability of Living Systems: Ion Cyclotron Resonance-Like Interactions. *Electromagnetic Biology and Medicine*, *28*(2), 124–134. doi:10.1080/15368370902729293

Liboff, A. R., & McLeod, B. R. (1988). Channel ion helicity and inverse cyclotron-resonance eigenfrequencies. *Biophysical Journal*, *53*(2), A632–A632.

Liboff, A. R., McLeod, B. R., & Smith, S. D. (1989). Rotating magnetic-fields and ion-cyclotron resonance. *Journal of Bioelectricity*, *8*(1), 119–125.

Liboff, A. R., & Parkinson, W. C. (1991). Search for ion-cyclotron resonance in an Na+-transport system. *Bioelectromagnetics*, *12*(2), 77–83. doi:10.1002/bem.2250120203

Liboff, A. R., Smith, S. D., & McLeod, B. R. (1995). Clarification and application of ion parametric resonance model for magnetic-field interactions with biological-systems - comment. *Bioelectromagnetics*, *16*(4), 272–273. doi:10.1002/bem.2250160412

Machlup, S., Blackman, C. F., & Blanchard, J. P. (1996). Biological effects of extremely-low-frequency (ELF) magnetic fields may go linearly (not quadratically) with field amplitude. *Biophysical Journal*, *70*(2), MP419–MP419.

Markov, M. S., & Pilla, A. A. (1997). Weak static magnetic field modulation of myosin phosphorylation in a cell-free preparation: calcium dependence. *Bioelectrochemistry and Bioenergetics*, *43*(2), 233–238. doi:10.1016/S0302-4598(96)02226-X

Markov, M. S., Wang, S., & Pilla, A. A. (1993). Effects of weak low-frequency sinusoidal and dc magnetic-fields on myosin phosphorylation in a cell-free preparation. *Bioelectrochemistry and Bioenergetics*, *43*(2), 233–238. doi:10.1016/S0302-4598(96)02226-X

Mayrovitz, H. N., Groseclose, E. E., Markov, M., & Pilla, A. A. (2001). Effects of permanent magnets on resting skin blood perfusion in healthy persons assessed by laser Doppler flowmetry and imaging. *Bioelectromagnetics*, *22*(7), 494–502. doi:10.1002/bem.78

McLean, M. J., Engstrom, S., Holcomb, R. R., & Sanchez, D. (2003). A static magnetic field modulates severity of audiogenic seizures and anticonvulsant effects of phenytoin in DBA/2 mice. *Epilepsy Research*, *55*(1-2), 105–116. doi:10.1016/S0920-1211(03)00109-8

McLeod, B. R. (1983). Electromagnetic signal analysis applied to controlling cell functions electrically. *Journal of the Electrochemical Society*, *130*(3), C122–C122.

McLeod, B. R., Liboff, A. R., & Smith, S. D. (1992). Biological-systems in transition - sensitivity to extremely low-frequency fields. *Electro- and Magnetobiology, 11*(1), 29-42.

McLeod, B. R., Smith, S. D., & Liboff, A. R. (1987). Calcium and potassium cyclotron-resonance curves and harmonics in diatoms (amphora-coffeaeformis). *Journal of Bioelectricity*, *6*(2), 153–168.

Moten, K., Durney, C. H., & Stockham, T. G. (1991). Electromagnetic pulsed-wave radiation in spherical-models of dispersive biological substances. *Bioelectromagnetics*, *12*(6), 319–333. doi:10.1002/bem.2250120602

Muehsam, D. J., & Pilla, A. A. (1996). Lorentz approach to static magnetic field effects on bound-ion dynamics and binding kinetics: Thermal noise considerations. *Bioelectromagnetics*, *17*(2), 89–99. doi:10.1002/(SICI)1521-186X(1996)17:2<89::AID-BEM3>3.0.CO;2-1

Muehsam, D. J., & Pilla, A. A. (1999). The sensitivity of cells and tissues to exogenous fields: effects of target system initial state. *Bioelectrochemistry and Bioenergetics*, *48*(1), 35–42. doi:10.1016/S0302-4598(98)00149-4

Panagopoulos, D. J., Chavdoula, E. D., Karabarbounis, A., & Margaritis, L. H. (2007). Comparison of bioactivity between GSM 900 MHz and DCS 1800 MHz mobile telephony radiation. *Electromagnetic Biology and Medicine*, *26*(1), 33–44. doi:10.1080/15368370701205644

Panagopoulos, D. J., Chavdoula, E. D., Nezis, I. P., & Margaritis, L. H. (2007). Cell death induced by GSM 900-MHz and DCS 1800-MHz mobile telephony radiation. *Mutation Research/Genetic Toxicology and Environmental Mutagenesis*, *626*(1-2), 69–78. doi:10.1016/j.mrgentox.2006.08.008

Panagopoulos, D. J., Karabarbounis, A., & Margaritis, L. H. (2004). Effect of GSM 900-MHz mobile phone radiation on the reproductive capacity of Drosophila melanogaster. *Electromagnetic Biology and Medicine*, *23*(1), 29–43. doi:10.1081/JBC-120039350

Pilla, A. A. (1978). Interfacial electrochemical phenomena and control of living cell behavior. *Journal of the Electrochemical Society*, *125*(3), C171–C171.

Shuvalova, L. A., Ostrovskaya, M. V., Sosunov, Y. A., & Lednev, V. V. (1991). Effect of parametric resonance magnetic-field on the rate of Ca2+-calmodulin dependent myosin phosphorylation. *Doklady Akademii Nauk SSSR*, *317*(1), 227–230.

Smith, S. D., McLeod, B. R., & Liboff, A. R. (1991). Effects of resonant magnetic-fields on chick femoral development invitro. *Journal of Bioelectricity*, *10*(1-2), 81–99.

KEYTERMS AND DEFINITIONS

Electromagnetic Fields: This consists of both electric and magnetic field components. The motion of electrically charged matter produces an electromagnetic field. A changing magnetic creates an electric field and vice versa.

Extremely Low Frequency (ELF): Electromagnetic fields with a frequency between 1 - 300 Hz.

Electromagnetic Radiation: Energy propagation of electromagnetic waves through space.

Exposure: When a person is exposed to electric, magnetic or electromagnetic fields other than those naturally arising from physiological procedures in the body.

Frequency (Hz): The number of complete cycles per second, measured in Hertz (Hz). Frequency is inversely proportional to wavelength, which is the distance between identical points in the adjacent cycles of a waveform.

Ionizing radiation: The electromagnetic waves that have energy to remove an electron from an atom or molecule, thus creating an ion.

Non-Linear: A non-linear system gives an output which is not proportional to input. This occurs as a result of signals that are not linear. In nonlinear systems the effect of external factors are not purely additive.

Oscillation: Cyclic variation, usually in time, of some measure relative to central value or between two or more dissimilar states.

Viscosity: The resistance of fluid to its flow.

Chapter 3
Social and Ethical Concerns of Biomedical Engineering Research and Practice

Snehasish Mishra
KIIT University, India

ABSTRACT

Biomedical engineering is an advanced and relatively new field in the healthcare sector. Owing to the very nature of the various professional challenges faced by healthcare professionals, the moral and ethical values seem to have taken the backburner. The factors contributing to it may include a sound knowledge of the healthcare professional on the legally-permissible ethical values, and the desperate situations requiring precise split-moment decision-making. No technological advancement without a human face is worth it, and hence, during the course of the degree, a biomedical engineering student needs to be exposed to various ethical issues through theory, live cases and demonstrations. Being intrinsically multi- and inter-disciplinary, biomedical engineering lacks precise ethical rules that delineate and delimit professional responsibility, thus blurring the ethical understanding of biomedical engineering. The solution seems to lie in giving due place to human virtues. In the coming days, bioethical issues are expected to be increasingly complicated and dominating the decision-making process owing to the advancements in sciences, and the ever-complicated cases handled by healthcare professionals. A global healthcare and ethics-related online open-access portal may serve as a common platform for all the stakeholders in the interest and ethical growth of biomedical engineering in particular and medical sciences in general.

INTRODUCTION

Technology and ethics are neighbours, not foreigners, facing rather than interfacing each other in the world of human accomplishment. Personal face of ethics looks at the impersonal face of technology to comprehend the latter's potential and limits directed at human purposes and benefits. Technology is a human achievement of extraordinary ingenuity and utility, and is far-off from the human accomplishment of ethical values. In an effort to make one face the other, it is important

DOI: 10.4018/978-1-61692-004-3.ch003

to examine critically-accepted views, evaluate and draw universally-acceptable conclusions.

Biomedical engineering is an integrating medium for two dynamic professions, Medicines and Engineering, and assists in the struggle against illness and disease by providing effective tools for research, diagnosis and treatment by healthcare professionals. They are relatively new members in the healthcare delivery team seeking effective solutions for the difficult problems the modern society faces. Artificial limbs, heart valves, blood vessels, biosensors, biomaterials, respirators, pacemakers and artificial kidneys ('spare-parts' surgery) have redefined medical sciences. Numerous routine diagnoses now use wide-ranging highly sophisticated life-saving image processing and artificial intelligence devices.

These various advancements albeit, have not been entirely benign, having significant moral consequences, be it the cardiovascular assist devices to maintain breathing/heartbeat, or organ transplants in the terminally-ill patients. Society is forced to revaluate the meaning of such terms as death, quality of life, heroic efforts and acts of mercy, and consider such issues as the patients' right to refuse treatment (living wills) and participating in experiments (informed consent). As a result, these advancements have added complex moral dimensions of healthcare more and pose new, troubling moral dilemmas for the society at large. Healthcare system continually relies on researchers to produce improvements in patient therapy. New technology has a large social impact and is setting the new treatment standards. In this light, the society increasingly expects a researchers' moral responsibility to uphold those virtues that ensure good ethical conduct. It is disturbing that bioengineering health professionals, as they represent new medical innovations, had relatively little contact with moral and legal theory in light of developments (Naurato and Smith, 2003).

Biomedical engineering involves various scientific disciplines, viz., tissue engineering, neural engineering, biomedical instrumentation, nanotechnology, physiological modelling, rehabilitation engineering, medical bioinformatics, clinical engineering, biosensors, biomedical analyses, biomechanics, prosthetic devices and artificial organs, medical imaging, biomaterials and biotechnology. Biotechnology for instance, further, is a multi-disciplinary science encompassing many applied sciences together (Mishra, 2007). This calls for 'engineering ethics' oriented towards protecting the public from professional misconduct by engineers and the harmful effects of technology, promulgated by negative rules. Some aspects like sensitivity to risk, awareness of the social context of technology, respect for nature and commitment to the public good cannot be adequately accounted for in terms of rules, certainly not the negative rules (Harris, 2008). The importance of humanities and social sciences in promoting these are crucial in the professional education of engineers.

With an increasing focus on molecular biology and concern for increasing human health and longevity, modern biotechnology, an integrated component of Biomedical Engineering, is about the future. This 'biotechnology-of-tomorrow' presses in sparking imaginations daily, and elicits wariness or even fear that humanity is gaining too much power or too little choice over human evolution and destiny. Some ethicists explain it as transgressing in to the God's domain. Permeated as it is by a ferocious 'moral approach' to science policy, political climate has heightened this public concern, thus seeming to have the researchers lost their capacity for rational discourse in the public arena. For better or worse, science is political. Advancements in research and development in biotechnology has been adversely affected in the recent past attributable less to the lack of funding or skilled workforce, and rather more to the embattling social, ethical and legal issues (in short, SELI). The challenge of the new-breed researchers in biotechnology in general, and a touchy focus area as medical bioengineering in particular, is to address these issues in greater detail by indulging in responsible and transparent research practices. Bioindustry has increasingly realised that not only regulatory schemes but also contentious public and political debate can impact the future biotechnological research and development.

Dolly's birth opened up technical possibilities to clone a human child into existence, a sense that science is unstoppable. Science seemingly, is not a subject of ethical concern where it either takes a quietist turn or becomes completely irrelevant. A mantra of 'if we can, we inevitably will' (a possibility, however captivating and daunting, is not inevitable) places troubling limits on the critical thinking and moral imagination. It's imperative thus, to enlist the ethical issues that are of interest to medical bioengineers and a programme outline to integrate these in education. The objectives of this chapter are to describe some of the moral and ethical questions on biomedical engineering and technology, intending to demonstrate that each technological advance has consequences that affect the very core of human values, but not to provide solutions or recommendations for these.

Scientist and layperson alike have the opportunity to deliberate about the ethical ramifications of the possible futures opened by scientific research in human biotechnology. Ethics asks us to justify our actions and account for our intentions. Just intending good or doing something to bring it about is not enough, but rather giving good reasons why we envision to do what we intend. In the realm of (human) biotechnology, our reasoning needs to address Incentives: ways to encourage scientists to do a particular research, Intentions: the research goals, and Actions: potential applications of the research results (McLean, 2003).

UTILITARIANISM *VS* KANTIANISM & BENEFICENCE *VS* NONMALEFICENCE

The Greeks, being seafarers and colonisers, had close contact with many different peoples, cultures, customs, laws and institutions that prevailed in the societies. They began to examine and compare all the various human conducts as a part of philosophy which they called as ethics (Greek ethos means custom). Kant's theory (German philosopher Immanuel Kant; 1724–1804) states that, humans have certain rights that do not apply to other animal. The moral judgments that we should not kill and eat each other for food or hunt each other for sport or experiment on each other for medical science are all based on this view of human rights, thus bestowing a special kind of respect.

Though often used interchangeably, both ethics (from Greek 'ethos') and morality (from Latin 'mos') are distinct terms. Philosophers define ethics as a kind of study and morality, its subject matter. Morality encompasses what people believe to be right and good, and the reasons they give for it. Individuals who disregard these accepted codes-of-conduct are considered deviants and, often are punished for engaging in a socially unacceptable activity. These codes-of-conduct are flexible and undergo continual modification to fit to changing conditions and thereby avoid the trauma of revolution as the vehicle for change. In contrast, ethics is the study of right and wrong, of good and evil in human conduct. Ethics is not about providing any judgments or specific rules for human behaviour but an objective analysis about what individuals ought to do. Precisely, it represents the philosophical view of morals, and, therefore, is often referred to as moral philosophy.

Should badly deformed infants be kept alive? Should treatment be stopped to allow a terminally-ill patient to die? Should humans be used in experiments? All these inquiries are questions of moral judgment. Philosophers argue that all moral judgments can be considered normative judgments to be recognised simply by their characteristic evaluative terms (good, bad, right or wrong): what is natural is normal, and above being judgemental. Each judgment expresses an evaluation, intended to play an action-guiding function, and conveying a negative or positive attitude toward some states of affair. Facts describe what is and ethics deals with what ought to be. Moving responsibly from what is to what ought to be is the job of philosophical ethics which provides standards to help us identify what ought to be done. Though biomedical engineering has dramatically advanced modern medicine, bioengineers often lack adequate training to face moral and ethical problems, including clash of interest, allocation of scarce resources, research misconduct, animal experimentation and clinical trials for new devices (Saha and Saha, 1997). Thus, there is a need for ethics training vis-à-vis bioengineering education and adoption of a code of ethics.

A biomedical engineer often encounters ethical crossroads, such as, what aspects to consider; what are the personal and social impacts; what are its potential impacts on human values, virtues and relationships; does an application protect or endanger human or individual rights; are the benefits and burdens distributed fairly; does it advance or impede the common good; what are the risks, burdens and benefits; on whom do they fall and how do they distribute; what is an acceptable way to achieve a given benefit; may we do anything, as long as the outcome is good on balance; are there limits on what we do, even in the name of human health; and, what (or whom) have we not thought about. Answering these is quite difficult for the informed/learned and impossible for people not well-versed in human biology and genetics. Many disagreements originate from not grasping the facts-of-matter. It is impossible to make sound judgments about the appropriate uses of, say, genetic testing without understanding genetic science and the nature of information-gathering in it. It is incumbent upon the scientists and other stakeholders in biomedical engineering to educate the general public and the media about the scientific method and the experimental results.

Arriving at moral judgments, however, requires knowledge of socially-acceptable moral and ethical standards. How is such knowledge obtained? The efforts to answer this question lie in two competing schools of ethical-thought: utilitarianism (consequentialism) and Kantianism (nonconsequentialism). The former holds that the morally right action is always the one among the available options for best consequences. No specific actions or courses of conduct are automatically ruled out as immoral or ruled in as morally obligatory, but the rightness or wrongness of an action. It proposes to determine the courses of action that are open, and then determine the consequences of each alternative. Upon accomplishing this, the morally right course of action is the one that maximises pleasure, minimises pain or both: the one that does the greatest good for the greatest number. Utilitarianism, thus, advocates that 'the end justifies the means'. As long as any form of treatment maximises good consequences, it should be used. Because the central motivation driving the design, development and use of medical devices is improvement of medicine's capacity to protect and restore health, an obvious virtue of utilitarianism is that it assesses medical technology in terms of what many believe makes health valuable - attaining well-being and avoiding pain.

Nonconsequentialism, in contrast, is a moral evaluation beyond determining the consequences of human conduct. It agrees that other considerations are relevant to moral assessment and so rejects the view that morally right conduct is whatever has the best consequences. Based largely on the views of Kant, it insists unique preciousness about human beings from moral viewpoint. These two ethical schools of thought provide some rationale for moral judgments, but also moral dilemmas in many situations where there is no clear moral judgment. 'Is it more important to preserve life or prevent pain', 'Is it right to withhold treatment when doing so may lead to a shortening of life', 'Does an individual have the right to refuse treatment when refusing it may lead to death': neither choice seems to be a satisfactory solution to the problem, and no clear-cut imperative based on our present set of convictions about right and wrong. That is the dilemma raised by Kant: what ought I do?

Beneficence and nonmaleficence are increasingly being accepted as fundamental principles of morally and ethically sound medical practice. Although beneficence and nonmaleficence were regarded merely as concomitant to the craft of medicines in classical Greece and Rome, emphasis on compassion and universal brotherhood (Vasudheywa kutumbakam) increasingly made these the only acceptable motives for medical practice. The provision of benefits and the avoidance of doing harm are stressed in virtually all contemporary codes-of-conduct for health professionals, similar to the oaths and codes that guided past healthcare providers. Traditionally, healthcare ethics have given greater prominence to nonmaleficence than to beneficence, grounded in the fact that the harmful side-effects of medicines far exceeded its capacity to protect and restore health in the past. Healthcare providers possessed many treatments that posed clear and genuine risks and offered little prospect of benefit to patient. In recent times also, many popular allopathic treatments are infamous for their multi-side-effects. In this context, it is rational to give substantially higher priority to avoiding harm than providing benefits.

In modern times, acquiring knowledge in the laboratories, testing in clinics and verifying by statistical methods has increasingly dictated medicines practice. Ongoing alliance between medicines and science became a critical source of the plethora of technologies that now pervade healthcare, many in the form of bioengineering marvels. Impressive increases in therapeutic, preventive and rehabilitative capabilities today have pushed beneficence to the forefront of medical morality. Old medical ethic of, 'Above all, do no harm,' needs to be replaced with the dictate 'The patient deserves the best'. However, the rapid advances in medical technology capabilities have also produced great uncertainty as to what is most beneficial or least harmful for patient. Along with increases in the ability to be beneficent, medicine's technology has generated much debate about what actually counts as beneficent or nonmaleficent treatment. The many recognised approaches in morality and ethics are, utilitarianism, rights, the justice approach, common good and virtue consideration.

Utilitarianism

One way to think about ethical approach (the ought) is through the lens of utility looking at various options for action, who will be affected and to what extent each stakeholder benefits or harms. An ethical action is the one that produces greatest balance of good over harm or the greatest good for the maximum population. In human molecular genetics research, for instance, a utilitarian might argue that the potential benefit of relieving human suffering outweighs the possible dangers of manipulating human genes and evolution through germ-line intervention.

Rights

What makes human beings more than mere things is the ability to choose the type of lives to lead freely as per individual taste, choice and preference. This view describes an ethical action as that which protects people from being used in ways that they do not choose. Humans have a right not to be treated as a means to another's end, even an undeniably good end. The right not to be used encompasses other rights, such as, the right to be told the truth, right to privacy, and the right not to be harmed. Respecting rights may set limits on research in human molecular genetics by requiring adequate informed consent, an honest assessment of risks and benefits, or it may require experimental gene transfer therapy be undertaken only as a last resort. Thus, actions that violate individual or human rights are wrong.

The Justice Approach

This approach is rooted in the principle of 'treating equals equally and unequals unequally'. Justice mandates fairness in that people must be treated the same way unless they differ in ethically relevant ways. When two runners crossing the finish line at the same time, for instance, it is unfair to award one. Primary form of justice in medicine and medical research is distributive justice - fair distribution of benefits and burdens across society. It seeks clarity regarding those aspects of individuals and society that may justify drawing distinctions in how benefits and burdens are allocated. It seeks to identify the justified conditions to treat unequals unequally. Such conditions could include distribution based on determinations of need, social worth, contribution or effort. The principle of need would support mechanisms for providing access to cutting-edge treatments to all who would tangibly benefit irrespective of their ability to pay for them. A principle of contribution might suggest that a family who sponsored research into an illness might have more influence on the direction of the research and greater access to its fruits than the rest.

The Common Good

It rests on society's vision for common pursuit of values and aims. As individual good is inextricably woven into the good of the whole community, pursuing the common good includes creating a set of generally applicable conditions to the advantage of all. Together with respecting individual rights and freedoms, the common good approach requires that common goals of human health and well being be pursued through innovation and a stable healthcare infrastructure.

Consideration of Virtue

This assumes that certain ideals allow for the complete development of humanity. A person who has inculcated these core ideals or virtues will do what is right when faced with an ethical choice. Virtues are dispositions that facilitate acting in ways that develop human potential and allow human flourishing. Virtues are good habits in that they are acquired through repetition and practice and, once acquired, they become characteristic of a person. Honesty, integrity, prudence, courage, wisdom and compassion are examples of virtues. Once a person has developed a virtuous character, he/she is inclined to ethically consistent acts, such as telling the truth, and acting with compassion and courage. Emphasising on character and ideals, virtue ethics captures the idea of the 'good scientist' - intelligent, honest, compassionate, determined - much more so than principle-based approaches of utility, justice and rights. Harris (2008) qualifies virtue ethics as a more appropriate vehicle for expressing the aspects of engineering professionalism that gives greater place for discretion, judgment, inner motivation and commitment. Developing pharmaceuticals and drugs for 'compassionate use' is an example of ethics of virtue.

REDEFINING DEATH: THE TERMINALLY-ILL PATIENT AND EUTHANASIA

Although medicine has long been involved in observing and certifying death, many of its practitioners have not always expressed philosophical concerns regarding the beginning and the onset of end of life. Since medicines is clinical and empirical science, it would seem that health professionals had no medical need to consider the concept of death, and rather the fact of death was sufficient. Life and death are differentiated by the comparison of two extreme conditions separated by an infinite chasm. This notion entails reviewing with the technological advancements in medicine to assist health professionals to prolong life. In India, the average life expectancies for males and females at present (CIA, 2008) are 66.28 and 71.17 years respectively (average, 68.59). In the US similarly, the figures for males and females are 75.15 and 80.97 years respectively (average, 78.06) compared to the average life expectancy figure of 47 years in 1900. Macau tops the list with average figures at 84.379. The infant mortality has significantly reduced in developed nations where technology is an integral part of the culture. Thanks to the provision of an incubator, premature births no longer constitute a threat to life. Technology has been effective in delaying the inevitable, enabling the individuals to add many more productive years to their lives. Such is the success that health professionals have been able to hold the 'vital signs of life' of critically-ill patients for an extended period. The quality of the life provided in such circumstances has, however, raised serious moral philosophical questions. Advancements in medical technology that delayed death, the extent of medical knowledge and available technology, and the increasing occurrence of dilemmatic situations have all stimulated health professionals to revisit the definitions of life and death.

For centuries, death was defined solely as the absence of breathing, since it was felt that the human spirit resided in the spiritus (breath). With continuing proliferation of scientific information regarding human physiology and the development of techniques to revive a non-breathing person, attention turned to the pulsating heart as the focal point in determining death. However, this view changed through additional medical and technological advances in supportive therapy, resuscitation, cardiovascular assist devices and organ transplantation. Oxygen was acknowledged as a primary constituent of the blood and that an oxygen-deprived organ would cease to function beyond a period of time and eventually die. Particularly vulnerable to this type of insult is the highly active brain cells. Removing oxygen from the blood supply even for a couple of minutes produces irreversible damage to these. Thus, the evidence of death shifted from the pulsating heart to the brain. Once the brain's activity could be monitored (by EEG), another chapter was introduced in defining death. The concept of brain-death argues that the human brain is truly essential to life, and its damage leads to dysfunctions that are identified with humanness, viz., memory, feeling, thinking and knowledge. It is widely accepted in clinical death that there is irreversible cessation of functioning of all three major organs (i.e., heart, lungs and brain) before pronouncing death.

The movement to redefine death received considerable impetus by the Harvard Medical School publication (Anon., 1968), wherein death was redefined based on the functioning of the brain. A total and irreparable loss of brain function (brainstem death) or whole brain death or simply brain-death is a legal standard for death now. This means, an individual in a state of brain-death is legally indistinguishable from a corpse and may be treated as one even though respiratory and circulatory functions are sustained through life-support system. Well-equipped Modern respirators maintain a patient with irreversible brain damage almost indefinitely. This exercise is merely postponement of the inevitable and sustains nothing of a personality, character or conscious individuality. Once destruction of the brainstem has occurred, the brain cannot function at all, and the body's regulatory mechanism fails unless artificially sustained. Many take this legal standard to be the morally appropriate one, stating that a mechanically ventilated corpse is a corpse nonetheless. It takes much more than just a biological life to be a human person, a mere vegetative human life is not one.

An otherwise intact and alive but brain-dead person without an 'intact functioning brain' is not a human person. Precisely this issue was at stake in the gradual movement from using heartbeat and respiration as indices of life to using brain-oriented indices instead. Even with a consensus that a brain-dead is dead and indeed a corpse, difficult cases remain. Neocortical death where an individual is in a persistent vegetative state is one such case, where brain is functional enough to respond to mechanically-sustained respiration and circulation without any purposeful response to external stimuli and self-awareness. Some patients yawn, make chewing motions, swallow spontaneously, or open eyes periodically exhibiting sleep-wake cycles. Unlike complete unresponsiveness of the individuals in a state of brainstem death, a variety of simple and complex responses can be elicited from an individual in a persistent vegetative state. Nonetheless, the chances that such an individual will regain consciousness are remote. Artificial feeding, kidney dialysis and the like make it possible to sustain an individual in a state of neocortical death for decades.

Then, is neocortical death also death? Specifying features of living individuals distinguishing them from corpse and making treatment as one morally impermissible, makes the issue a crooked factual matter. Irreparable cessation of respiration and circulation, classical criterion for death, would entail that an individual in a persistent vegetative state is not a corpse and so, morally speaking, must not be treated as one. The brainstem death criterion for death also entails that a neocortically-dead person is not yet a corpse. What is crucial here is that, brain damage should be severe enough to cause failure of the regulatory mechanisms of the body. Is a neocortically-dead individual, one whose respiration and circulation are mechanically maintained, any less in possession of characteristics distinguishing the living from cadavers? It is a matter that society must decide. And until society decides, it is not clear what counts as beneficent or nonmaleficent treatment in such a situation. Terminally-ill patients today often find themselves in a strange world of institutions and technology assisting them in their fight against death. This modern medical system may cause patients and their family considerable economic, psychological and physical pain. While prolonging life, modern technology has in many cases made dying slower and more undignified which leads to a moral dilemma in medicines. Is it right or wrong for medical professionals to stop treatment or administer a lethal dose to a terminally-ill patient?

Although death is all around us in the form of accidents, drug overdose, alcoholism, murder and suicide, a dignified death is in growing older and succumbing to some chronic illness. As the aged approach the end, s/he may eventually wish for the day when all troubles can be brought to an end. Such a desire, frequently shared by a compassionate family, is often shattered by therapies provided to prolong life without other concerns. For many, the fight for life is a correct professional view believing that the forces of medicine should always be committed to using innovative ways of prolonging life. However, this cannot be the only approach to caring for the terminally-ill. Thus, many opine that a dignified death is often not compatible with today's standard medical view.

Moral judgements on intentional termination of life requires decision on the capacities and qualities that make life worth living, which qualities are sufficient to endow it with value worth sustaining, and whether their absence justifies deliberate termination of a life, at least when this would be the wish of the concerned individual. Else, the norms of beneficence and nonmaleficence provide no guidance. Whether termination of life support is a benefit or harm to the patient cannot thus be determined. Thus, to preserve individual's rights, moral questions regarding the extent to which physicians engage in heroic efforts to prolong life must be addressed. The healthcare professionals' goal for patient-care should not solely be to prolong a compromised life through extensive use of drugs, operations, respirators, haemodialysers, pacemakers, and the like, but rather providing a reasonable quality of life. Out of this new concern, euthanasia (from Greek words meaning 'good' and 'death') has once again become a controversial issue in the practice of medicines.

THE MORAL STANDPOINT ON EUTHANASIA

Euthanasia implies to many in today's world as 'death with dignity', a practice to terminate a machine-supported life seemingly without any life-values left. Thus, it means a contract to terminate life to avoid unnecessary suffering at the end of a fatal illness and, therefore, has the connotation of relief from pain. Euthanasia was practiced in societies since eternity. Aristotle advocated euthanasia for gravely deformed children. Ancient Greeks assembled the elderly and sick at an annual banquet and served a poisonous potion. Others abandoned their aged when they felt these individuals did not serve any useful purpose.

'Moral-euthanasia' often distinguishes active from passive euthanasia resting on the difference between the acts of commission and omission. Failure to take steps to effectively forestall death resulting in an individual's demise is an act of omission. When a death of a person is the result of hastening the process (e.g., giving a lethal injection) it is an act of commission and thus, is a case of homicide. In passive euthanasia, the physician does not do anything to bring about the patient's death and it results due to whatever illness s/he is afflicted with. In active euthanasia, the physician has a proactive role in the patient's death. A physician giving a lethal injection to the cancer-patient causing the death is the active type, whereas ceasing to treat so that the cancer causes the death is the passive type. The physician attempts self-exoneration in the second case by saying, 'the death was the result of illness. I was not the cause of death. I did nothing'. Such a response would have any credibility, neither legally nor morally. The physician would be blameworthy for the death, similar to active killing. Thus, a physician continuing to treat to the very end is understood.

Euthanasia can also be classified as involuntary or voluntary. In voluntary euthanasia, when a prior consent exists, the decision to hasten death would be morally justified. When death is hastened against an individual's wish it is involuntary, and is no morally-relevant different way from unjustifiable homicide. What happens when say, an unconscious terminally-ill can't express personal wishes? Is hastening death in such case permissible?

Those favouring euthanasia stress the importance of individual rights and freedom of choice and a means of kindness to allow dignified death. Dignified death is much more preferable than continuous suffering and gradual decay into nothingness, without possession of a unique mind and personality. Those opposed to euthanasia demand to know whose right it is to end the life of another. Moral judgments stress that euthanasia-killing was considered a sin, and a decision on whether someone should live or die was viewed solely as God's responsibility. Anyone practising euthanasia is essentially acting in the place of God, and no human should ever dare that.

Health professionals responsible for patient-care must do everything to save a life. They cannot honour their pledge and still believe that euthanasia is justified. If a patient is kept alive, there is at least a chance of finding a cure that might be useful to them. Opponents of euthanasia feel that legalising it would destroy the bonds of trust between doctor and patient. How would sick individuals feel if they were not sure that their physician and nurse would try everything possible to cure them, knowing that if their condition worsened, they would just lose faith and decide that death would be better? Opponents of euthanasia also question that the exercise benefits less to the suffering person and is used more as a means to relieve the agony of the family. They believe that destroying life (no matter how minimal) merely to ease the emotional suffering of others is indeed unjust.

Once euthanasia is legalised, it will be difficult to define and develop clear guidelines to serve as the basis for carrying it out. Once euthanasia is accepted by society, its detractors fear the rise of many other problems. Passive euthanasia could be applied in state hospitals and institutions for the mentally retarded and the elderly. Its legalisation could prompt an increased number of suits by parents seeking to end the agony of an incurably-afflicted child or by children seeking to shorten the suffering of an aged and terminally-ill parent. Clearly, the situation is delicate and thought-provoking.

TAKING CONTROL

Flexman and Lazareck (2007) opined that the regulation and research funding has the potential to dramatically affect biomedical engineering research and commercialisation, and commercial funding is critical for developing new biomedical technologies. This dependence, however, carries certain risks from ethical standpoint. Adherence to basic ethical norms is of vital importance for biomedical engineering (Persson, 2006). New developments may affect society in new ways, and necessitates discussion between scientists, engineers, policy-makers and the public. Healthcare decisions often involve unpleasant topics and arise at emotionally and physically most vulnerable situations, and thus can be tremendously difficult. Almost always these choices involve new medical information that feels alien and can seem overwhelming. In an attempt to assist individuals in decision-making, it is helpful to first obtain all the relevant medical facts, understand all options and consequences, and finally, place a value on each option based on a set of personal values. These three-step facts-options-values path concerns the 'how' of decisions, but equally important is the 'who'. Someone must make every single medical decision, and ideally by the person most intimately involved: the patient. Very often, however, they are made by someone else: spouse, family, physician or a group on behalf of the patient. It is, hence, important to recognise the four concentric circles of consent (See Figure 1.). The primary circle is the patient, second is the use of advance directives (choosing in advance through the use of such documents as 'living will'), third is others deciding for the patient (i.e., the move from personal to surrogate control), and the fourth and final circle is the courts and bureaucrats.

As the last resort, the society decrees the patient incapacitation, when there is no clear advance directive, and the decision-maker is not clear. This 'three-steps-four-circles' is an attempt to impose some order on the chaos in medical decision-making (Enderle et al., 2005). Monzon and Monzon-Wyngaard (2008) presented certain rules of practice and obligations emerging from accepted fundamental canons of ethics for engineers, including the basic recommendations dissenting on ethical grounds. These can help individuals take control.

HUMAN EXPERIMENTATION

Biomedical engineering research has long held an exalted position in modern society, acclaimed for its significant achievements ranging from the development of Salk-Sabin polio vaccines to the development of artificial organs. To determine their effectiveness and value, however, these new drugs and devices eventually are used on humans. Hence, the issue is not only whether humans should be involved in such studies designed to benefit them or their fellow humans but also clarifying and/or defining precisely the conditions for such studies.

What guidelines need to be followed for experimenting with drugs/devices that may (not) help an aged suffering from severe coronary artery disease? Should only procedures viewed as potentially beneficial be tried? Should diagnostic procedures or equipment be tested on the subject instead of more accepted techniques, even though they will not be directly beneficial to the patient? Similarly, should conducting research on human foetus be considered? Such research is possible resulting from the legalisation of abortion and

Figure 1.

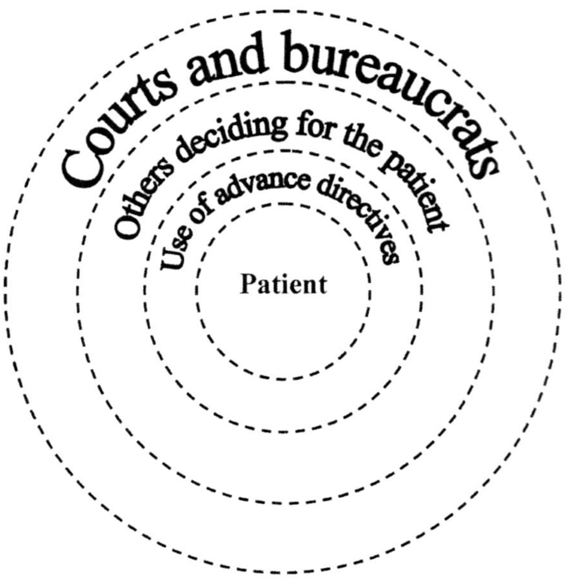

technological advances that have made foetal studies more practical now-a-days. Under what conditions should research in medical sciences be conducted on these subjects then? Should potentially hazardous drugs be given to planning-to-abort women to determine neonatal effect? Should aborted foetus be used in experimental studies? How ethical and medically-effective the tests done on laboratory mammals will be? Clinical researchers responsible for the patients' well-being must face these moral issues while safeguarding individual rights for trials. Dilemma lies between the potential harm to participating volunteers and the knowledge envisaged to be gained to benefit the society in general. Such research in developing countries by the US and other industrialised countries give rise to unique challenges owing to differences in history, culture, politics, wealth and power between the countries. Page (2004) identifies several ethical issues to be considered in such cases and provides possible legal and ethical framework for resolving them.

Purpose of Such Experimentation

Although experimental protocols vary, it is generally accepted that human trials occur whenever clinical situation of an individual is consciously manipulated for information gathering. Human experiments have been classified as either therapeutic (direct benefit to the patient) or nontherapeutic (providing additional domain knowledge without direct benefit). The central difference is a matter of intent or aim rather than results. Medical sciences have abundant examples of therapeutic research projects historically, viz., nonconventional radiotherapy against malignancy, pacemakers to facilitate proper heart function, and artificial kidneys to mimic nature and remove poisons from blood. At one time, these were considered novel approaches having some value for the patient, were tried and found beneficial for them, as also for humankind. In nontherapeutic research, trials on the impact of hepatitis virus and malaria parasite infection or cardiac catheterisation significantly affected medical science, paving the way for developing appropriate medical procedures.

In mid-1970s (1974-78), the National Commission for protection of human subjects of biomedical and behavioural research in the US (Anon., 1979) offered the terms 'practice' and 'research' to replace the conventional therapeutic and nontherapeutic distinction, respectively. In medical sphere, 'practice' usually involves diagnosis, preventive treatment or therapy. By contrast, 'research' designates a designed activity to test a hypothesis, draw conclusions, and develop or contribute to generalisable knowledge (theories, principles or statements of relationships). Practice uses a proven technique in an attempt to benefit one or more individuals, while research studies attempt to increase the knowledge-base.

Moral dilemma in healthcare has affected biomedicine engineers, physicians, other healthcare professionals and society. Professionals must update on their responsibilities for complete testing and review during the complete R&D process.

A kidney dialyser or NMR diagnostic scanner demonstrate state-of-the-art capabilities but come with a price-tag, thus changing the past healthcare standards and resource allocation (Saha et al., 1985) in terms of product liability and clash of interests. There is, thus, a strong need for proper awareness and education in ethics and professional responsibilities.

Although the practice and research dichotomy has the advantage of not implying that therapeutic activities are the only clinical procedures intended to benefit patients, it is based on intent, not outcome. Interventions employing proven techniques to benefit the patient are practices, but to increase generalisable knowledge constitute research. What about those not happily fitting into either category (e.g., nonvalidated practice encompassing prevention and diagnosed therapy). The primary purpose of a nonvalidated practice is to benefit patient while emphasising its non-validity on safety and efficacy. Nonvalidated practice requires informing the human subject and obtaining consent.

In 1964, World Medical Association (WMA) endorsed and provided guidelines on the code-of-ethics for human experimentation, revised in 2000 (WMA, 2000). For ethically-sound human experimentation, the guidelines converge on six basic requirements. First, prior research based on laboratory and nonhuman subjects, and on established scientific fact, so that the point under inquiry is well focused and has been advanced as far as possible by nonhuman means. Second, research on humans should use tests and means of observation reasonably believed to be able to provide the research information being sought, lest it should rob the research of its scientific value. Third, research should be conducted only domain experts. Fourth, all foreseeable risks and reasonably probable benefits to each stakeholder must be carefully assessed, and the comparison must indicate the latter clearly outweighing the former. The probable benefits must not be obtainable through other low-risk means. Fifth, research participation should be based on informed and voluntary consent. Sixth, a voluntary participation should be halted immediately if desired so by the subject, or the investigator believes that the experiment may result in injury, disability or death to the subject. Clause Five is widely regarded as an important protection of all these conditions.

Conforming to all conditions probably limits the pace and extent of medical progress, but insistence on these conditions means that the only medical progress truly worth having must be consistent with high respect for human dignity. Strict interpretation of the criteria rules out many individuals from participating. Children and the mentally-compromised are excluded due to their inability to comprehend experimental nuts-n-bolts. Exclusion also applies to individuals having a dependent relationship to the investigator including his/her patients and students. Since mental capacity includes the subjects' ability to appreciate the seriousness and consequences of a study, this means that even though some minors have the right to give consent for certain treatment, they must be able to figure out all involved risks. Here, the risks involved are well-defined and shared. In the past, such evaluations in many situations belonged to the medical professional alone but not valid today. The medical staff weighs the medical-soundness of the procedure, and the risks and benefits involved in a suggested procedure as that requires more medical expertise than what an average individual possesses. But, the right to make a final determination lies with subject. Once recommended, enough information is shared with the patient to help decide whether the hoped-for benefits are sufficient to risk the hazards, a sort of the economist's cost-benefit analyses. Then, a valid consent is obtained with additional bipartite legal protections as follows:

- Authorisation to proceed with study: subject cannot later claim assault and battery.
- Authorisation to use the generated data for professional/research purposes: invasion of privacy cannot later be claimed.

- Elimination of any claim in case the subject fails to benefit from the procedure.
- Defense against a claim of injury when the procedural risk is understood and consented to.
- Protection to the investigator against a claim of injury resulting from the subject's failure to follow safety instructions if the orders were well explained and reasonable.

Can the aims of research ever be reconciled with traditional moral obligations of physicians? Is the researcher/physician in an untenable position? Informed voluntary consent once again is the key with the wilful participation. What happens then during and after the experiment becomes a product of their own decision, not something imposed on them but whatever they elected to have done to themselves consensually. As their autonomy is thus respected, they are not made a mere resource for others' benefit. Although they may suffer harm for the benefit of others, they do so of their own volition, as a result of exercising their own autonomy, and not as a result of having limited or diminished autonomy.

For consent to be genuine it must be truly voluntary and not the product of coercion. Not all sources of coercion are as obvious and easy to recognise as physical violence. A subject may be coerced by fear that there is no other recourse for treatment, by the fear that no consent will alienate the physician on whom the subject depends for treatment, or even by the fear of disapproval of others. This sort of coercion is often difficult to detect and remedy. Individuals must understand what they are consenting to, for which they are given sufficient information to arrive at an informed intelligent decision. Although a subject may not require all the information a researcher has, determining how much should be provided and what can be omitted without compromising the validity of the subject's consent is critical.

Ascertaining the subject's competence to understand the provided information and render an intelligent opinion is another difficulty. These are matters of probably no-precise and uncertain judgment, but efforts in good faith to prevent gross violations of human dignity. When the bottom-line is good faith, it is the understanding and appreciation of human value by the team of investigators, which again trickles down to morals and ethics. Engineering ethics emphasises professional codes of ethics, business ethics and technology studies, neglecting the not-mandatory personal moral commitments, personal aesthetic, religious and other values. Martin (2002) opines that personal moral commitments motivate, guide and give meaning to the work, contributing to both self-fulfillment and public good. It is the duty of the concerned medical practitioner to protect the life and health of volunteer. The basic criterion for a subject to volunteer is that s/he should be an otherwise (with unrelated illness, if any) healthy person for the experimental design. The investigator (investigating team) should discontinue research upon suspicion of harm to the individual.

Informed Consent

Informed consent is one of many patient protection safeguards. A research precedes a plan-of-action (protocol) for the study, outlining the number of subjects in the study, medical tests to receive, frequency and the treatment plan. Before a study proceeds, the protocol is reviewed and approved by the competent team that includes doctors, ethicists and local community members, to comply with the safety and ethical issues.

Considered to be a critical moral issue in human experimentation, informed consent is the principal lawful and ethical precondition. All adults (not minors) have the legal capacity to give medical consent (unless specifically legally denied). It is an attempt to preserve rights by giving the opportunity for self-determination to whether one wishes to participate in an experimental effort. In the beginning of a formal process, before agreeing to become a subject, one is educated about the study, receiving information about the key aspects including the treatment expected to receive. In addition to discussing the study with competent authority, a copy of the written consent form can be taken home to read and discuss with family and friends. This includes the study approach, the intervention (new drug or treatment) intended, possible risks and benefits, and the tests one might be subjected to.

Human research must conform to generally-accepted scientific principles, based on adequately performed laboratory and animal experiments, and credible knowledge obtained. The design and performance of such experiment is clearly formulated as a protocol and transmitted to an independent committee for consideration, comment and guidance. Such research is conducted only by qualified persons and supervised by competent medical personnel. It cannot legitimately be carried out unless the importance of the objective is in proportion to the inherent risk. Such research projects should ensue after careful assessment of predictable risks compared with foreseeable benefits. Concern for the subject's interests must always prevail over any other interests. The subject's integrity with regard to his/her privacy and the impact of the study on the physical/mental integrity and personality is respected. Doctors may abstain from engaging in such research projects before satisfying themselves that the hazards involved are believed to be predictable, and further, cease any investigation upon discovering that the hazards outweigh the potential benefits.

Upon deciding to participate in the study, one signs the consent form followed with an ongoing conversation with the patient-care team to make educated decisions about whether to participate, or continue participating, without hesitating to ask questions at any time about any aspect of the study or care. The research team obliges by keeping informed, helping understand the information and answering questions, understanding well that the subject is making the research possible through wilful participation.

The doctor obliges to preserve the accuracy of results while publishing. Experimental report non-accordance with the principles laid down in declaration should not be published. In such study, a potential subject is adequately informed of the aims, methods, anticipated benefits and potential hazards and the discomfort it may entail. He/she is informed that he/she is at liberty to abstain from participation in the study and that he/she is free to withdraw his/her consent to participate at any time unconditionally. The 'freely-given' informed consent of the subject is obtained preferably in writing, which must include confidence of the dependents as well, obtained by a doctor completely independent of official relationship and the investigation. In case of legal incompetence, informed consent is obtained from legal guardian. If obtaining written informed consent is impossible (due to physical or mental incapacity), or when the subject is a minor, permission is obtained from responsible relative. Research protocol should always contain a statement of the ethical considerations involved and should indicate that the principles enunciated in the declaration are complied to.

CLINICAL RESEARCH: RESEARCH COMBINED WITH PROFESSIONAL CARE

Clinical trials carry potential benefits and risks. Potential benefits include, provision of health-care by leading specialised physicians allowing one to access to the most advanced care, before they are widely available. The volunteer takes a proactive role in own healthcare, and may be among the first to benefit. In the process, one has an opportunity to contribute valuably to medical research. Potential risks in the trial include, new drugs and procedures may be not or less effective than currently available ones. The benefits may not work for all. These may have latent side-effects or risks hitherto unknown.

The clinical trials conducted could be of many types, viz., treatment trials, prevention trials and others. Treatment trials are usually the first type of clinical trial that comes to mind when mentioned. New treatments, viz., new drug, approaches to surgery (or radio-/chemo-) therapy, cocktail treatments or new methods, such as gene therapy are tested. Prevention trials study the effects of doing a particular exercise, viz., quitting smoking or taking a particular medicine or nutritional supplement, to find out whether it helps prevent a disease. Other trials study the ways to reduce the risk of getting a particular disease, find better ways to detect it and improve quality of life for such patients and survivors.

The first two methods progress in an orderly series of phases to protect patients and ensure that the researchers ask and answer questions in a way resulting in reliable and reproducible information. There are usually three phases: **Phase 1:** Evaluation of how a new drug should be administered (oral, intravenous, intramuscular or a device), how often and at what dose. As the possible risks and benefits at this stage is less known, these studies involve a limited number of patients unresponsive to other known treatments. **Phase 2:** This phase continues to test drug safety and begins to evaluate its efficacy. Here, studies usually focus on a particular type of disease symptom and involve a small number of people due to the latent risks and unknowns involved. **Phase 3:** Trials at this stage test a new drug, drug cocktails or surgical procedure with current standard as a control, ensuring equal receipt of the treatments. A participant usually is assigned to a particular group at random without any bias or human factors, to ensure dependability and repeatability of the finding. Phase 3 trials often enrol many people and conducted at many doctors' offices, clinics and hospitals spread over a wide geographical region.

After each phase, researchers examine the data and decide on the next stage based on the safety and efficacy of the treatment, comparing between the new and the 'control' (if at all there is one) approaches. As an alternate approach, researchers may wish to compare the effectiveness of the new approach against a placebo (dummy pill without active ingredients). The subject is notified, then, that he/she may receive a placebo, rather than active treatment, before enrolling as a participant. When Phase 3 study is completed, researchers decide on the medical importance of the results and publish it in peer-reviewed journals. Important findings may be featured in the news media. If an intervention is proven safe and effective, it may redefine healthcare standard. Clinical trials are, thus, tools to build on what we already know to progressively improve the quality of care and prevention available.

Responsibilities of medical engineers towards patients, physicians and institutions have increased with the increasingly important roles within the healthcare system (Saha and Saha, 1986), with clearly defined roles and authority, acknowledged and supported by other line professionals. They must self-recognise the seriousness and contribute to the design, use and maintenance of equipment responsibly, and fulfill roles in administration, management and research. They must also be prepared to face ethical issues arising from defective or inadequate equipment, hazards and incidents, scarcity of resources, conflict of interest, confidentiality, clinical research, truth-telling, and caring for the terminally-ill.

Doctors 'practise' medicines, which means that a doctor is free to use a new diagnostic and therapeutic measure, if in his/her judgment it offers hope of saving life, reestablishing health or alleviating suffering. Potential benefits, hazards and discomfort of a new method, albeit, should be weighed against the advantages of the best current diagnostic/therapeutic methods. A patient (including control group) should be assured of the best-proven diagnostic and therapeutic method. The refusal of the patient to participate in a study must never interfere with the doctor–patient relationship. If the doctor considers it essential not to obtain informed consent, specific reasons for this need to be stated in the protocol while submitting for approval. The doctor can combine medical research with professional care, the objective being the acquisition of knowledge justified by potential diagnostic/therapeutic value.

BIOTECH-BASED BIOMEDICAL ENGINEERING

Biotechnology-based biomedical engineering emphasises five ethics-related questions that a domain-specialised engineer must be accountable for:

1. *What benefits and harms can be predicted for biotech innovations* in both the research and application phases? Which course of action may result in overall best consequence, though it is more-or-less a guessing game? While weighing benefits-risks in profound uncertainty and sizable risk, without overdoing hopes or fears, it is best to err on the side of caution.
2. *Who are the ethically relevant stakeholders*? What rights do they have and which course of action protects them? Is human dignity respected? The consideration of specific individual and group rights requires coming to grips with the right to healthcare.
3. *Which option treats everyone the same* unless there is an ethically justified reason to treat one differently? Justice may hold up 'need' as a criterion for accessing innovative treatment.
4. *Which course of action seeks the common good*? Recent disease-outbreaks have heightened the concern for health and creation of conditions that maximise societal good health.
5. *Which option best develops virtues*? Which virtues, such as trust and compassion, might be particularly relevant to biotechnology development and human health?

This framework does not offer an easy or automatic solution to ethical dilemmas, and that is not the goal either. It stresses that ethics needs to consider benefits and burdens, rights and justice, and virtues and the common good. Each approach gives key information about situation-specific ethical options. Each informed stakeholder contributes to the moral judgment, considering carefully the right-making and wrong-doing. With a brainstorming by these stakeholders, a healthcare social vision could be developed providing necessary determining criteria. As biotechnology innovations may eventually involve germ-line manipulation, actions taken today may affect future human generations, making them stakeholders in our ethical analysis. Consideration of trans-generational consequences imposes limits on what we do now in the interest of generations to follow. Many including India speak of responsibilities extending to the next seven generations. Minimally, we should not knowingly inflict harm. As we approach cutting-edge biotechnology, this ancient moral wisdom ingrained in the form of virtues can serve well.

REGULATING MEDICAL DEVICE INNOVATION AND MARKETING

According to the USFDA, a medical device is an instrument, apparatus, machine, contrivance, implant, *in vitro* reagent or other similar or related article intended for diagnosis of disease or other conditions, or in the cure, mitigation, treatment or prevention of disease in humans and animals OR intended to affect the structure or function of the human body or animals which does not achieve any primary intended purposes through chemical action or is not dependent upon being metabolised. Thus, a manufacturer-claimed medical product is considered a device. The FDA is the sole federal agency to regulate the safety and efficacy of medical devices in the US since 1938. Initially restricted to ensuring legitimate and truthfully labelled (not misbranded) medical devices in the marketplace the scope has evolved over time with technology. Attempt to broaden the scope was to address premarket review through the Medical Device Amendment (1976; Pub. L. No. 94-295, 90 Stat. 539) act. It statutes FDA approval before a new device reaches market and imposes clinical investigation requirements (http://www.fda.gov/). The principal route to market particularly Class III (high-risk) medical devices under the regulatory authority is premarket approval (PMA). It allows determination of the safety and efficacy by the regulatory body which is a costly affair. The timeline for a PMA applicant for requisite data collection could be several years. Once approved, it is a private license to market a medical device.

Morsy and Flexman (2008) discuss a case of an artificial heart valve failing at unexpected rates and the critical role of bioengineers involved, their education and training. Based on the risk-level, the FDA categories devices into significantly risky (*e.g.*, orthopedic implant, artificial heart and infusion pump), and insignificantly risky (*e.g.*, dental devices and daily-wear contact lenses). Clinical research on the former cannot begin until an institutional review board (IRB) approves the protocol and the informed consent form. This requirement is waived in case of the latter, where the regulatory body requires that approval from an IRB be obtained certifying that the device in question poses only insignificant risk. In deciding approval of a proposed clinical investigation, the regulatory authorities confirm minimal risk to subjects, anticipated benefits and knowledge gained, equitable subject selection, adequate informed consent materials and procedures, and acceptable provisions to monitor the study and protect patient information. The FDA allows the use of unapproved device in three situations: feasibility study, emergency and treatment, each having typical ethical concerns.

Feasibility Study

It is a limited investigation involving new or modified use of existing devices at a single institution with a relatively small subject pool of about ten human subjects, so that harm due to ethical lapses would affect fewer people. The sponsor submits a 'Notice of Limited Investigation' describing the device, summary-of-purpose, protocol, sample informed consent form, and an approval certificate by the responsible medical board. The goal of the study makes it an instance of research, not practice. Manufacturers seek to determine the performance (efficacy and safety) of a device with respect to a particular target population, whether further animal/human studies are required, whether device modification is needed before use, etc. The responsibility on ethically-sound practice falls primarily on the IRB who scrutinises scientific soundness of the trial and respecting the volunteer's rights. Decreased scrutiny will increase the unlikelihood of either or both conditions not being met.

The ethical concern posed here is best comprehended with a clear understanding of research justification. Basic research and animal experimentation on a given device cannot adequately determine the risks and benefits it poses for humans without actual human use. The human benefit thereof lies primarily in the provided generalisable information crucial to medical science's ability to generate new efficacious and safe modes of medical treatment. So, a condition for ethically-sound experimentation is that it must be scientifically sound. Though scientific soundness is a necessary condition of ethically-sound human research, it is not of and by itself sufficient. Volunteers are at risk of being mere research resources having value only for the ends of the research. Humans are valuable simply by being the kinds of entities they are, and to treat them as such is to respect them and their autonomy. This requirement is met by ensuring prior voluntary informed consent before clinical intervention.

The device manufacturer is a commercial enterprise, and is motivated to maximise profit by launching the device in market sooner with least possible delay and costs. Profit is not the only motive to induce manufacturers to contravene ethically-sound research needs. A manufacturer may sincerely believe that its product offers great benefit to people and be prompted to take shortcuts. Whether the consequences being sought are desired for reasons of self-interest, altruism or both, the ethical issue is the same: treating volunteers as mere objects. What about the circumstances under which feasibility studies would take place? Are these not sufficiently different from 'normal' research scenario to warrant reduced scrutiny?

Although a fewer subjects are harmed in a single feasibility study, still the harm is ethically wrong nonetheless. Are ethical lapses more likely to occur in feasibility studies? It is a question of high priority the answer to which might be quite different when the device is a temporary or permanent implant than when it is an already approved device being put to new or modified use. Whatever the contemplated use under feasibility studies mechanism, regulatory body must not allow such exception without a reasonably high certainty that the subject would not be placed in greater danger than in 'normal' research circumstances.

Emergency Use

Emergency use is authorised administration of unapproved device as the last resort to save a life. FDA insists that emergencies are circumstances that reasonable foresight would not anticipate. It constitutes practice rather than research, aiming primarily to benefit patient. As such use is before completion of clinical investigation, it constitutes nonvalidated practice. Although the aim of the use is to save the life of the patient, the nature and likelihood of the potential benefits and risks ingrained by use of the device are far more speculative than intervention by a validated one. Should emergency use of an unapproved device be regarded as immoral, as an assessment of the risks and benefits of the use is non-substantive. The involved physician must have enough reasons to believe the existence of benefits. There should be a preclinical and animal tests body to predict human benefits.

Although the benefits and risks posed in emergency use are highly speculative, they are not entirely speculative. Although validation requires research on humans at some point, all nonvalidated technologies are not equal. Assessing risks and benefits will be almost wholly speculative in the largely noninvestigated ones. Others shall have the support of preclinical and animal tests to justify as desperate (not reckless) actions in desperate circumstances. Ethical soundness in the support of emergency use of the unapproved device by solid results from preclinical and animal tests is warranted. Desperate circumstances though may legitimatise desperate actions, the onus to such actions rest on the informed consent. A physician should not 'create' an emergency to circumvent IRB and avoid requesting sponsor's authorisation of unapproved use of a device.

The nature of the consent especially in such vulnerable situation is important. Greater protection measures than otherwise essential is thus necessary. One measure is to ensure that the patient (or proxy) knows the highly speculative nature of the offered intervention. The patient must not be made to believe that the risks and benefits of the intervention are not better understood than they in fact are. Other point is to ensure patient's understandings of all the options, including a compromised life. The clinician involved must recognise that the activities constitute a nonvalidated practice (not research), and the patient wellbeing is the primary obligation. The patient enters into a relationship with same trust as in any normal clinical situation. To treat this sort of intervention as research and justifying by its benefits to science and society would be an abuse of this trust.

Treatment Use

USFDA has adopted regulations that authorise the use of investigational treatments in circumstances where a patient has not responded to approved therapies. This treatment-use of unapproved new drugs is extended also to treat serious diseases and conditions, but not extended to the approved treatment use of unapproved medical devices. A manufacturer could obtain approval by establishing specific protocol for this kind of use within the context of an IDE (Investigational Device Exemption). The conditions for treatment-use of devices are, the device is intended to use where there is no comparable or satisfactory product available, the device is under or received an IDE or all clinical trials have been completed awaiting approval, and the sponsor is actively pursuing marketing approval of the device. The treatment-use protocol is submitted as part of the IDE and must describe the intended use of the device, the rationale for the use, available alternatives and the reason for preferring the product, criteria for patient selection, measures to monitor the use and to minimise risk, and relevant technical information on safety and efficacy for the intended treatment.

What are the ethical issues in approving treatment-use of unapproved devices? Because such use is after the failure of validated interventions to alleviate patient's suffering adequately, it is practice and not research. Since the device is unapproved, such practice is a nonvalidated one, and should be subject to the regulatory requirements of preclinical/animal tests providing substantial reason to believe in the resultant benefit. As with emergency use, although this does not prevent assessment of the intervention's benefits and risks from being highly speculative, it does prevent from being totally speculative. The circumstances for treatment-use involve serious health impairment rather than homicide threat. The issue is the seriousness of the impairment to justify an intervention whose risks and benefits are yet to be solidly established. It thus necessitates that the patient is informed of the speculative nature of the intervention and of the possibility of risking little to no benefit.

Healthcare institutions such as hospitals, ambulatory-surgical facilities, nursing homes and outpatient treatment facilities need to report reasonably suggestible information on treatment malfunction. When it is device-related, the regulatory authority and device-manufacturer must be directly reported. Medical device reporting (MDR) regulations (1984) require that the manufacturers/importers submit reports of device-related deaths and serious injuries (www.fda.gov/MedicalDevices/Safety/ReportaProblem/default.htm) to regulatory authority in the US. Revisions in 1990, 1996 and 2000 have expedited the reporting of the medical-devices related problems involving the users in the process (www.fda.gov/MedicalDevices/DeviceRegulationandGuidance/PostmarketRequirements/ReportingAdverseEvents/default.htm), giving the authority more teeth over device-user facilities. Such exercise increases patient-protection. The controversy however is essentially utilitarian in nature, centring on the worry that patient-benefits are marginal and far outweigh the costs.

CONCLUSION

The guidelines outlining ethical conduct in human and animal research have evolved into large complex documents, making the approval process a complicated task (Shankar and Simmons, 2009). Biomedical engineers need to update on the societal mechanism to control improper, unethical practices, through various regulatory bodies, their regulations and the approval process in medicines. An interface for scientists, policymakers and the public at large (www.fosep.org) was started by students and fellows which has reportedly received support from the administration (Flexman and Lazareck, 2007) as well, an example of influencing science policy and ethics in early careers.

New researchers in the field can struggle to understand the parts of the guideline that apply to them and the ethical obligations. These guidelines will only increase in complexity and number in future. Shankar and Simmons (2009) discuss on the possible solution in an internet-based expert system capable of distributing the information to individual researchers, intelligently and interactively. One such system for Australian medical research ethics guidelines has already been designed and tested. The need is, thus, to educate, empower, and make ethics-related information easily and timely accessible to the biomedical engineering personnel. There is a need for ethics training vis-à-vis bioengineering education and adoption of a code of ethics in line with medical ethics.

REFERENCES

Anon., (1968). A definition of irreversible coma. Report of the ad hoc committee of the Harvard Medical School to examine the definition of brain death. *Journal of the American Medical Association*, *205*(6), 337–340. doi:10.1001/jama.205.6.337

Anon., (1979). *National Commission for the Protection of Human Subjects of Biomedical and Behavioral Research (National Commission). Belmont Report: Ethical Principles and Guidelines for the Protection of Human Subjects of Research*. Washington, DC: US Government Printing Office.

CIA. (2008) *World Factbook*. Retrieved July 21, 2009 from https://www.cia.gov/library/publications/the-world-factbook/fields/2102.html

Enderle, J. D., Blanchard, S. M., & Bronzino, J. D. (Eds.). (2005). *Introduction to Biomedical Engineering* (2nd ed.). Oxford: Elsevier Academic Press.

Flexman, J. A., & Lazareck, L. (2007). Biomedical engineering and society: policy and ethics. In *Proceedings of IEEE Eng. Med. Biol. Soc., 6156-6158*.

Harris, C. E. Jr. (2008). The good engineer: giving virtue its due in engineering ethics. *Science and Engineering Ethics*, *14*(2), 153–164. doi:10.1007/s11948-008-9068-3

Martin, M. W. (2002). Personal meaning and ethics in engineering. *Science and Engineering Ethics*, *8*(4), 545–560. doi:10.1007/s11948-002-0008-3

McLean, M. R. (2003). A framework for thinking ethically about human biotechnology. *BioProcess International*, *1*(6), 26–29.

Mishra, S. (2007). Biotechnology: An Indian prospective. *Bioimpulse*, *1*(1), 12–15.

Monzon, J. E. (1999). Teaching ethical issues in biomedical engineering. *Int. J. Eng. Ed.*, *15*(4), 276–281.

Monzon, J. E., & Monzon-Wyngaard, A. (2008). Professional ethics in biomedical engineering practice and research. In *Proceedings of IEEE Eng. Med. Biol. Soc.* (pp. 2893-2896).

Morsy, A., & Flexman, J. (2008). Ethics in biomedical engineering. In *Proceedings of IEEE Eng. Med. Biol. Soc.* (p. 3823).

Naurato, N., & Smith, T. J. (2003). Ethical considerations in bioengineering research. *Biomedical Sciences Instrumentation*, *39*, 573–578.

Page, A. K. (2004). Ethical issues in international biomedical research: an overview. *Journal of Health Law*, *37*(4), 629–665.

Persson, A. (2006). Research ethics and the development of medical biotechnology. *Xenotransplantation*, *13*(6), 511–513. doi:10.1111/j.1399-3089.2006.00352_5.x

Reiss, J. (2001). *Bringing Your Medical Device to Market*. Washington, DC: FDLI Publ.

Saha, P., & Saha, S. (1986). Ethical responsibilities of the clinical engineer. *Journal of Clinical Engineering*, *11*(1), 17–25.

Saha, S., Misra, S., & Saha, P. (1985). Bioengineers, health-care technology and bioethics. *Journal of Medical Engineering & Technology*, *9*(2), 55–60. doi:10.3109/03091908509028765

Saha, S., & Saha, P. S. (1997). Biomedical ethics and the biomedical engineer: a review. *Critical Reviews in Biomedical Engineering*, *25*(2), 163–201.

Saha, S., & Saha, P. S. (2000). Ethical issues of animal and human experimentation in the development of medical devices. In Bronzino, J. D. (Ed.), *The Biomedical Engineering Handbook* (2nd ed.). Boca Raton: CRC Press LLC.

Seebauer, E. G., & Barry, R. L. (2001). *Fundamentals of ethics for scientists and engineers*. New York: Oxford Press.

Shankar, G., & Simmons, A. (2009). Understanding ethics guidelines using an internet-based expert system. *Journal of Medical Ethics*, *35*(1), 65–68. doi:10.1136/jme.2007.023358

WMA (World Medical Association). 2000. Declaration of Helsinki Ethical Principles for Medical Research Involving Human Subjects, Adopted by 18th WMA General Assembly, Helsinki, Finland, June 1964. Amended by the 29th WMA General Assembly, Tokyo, Japan, October 1975; 35th WMA General Assembly, Venice, Italy, October 1983; 41st WMA General Assembly, Hong Kong, September1989; 48th WMA General Assembly, Somerset West, Republic of South Africa, October 1996 and the 52nd WMA General Assembly, Edinburgh, Scotland, October 2000.

KEY TERMS AND DEFINITIONS

Ethics: A study where morality is the subject matter. It is the study of right and wrong, of good and evil in human conduct. It is not about providing a judgment or specific rules for human behaviour but an objective analysis about what individuals ought to do.

Morals: Customs that result from some abiding principal human interaction in our society are called morals. Most of us usually consider such conduct not only customary but also correct or right. These codes-of-conduct are flexible and undergo continual evolution to fit to changing conditions and thereby avoid the trauma of revolution as the vehicle for change.

Clinical Trial: Before a drug or medical device is released into the market for intended human use it undergoes a three-tier (Phases I, II & III) trial-run, known as clinical trial. It could be further categorised into three forms based on the intent/objective, treatment trial, prevention trial, and other trials.

Informed-Consent: An exercise to obtain a signed consent form after a volunteer decides to participate in a clinical trial/study. This is done only after a transparent conversation with the patient-care (clinical trial) team to help the volunteer make educated decisions about whether to participate, or continue participating, without hesitating to ask questions at any time about any aspect of the study or care.

Virtue-Consideration: Dispositions that facilitate actions in ways that develop human potential and allow human flourishing. Inculcating virtues facilitates doing the right thing when faced with an ethical choice. Virtues are acquired through repetitive practice, and once acquired they become characteristic of a person. Honesty, integrity, prudence, courage, wisdom and compassion are examples of virtues.

Euthanasia: A practice of terminating a life which is merely being prolonged by machines and no longer seems to have 'human values' left, so that an individual has a 'dignified death'. It could be voluntary or involuntary, and active or passive.

Brain-Death: A total and irreparable loss of brain function, thereby incapacitating an individual to respond any form of external stimuli. It is a state when voluntary actions are completely ceased, and involuntary actions are seriously compromised.

Spare-Part Surgery: Medically-defined certified devices that assist in the struggle against illnesses through provision of research, diagnosis and treatment by healthcare professionals. Artificial limbs, heart valves, blood vessels, biosensors, biomaterials, respirators, pacemakers and artificial kidneys are some of the examples of 'spare-parts' that have redefined healthcare.

CASE STUDY I: ETHICAL CONCERNS ON EMBRYONIC STEM CELLS

Five-day-old embryo has hundreds of cells forming tight junctions of a compact epithelium, arranged around a central cavity (blastocyst stage). A mass of cells exists within the cavity protruding inward destined to become the embryo. The exterior cells (trophoblast) eventually form the placenta. When isolated and grown in a culture, the cells from inner cell mass of the blastocyst are identified as embryonic stem cells (Figure 2.). Is the embryo a living human being, entitled to all of the same rights that a human at any other age would be granted? Should any research that is potentially beneficial to the well-being of mankind be pursued? Should such research be supported by the government?

Figure 2.

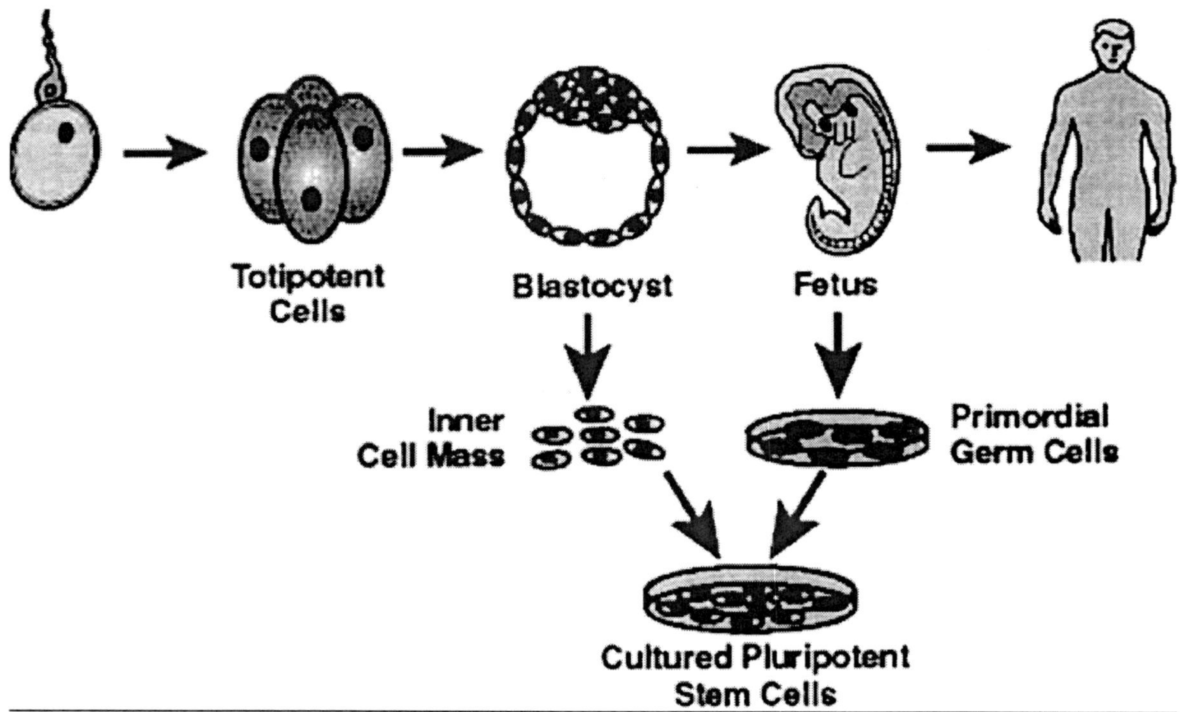

CASE STUDY II: ETHICAL VIEWS ON SPARE-PART BIOMEDICAL ENGINEERING

In August 1985 at the Medical Center of Arizona University, Jack G. Copeland implanted the Jarvik-7 artificial heart (Figure 3.) in Michael Drummond which kept him alive until a donor organ became available one week later. The medical center offered this to the Smithsonian as a successful example of 'spare parts' devices or machines.

Figure 3.

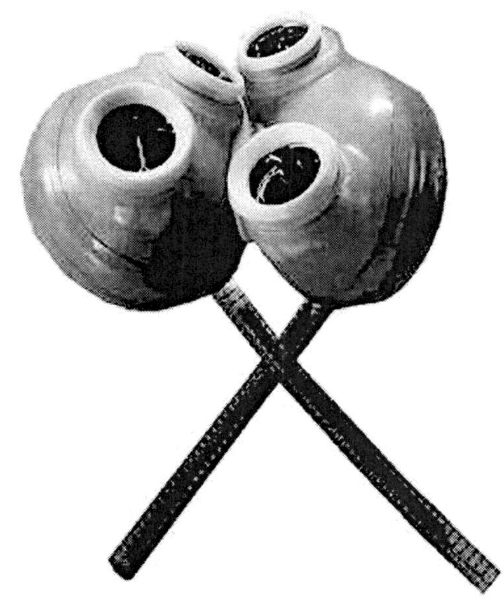

CASE STUDY III: RELEVANCE OF DATA ACQUISITION AND RETRIEVAL IN HEALTHCARE

A major problem associated with a continued medical advice is the absence of any record at the hospital and the same patient is treated by another clinician. Establishment of healthcare network is proposed to enable and inform clinicians better. This requires computer software to maintain medical records to be accessed and updated by the clinicians (Figure 4.). Apart from helping individual patients, this shall provide relevant information that may be useful from ethical standpoint as well.

Figure 4.

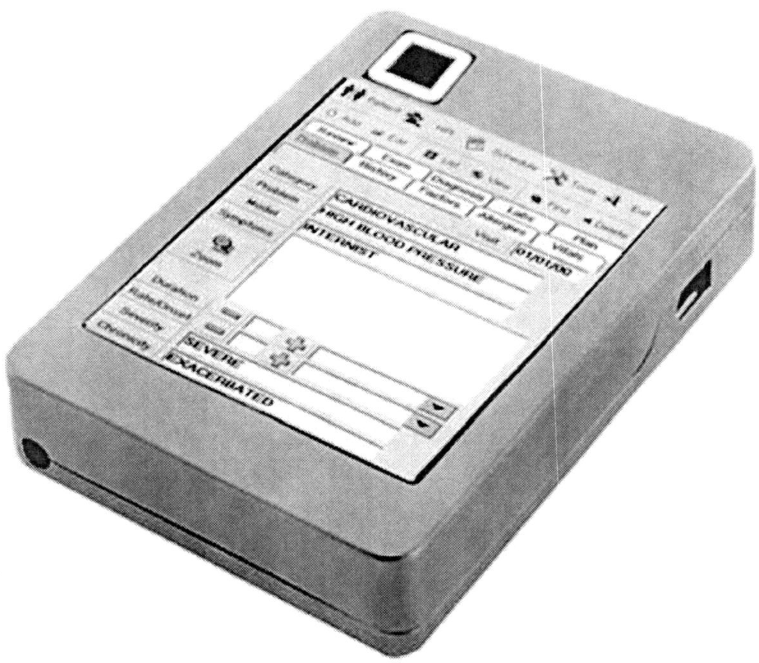

CASE STUDY IV: AN EXAMPLE OF THE PROCESS EMPLOYED BY THE MEDICAL REVIEW TEAM

Figure 5 shows a model showing the medical-device review process which is the purpose of the regulatory process. The process conducts product reviews to assure device safety and effectiveness, assure quality of design, and provide surveillance to monitor device quality, thus verifying and validating the medical device.

Figure 5.

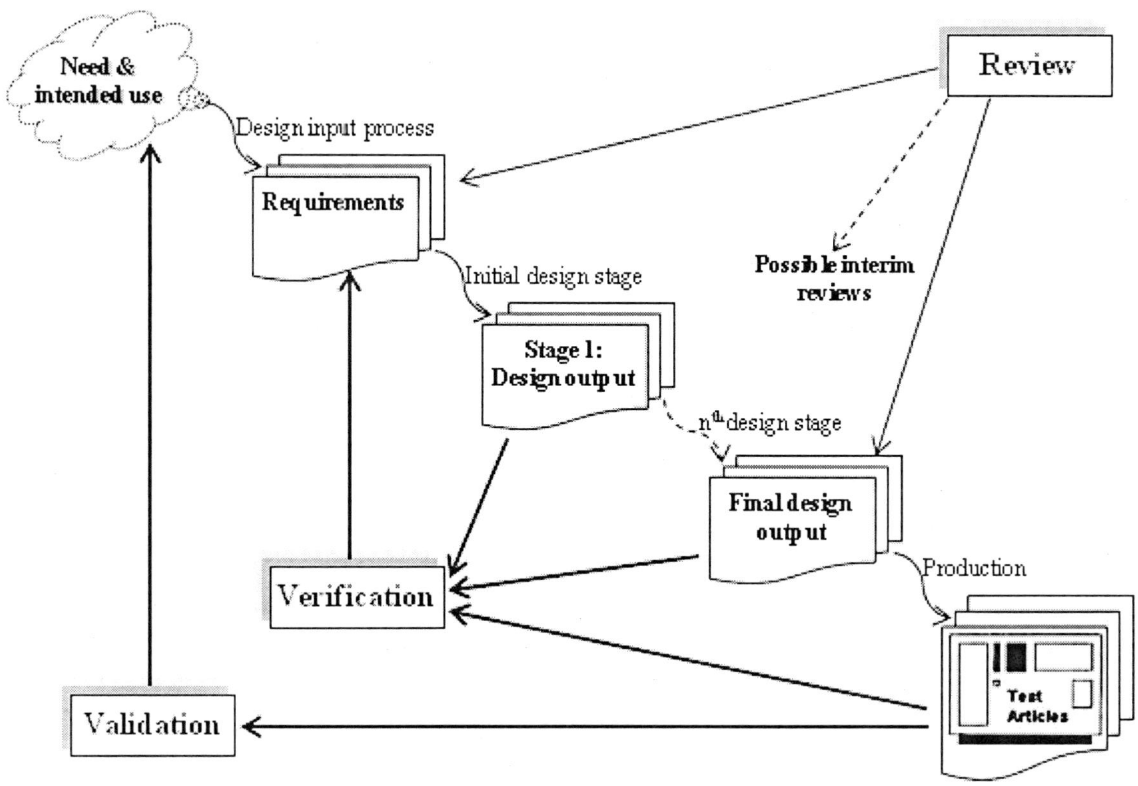

CASE STUDY V: AN EXAMPLE OF FLOW-DIAGRAM OF THE PROCEDURE FOLLOWED IN CLINICAL TRIALS

Figure 6 shows sample protocol followed to carry out medical treatment procedure for monitoring drug treatment in a psychiatric clinic. Designed and implemented by biomedical engineers with clinicians, the system begins by the entry of a specific diagnosis and recommends appropriate drugs to consider for the treatment of the mentally-disabled. The physician selects one of the recommended drugs and conducts a patient-specific dose regimen to determine the efficacy of the drug. During the treatment, blood tests are conducted to ascertain the drug persistence, and other psychiatric measures to determine if the drug is having the desired effect. As data are entered they are compared with standard expected outcomes and if the outcomes are outside the expected limits, an alert is sent to the physician for corrective action.

Figure 6.

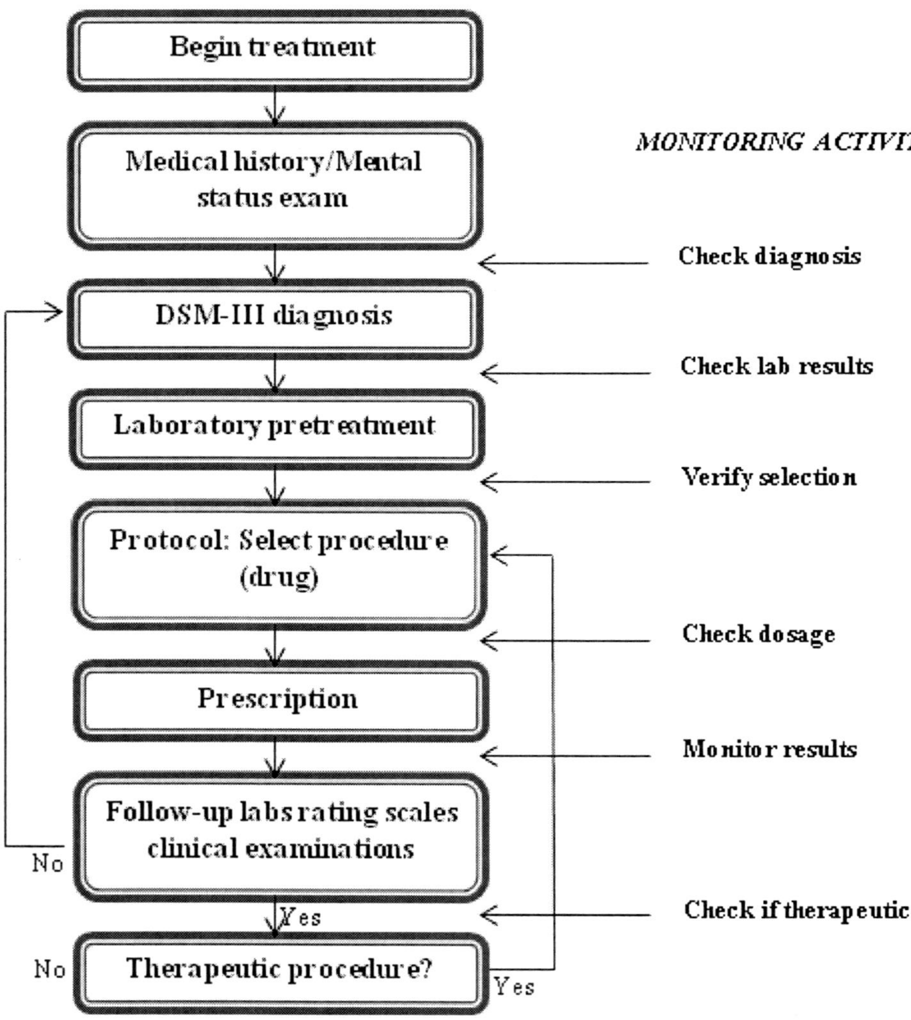

Chapter 4
Biomedical Watermarking

Subir Kumar Sarkar
Jadavpur University, India

Tirtha Sankar Das
Future Institute of Engineering & Management, India

ABSTRACT

The current work presents a medical watermarking method through contour detection and recovery for the authenticity of bio-medical images, which uses the region growing algorithm and human visual system (HVS). The proposed scheme makes the use of neighbourhood region for converting non-specific discontinuous region into specific continuous contour data. This contour as a fragile watermark is embedded in the perceptually insignificant, spatially selected detail coefficients using sub band adaptive threshold scheme along with the EPR as a robust one. Here, a new type of non-oblivious detection method is also proposed. The improvement in performance is supported through experimental results. The reported result shows improvement in visual and statistical invisibility of the hidden data. Moreover, this algorithmic architecture utilizes the existing allocated bandwidth in the data transmission channel in a more efficient manner.

INTRODUCTION

Modern health care infrastructure is based on the Digital Information Management (DIM) in hospitals as well as in Telemedical Information System (TIS). The main attributes of these systems are PACS (Picture Archiving and Communication System), HIN (Health information network), HIS (Hospital Information System), and its special cases of RIS (Radiology Information System) according to the DICOM (Digital Imaging and Communication in Medicine) standard (Coatrieux *et al,* 2000). This Standard is a set of rules or protocols that allow medical information to be transmitted between instruments and computers of health care units and users in network. Recently the advent of DIM has boosted the potential of telemedicine applications ranging from Teleconsulting, Telediagnosis etc. to cooperative working session and Telesurgery (Zain & Malcolm, 2007).

DOI: 10.4018/978-1-61692-004-3.ch004

These technologies provide new ways for long-term storage in database, easy access and distribute medical data, and introduces new practices for the profession, as well as the patient themselves by accessing to their own medical files known as Electronic Patient Records (EPR) for a better diagnosis. The medical information records are a complex set of clinical examinations, diagnosis annotations and other findings and images centered in its EPR. With these benefits there are parallel risks for EPR and strictly personal documents circulating in open networks, and being accessible, e.g., via Internet. Thus it is a widely shared point of view that there is an urgent need for network level security measures and protocols in medical information systems. It is well known that confidentiality, reliability (integrity & authenticity), availability as well as traceability of Medical Information Systems (MIS) are critical issues for ethical as well for legal reasons. To achieve these objectives, newly emerging technologies such as cryptography, steganography, digital watermarking etc. may be employed (Cox *et al*, 2003). Cryptography is probably a very efficient tool, but once the sensitive data is decrypted, the information is not protected any more. Furthermore the file headers are in the plain text format and can be usurped by a pirate. In case of, Cipher text, unless it is protected by error correction facility, is very sensitive to bit errors occurring during storage and transmission. On the other hand, Steganography always requires a covert channel resulting in complex as well as costly system. In this context digital watermarking is the most suitable scheme for multimedia data authentication as well as copyright protection. Copyright protection is achieved by robust watermarking while image authentication is usually achieved by fragile schemes. A fragile watermarking scheme detects any manipulation made to a digital image to guarantee the content integrity while a robust scheme prevents the removing of watermark from the stego unless the quality of that image is greatly reduced (Chao *et al*, 2002). In general, fragile schemes modify the LSB planes of the original image in an irreversible way. This is not acceptable in medical imagery where the least modification can lead to an erroneous diagnosis as well for legal reasons. HVS (Human Visual System) watermarking is a new paradigm which enables the exact recovery of the original image upon extraction of the embedded information. In this work, the scanned raw data (X-Ray, CT, MRI, USG etc.) having nonspecific infected region is converted into a continuous contour for improved detection. Latter the diagnosis reports, in the form of contour data and patient information including brief case history, are embedded in perceptually significant and insignificant biomedical image coefficients, respectively, in order to ensure greater security. The literature survey strongly suggests that in most of the watermarking, the ROI (region of interest) is required for inserting the medical watermarks such as EPR (electronic patient record) etc. In addition to that, distinct fragile as well as robust watermarks are necessary to provide the tamper detection and authenticity, respectively. Finally the information embedded by earlier medical watermarking schemes does not help to readily decide the diagnostics measures.

One of the major concerns throughout the world today is to make high quality health care available to all. Traditionally, part of the difficulty in achieving equitable access to health care has been that the provider and the recipient must be physically present in the same place. Recent advances in information and communication technologies have increased the number of ways health care can be delivered to reduce these difficulties. Telemedicine, the area where medicine and information and telecommunications technology meet, is probably the part of this revolution that could have the greatest impact on health care delivery. The prefix 'tele' derives from the Greek 'at a distance', and therefore, more simply telemedicine is medicine at a distance. The information infrastructure of modern health care is based on digital information management. While the recent advances in information and communication technologies provide new means to access, handle and move medical information, they also compromise their security due to their ease of manipulation and replication. All patients records, electronic or not, linked to medical secrecy, must be confidential. The digital handling of EPR (Electronic Patient Record) on network requires a systematic content validation that is aimed at quality control: actuality (precise interest of the information at a given instant) and reliability (authentication of the origin and integrity).

Medical image sharing participates to a wide variety of applications ranging from tele-diagnosis to telesurgery, and promotes also applications like remote diagnosis aid and e-learning. These two last applications are being possible through the ability of comparing images to already treated examinations. Beyond image comparison, similarity research between examinations implies a medical knowledge representation. In earlier works, inspired by medical practice, a bi-leveled is defined–disease and lesion–description language of diagnostic information in endoscopy in order to unify the representation of pathologies and of cases. Upon this analysis of the diagnostic reasoning process, all the elements were joined to a system of decision aid which suggests consistent diagnostic hypothesis and relevant cases according to the problematic case description. This system leans on two bases, one defines the endoscopic knowledge and the second corresponds to a case iconography. To identify potential cases within the same class than the problematic case, the similar case retrieval consists in a classification process upon the endoscopic knowledge. Potential cases are then sorted according to their similarity with the problematic case. Such a system is at the midpoint of the Pattern Recognition and Case Base Reasoning paradigms. Now, it is the matter of promoting the knowledge base, in particular the finding level which represents semiology in the case of an e-learning application demonstrator project in order to share and teach this endoscopic semiology. The basic principle of this approach is to share with a medical image a knowledge digest (KD) that gives a medical synthetic description and interpretation of the image content. Such a digest will constitute the distributed knowledge and is thereafter exploited: (i) to update user's case and knowledge bases and, (ii) to provide the means allowing similar images retrieval with either the same findings or differential diagnoses. To share with medical images some concomitant data, one approach consists in adding, when allowed by the image file format, some extra header information. Here, people have opted for watermarking. Watermarking is the insertion of a message in a host document which in our case corresponds to an image. Embedded at the pixel gray level of the image, it means independently of the image file format, it is usually required that the watermark information remains hidden to any unauthorized user (as for data encryption, a secret key is needed to access the watermark content), non-interfering with the use of the watermarked document, that is in our case not modifying image interpretation. Between the different approaches proposed for watermarking medical images, we have retained reversible watermarking. The reversibility property allows the removal of the watermark from the image retrieving exactly the original image. In this work, we extend to JPEG compressed image a reversible watermarking method we have proposed for raw image. Suggested KD and watermarking are jointly exploited at the database level of an e-learning demonstrator of endoscopic semiology. Watermarking makes the image more usable by inserting KD in the image and provides also data integrity control by embedding a digital signature computed on both image and KD.

Hiding patient data in the medical image is one of the applications of digital image watermarking. The patient data in the electronic format is called Electronic patient record (EPR). All works reported in data hiding in medical image are watermarking for authentication and EPR hiding. The medical images of different modalities with EPR attached to them can be sent to the clinicians residing at any corner of the globe for the diagnosis. Embedding of EPR with medical images will save storage space of the Hospital Information System, enhance confidentiality of the patient data and save the bandwidth required for transmission. Obviously this will reduce the cost of diagnosis. This kind of a system requires a high level of security, which can be ensured by using digital watermarking techniques. Literature is devoid of a systematic norms or regulations for watermarking medical images. Medical image watermarking communities around the world need a standard benchmark for the exchange of information globally. The currently popular benchmarks focus on evaluating imperceptibility and robustness under typical non-medical image degradation processes. They do not provide an evaluation scheme applicable for specific medical image types, or for typical degradations arising from medical image processing. Image watermarking has become an increasingly popular research area with applications in data security, content verification and image integrity. Medical image watermarking is a particular subset of image watermarking whereby medical images are embedded with hidden information that may be used to assert ownership, increase the security, and verify the numerical integrity of medical images. Unlike most images, medical images require particular care when embedding additional information within them because the additional information must not affect the reading of the images. Medical imagery is a field where the protection of the integrity and confidentiality of content is a critical issue due to the special characteristics derived from strict ethics, legislative and diagnostic implications. It is very important to prevent unauthorized manipulation and misappropriation of such digitized images. The risks are increased when dealing with an open environment like the internet. Medical images should be kept intact in any circumstance and before any operation they must be checked for:

- **Integrity:** the image has not been modified by non authorized people.
- **Authentication:** the image belongs indeed to the correct patient.

Before applying watermarking techniques developed for multimedia applications to medical imagery applications, it is important that the requirements imposed by medical images are carefully analyzed to investigate whether they are compatible with existing watermarking techniques. Different watermarking schemes have been proposed to address the problems of medical confidentiality protection and both origin and data authentication.

For the purpose of diagnosis, medical images must be utilized in association with ancillary data, such as demographic information (patient identity, age, gender, etc.), data acquisition parameters, and comments and notes from medical personnel. Solomon provided standard of image, called DICOM, which can integrate patient information onto the image data header section. On the other hand, the advances in communication technologies provide a new ways to store and distribute medical data in a digital format. But these advances have introduced new risks for inappropriate use of medical information circulating in open networks, and then use of DICOM standard presents a high risk of tampered with, because the information can be easily obtained from the image file. Classical encryption technology is an important tool that can be used to protect data transmitted over computer networks but it does not solve all digital data protection problems. Nowadays, digital watermarking appears as an efficient mean of authentication and copyright protection. Robust watermarks are designed to be hard to remove and to resist common image-manipulation procedures. They are useful for copyright and ownership assertion purposes. Unlike robust watermark, fragile watermarks are designed to be easily destroyed if the watermarked image is manipulated in the slightest manner. This property is ideal for image authentication applications (in our case medial images), where the objective is to determine if the watermarked image has been tampered with or modified. Early fragile watermarking systems embedded checksums or pseudo-random sequences in LSB bitplane of an image.

Medical image watermarking has not been the subject of as much research as generic image watermarking, however some methods have been specifically tailored for medical images. These methods are briefly reviewed here, with particular focus on the perceptual degradation caused to images. Traditional methods embed checksums or pseudorandom sequences in the Least Significant Bit (LSB) plane (Johnson, 2001). More recent works have employed increasingly sophisticated embedding techniques such as cryptographic hash functions (Lin *et al*, 2000). Fragile invertible authentication schemes have been proposed for medical images, whereby a watermark can be removed from a watermarked image, thereby results into the exact original image (Macq and Dewey, 1999). Another medical image watermarking system embeds information in bit planes, which results in watermarked images with very low normalized root mean square errors (NRMSEs), indicating that the watermark is practically invisible (Jagadish *et* al, 2004). A number of robust medical image watermarking systems have been developed. For example one system uses a spread spectrum technique to encode copyright and patient information in images (Tachibana, *et al* 2002). Another embeds a watermark in a spiral fashion around the Region of Interest (ROI) of an image 9 (Wakatani, 2002). Any image tampering that occurs will severely degrade the image quality. The Gabor transform has also been applied to hide information in medical images (Kong, 2001). Jagadish *et al.* investigated interleaving hidden information in the Discrete Cosine Transform (DCT) and the Discrete Wavelet Transform (DWT) domains (Jagadish *et al*, 2004). Multiple watermarking systems have the advantages that different watermarks can be applied for different purposes (for example, copyright, authentication, data integrity) (Giakoumaki *et al*, 2003). Anand and Niranjan proposed to embed an encrypted version of the Electronic Patient Record (EPR) in the least significant bit (LSB) plane of the image (Anand and Niranjan, 1998). Miaou et al similarly proposed a LSB technique where the host image authenticated the transmission origin with an embedded message composed of various patient data (e.g. ECG record), the diagnosis report and the doctor's signature (Miaou *et al*, 2000). Macq and Dewey proposed a trusted header scheme by embedding the hash of the file header of medical standard image in the image raw data (Macq and Dewey, 1999). Coatrieux et al proposed Region of Interest (ROI) to preserve the diagnostic zone and Region of Non Interest (RONI) whose integrity need not be preserved and served as the watermark carrier (Coatrieux *et al*, 2001). Wong described a fragile marking technique in which a digest was obtained using a hash function. The image, image dimensions, and marking key were hashed during embedding and used to modify the least-significant bit plane of the original image (Wong, 1998). However, Holliman and Memon presented a vector quantization (VQ) counterfeiting attack that could construct a counterfeit image from a VQ codebook generated from a set of watermarked images (Holliman and Memon, 2000). Celik et al then presented an algorithm based on Wong's scheme and demonstrated that their algorithm could thwart the VQ codebook but compromised on the accuracy of localization (Celik,).

In view of the above discussion the proposed method is completely different in various aspects. As the process is based on HVS, it does not require finding any ROI for data hiding. In medical diagnosis, several image based investigations like X-ray, CT-scan, MRI etc., are available. Each and every process provides a non-specific raw scanned data (discontinuous contour) from which exact diagnosis is very difficult. The proper diagnosis is possible if and only if a continuous contour data is available. This establishes the novelty of the present work. The embedding operation is associated with a contour detection section which converts the non-specific region into a specific continuous contour data. This can help to take a right diagnostic decision instantly. Moreover it can be used as fragile watermark because any little bit tempering over bio-medical image makes it non-specific and discontinuous. Secondly, as the EPR is redundantly hidden inside the image can act as a robust watermark. In this way, the proposed algorithm discards the additional data hiding for fragile and robust watermark. Therefore, the proposed method minimizes the possibility of the image degradation and increases the security to a large extent.

CONTOUR DETECTION USING REGION GROWING

The terms segmentation means partitioning an image into its constituent's parts or regions. Boundary is the difference between two regions depending on their intensity levels. Here our objective is to find the accurate boundary of the infected regions very precisely. To get the appropriate boundary and also to make it continuous contour, region growing algorithm is used. Region growing is a procedure that groups pixels to form a region based on predefined criteria for growth (Gonzalez). The predefined criteria may be intensity level or gray level, color, texture etc. Here the intensity or gray level property is used to group the pixels to form a region of interest (ROI). In this algorithm first a seed point (position: r, c) is taken which can be selected from the any part of the medical image. Generally the seed point is selected by clicking the mouse pointer on the ROI or the affected part of the medical image from the clinic. This point is called seed point because it is the starting point from where the region starts to grow. In region growing algorithm, the surrounding pixels are compared with intensity level of the seed point depending on the threshold which can also be set by the user. The threshold is used to make the intensity level of the surrounding pixels into a certain acceptable range. In this process the seed point is compared with the neighboring pixels (4 neighbors) and it groups the pixels having the same or nearby intensity levels, thus forming the region of interest if they satisfy the homogeneity property of that region (Chanda B, Majumder, 2002). The homogeneity property Prop (R) can be mathematically expressed as follows:

$$\Pr op(R) : (\frac{1}{Card\ R}) \sum_{(r,c)\varepsilon R} \{g(r,c) - \exp[g]\}^2 = T_h \quad (1.01)$$

where Card R is the number of pixels in the region R and exp[g] is the mean gray level of pixels lying in that region, i.e.

$$\exp[g] = (\frac{1}{Card\ R}) \sum_{(r,c)\varepsilon R} g(r,c) \quad (1.02)$$

and T_h is the predefined threshold. This process goes on recursively till the current region is marked with unique label. To make the region more accurate we have to choose the threshold carefully. After getting the region of the affected part of the medical image, to separate the region we have to find the edge of the corresponding region. Now if we draw or plot the edge of the affected region in the original image we can easily find out the ROI or the affected region in that medical image. If we can make the boundary perfect the treatment will be more accurate and the patient will have greater chance of complete recovery.

WATERMARK EMBEDDING AND DETECTION

This section explains the embedding and detection operations of the proposed watermarking scheme.

Figure 1. Results for PSNR, SSIM, Security Values

Image	PSNR (dB)	SSIM
Brain I	69.191292	1
Fetal (6 weeks)	75.576782	1
Brain II	75.764816	1
MRI of Coitus	75.881676	1
Fetal (22 weeks)	69.103629	1

Figure 2. Results for BER, NCC, Mutual Information

Image	BER	NCC	Mutual Information
Brain I	0	1	0.0604
Fetal (6 weeks)	0	1	0.0160
Brain II	0	1	0.0144
MRI of Coitus	0	1	0.0138
Fetal (22 weeks)	0	1	0.0126

Actually, there are two watermarks, one fragile and another robust, in this biomedical data hiding technique. The continuous contour obtained from the region growing algorithm acts as a fragile watermark whereas EPR is being considered as robust one. Both the watermarks are to be hidden inside the original raw scanned image as a cover intended for the diagnosis. The EPR is converted into its binary counterpart which further will be considered as the robust watermark. The fragile watermark is made from binary continuous contour having a dynamic size. Then it is split into three segments, each having almost equal number of elements. During this process of segmentation, four distinct indices are determined in the binary form from the original contour. These indices latter solve the purpose of retrieving the contour data by concatenating individual recovered segments. Now the original image is decomposed by L levels using Discrete Wavelet Transform (DWT) through Daubechies 2pt analysis wavelet filter bank (Daubechis, 1988). The HVS is sensitive for the changes in smooth parts of the image, not for small changes in high frequencies. So the robust and fragile watermarks are embedded in perceptually significant and insignificant coefficients of each of the 3 sub bands in 1st level respectively. The hiding process embeds the individual segments of the entire fragile watermark in three respective sub bands. The robust watermark is embedded in each of the 3 sub bands in 1st level excluding the LL sub band. Finally, the binary indices are also concealed but in the LL sub band only. The coefficients selection and data hiding algorithm is now explained as follows:

The maximum of the coefficients from each sub band are computed as given by the equation:

$$M_{s,l} = \max(\max(C_{s,l})) \qquad (1.03)$$

where $M_{s,l}$ is the maximum of the coefficients from the respective detail image, C is the original cover image, s ∈ {h, v, d} (h, v, d stands for "horizontal", "vertical" and "diagonal", respectively) and l = 1,…..,L. Now for each level (except for the LL sub band), the largest coefficient C_l is computed as:

Figure 3. Original Scanned Image, Original Detected Contour (Watermark), Recovered Watermark and Superimposed Image

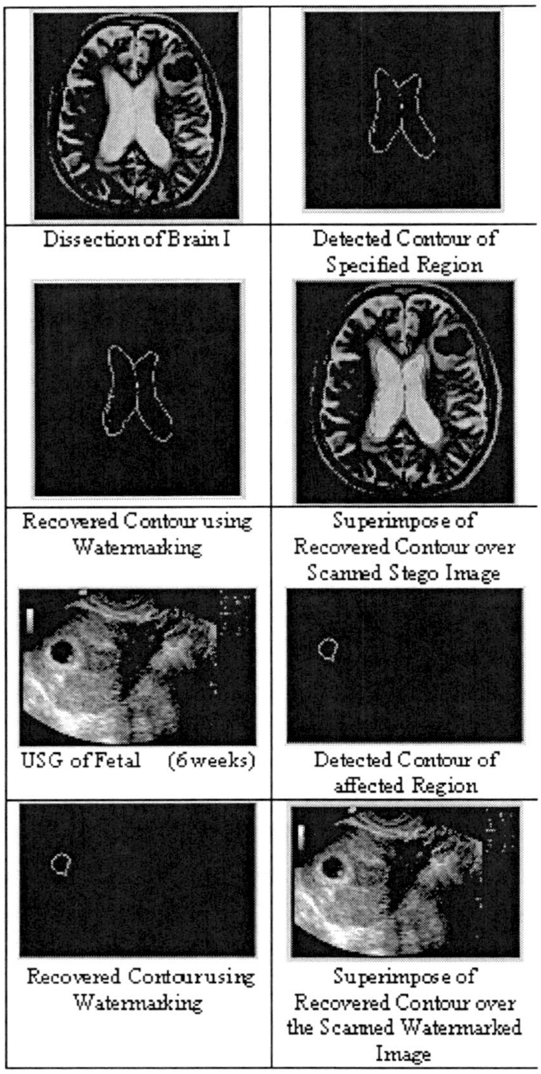

Figure 4. Original Scanned Image, Original Detected Contour (Watermark), Recovered Watermark and Superimposed Image

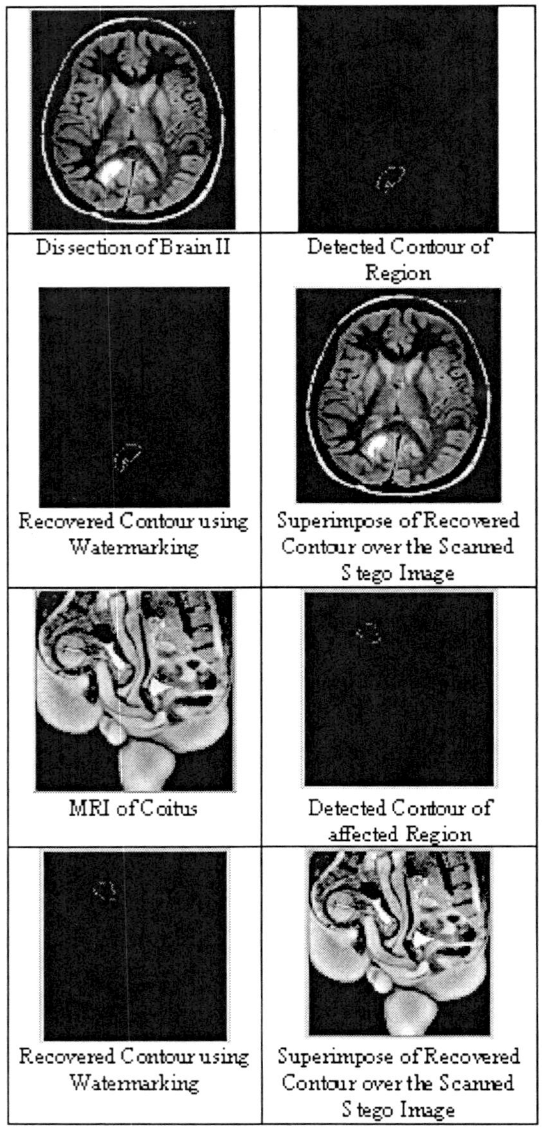

$$C_l = \max(M_{s,l}) \tag{1.04}$$

where C_l is the maximum of the coefficients from the l level subbands (HH_l, HL_l, LH_l). Now for each level we compute the threshold T_i as:

$$T_i = [\log_2 C_l] - 1 \tag{1.05}$$

If the wavelet coefficient seems to be less or equal than the computed threshold, the coefficients are modified for the fragile bit stream. On the other hand, the coefficients which are above the threshold are modified for the robust watermark. The watermark embedding modulation function is mathematically expressed using the negative modulation function as:

$$c^{w}_{s,l}(m,n) = c_{s,l}(m,n)[1 - \alpha.b(m,n)] \qquad (1.06)$$

where $c^{w}_{s,l}(m, n)$ denotes the watermarked image, $c_{s,l}(m, n)$ denotes the DWT coefficients of the original image, b is the fragile or robust watermark bit stream and α is a parameter, $\alpha \in (0,1)$, controlling the level of the watermark. The negative sign implies that when the watermarked bit is negative it is added with image coefficient and vice versa. This ensures the better robustness efficiency than being used with the positive modulation.. The higher the strength of the mark α and the lower the parameter q_l are the more robust yet visible the watermark will be. The watermarked image C^w is thus computed from the newly modified coefficients using the Daubechies 2pt synthesis wavelet filter bank.

The detection process is the inverse procedure of the insertion process. The detection scheme is a non- blind watermarking scheme. So the original image is required in the decoder side to extract the watermark. To detect the watermark from the watermarked distorted image C', first the original and the received images are transformed using DWT using the same analysis filter. Then once again the threshold is calculated from the original image by the same process as in the embedding process.

$$M_{s,l} = \max(\max(C_{s,l})) \qquad (1.07)$$

$$C_l = \max(M_{s,l}) \qquad (1.08)$$

$$T_i = [\log_2 C_l] - 1 \qquad (1.09)$$

If $C_{s,l}(m, n) > T_{s,l}$, then we extract the robust watermark wheras if $C_{s,l}(m, n) \leq T_{s,l}$, the fragile watermark is extracted using the equation as:

Figure 5. Electronic Patient Record (EPR)

> Patient Reference Number: 1437205
> Name of the Doctor: Dr. Ananta Majhi
> Name of the Patient: Mrs. G.Ganguly
> Age in years: 47
> Residential Address: # 27, Mandir Para, Sodpur, Kolkata 700114
> Case History: Date of admission: 17.7.07
> Acute Headache and vision Problem having Vomiting Tendency, Patient had a similar symptom 3 months ago.
> Tests Performed: CT scan
> Diagnosis: Suspected Brain Tumor or cyst
> Treatment: Sublingual Nitroglycerin.
> Required Tests: MRI
> Referred to: Dr. Sanjay Nath, PGI Hospital, Sector IV, Chandigar.

$$\tilde{b}(m,n) = \operatorname{sgn}\left[\frac{c'_{s,l}(m,n) - c_{s,l}(m,n)}{c_{s,l}(m,n)}\right] \qquad (1.10)$$

where $\tilde{b}(m,n)$ is the recovered watermark bit.

By this way the watermarks are extracted from all 3 sub bands at first level of decomposition. The final fragile watermark is computed from these 3 sub bands by properly concatenating them with the recovered indices. Moreover, the robust watermark is determined from these 3 sub bands watermarks by making a comparison using the majority rule defined as follows: the most common bit values from the recovered sub bands are assigned to the final watermark. This detector structure is modified by taking various combinations of sub bands in order to improve the robustness performance. The EPR is given in Figure 5. The Proposed architecture is shown in details as a block diagram in Figure 6.

RESULTS AND DISCUSSION

The proposed algorithm is tested over various numbers of bio-medical images having dimension 256 X 256. The robust and fragile watermarks

Figure 6. Block Diagram of the Proposed Algorithm

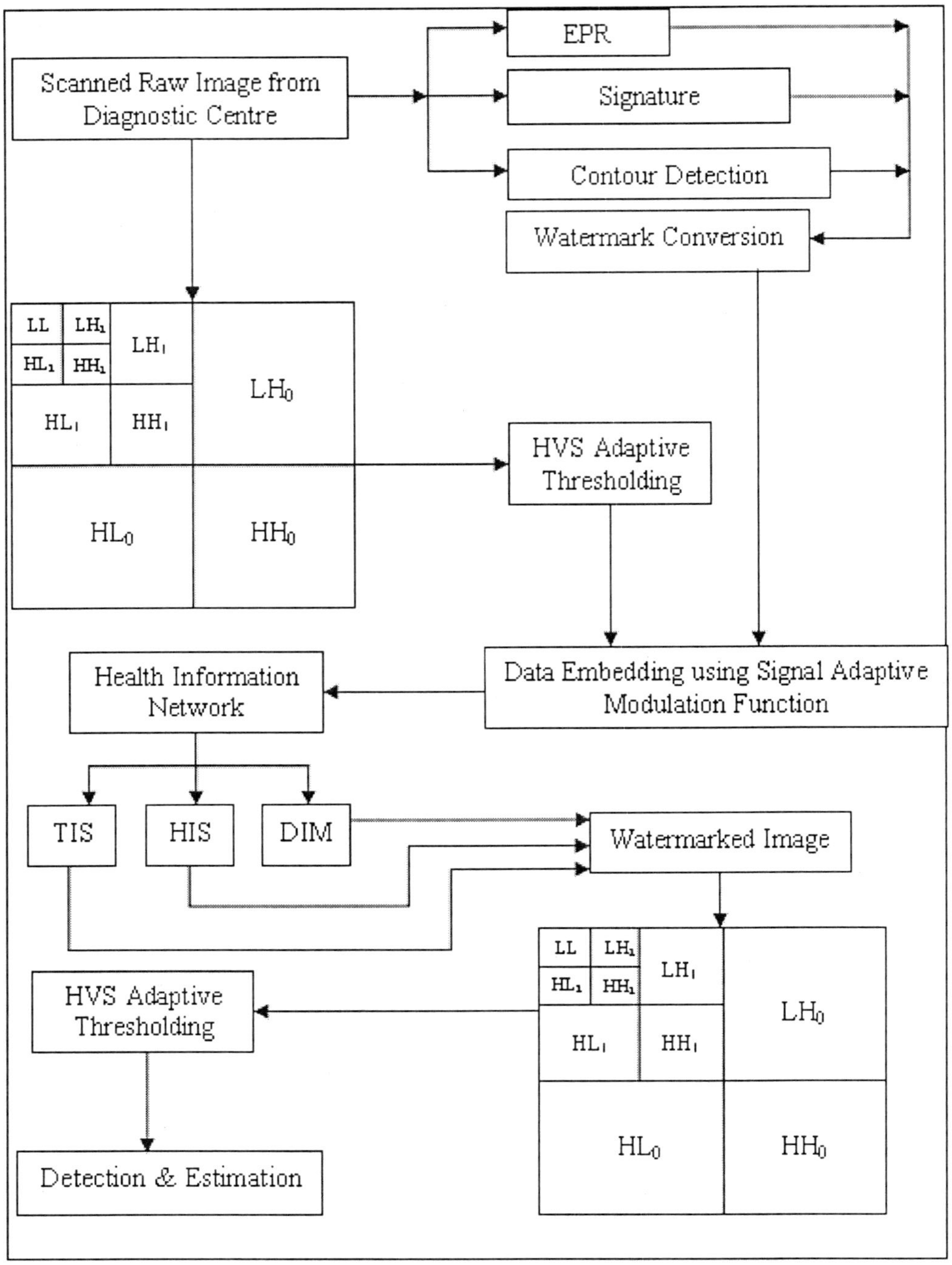

have a dynamic size limited to the maximum 256 X 256. The Daubechies 2pt (db2) wavelet is used to produce the wavelet coefficients. The various parameters used in the present algorithm are as follows: the number of resolution levels L = 1; the strength of the watermark $\alpha = 0.4$ for the coarsest bands and $\alpha = 0.5$ for the other 3 sub bands. The robust watermark is extracted by a majority rule being used with different types of detector structures. The fragile watermark is recovered using the above specified non-oblivious detection process. The results obtained by several structures motivated us to select the two best-optimized watermark decoders.

The distortion caused by both the watermarks can be measured by the peak signal-to-noise ratio (PSNR) and Structural Similarity Index Measurement (SSIM) respectively. Moreover, the detection efficiency is supported by bit error rate, normalized cross-correlation and mutual information. The experimental results of visual transparency and robustness performances are given in Figure 1 and Figure 2 as well as in Figure 3 and Figure 4.

The proposed method shows better robustness against different image impairments. Specific subjective watermarks are being used and the computational cost and complexity is comparatively low. Moreover, the proposed method extracts the watermark image in both subjective and objective manners in single pass with better robustness which is shown.

REFERENCES

Anand, D., & Niranjan, U. (1988). *Watermarking Medical Images with Patient Information.* In *Proceedings of the IEEE/EMBS Conference*, (pp. 703-706).

Celik, M., Sharma,U. G. Saber, E. Tekalp, A. M. (n.d.). Hierarchical Watermarking for Secure Image Authentication with Localization. *IEEE Trans. Image Processing, 11*(6), pp.585-594.

Chanda, B., & Majumder, D. D. Digital Image Processing.(2002), Prentice-Hall of India, ISBN-81-203-1618-5, 2003.

Chao, H. M., Hsu, C. M., & Miaou, S. G. (2002). A Data-Hiding Technique with Authentication, Integration, and Confidentiality for Electronic Patients Records. *IEEE Transactions on Information Technology in Biomedicine*, *6*(1), 46–53. doi:10.1109/4233.992161

Coatrieux, G., Maître, H., Sankur, B., Rolland, Y., & Collorec, R. (2000) *Relevance of watermarking in medical imaging.* In *Proceedings of 22nd International Conference of IEEE EMBS*, (pp 250–255).

Coatrieux, G., Sankur, B., & Maitre, H. (2001). *Strict Integrity Control of Biomedical Images*. In Proceedings of SPIE Conf. 4314: Security and Watermarking of Multimedia Contents III.

Cox, I., Miller, M., & Bloom, J. (2002). *Digital Watermarking*. San Francisco: Morgan Kaufmann Publishers.

Daubechis, I. (1988). Orthogonal bases for Compactly Supported Wavelets. *Communications on Pure and Applied Mathematics*, *41*, 909–996. doi:10.1002/cpa.3160410705

Giakoumaki, A., Pavlopoulos, S., & Koutsouris, D. "*A Medical Image Watermarking Scheme Based on Wavelet Transform*", (Sept. 2003), In *Proceedings of the 25th Annual Int. Conf. of the IEEE-EMBS*, (pp. 856-859).

Gonzalez, Woods. "Digital Image Processing", *Prentice-Hall of India*, ISBN-81-7808-629-8,.

Holliman, M., & Memon, N. (2000). Counterfeiting Attacks on Oblivious Block-Wise Independent Invisible Watermarking Schemes. *IEEE Transactions on Image Processing*, *9*, 432–441. doi:10.1109/83.826780

Jagadish, N., Subbanna Bhat, P., Acharya, R., & Niranjan, U. C. (2004, June). Simultaneous storage of medical images in the spatial and frequency domain: a comparative study. *Biomedical Engineering Online*, *3*(1).

Johnson, N. F., Duric, Z., & Jajodia, S. (2001). *Information Hiding: Steganography and Watermarking - Attacks and Countermeasures*. Amsterdam: Kluwer Academic Press.

Kong, X., & Feng, R. (2001, September). Watermarking Medical Signals for Telemedicine. *IEEE Transactions on Information Technology in Biomedicine*, *5*(3), 195–201. doi:10.1109/4233.945290

Lin, T., Podilchuk, C. I., & Delp, E. J. (2000, January). Detection of image alterations using semi-fragile watermarks. In *Proceedings of the SPIE Int. Conf. on Security and Watermarking of Multimedia Contents II*, (vol. 3971, pp. 152-163).

Macq, B., & Dewey, F. (1999, October). Trusted Headers for Medical Images. In DFG VIII-D II Watermarking Workshop.

Miaou, S., Hsu, C., Tsai, Y., & Chao, H. (2000, July, 23-28). A Secure Data Hiding Technique with Heterogeneous Data-Combining Capability for Electronic Patient Records. In *Proceedings of the 22nd Annual International Conference of the IEEE Engineering in Medicine and Biology Society*, (pp. 280-283).

Tachibana, H., Harauchi, H., Ikeda, T., Iwata, Y., Takemura, A., & Umeda, T. (2002, December). Practical Use of New Watermarking and VPN Techniques for Medical Image Communication and Archive. In *Proceedings of the RSNA 88th Scientific Assembly and Annual Meeting.*

Wakatani, A. (2002, January). Digital Watermarking for ROI Medical Images by using Compressed Signature Image. In *Proceedings of the Annual Hawaii Int. Conf. on System Science*, (pp. 2043-2048).

Wong, P. W. (1998, October). *A Public Key Watermark for Image Verification and Authentication.* In *Proceedings of the IEEE International Conference on Image Processing*, (pp. 455-459).

Zain, J. M., & Clarke, M. (2007, September). Reversible Region of Non-Interest (RONI) Watermarking for Authentication of DICOM Images. *International Journal of Computer Science and Network Security*, *7*(9), 19–28.

KEY TERMS AND DEFINITIONS

Digital Watermarking: It is a process by which the copyright information is embedded invisibly inside the original entity, which is to be protected from the illegal replication and distribution, is known as digital watermarking.

Medical Watermarking: Medical watermarking is a signal processing technique in order to achieve the objectives e.g. confidentiality, reliability, availability as well as traceability of medical information systems.

Region Growing: Region growing is a procedure that accumulates pixels to form a region based on intensity level or gray level, color, texture etc. which is used to group the pixels to form a region of interest.

Human Visual System: Human visual system is an image masking process where the characteristics of the pixels are being modified depending on visual systems obtained from the image.

Bio-Medical Images: Bio-Medical images are the image obtained from the data acquisition devices applied in telemedical information system.

EPR: It is data base system for modern day health care known as electronic patient record.

Contour Detection: The usefulness of this technique has been critically analyzed about for proving the authenthenticity of bio-medical images along with some other medical information and utility. The proposed method does not require any additional robust or fragile watermark for content protection and integrity control, respectively. This is because the contour data itself is a fragile watermark in selected image coefficients followed by HVS system along with the electronic patient record as a robust one.

Chapter 5
Methods for Improving Foot Displacement Measurements Calculated from Inertial Sensors

Edgar Charry
The University of Melbourne, Australia

Daniel T. H. Lai
Victoria University, Australia

ABSTRACT

The use of inertial sensors to measure human movement has recently gained momentum with the advent of low cost micro-electro-mechanical systems (MEMS) technology. These sensors comprise accelerometer and gyroscopes which measure accelerations and angular velocities respectively. Secondary quantities such as displacement can be obtained by integration of these quantities, a method which presents challenging issues due to the problem of accumulative sensor errors. This chapter investigates the spectral evaluation of individual sensor errors and looks at the effectiveness of minimizing these errors using static digital filters. The primary focus is on the derivation of foot displacement data from inertial sensor measurements. The importance of foot, in particular toe displacement measurements is evident in the context of tripping and falling which are serious health concerns for the elderly. The Minimum Toe Clearance (MTC) as an important gait variable for falls-risk prediction and assessment, and therefore the measurement variable of interest. A brief sketch of the current devices employing accelerometers and gyroscopes is presented, highlighting the problems and difficulties reported in literature to achieve good precision. These have been mainly due to the presence of sensor errors and the error accumulative process employed in obtaining displacement measurements. The investigation first proceeds to identify the location of these sensor errors in the frequency domain using the Fast Fourier Transform (FFT) on raw inertial sensor data. The frequency content of velocity and displacement measurements obtained from integrating the inertial data using a well known strap-down method is then explored. These investigations

DOI: 10.4018/978-1-61692-004-3.ch005

revealed that large sensor errors occurred mainly in the low frequency spectrum while white noise exists in all frequency spectra. The efficacy of employing a band-pass filter to remove a large portion of these errors and their effect on the derived displacements is elaborated on. The cross-correlation of the FFT power spectra from a highly accurate optical measurement system and processed sensor data is used as a metric to evaluate the performance of the band-pass filter at several stages of the processing stage. The motivation is that a more fundamental method would require less computational demand and could lead to more efficient implementations in low-power and systems with limited resources, so that portable sensor based motion measurement system would provide a good degree of measurement accuracy.

INTRODUCTION

Gait is one of the most essential and common form of human movement, as it allows the movement from one destination to another. This entails the quasiperiodic movement of the limbs and the appropriate positioning of the feet on the floor. Depending on the walking style, terrain conditions and speed, gait can have different forms and features. Excluding the evident linkage between this activity to the effects on public health risks such as obesity, diabetes and cardiac disease, the analysis of these features in a biomechanical context has also provided answers to pathological aspects related to the task of walking. This can also include the research of gait functionality deviations, such as musculoskeletal disorders (amputation and osteoarthritis), and neurological disorders such as cerebral palsy and stroke, that may considerably affect gait functionality. Many hospitals and research institutions now possess gait laboratories, where patients with pathological diseases are examined with statistical methods that provide means for further understanding and identifying causes and effects of these deviations. This is where progress in gait analysis has the greatest impact, in deciding on overall treatments, preventive measures and also modified surgery procedures (Begg et al., 2007)

Recent research of human motion has turn to the developments of low-cost and small sensor devices, set to replace the current reliance on bulky, laboratory constraining optical video systems such as Vicon and Optotrak NDI. These low powered sensors can be used to develop portable systems which would extend motion analysis to the outdoor environment as opposed to the optical systems. Secondary quantities such as limb velocity and displacement and joint instantaneous angles can be inferred by numerically integrating the primary signals. Early work directly used the raw inertial signals to track physical quantities such as limb or upper body accelerations, and joint orientations and inclinations. Baten et al. (1996) assessed accelerometers and gyroscopes to compute low-back angles against a 3D video system with errors around ±10%. These results were extended to using EMG signals to track trunk muscle activities during lifting, achieving estimation errors below 5° (Baten et al., 2000). Gyroscopes have been used by Najafi et al. (2002) to detect postural transitions and hence determine potential elderly fallers. A Discrete Wavelet Transform (DWT) successfully denoised the signal and left the integrated trunk tilt, which is the angle between the vertical axis and the thorax wall, reasonably intact to measure transitions, such as sit-stand or stand-sit. Zijlstra et al. (2003) also measured lower trunk acceleration to detect spatio-temporal gait events such as walking speed, foot contact and step length. Using Ground Reaction Forces (GRF) to compare, it was shown that accelerometry had small biases but reasonable accuracy to estimate mean step length and walking speed. Bourke et al. (2008) extended this work by using Vertical Velocity Thresholding (VVT) to detect potential falls in the elderly. The authors used tri-axis accelerometers and gyroscopes to monitor vertical trunk speed and avoided integration drift errors by using a strap-down method, assuming speed was 0m/s before and after each activity period. The authors claimed achieving 100% precision to detect potential falls with an average lead-time of 323ms prior to trunk impact. Dejnabadi et al. (2005) studied the knee extension and flexion angles using also accelerometers during walking, measuring the angles without gyroscope integration and hence avoiding cumulative errors. Good performance (1.3° RMS error) was reported when compared with a reference motion measurement system. More specifically in human gait, as it is the goal of this study, early work by Miyazaki (1996) monitored stride length and walking velocity using a piezoelectric gyroscope and a data logger in 20 healthy and 17 gait impaired patients. The difficulties in accurate measurements due to gyroscope drifts was pointed out, when a modest 15% error was achieved. Pappas et al. (2001) proposed a real-time gait phase detection shoe using the gyroscope integrated angular speeds and three FSRs (force sensitive resistors) on the sole of ten healthy and six gait impaired subjects. Results achieved 99% reliability against a video system on different walking activities, making possible the gait disabilities tracking and bio-feedback on impaired gait walking subjects. The signals sampled at 100Hz and the angular speeds were band-pass filtered with a 3rd-order, 0.25-25Hz cut-off filter. Morris et al. (2002) also studied heel strike and heel off events, by designing a Wireless Gait Shoe with a 3D gyroscope and accelerometer, Force Sensitive Resistors (FSR) to track the sole's pressure and Polyvinlylidine Fluoride (PVDF) pads to provide information on the heel-strike and toe off. Although only the primary signals were analysed, it was pointed out that ideally the subject should be analysed outside the laboratory to guarantee the natural gait pattern.

More recent work deployed wireless data transmission for sensor data transmission which reduced the need for a wire harness and cumbersome setups, whilst providing real-time data collection for further processing or storing. Gafurov et al. (2006) proposed gait pattern recognition for security purposes through acceleration measured from the ankle, achieving 5% and 9% errors rates with cycle length and a normalised histogram method respectively. The author concluded that these values are promising to increase security with other methods such as PIN numbers, but not for high security applications. Also in the security research field, Rong et al. (2007) proposed an individual recognition system based on gait vertical acceleration using wavelets denoising and Dynamic Time Warping (DTW) to take into account natural gait variations. The author divided the vertical acceleration into gait cycles using local maximum and minimum points and achieved satisfactory results in identifying 35 subjects. Previously, frequency analysis correlation was used by Rong et al. (2007) to improve the recognition of walking patterns from different subjects and it was found the method robust to changes in gait speed. Later in the rehabilitation field, Lau et al. (2008) used one dual-axis accelerometer, one single-axis gyroscope and Force Sensitive Resistors (FSR) to detect gait events during the swing phase on 10 people with dropped foot and 3 without impairments, achieving better performance for the threshold method at higher walking speeds. While most previous work used directly the raw inertial signals, recent attempts have used integration techniques to obtain secondary measurement quantities, particularly in the assessment of foot motion. Pappas et al.(1999) attempted to exploit the gait characteristics to compensate numerical integration errors arising from sensitivity and bias temperature drifts. It was proposed to calibrate the bias during each stance phase using the accelerometers tilting capabilities, but this was not feasible in faster walking speeds due to the shorter stance phase. Also exploiting the gait periodicity to bound errors, Sabatini et al. (2005) studied velocity and displacement quantities obtained through a strap-down integration method between detected gait events and known initial conditions of speed and displacement. Estimated treadmill speed and inclination was estimated with good accuracy, although the displacement error was not verified against a video-based device (Lai et al., 2008).

In this chapter, we investigate the effectiveness of static filtering methods for reducing the errors obtained from inertial sensor integration to obtain limb displacements. The application of interest is in measuring foot motion or more precisely minimum toe clearance (MTC), which is the minimum vertical displacement during the mid-swing phase (Figure 1). This variable has been shown to be a sensitive predictor of tripping falls risk. Research in automated detection and diagnosis of those at risk of falling has been undertaken so that preventive measures can be developed to reduce trip-related falls. Automated detection systems based on signal processing and computational intelligence techniques, such as fuzzy logic (Hassan et al., 2006) and support vector machines (Begg et al., 2005), have demonstrated high accuracies at detecting the elderly susceptible to tripping. However, most data has been based on measurements made in a gait laboratory where gait studies may potentially induce controlled walking environments not truly indicative of tripping gait in the natural environment.

In the next section, an investigation on the sensor errors is undertaken in the frequency domain. It is hypothesized that comparing the motion power spectra from the sensors and video-based devices, namely the Optotrak NDI, would provide clues to the location of sensor errors in the frequency domain and allowing more targeted static filtering methods to be applied.

SPECTRAL INVESTIGATIONS OF INERTIAL SENSOR DATA

Analysing the sensor errors and limitations from the fundamental view and its internal mechanisms, it was hypothesized that a large part of the sensor errors arise from low frequency bias drifts, as the

Figure 1. Gait swing phase showing the Minimum Toe Clearance.

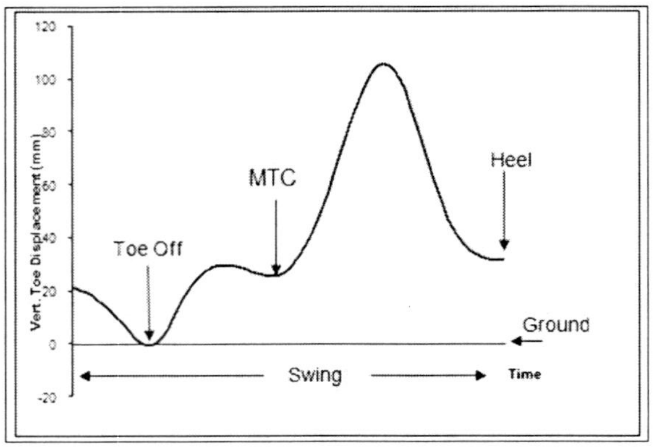

integration error rate increases at T^2 if double integrated, T being the period of integration. To investigate the effect of sensor errors on the frequency components in motion measurements, the Fast Fourier Transform (FFT) was employed to analyze the accelerometer and gyroscope raw signals, vertical acceleration, speed and displacement. The main assumption was that the spectra obtained from video data would contain high frequency noise due to differentiation, but provide a very accurate representation of low frequency information in which motion occurs.

Experimental Methods

The inertial sensors used were available on a single chip implementation known as the IMU 5DOF from Sparkfun. The IMU consisted of a Sparkfun breakout board containing the inertial sensors IDG300 and ADXL330. The board included low-pass filtered accelerometer outputs with passband at 500Hz. The ADXL330 is a polysilicon surface micro-machined sensor capable of measuring ±3g with a ratiometric sensitivity of 330mV/g, 1.65V of DC offset at 3.3V of voltage reference. The dual axis gyroscope (IDG300) was an integrated x- and y-axis gyroscope also with integrated low-pass output filters at 140Hz, sensitivity of 2mv/°/s and required a 3V minimum supply source. A

Figure 2. Prototype with inertial sensors and Optotrak markers

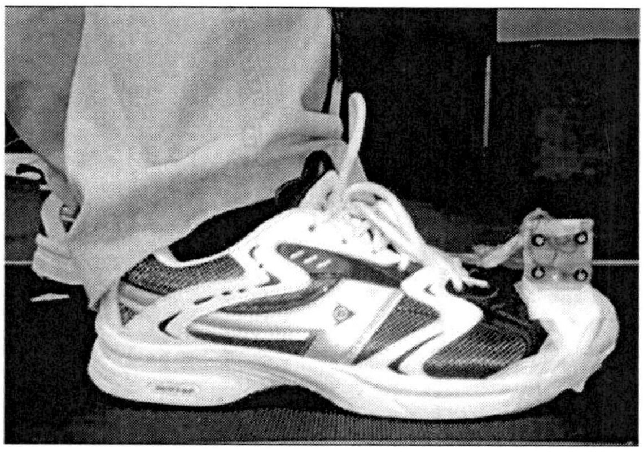

DAQ-Board from National Instruments was employed, containing 16 analog inputs (maximum 250 Ksamples/s) and 4 digital inputs and outputs. The board is USB Bus-powered and has driver compatibility with Labview. The sensors were placed on the toe with the Optotrak markers as described in Figure 2.

The Graphical-User-Interface(GUI) was programmed in Labview 8.0, where sensor data collection was monitored. The DAQ-Board provides limited memory (256kbytes), where the samples are stored before the USB transmission and processed by the Labview interface on the laptop. During this transmission, no further data is recorded, making necessary the measurement of larger windows by the recording loop in Labview to achieve more continuous data. Thus, the interface shows the collection and monitoring of signals in windows of 10 seconds at 1Khz yielding 10Ksamples/window. The Optotrak system was set to 500Hz sampling rate which was the maximum rate for each marker. The sensor outputs were sampled at 1Khz before being down-sampled to 500Hz.

Experiments were performed on five healthy subjects with no record of gait impairments. The subjects were made to walk on a treadmill for 30 seconds at 3 separate speeds, namely 2.5, 3.5 and 4.5km/h so that an average of 30 gait cycles could be collected. Sensor data and video data were manually synchronized, allowing 10 seconds of static position for off-line data synchronization and gyroscope bias estimation.

Data Processing for Optical Motion Measurement System

Although gait motion is considered a low-frequency activity, it was assumed that the variation of walking speeds and inter-subject walking styles would not match singularly a fixed pass-band in the frequency domain. It has also not been reported in the literature that high frequency components with low power contribute to the overall main reconstruction of the gait signal using sensors through the Direct-Cosine-Matrix (DCM). Therefore, the IMU raw signals were initially not filtered, to investigate this question during the comparison against the 'gold standard' signals provided by the Optotrak device. Hence, for each walking speed, three resultant vertical accelerations of the toe were calculated as:

1. Acceleration by double differentiation of Optotrak toe clearance;
2. Unfiltered IMU acceleration calculated using the rotation matrices and without drift correcting;
3. Acceleration using Sabatini's technique (Sabatini et. al., 2005)

This was followed by the spectral analysis using the Fast Fourier Transform (FFT) functions from the Matlab *Signal Processing Toolbox.*

The Optotrak vertical trajectories were differentiated twice to obtain the respective accelerations. Let s_{op}, v_{op} and a_{op} be the Optotrak measurements of vertical toe displacement, velocity and acceleration respectively, for $k = 1, 2, \ldots, N$, N being the total number of digital samples, and sampling frequency f_s(Hz) then:

$$v_{op}(k+1) = f_s\,[s_{op}(k+1) - s_{op}(k)]$$

Figure 3. Orientation of medio-lateral and sagittal planes on top; accelerometer's response to tilt on the sagittal (left bottom) and medio-lateral (right bottom)

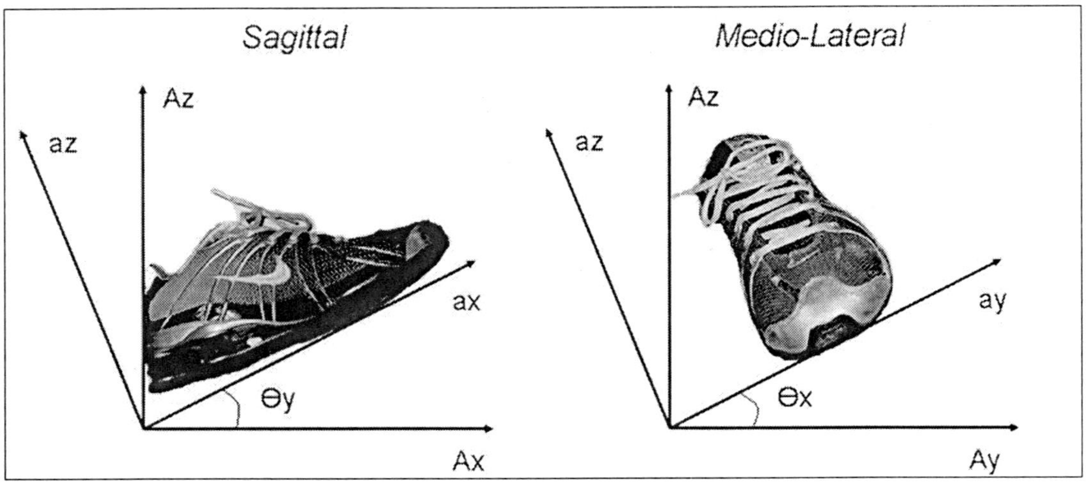

$a_{op}(k+1) = f_s\,[v_{op}(k+1) - v_{op}(k)]$

Filtering has been previously reported as a satisfactory method for smoothing noisy-differentiated signals, especially as the human gait is predominantly a low frequency activity (Shukla et al., 1985, Begg et. al., 2007). Therefore, high frequency noise due to the Optotrak signal differentiation is removed from the gait motion of a_{op} by a qth order low-pass filter. The type and cut-off frequency of the filter is decided upon the level of experimental differentiation noise in the signals.

Data Processing for Inertial Sensor System

The sensor data processing scheme initially converted IMU readings units into engineering units and then projected upon the earth's coordinate frame to obtain the vertical acceleration through the use of rotation matrices (Figure 3). The rotation matrices R_x (medio-lateral rotation) and R_y (sagittal rotation) were used to calculate the resultant acceleration a_{IMU} because the orientation of the sensors with respect to the earth's frame is the same. This is summarized in Figure 4:

a) w_x and w_y are not filtered (filter $H1$ is bypassed).
b) For k = 1,..., N, the gyroscope outputs are integrated to obtain 0_j according to:

$$\theta_j = \frac{1}{f_s^2}\left\{\sum_{k=2}^{N}(N-k)w_j(k)\right\} + \frac{1}{2f_s^2}(N-1)w_j \qquad (1)$$

c) a_{IMU} is not filtered (filter H2 is bypassed).
d) Obtain $a_{Global} = \{a_{Gx}, a_{Gy}, a_{Gz}\}$ from the sensor accelerations by:

$a_{Global} = R_x R_y a_{IMU}$

e) After subtracting the effect of gravity, a_R is analysed in the frequency domain by the FFT.
f) The strap-down method (Sabatini et. al., 2005) is implemented in parallel and the calculated acceleration spectra content is compared.

Figure 4. Block diagram depicting the computation of the power spectra of the vertical acceleration

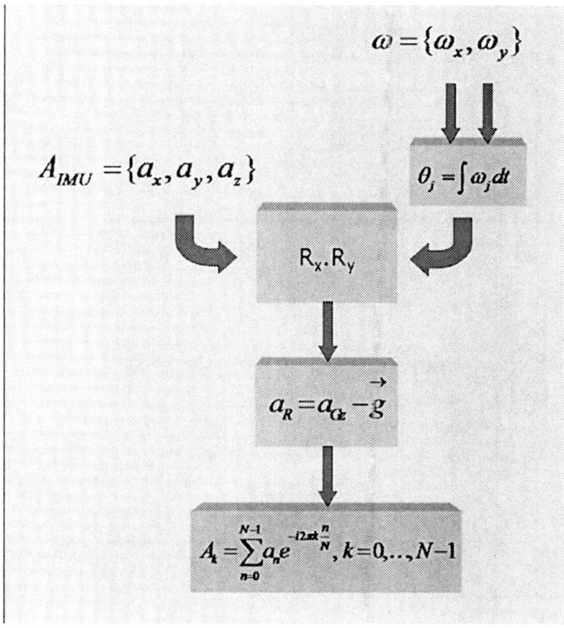

Experimental Results

A sample of the raw signal frequency content pertaining to the x- and y-axis of the gyroscope and x- and z-axis of the accelerometer from two subjects at the walking speed of 4.5km/h is depicted in Figure 5. Raw IMU accelerations (before the DCM transformation) were found to possess large DC components as expected, because of the intrinsic accelerometer response to gravity. The medio-lateral and sagittal angular speeds also showed DC components in subject A of 8.9×10^5 and 9.1×10^5 and in subject B of 1.9×10^4 and 3.5×10^5 respectively. However, for subject A the sensor signals frequencies were overall differently scattered than for subject B. For example, in the medio-lateral rotation (x-axis Gyroscope), the first three most significative harmonics were found at 1.9, 2.9 and 3.9Hz, whereas for subject B they were slightly shifted to 1.9, 3.0 and 3.9Hz. In addition, power was also differently distributed, as for example in the frontal acceleration (x-axis), where the 0.9Hz and the 1.0Hz harmonics showed 1.7×10^5 power and 1.1×10^5 for subject A and B respectively. Also, the power spectra envelope of the medio lateral angular speed was significantly smaller for subject A than for B as seen in Figure 5.

The Optotrak spectra of the vertical displacement and speed for subjects A and B is illustrated in Figure 6. In the displacement and speed, most significant harmonics were found at the same frequencies as in the raw signals from the sensors (1, 2,...,8Hz), but their power envelope was differently distributed between subject spectra. In addition, the power amplitude from the displacement was found to be an order lower in magnitude from the speed and a large bias in the Optotrak's displacement was observed for both subjects.

Figure 7 depicts a sample of differentiation noise from one subject's vertical acceleration from Optotrak in the time and frequency domain at the walking speed of 2.5km/h. The right column plot reveals approximately 20Hz a significant increase of noise with power amplitudes of approximately $500 m/s^2$ in the time domain, which is usually removed under the assumption that it does not contribute to the motion information. This value was found constant among all 5 subjects for the same speed and varied slightly as walking speed increased. Based on these observations, the cut-off frequency of a 4th order Butterworth low-pass filter was set to 20Hz.

The resultant accelerations respectively derived from the filtered Optotrak signal, unfiltered IMU data and Sabatini's technique with drift correction, are depicted in Figure 8 for the first 5 seconds of each walking speed. It was found that the amplitude was larger at higher walking speeds for all subjects but no conclusive visual differences were apparent in the time domain.

The corresponding power spectra derived for the entire 30 seconds of recording for each walking speed is shown in Figure 9. The Optotrak spectra revealed that more than 90% of signal power was contained in the 1-8Hz frequency band for all three walking speeds. This overall trend was found to be similarly captured by the sensors as seen in both

Figure 5. Comparison of the raw signals FFT between two subjects

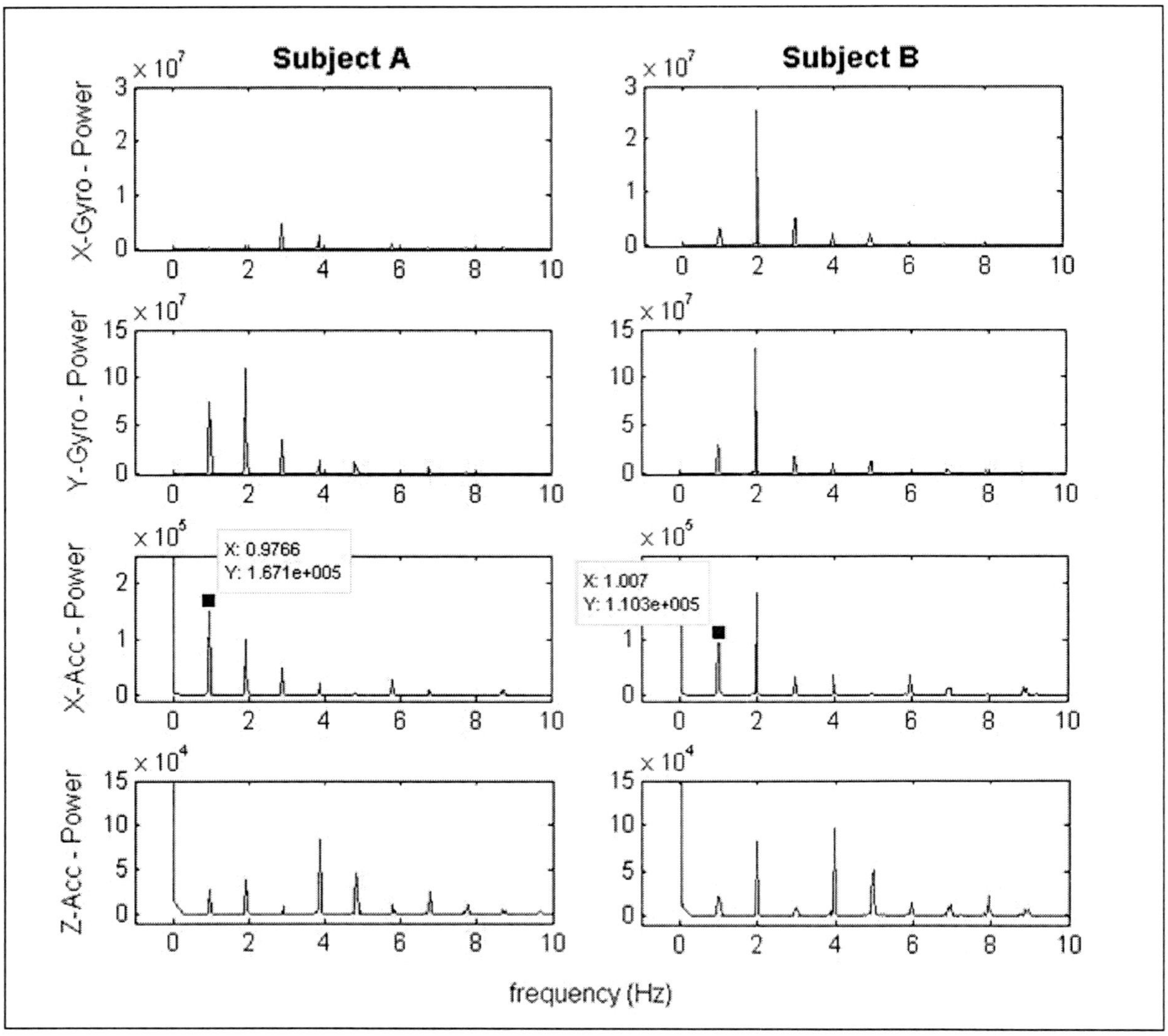

the unfiltered resultant acceleration from IMU data and the resultant acceleration computed using Sabatini's method. Several distinct differences in the power spectra envelope were found.

Firstly, the Optotrak acceleration was found to have zero DC component for all three speeds. In contrast, the unfiltered IMU acceleration was found to possess a large DC component of magnitude 2.9×10^5, 9.5×10^5 and 23×10^5 for walking speeds of 2.5, 3.5 and 4.5km/h respectively. Sabatini's technique reduced this DC component, but did not eliminate it completely where the attenuated DC components were 1.9×10^3, 30.9×10^3 and 49.7×10^3 respectively. Secondly, Sabatini's technique was observed to result in spectra with attenuated low frequency components (1-3Hz) as opposed to the Optotrak acceleration. The unfiltered IMU acceleration, however, had large peaks at these frequencies where, for example, the 3.5km/h speed possessed 6.3×10^4 and 6.2×10^4 peaks at the 1 and 2Hz frequencies, while the equivalent Optotrak peaks were only 1.8×10^3 and 11.3×10^3.

Figure 6. Comparison of the displacement and speed FFT of two subjects

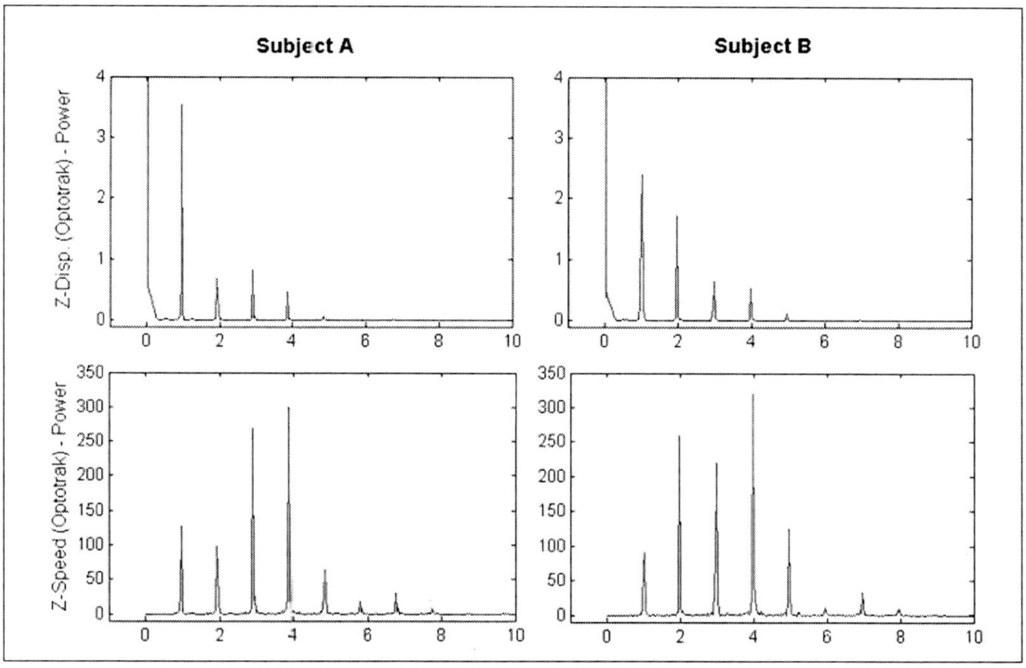

Figure 7. First column shows the unfiltered and low-pass filtered vertical acceleration at the treadmill speed of 2.5km/h; second column on top indicates the Optotrak vertical acceleration spectra and, at the bottom, its zoomed-in version over 0-50Hz

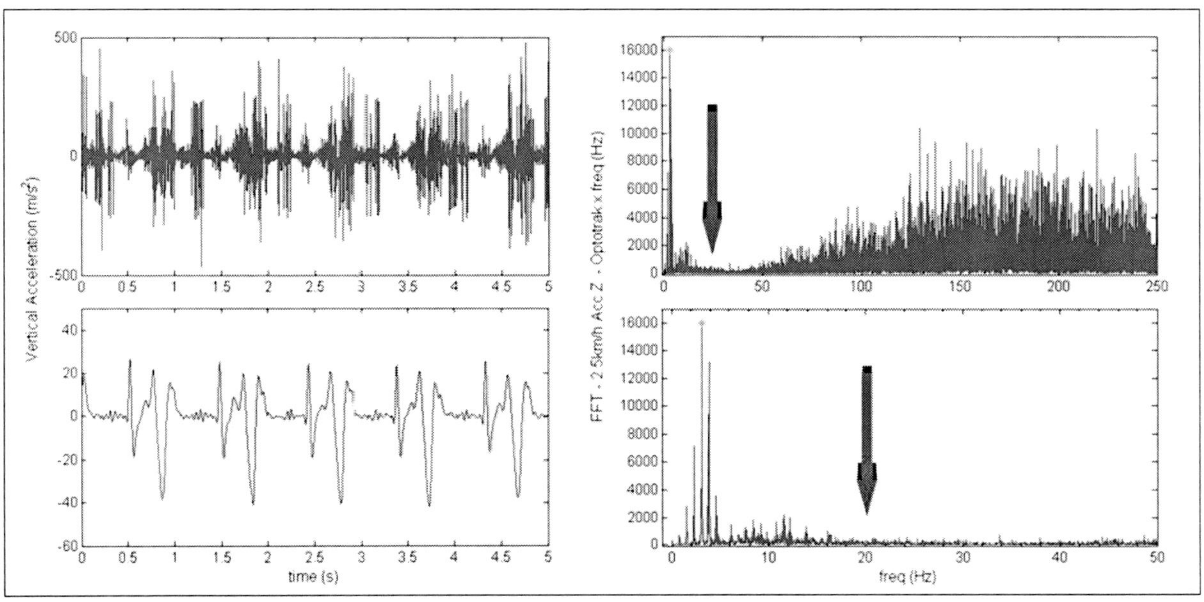

Figure 8. Left to Right: Graphs of resultant acceleration in Z direction derived from Optotrak, IMU data and the technique due to Sabatini et al. [6]. Top to Bottom: Treadmill speeds of 2.5, 3.5 and 4.5km/h

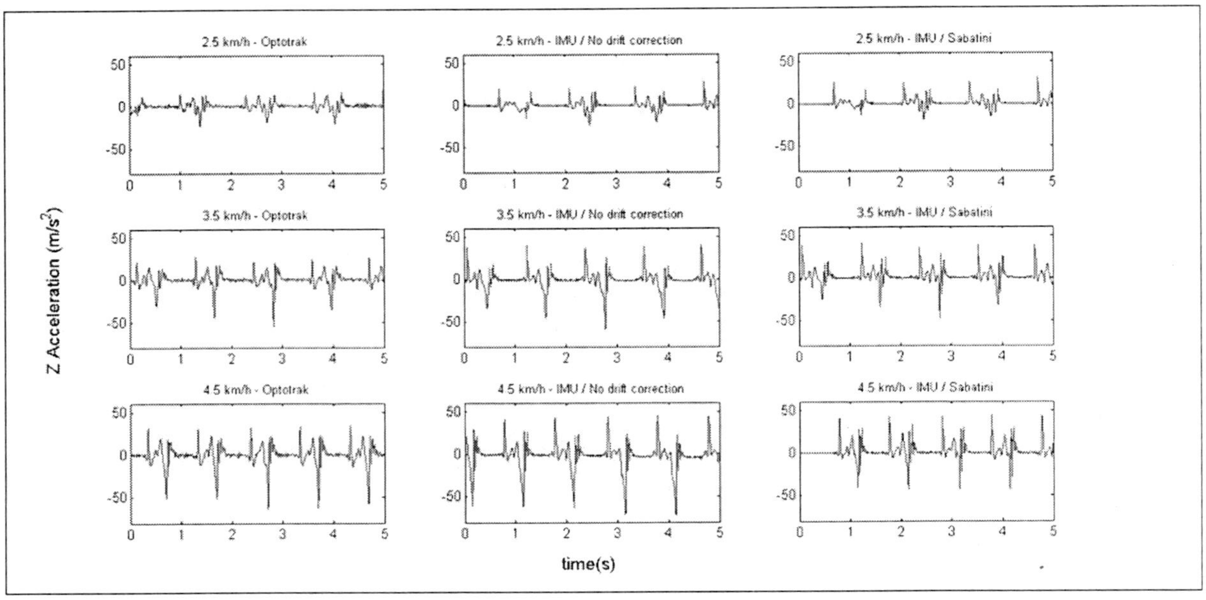

Figure 9. Spectral comparison obtained by the Optotrak, Unfiltered IMU signals and employing the Strap-Down method by Sabatini

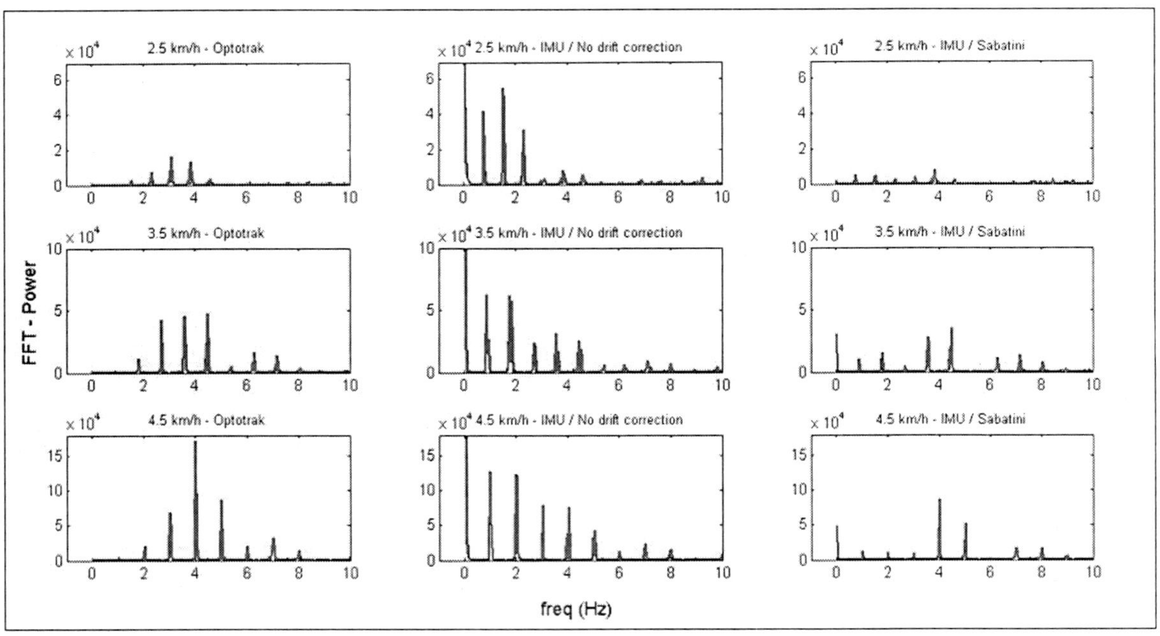

Figure 10. The left column shows the resultant IMU Z-acceleration after application of a bandpass filter (BPF) with passband of 1-20Hz, for the treadmill speeds of 2.5, 3.5 and 4.5km/h. The right column depicts the corresponding FFT power spectra

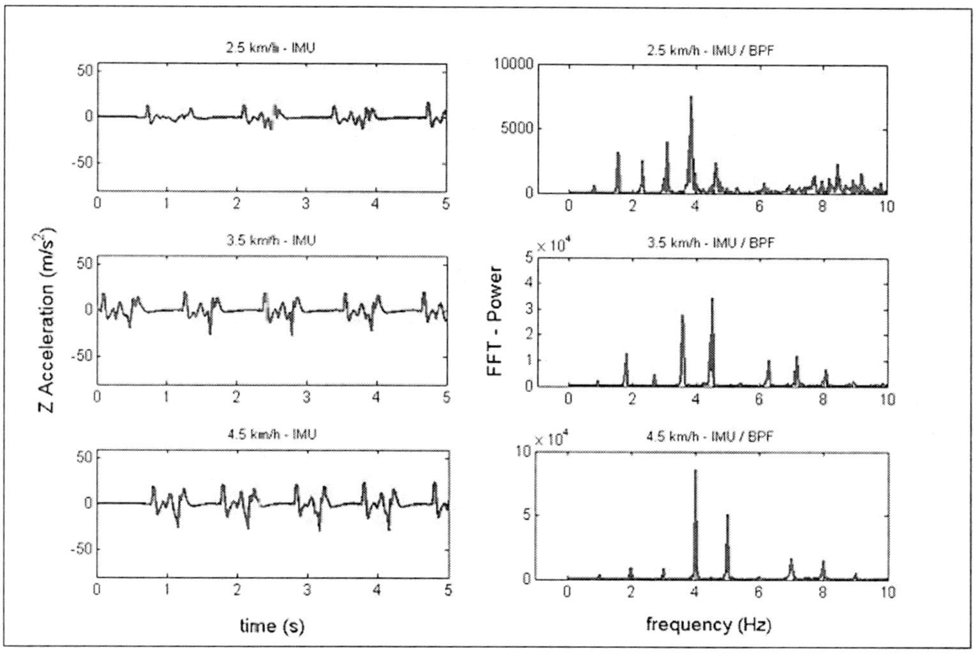

Given the revealed large bias from the unfiltered IMU case in the vertical acceleration, it was deemed to add an extra step in the experimental methodology to reduce this effect. The band-pass filter was investigated to reduce bias or 'couple' the AC components on a DC (or zero bias) (Summit Instruments, 2005, Pfau et. al., 2005). After this method was applied, the acceleration was then double integrated to achieve the displacement.

The unfiltered resultant acceleration from the IMU data for all subjects was then bandpass filtered based on the previous results, at all walking speeds with 1-20Hz passband (Butterworth and Order = 4) to remove the DC bias, as acceleration gait is predominantly a low-frequency activity (< 20Hz). In addition, this matched the higher passband specification from the derived acceleration of the Optotrak, with its 4th Butterworth filter and cut-off frequency of 20Hz. Figure 10 depicts the filtered acceleration signals and corresponding power spectra, which had some harmonics attenuated by the band-pass filter. Note now that the filtered IMU acceleration from this single subject has no DC component and the trend resembles the Optotrak trend for a single gait cycle.

Finally, the resultant acceleration obtained from the Optotrak, band-pass filtered IMU data and Sabatini's methods are compared in greater detail in the time domain for all subjects. Figure 11 shows at the walking speed of 2.5km/h that the simple technique of band-pass filtering (dashed line) provides an acceleration signal which shows higher correlation with the Optotrak acceleration (solid line) and smoother than Sabatini's technique (dotted line). Both filtered and Sabatini's acceleration appear phase shifted from the Optotrak acceleration due to the inherent phase shift of digital filters.

On the bottom, the speed processed by the band-pass filter more clearly resembles the one derived by the Optotrak as opposed to Sabatini's and finally, on the right plot, a comparison between

Figure 11. Comparison of Optotrak (solid line) measurement, Sabatini's method [22] (dotted line) and Band-Pass filtering (dashed line) in estimating vertical acceleration, speed and displacement

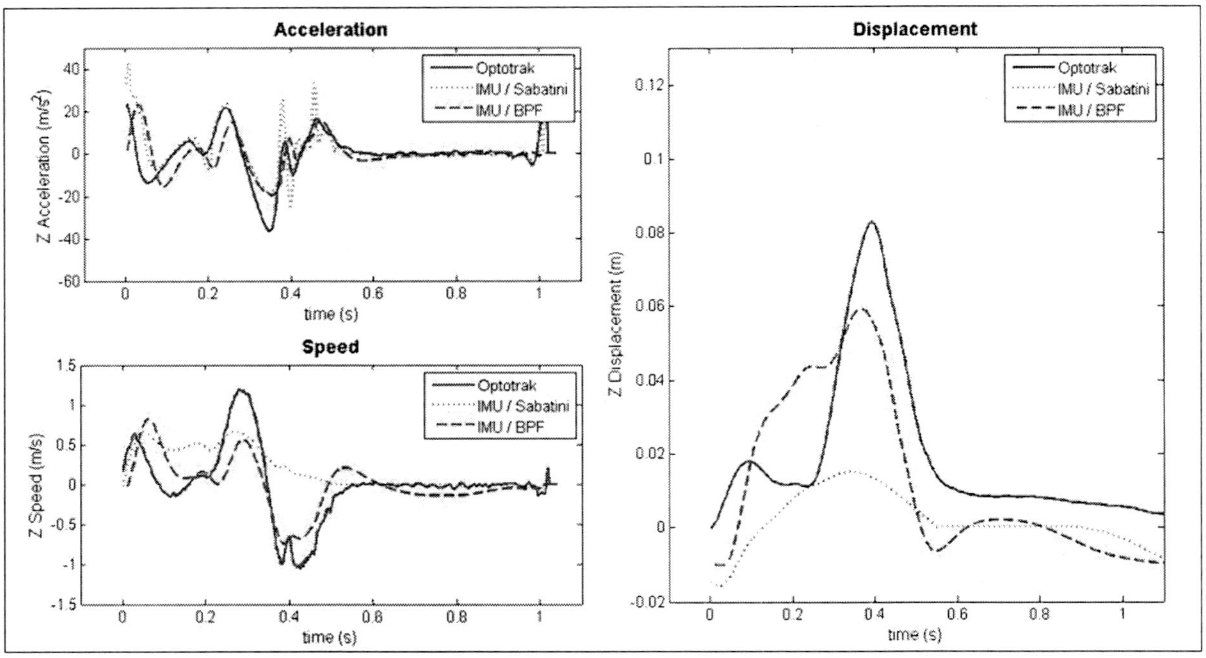

the derived toe clearance of the three techniques is shown. It can be seen that the displacement was greatly improved in comparison to Sabatini's method, where the amplitude of gait in the mid-swing phase (highest peak) is only 2cm off and in addition the toe clearance could be detected. The displacement was computed by double integration without observed drift after the band-pass filtering.

Discussion

In this section, the frequency content of the IMU vertical acceleration was analysed and frequency spectra of unfiltered raw IMU signals and the strap-down method were compared from the perspective of their Fourier Spectra. The spectral harmonics of the gyroscope and accelerometer raw signals, showed more power in the low frequency range for all subjects at each walking speed. Slight variances in the harmonics among the subjects were due to specific biomechanical dynamics of each subject. For example, taller subjects with longer lower limbs would need less strides to achieve the same speed than shorter subjects with smaller lower limbs. This could be translated in the frequency domain as a trade-off between higher frequency harmonics with lower power and vice-versa. In comparison against those from the Optotrak's displacement and inferred speed, the frequencies from raw signals matched, confirming that the IMU's dynamic response was suitable for this application. However, in terms of the harmonics power, the raw signals showed significant differences between subjects, suggesting the walking style and inter-subject features were sensitive to the IMU. For example, the medio-lateral motion had less contribution for subject A than for B. However, at this point, it is unclear how each significant harmonic of the accelerometer and gyroscope contributes to the resultant vertical acceleration.

Further analysis of the acceleration spectra obtained from Optotrak data revealed that it was similar to that obtained by Meng et al. (2006) for foot motion. This reinforces the method of using the Optotrak system and resulting spectra as a gold standard for comparison when performing experiments with the IMU sensors. The major finding in the previous analysis is that inertial sensors possessed a large DC bias as well as larger low frequency harmonics which are absent from Optotrak data. The hypothesis here is that these differences are mainly due to sensor measurement errors. This is reinforced further by the finding that the DC component was reduced in Sabatini's technique (Figure 9 right column) which in addition attenuated harmonics in the low frequency range. It is difficult to know for certain if the observation is due to the strap-down method or due to the approximation of the resultant vertical acceleration made by the linear correction algorithm.

We then proposed the application of a 4-th order Butterworth band-pass filter with a passband of 1- 20Hz to investigate the removal of this DC bias. The filtered resultant acceleration had zero DC bias (Figure 10) but suffered further attenuation in the low frequency region of 1 - 3Hz when compared to the Optotrak spectra. Comparisons of plots in Figure 9 show a substantial presence of low frequency signal information in the Optotrak data indicating movement information. The same peaks were larger in the unfiltered IMU acceleration providing evidence that a slow varying sensor error (low frequency signal) was present together with the low frequency movement information. This phenomenon could be mainly due to thermo-mechanical noise, temperature drift or impurities in sensor manufacturing; however, verification of these hypotheses entails more complex empirical investigations.

The existence of these low frequency sensor errors poses a difficult filtering task. Since the conjectured errors occur in the same frequency band, it is unknown how effective static filters will be at removing them, without losing motion information. For a fixed band pass filter, evidence of its effectiveness can be seen in Figure 11 where the estimated toe clearance resembled the Optotrak trend. The results indicate that bandpass filtering instead of lowpass filtering (Pappas et al., 2001, Sabatini et al., 2005) should be advocated as a first preprocessing step to remove a large source of sensor error. This should be applied before attempting more complex methods such as gait event detections and strap-down integration.

EVALUATING THE EFFECTIVENESS OF THE BAND-PASS FILTER

In the previous section, it was observed that inertial sensor measurements contained large differences in the lower frequency ranges compared to video data of the same motion (Lai et. al., 2008). These results suggested that a major portion of sensor errors resides in the low frequency region while sensor datasheets suggest the presence of gaussian noise in all frequency bands. We hypothesize that a majority of these errors could be removed by band pass filtering. Limited studies have applied band-filtering to monitoring trunk motion in a horse (Pfau et. al., 2006), however, to our knowledge, no thorough experiments have been reported on the effectiveness of band-pass filtering to remove sensor errors for human gait measurements.

The aim of this section is to investigate the effectiveness of band-pass filtering on the vertical toe acceleration and displacement. The FFT will be used as a spectral analysis technique to motivate our selection of passband frequencies, order and type of the filters by using the correlation coefficient ρ between the acceleration spectras, over a range of 4 different walking speeds from sensor and video data from the Optotrak NDI Certus system. Taking the latter as an accurate measurement of the motion, the Normalized Root Mean Squared Error (RMSE) of acceleration and displacement signals are used to assess the practical accuracy of the filters for improving displacement measurements calculated from inertial sensors from a group of healthy subjects.

Hardware and Software

The system setup is the same used as in the last section. A DAQ-Board digitized the inertial sensors (ADXL330 and IDG300) analog signals through a wired link and the data was visualized and stored for off-line processing using the interface programmed in Labview 8.0. The sensors were mounted at the distal end of the shoe together with a rigid body containing 4 Optotrak markers and a virtual point corresponding to the center of the IMU was positioned. Signals from the Optotrak and IMU were sampled at 500Hz and the recordings were manually triggered simultaneously.

Video Data Processing

The Optotrak vertical trajectories were differentiated twice to obtain the respective accelerations. Let S_{op}, V_{op}, and a_{op} be the Optotrak measurements of vertical toe displacement, velocity and acceleration respectively, for $k = 1, 2, \ldots, N$, N being the total number of digital samples, and sampling frequency f_s (Hz) then:

$$V_{op}(k+1) = f_s\,[S_{op}(k+1) - S_{op}(k)]$$

$$a_{op}(k+1) = f_s\,[V_{op}(k+1) - V_{op}(k)]$$

As previously described in Figure 7, differentiation noise was smoothed a_{op} by a qth order low-pass filter, as gait is predominantly a low frequency activity. The type and cut-off frequency of the filter is decided upon by the level of experimental noise differentiation in the signals.

Sensor Data Processing

The sensor data processing scheme follows section 1.2.3, where initially the IMU readings units were first converted to engineering units and then projected upon the earth's coordinate frame to obtain the vertical acceleration through the use of rotation matrices (Figure 3). The angles of the rotation matrices $\mathbf{R}_x$ (medio-lateral rotation) and $\mathbf{R}_y$ (sagittal rotation) were band-pass filtered to remove DC bias and avoid integration drift. The signal processing flow is described in Figure 12 as:

a) Filter ω_x and ω_y with a qth-order bandpass digital filter H1 and passband $[fH1_L, fH1_H]$.
b) For $k = 1, \ldots, N$, the filtered gyroscope outputs are integrated to obtain θ_j according to:

$$\theta_j = \frac{1}{f_s^2}\left\{\sum_{k=2}^{N}(N-k)w_j(k)\right\} + \frac{1}{2f_s^2}(N-1)w_j \quad (1)$$

where ω_j is the angular velocity about a particular axis of choice.

c) Filter $\mathbf{a}_{IMU}$ using a qth-order low-pass filter with $H2$ and cut-off frequency $fH2_L$.
d) Obtain $\mathbf{a}_{IMU} = \{a_{Gx}, a_{Gy}, a_{Gz}\}$ from the sensor accelerations by:

$$\mathbf{a}_{Global} = \mathbf{R}_x \mathbf{R}_y \mathbf{a}_{IMU}$$

e) As we are interested in the vertical acceleration and displacement, after subtracting the effect of gravity, it is filtered with a qth-order bandpass digital filter with $H3$ and passband $[fH3_L, fH3_H]$ to obtain IMU measurements of the vertical toe acceleration a_R.

Under the assumption that differentiation noise from the video-device could reduce the ineffectiveness of the spectra correlation, the BPF's $fH3_H$ was chosen to match the low-pass filter's cut-off frequency from the Optotrak's acceleration, to provide equivalent spectral conditions for comparisons. In addition, the root mean square error (RMSE) and normalized RMSE (NRMSE) between the Optotrak and sensors were calculated. These values would be affected by the phase effect caused by the digital filters, however, phase was considered less significant in our case, because

Figure 12. Sensor signal processing flow chart; R_x and R_y represent the rotation matrices

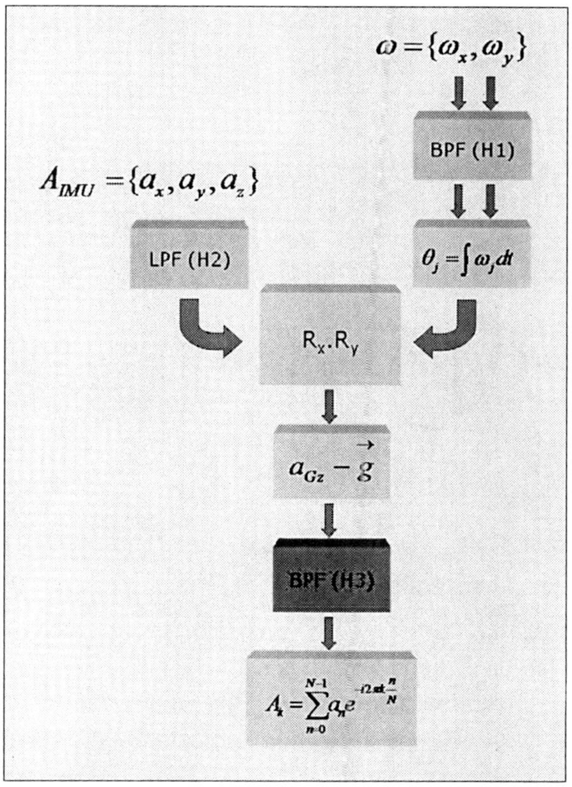

both signals were manually synchronized using the static motion phases and filtered in the forward and backwards direction to minimize any phase effects. As such the RMSE and NRMSE are normally defined as:

$$RMSE(A_{IMU}, A_{OP}) = \sqrt{\frac{\sum_{i=1}^{N}(A_{IMU}(i) - A_{Op})(i)^2}{N}}$$

$$NRMSE(A_{IMU}, A_{OP}) = \frac{RMSE(A_{IMU}, A_{OP})}{(A_{OpMAX} - A_{OpMI}}$$

where A_{IMU} and A_{Op} represent the vertical toe acceleration calculated from IMU data and video data respectively and A_{OpMAX} and A_{OpMIN} correspond to the maximum and minimum Optotrak acceleration values found in each experimental trial. Also, the displacement RMSE is calculated for all gait cycles over the complete motion (RMSE 1) and only from the toe-off time and maximum peak (RMSE 2) during the swing phase of the recorded data for all trials.

Experiment Methodology

As the filters $H1$, $H2$ and $H3$ influence the resultant vertical toe acceleration a_R, they were compared against the baseline condition (no filtering) and the strap-down integration method (Sabatini et. al., 2005). In all experimental conditions, $H1$, $H2$ and $H3$ were the same filter type, (i.e. homogenous filter system). The filter parameters were varied according to the following experiments:

- **H1 and H2 filter type effect:** Two filter types were tested, namely the Butterworth and Ellipic. In each case, $H3$ was fixed with parameters: order = 4, $f\,H3_L$ = 0.7Hz, $f\,H3_H$ = 35Hz. $H1$ was fixed with $f\,H1_L$ = 0.1Hz. $f\,H3_H$ is the same value as the lower-cut off frequency of the video differentiated displacement (Subsection 1.4.2) while $f\,H1_L$ = 0.1Hz was empirically found to be the highest effective cut-off frequency, i.e., lower values did not alter the results further. $f\,H1_H$ and $f\,H2_L$ were then varied monotonically from 8Hz to 50Hz in steps of 1Hz.
- **H1 and H2 filter order effect:** Three filter orders were tested q = 2, 4 and 6. In each case, $H3$ was fixed with parameters: $f\,H3_L$ = 0.7Hz and $f\,H3_H$ was chosen upon the frequency analysis of the acceleration. $H1$ was fixed with $f\,H1_L$ = 0.1Hz. $f\,H1_H$ and $f\,H2_L$ were varied from 8Hz to 50Hz in steps of 1Hz.
- **H3 effect:** Filter parameters were fixed with $f\,H1_L$ = 0.1Hz and $f\,H3_H$ was chosen upon the frequency analysis of the acceleration. $f\,H1_H$ and $f\,H2_L$ were set to the average cut-off frequencies $\{f\,H1_H, f\,H2_L\}$ which produced the highest ρ for all subjects in the previous section. The cut-off frequency $f\,H3_L$ for Butterworth and

Figure 13. First and second columns show contours over different accelerometer and gyroscope cut-off frequencies for a 4th-order Elliptic and Butterworth filter obtained by subject 1 respectively; rows indicate the walking speeds of 2.5km/h and 5.5km/h

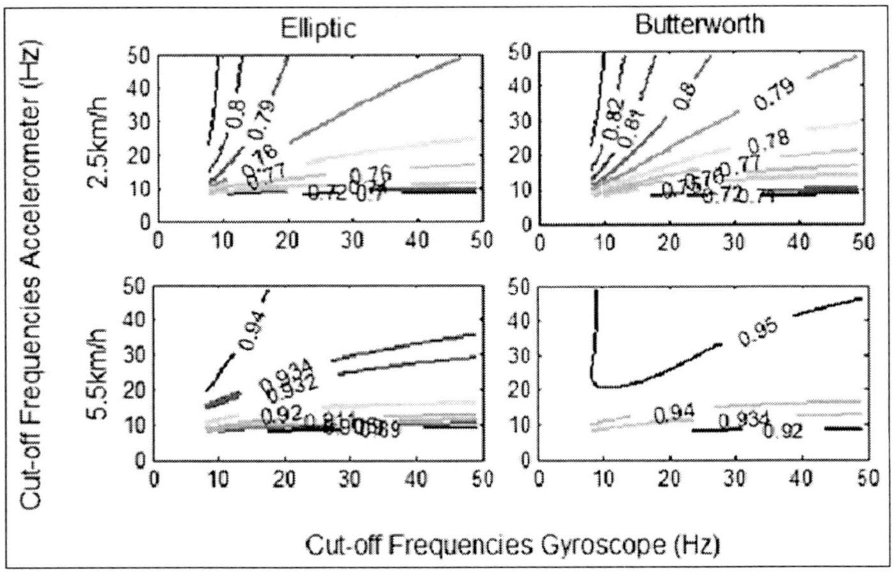

Elliptic filter was varied in steps of 0.1Hz from 0.1Hz to 4.5Hz.

- **Subject Trial Protocol:** Five healthy adults participated in experimental trials. The experiments were carried out over 4 different walking speeds of 2.5km/h, 3.5km/h, 4.5km/h and 5.5km/h. The position of the IMU was determined in 10 seconds before each trial, so that the gyroscope bias could be estimated. Subjects were then allowed to walk for 30 seconds so that at least 30 gait cycles could be obtained.

Experimental Results

- **The effect of differentiation noise:**Figure 7 depicted a sample of differentiation noise from one subject's vertical acceleration in the time and frequency domain at the walking speed 2.5km/h. In this case, the differentiation noise is removed with a cut-off frequency of 35Hz under the assumption that higher frequencies do not contribute motion information. This value was found constant among all 5 subjects for the same speeds a were 1.42Hz, 1.82Hz, 1.92Hz and 2.06Hz given the 4 walking speeds (WS) with best linear fit of $fH3_L = 0.202 \times WS + 0.997$, $R^2 = 0.9$ (R = correlation coefficient). As for the elliptic case, they were 2.16Hz, 2.66Hz, 2.84Hz and 3.32Hz with $fH3_L = 0.366 \times WS + 1.281$, $R^2 = 0.972$.
- Figure 14 depicts the power spectra of Optotrak on the left column and the spectra of the IMU signals from a single subject using the cut-off frequencies corresponding to the highest correlation at walking speeds 2.5, 3.5 and 4.5km/h and using the optimized parameters for $H1$, $H2$ and $H3$. At 2.5km/h the Optotrak and the IMU had maximum peaks of 1.6×10^4 and 1.25×10^4 at 3.3Hz respectively. This increased to 4.8×10^4 and 4×10^4 centred around 4.1Hz for 3.5km/h and achieved 17.5×10^4 and 14.1×10^4 at around 4Hz for the walking speed of 4.5km/h.

Figure 14. Accelerations power spectra from Optotrak and the IMU with optimized H1, H2 and H3 filter parameters

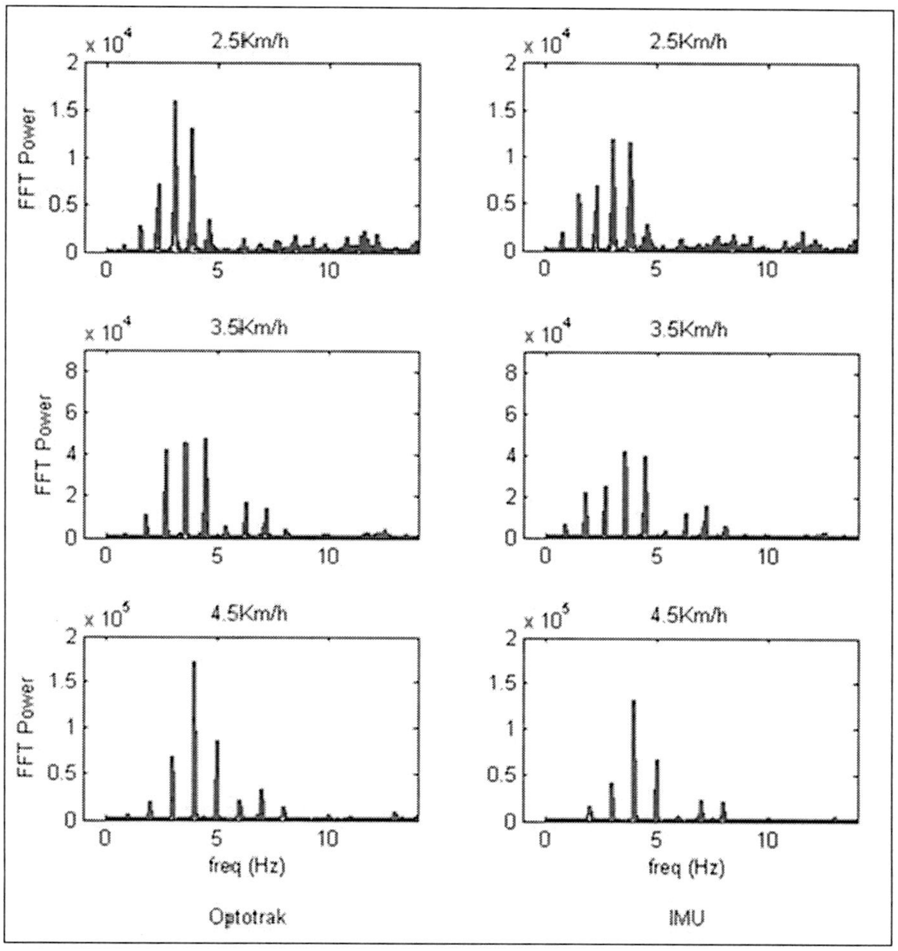

- **The effect of Medio Lateral contribution:**Figure 19 depicts 6 isoline plots of cross correlation coefficients as filter cut-off frequencies were varied for the raw accelerometer and gyroscope signals on the *x*-axis and the *y*-axis respectively. Rows indicate walking speeds of 2.5, 3.5 and 4.5km/h and the columns indicate the effect of the medio-lateral plane to the correlation of the acceleration. At 2.5km/h the highest isoline achieved was 0.6 on the left column and 0.2 on the right, which considerably increased to 0.8 and 0.65 respectively for 3.5km/h and to 0.95 for 4.5km/h in both cases. In the left column, the cut-off frequencies range for the highest isoline remains approximately constant over $fH3_H$ = 8-27Hz and at 2.5km/h the minimum $fH2_L$ reached 35Hz, whereas for 3.5km/h it reached 25Hz and finally, at 4.5km/h, 15Hz was the lowest value. For the right column, $fH2_L$ s range is approximately the same as on the left column; however, $fH3_H$ s range was reduced to 8-15Hz. The isolines reveal that, at each walking speed, the cross correlation was significantly higher when acceleration in the medio-lateral plane was included. This can be observed, for ex-

Figure 15. Comparison of vertical displacement RMSE 1 and RMSE 2 Errors at four walking speeds for 5 healthy subjects (S1, S2, S3, S4 and S5)

Speed (km/h)	RMSE1 (S1)	RMSE2 (S1)	RMSE1 (S2)	RMSE2 (S2)
2.5	3.06	7.19	3.86	5.34
3.5	3.11	7.41	4.69	8.91
4.5	3.54	2.71	3.83	8.19
5.5	2.96	3.55	3.56	7.23

Speed (km/h)	RMSE1 (S3)	RMSE2 (S3)	RMSE1 (S4)	RMSE2 (S4)
2.5	4.07	8.79	4.12	4.56
3.5	6.29	6.78	3.72	5.72
4.5	5.34	3.21	3.19	3.99
5.5	3.98	2.98	3.06	2.99

Speed (km/h)	RMSE1 (S5)	RMSE2 (S5)
2.5	7.12	7.01
3.5	4.30	5.87
4.5	3.33	4.12
5.5	4.01	4.22

ample, at 4.5km/h, where the area included by the isoline of 0.95 is significantly larger with the medio-lateral plane contribution than without it.

- **Comparison of Acceleration FFT spectra:** The Normalized RMSE is compared using the optimal filter parameters against the unfiltered case (*H*1, *H*2 and *H*3 absent) and the strap-down method (Sabatini et al., 2005). Figure 20 shows the normalized RMSE of acceleration of 5 subjects. Errors were reduced by up to 57.5% compared to the no filtering case and up to 18% against the Strap-down method among all subjects. The overall trend revealed higher normalized errors for slower walking speeds in the three methods and lower at the fastest of 5.5km/h. The inter-subject variability of the errors reached up to 15%, between 0.1 and 0.25, considering all walking speeds.
- **Comparison of the final foot displacement:**Figure 15 shows RMSE 1 and RMSE 2 in centimetres for the highest cross-correlation coefficients using the optimized parameters for 5 subjects. In general the overall trend was lower errors for higher walking speeds, where the highest was 8.91cm and the smallest 2.71cm. The displacement achieved at 5.5km/h for 2 subjects with the optimized cut-off frequencies of highest cross correlation is depicted in Figure 21. The plot on the right shows that the displacement was greatly improved in comparison to Figure 11 and the MTC event was clearly detected. However, the highest mid-swing peak was still lower against the Optotrak measurement and the ripple in the beginning of the stance phase was significant.

CHAPTER DISCUSSION

In this chapter, the use of static filters as a preprocessing method for reducing sensor errors in inertial sensor measurements was investigated

Figure 16. Normalized RMSE of vertical toe acceleration over different speeds with different methods for each subject

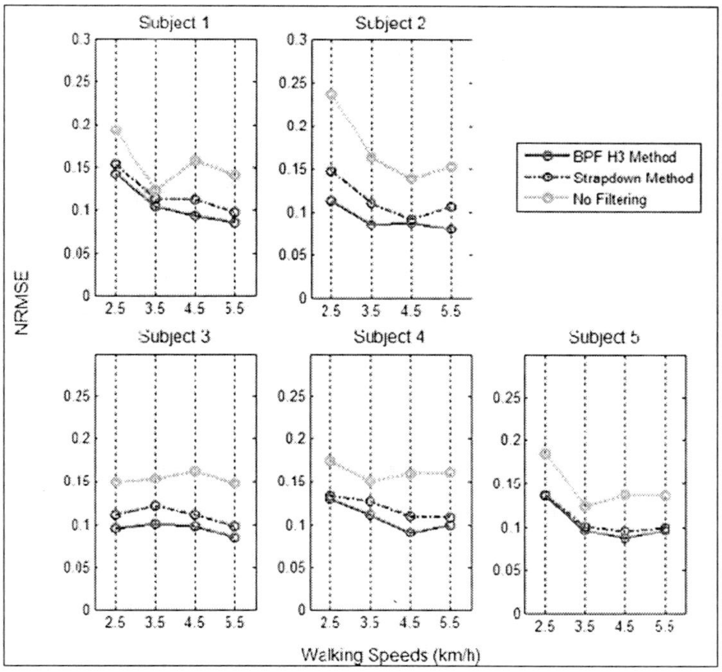

for gait analysis. The major results (Figure 20) showed up to 57.5% error reduction in vertical toe acceleration compared to the unfiltered case and 18% against the current popular strap-down method. For all subjects, errors were reduced consistently in all walking speeds, revealing a trend of smaller errors at faster walking speeds (Figure 16). This confirms our conjecture that the majority of sensor errors were slow time-varying bias drifts and these errors were superimposed on slower gait activity making the final filtering (*H*3 BPF) more difficult.

The Butterworth filter demonstrated better performance than the Elliptic (Figure 14), providing further evidence that the low frequency sensor errors were superimposed on the gait motion. The steep attenuation characteristics of the Elliptic filter meant that the frequency bands, where superposition occurred, were almost completely filtered out. The Butterworth response was less steep and averaged the frequencies in the superposition region. The better performance of the Butterworth configuration implies that the sensor errors superimposed at varying degrees in the frequency band. Figure 17 provides evidence that the errors were confined mostly to the lower frequency region, where the optimal Elliptic frequency cutoffs, $f\mathrm{H3}_{\mathrm{H}}$ were consistently higher than the Butterworth ones at each speed. At 5.5km/h (Figure 14) both trends achieved approximately the same ρ, indicating the high-frequency cutoff had minimal influence on the errors at this point. Furthermore, the average $f\mathrm{H3}_{\mathrm{H}}$ increased approximately linearly with walking speed, reinforcing the hypothesis that significant inertial sensor errors were mostly confined to the lower frequency spectrum.

In the frequency domain, different walking styles played a significant role for static filter specification at slower speeds. Note that the highest standard deviation of ρ at 2.5km/h on the left plot of Figure 16 and the lowest one at 5.5km/h. This was similarly observed in Figure 17, where the variation of ρ among subjects over [0.1-1.5]

Figure 17. Plots of the maximum ρ (bold circle) as a function of $f\,H3_L$ (Hz) given 5 subjects; first and second rows indicate the Butterworth and Elliptic filters respectively with $f\,H2_L$ = 49Hz, $f\,H1_H$ = 12Hz with q = 4

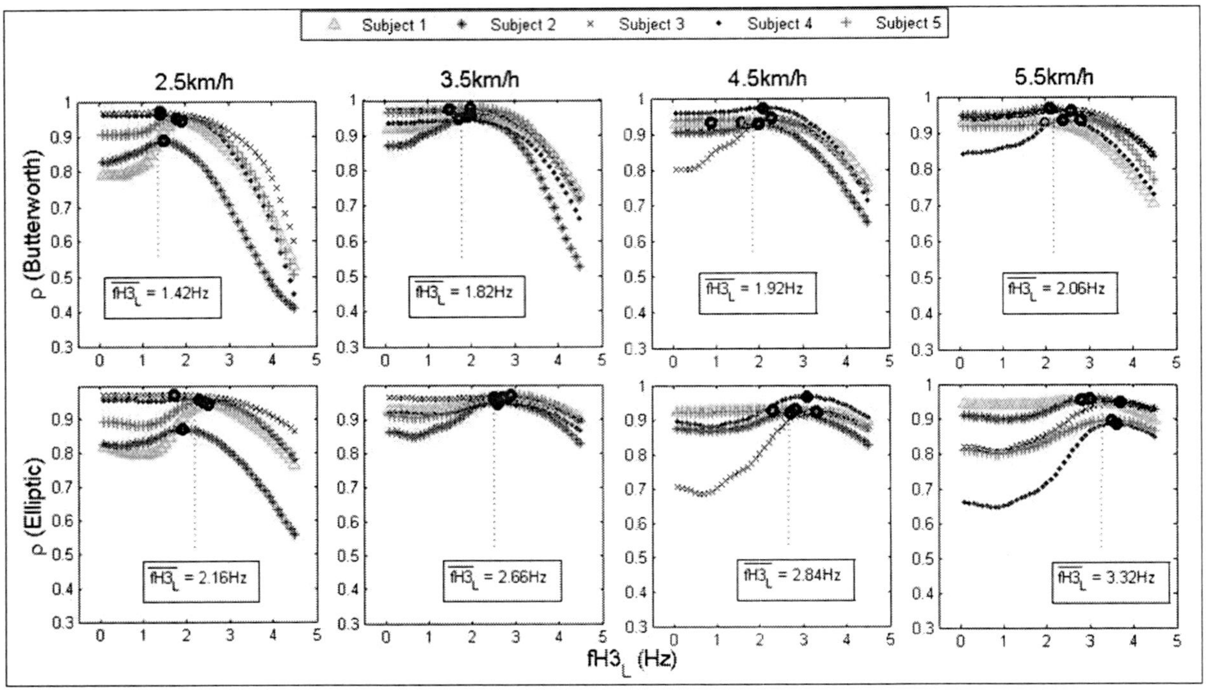

Hz at 2.5km/h, for example, suggested different noise levels in that band. However, the optimal filter parameters (highest ρ) were found to linearly cluster at each speed around a common range for all 5 subjects, which subsequently decreased for higher $fH3_H$, indicating the limit of high-pass filtering which increasing attenuates important motion information.

Most literature on inertial sensors tend to overlook the filtering of raw sensor data, focusing mainly on low-pass filtering noise attributed to high frequency electrical noise. This has been successful since most high frequency noise is well separated from frequencies of the gait activity. However, as the band-pass filter H3 used $f\,H3_H$ = 35Hz applied on the vertical acceleration and Figure 14 on the middle plot revealed the highest ρ at $f\,H2_L$ = 49Hz, higher motion frequencies captured by the accelerometer can be hypothetically important for the slower harmonics of the vertical acceleration a_z, independently whether they contain WGN in the same band. This suggests a necessary sampling frequency of at least 98Hz (Nyquist frequency). Lower values of $f\,H3_H$ showed opposite behaviour for the gyroscope. This implies that the rotation matrices also play an important role in sensor noise when they are used to translate the IMU data from local coordinates to the laboratory coordinate system i.e., obtain the vertical accelerations $\mathbf{a}_{Global} = \mathbf{R}_x\mathbf{R}_y\mathbf{a}_{IMU}$, for comparison against the optical motion measurement system, in this case the Optotrak.

The empirical results demonstrated that the acceleration contribution of the medio-lateral plane was significant as depicted by the cross correlation of the acceleration power spectra. A comparison of the two columns of Figure 19 shows that the combination of medio-lateral acceleration plays a more significant contribution to the resultant vertical acceleration during slower

Figure 19. Cross correlation difference with and without the medio-lateral rotation contribution in one subject's gait

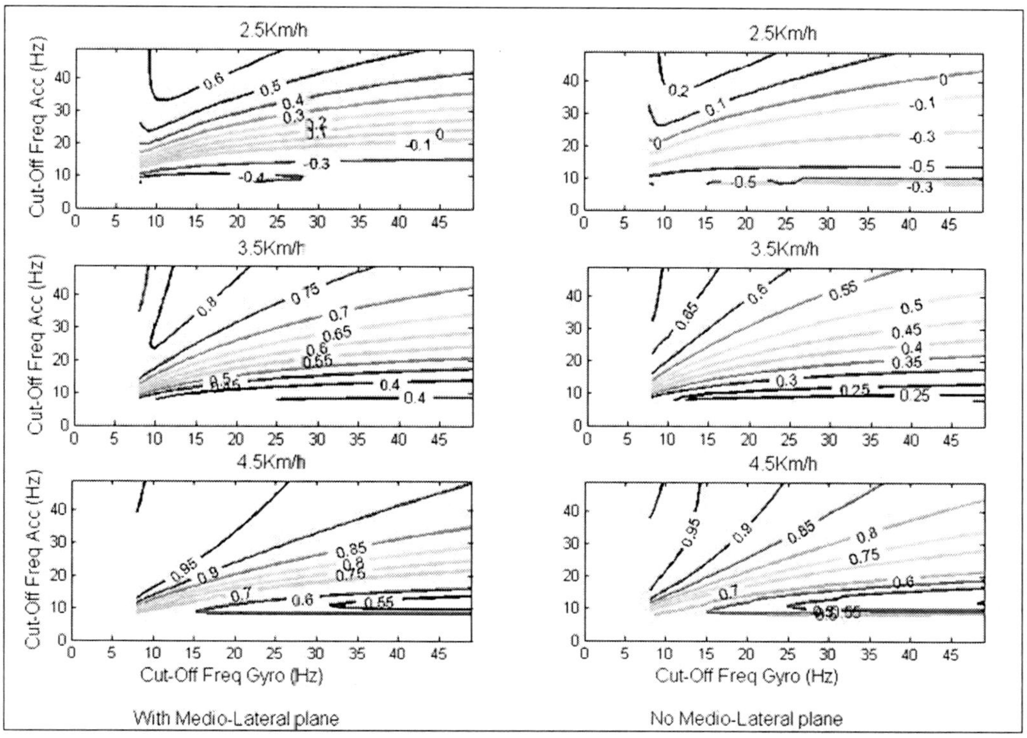

walking speeds. However, the medio-lateral toe rotation during strides becomes less significant at faster speeds indicating that more forward control is exerted on the foot during fast walking. This finding also suggests that the validity of assumption by Sabatini et al. (2005) is dependent on the speed of the walking activity.

The results in Table 1 indicate that band pass filtering is better applied to faster motion, in this case during the swing phase of the gait cycle, (i.e., from toe off to maximum displacement). Figure 21 depicts better displacement reconstruction in this phase than in the stance phase (less motion) where a large ripple in IMU measured displacement is observed as opposed to the stance phase measured by the Optotrak. The hypothesis is that the band-pass filter removes motion frequencies below the lower cut-off, causing a ripple due to the averaging effect of the recursive filter. This effect can be improved in the future by using adaptive filtering techniques such as adaptive Butterworth filters (Erer, 2007) which potentially reduce phase shift error.

As opposed to strap-down integration methods and Kalman filtering algorithms, bandpass filtering promises a more fundamental solution of minimizing sensor errors in gait analysis. This technique shows potential of reducing the need for additional 'correctional' sensors such as the magnetometers, provided the gait activity is sufficiently faster than the low frequency sensor errors. Future work will focus on the study of adaptive band-pass filters, and various non-periodic gait activities to further quantify the limitations and advantages of this technique.

Figure 21. Samples of vertical displacements at 5.5km/h from Optotrak and IMU for 2 subjects; dashed and solid lines indicate the Optotrak and IMU displacements

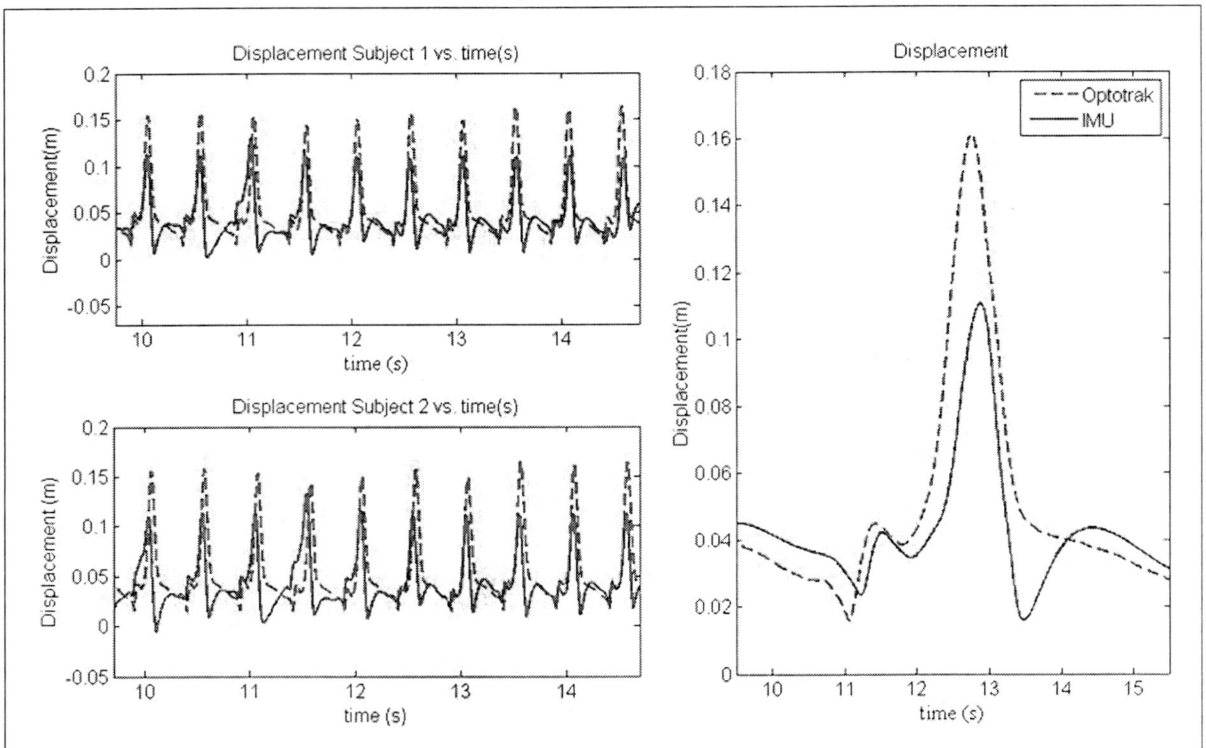

CONCLUSION

Inertial sensors are becoming an increasingly important part of human movement research due to their small physical size allowing research and continuous monitoring to be conducted outside restrictive gait environments. At this juncture, major challenges still exist for improving the accuracy of derived quantities from these sensors. Our contribution has been to study and investigate the sources of inaccuracy in these sensors from the perspective of the frequency domain. We showed by comparison with an optical measurement system, that inertial sensor measurements contained large discrepancies (errors) in the lower frequency spectra. Knowledge of these errors allowed the application of static bandpass filter for removing these errors by systematically altering the filter parameters and calculating the spectral deviations between optical and sensor systems. Results for toe accelerations demonstrated that proper filter parameters could significantly improve the accuracy of the acquired acceleration as well as the integrated foot displacements. Future work in this area will cover theoretical evaluations of the effect of the transformation matrices on the sensor errors when attempting to obtain a change of system coordinates, in particular when transforming from local sensor coordinates to the global laboratory coordinate system.

REFERENCES

Baten, C. T. M., Moerkerk, H. V., Kingma, I., Dien, J. V., Dolan, T., Veltink, P. H., & Hermens, H. J. (2000). Ambulatory low back load exposure estimation. In *Proceedings of the IEA 2000/44th Annual Meeting HFES 2000*, (4, pp. 609–612).

Baten, C. T. M., Oosterhoff, P., Kingma, I., Veltink, P. H., & Hermens, H. J. (1996). Inertial sensing in ambulatory back load estimation. In *Proceedings of the 18th Annual International Conference of the IEEE Engineering in Medicine and Biology Society*, (2, pp. 497–498).

Begg, R., Lai, D. T. H., & Palaniswami, M. (2007). *Computational Intelligence in Biomedical Engineering*. Boca Raton, FL: Taylor & Francis Books Inc.

Begg, R. K., Palaniswami, M., & Owen, B. (2005). Support vector machines for automated gait classification. *IEEE Transactions on Bio-Medical Engineering*, *52*(5), 828–838. doi:10.1109/TBME.2005.845241

Bourke, A. K., O'Donovan, K. J., & Olaighin, G. (2008). The identification of vertical velocity profiles using an inertial sensor to investigate pre-impact detection of falls. *Medical Engineering & Physics*, *30*(7), 937–946. doi:10.1016/j.medengphy.2007.12.003

Dejnabadi, H., Jolles, B. M., & Aminian, K. (2005). A new approach to accurate measurement of uniaxial joint angles based on a combination of accelerometers and gyroscopes. *IEEE Transactions on Bio-Medical Engineering*, *52*(8), 1478–1484. doi:10.1109/TBME.2005.851475

Erer, K. S. (2007). Adaptive usage of the butterworth digital filter. *Journal of Biomechanics*, *40*(13), 2934–2943. doi:10.1016/j.jbiomech.2007.02.019

Gafurov, D., Helkala, K., & Soendrol, T. (2006). Gait recognition using acceleration from MEMS. In *Proceedings - First International Conference on Availability, Reliability and Security, ARES*, (pp. 432–439).

Hassan, R., Begg, R., & Taylor, S. (2006). Fuzzy logic-based recognition of gait changes due to trip-related falls. In *Proceedings of the 27th Annual International Conference of the IEEE Engineering in Medicine and Biology Society (IEEE Cat. No.05CH37611C)*, (pp. 4970–4973).

Lai, D. T. H., Charry, E., Begg, R., & Palaniswami, M. (2008). Frequency analysis of inertial sensor data for measuring toe clearance. In *Proceedings of the International Conference on Intelligent Sensors, Sensor Networks and Information Processing - ISSNIP 2008*, (pp. 303–308).

Lau, H. Y., & Tong, K. (2008). The reliability of using accelerometer and gyroscope for gait event identification on persons with dropped foot. *Gait & Posture*, *27*(2), 248–257. doi:10.1016/j.gaitpost.2007.03.018

Meng, Q., Li, B., & Holstein, H. (2006). Recognition of human periodic movements from unstructured information using a motion-based frequency domain approach. *Image and Vision Computing*, *24*(8), 795–809. doi:10.1016/j.imavis.2006.01.033

Miyazaki, S. (1997). Long-term unrestrained measurement of stride length and walking velocity utilizing a piezoelectric gyroscope. In. *Proceedings of the IEEE Transactions on Biomedical Engineering*, *44*(8), 753–759. doi:10.1109/10.605434

Morris, S. J., & Paradiso, J. (2002). Shoe-integrated sensor system for wireless gait analysis and real-time feedback. In. *Proceedings of the Annual International Conference of the IEEE Engineering in Medicine and Biology*, *3*, 2468–2469.

Najafi, B., Aminian, K., Loew, F., Blanc, Y., & Robert, P. (2002). Measurement of stand-sit and sit-stand transitions using a miniature gyroscope and its application in fall risk evaluation in the elderly. *IEEE Transactions on Bio-Medical Engineering*, *49*(8), 843–851. doi:10.1109/TBME.2002.800763

Pappas, I., Keller, T., & Popovic, R. M. (1999). Experimental evaluation of the gyroscope sensor used in a new gait phase detection system. In *Proceedings of the 4th Annual Conference on the International Functional Electrical Stimulation Society, IFESS'99*, (pp. 23–27).

Pappas, I. P. I., Popovic, M., Keller, T., Dietz, V., & Morari, M. (2001). A reliable gait phase detection system. *IEEE Transactions on Neural Systems and Rehabilitation Engineering*, *9*(2), 113–125. doi:10.1109/7333.928571

Pfau, T., Witte, T. H., & Wilson, A. M. (2005). A method for deriving displacement data during cyclical movement using an inertial sensor. *The Journal of Experimental Biology*, *208*(13), 2503–2514. doi:10.1242/jeb.01658

Rong, L., Zhiguo, D., Jianzhong, Z., & Ming, L. (2007). Identification of individual walking patterns using gait acceleration. In *Proceedings of the 1st International Conference on Bioinformatics and Biomedical Engineering, ICBBE*, (pp. 543–546).

Rong, L., Zhiguo, D., Jianzhong, Z., Ming, L., & Xiangfeng, H. (2007). A wearable acceleration sensor system for gait recognition. In *Proceedings of the Second IEEE Conference on Industrial Electronics and Applications*, (pp. 2654–2659).

Sabatini, A. M., Martelloni, C., Scapellato, S., & Cavallo, F. (2005). Assessment of walking features from foot inertial sensing. *IEEE Transactions on Bio-Medical Engineering*, *52*(3), 486–494. doi:10.1109/TBME.2004.840727

Shukla, S. S. (1985). Comparison of methods for numerical differentiation. *TrAC –. Trends in Analytical Chemistry*, *4*(9), 229–233. doi:10.1016/0165-9936(85)85009-3

Summit Instruments (2005). Accelerometer offset drift reduction techniques, *Technical Note 404*.

Zijlstra, W., & Hof, A. (2003). Assessment of spatio-temporal gait parameters from trunk accelerations during human walking. *Gait & Posture*, *18*(2), 1–10. doi:10.1016/S0966-6362(02)00190-X

KEY TERMS AND DEFINITIONS

Gait Analysis: The study of human locomotion and mobility, usually based on measuring key parameters and data analysis of limb movement in a gait laboratory.

Minimum Toe Clearance: The minimum displacement of the toe from the ground during the mid-swing phase of the gait. Horizontal velocity is maximum at this point and tripping risk is high if the toe comes too close to the ground.

Inertial Sensors: Accelerometer and gyroscope sensors which measure linear acceleration and angular velocity respectively

Digital Filters: Functions implemented in software which attenuate specific frequency regions of a digital signal.

Fourier Transform: A signal processing tool which reveals the power of different components in a signal and its location in the frequency domain.

Chapter 6
Image Theory for Electrical Impedance Tomography

P.D. Einziger
Technion, Israel

M. Dolgin
Sea of Galilee College, Israel

ABSTRACT

Image reconstruction by electrical impedance tomography is, generally, an ill-posed nonlinear inverse problem. Regularization methods are widely used to ensure a stable solution. Herein, we present a novel electrical impedance tomography algorithm for reconstruction of layered biological tissues with piecewise continuous plane-stratified profiles. The algorithm is based on the reconstruction scheme for piecewise constant conductivity profiles, which utilizes Legendre expansion in conjunction with improved Prony method. This reconstruction procedure, which calculates both the locations and the conductivities, repetitively provides inhomogeneous depth discretization, (i.e., the depths grid is not equispaced). Incorporation of this specific inhomogeneous grid in the widely used mean least square reconstruction procedure results in a stable and accurate reconstruction, whereas, the commonly selected equispaced depth grid leads to unstable reconstruction. This observation establishes the main result of our investigation, highlighting the impact of physical phenomenon (image theory) on electrical impedance tomography, leading to a physically motivated stabilization of the inverse problem, (i.e., an inhomogeneous depth discretization renders an inherent regularization of the mean least square algorithm).

INTRODUCTION

The first step of medical treatment is the diagnosis. This investigation is focused on some fundamental mathematical and physical characteristics of such diagnostic tool, namely the Electrical Impedance Tomography (**EIT**), a subject of great scientific and public interest (Holder, 2005; Brown, 2003; Lionheart, 2004). The basic EIT's assumption is that different biological tissues can be distinguished by their conductivities. This knowledge allows one to acquire medical insight on the biological structure by **reconstruction** of its electrical characteristics. Many reconstruction techniques

DOI: 10.4018/978-1-61692-004-3.ch006

were developed during the last two decades. One of the most recently emerged techniques is the EIT. In this approach the, generally complex, conductivity profile of the tissues under reconstruction, is estimated by processing the quasistatic electromagnetic field data, and measured on the surrounding boundary.

EIT method is currently investigated for variable possible medical imaging and detection applications. For example, it appears appropriate for non-invasive cardiac stroke volume measurements, as the thoracic conductivity distribution is altered during the cardiac cycle (Zlochiver, 2006). Additional medical implementations include early breast and skin cancer detection (Assenheimer, 2001), biofilms thickness monitoring (Linderholm, 2007), and excitation with wireless (induced-current) electrodes (Zlochiver, 2003; Levy, 2002).

In spite of its advantages as a noninvasive, inexpensive, and potentially highly informative medical imaging modality, several factors limit the performance of EIT and prevent its adoptation as a clinically viable technique. These limitations can be classified into two groups: "physical" and "mathemtical". While the physical limitations may be addressed by improvements in instrumentation, the mathematical limitations are fundamental, and attempts to miligate them in the **reconstruction** procedure involve various, often undesirable performance compramises (Levy, 2002).

Herein, we are motivated to move one step forward in the process of incorporating analytic derivations into the solution of inverse problems. Specifically, we use the analytic solution of the forward problem associated with **plane stratified***n* layered media (Livshitz, 2001; Einziger, 2002; Einziger, 2005), for the solution of the EIT inverse problem. As it will be shown throughout the study, the pitfalls to be overcome in EIT **reconstruction** procedures rise in the presented media as well. However, the advantage of analytic solution, derived for this media, is exploited and enable to investigate the origin of the characteristic common failures of the existing EIT algorithms.

In applying EIT techniques (Dolgin, 2004; Dolgin, 2006) two crucially important issues have to be clarified and specified: (i) an explicit relation connecting the inverse procedure and the forward problem; (ii) a locality principle, linking between the electrical impedance spacial distribution and the corresponding quasistatic data, measured on the surrounding boundary. The first issue is resolved herein by utilizing a recently proposed image series expansion scheme for layered media, resulting in a novel reconstruction method. Furthermore, in the WKB limit leading to a one to one mapping between each image term and a corresponding layer the second issue is also resolved. For non-WKB image series expansion, however, where each image term corresponds to a specific layer and its neighborhood the novel **EIT** procedure can be readily modified as to account for a partial loss of the locality.

This work links between image theory (Einziger, 2002; Einziger, 2005) and an EIT model for reconstruction of **plane stratified** media. We begin with the **reconstruction** of piecewise constant layered media by a novel two step efficient algorithm utilizing Legendre transform and improved Prony Method (PM) (Dolgin, 2004). Computations based on this procedure, including noisy data, provide accurate, efficient and stable reconstruction, particularly, when relatively small data base and, consequently, shallow penetration are required. Furthermore, our methods holds promising for an efficient reconstruction of locally stratified media (relative to the Legendre window width). Then, the reconstruction procedure is extended as to incorporate piecewise continuous layered media. Each continuous layer is discretized and then reconstructed as a collection of a piecewise constant layers set. The algorithm provides accurate reconstruction results for moderate depths. This reconstruction procedure, which calculates both the locations and the conductivities, repetitively provides inhomogeneous **depth discretization**, (i.e., the depths grid is not equispaced).

Incorporation of this specific inhomogeneous grid in the widely used Mean Least Square (MLS) **reconstruction** procedure results in a **stable** and accurate reconstruction, whereas, the commonly selected equispaced depth grid leads to unstable reconstruction. This observation establishes the main result of our investigation, highlighting the impact of physical phenomenon (image theory) on EIT. In contrast, the conveniently selected conventional equispaced grid necessitates, in general, mathematical compensation, i.e., regularization techniques (e.g., Goharian, 2007; Kolehmainen, 1997) or extensive apriory knowledge on the reconstructed conductivity distribution (Isaacson, 2004).

In conclusion, this chapter focuses on reconstruction of **layered** biological **tissues** as a simplified prototype model for real-life **EIT** problems. It aims to gain physical and mathematical insight as well as to validate the feasibility of the reconstruction process via closed form direct solution for a simplified EIT measurement setup, rather than to develop a certain applicative system. In short, we tend to establish relations between both the physical-mathematical modelling of a simplified EIT model and the limitations on the accuracy and the resolution of a general three-dimensional EIT procedure.

BACKGROUND

The transimpedance measurements have been used for a long time to determine conductivity distribution inside a matter. Geophysicists have been using it as an aid in prospecting for minerals and oil, by identifying different layers (strata) close to earth's surface (Keller, 1966). It was realized that different tissues in the human body can be distinguished by their conductivity values, since each of them has its own distinct conductivity value. Recently, scientists seriously considered impedance imaging as an aid to medical diagnosis (Brown, 2003; Lionheart, 2004).

Electrical Impedance Tomography

EIT (or Imaging) is defined to be any technique which, from the knowledge of voltage and current conditions on the boundary of a region, determines the spatial distribution of conductivity therein. EIT is one of imaging techniques whose significant advantage is its noninvasive nature. Noninvasive nature of these imaging techniques make them very attractive for use in medical practice. It should be noted that EIT technique can't substitute totally existing imaging methods, since each of the above method provides some unique information usually unavailable (or available with low quality) in other methods, so it can be used as complementary or specific application oriented method.

Some techniques (like X-ray and nuclear particles emission techniques) is hazardous if over-used. In other methods (like MRI, PET) the equipment is very sophisticated and expensive. In view of the above, the EIT has several advantages: (i) cost-effective: it is a relatively cheap technique while providing valuable results; (ii) Healthy: there are no known hazards in applying this technique; (iii) Measurements process is fast, allowing for measurements of fast changing functions; (iv) lack of side effects makes it possible to perform long term medical monitoring; (v) Additional insight to tissue characterization can be obtained by performing the measurements at different frequencies. Thus, it is not surprising that this topic remains an area of intensive research for over 20 years, seeking for a working electrical impedance imaging system.

Methods and Measurements

The methodology of impedance imaging is similar in most imaging systems. Basically, there are two stages:

- The collection of a set of independent transimpedance measurements.
- Inverse problem solution, which determines conductivity distribution from the above measurements.

Given *N* electrodes one obtains up to *N(N-3)/2* independent transimpedance measurements, thus limiting the number of volume elements at which the conductivity can be determined (Brown, 2003).

There are two main classes of **EIT** system. The first class makes use of current injection through the surface electrodes (and is referred just as EIT in the following). This method had been thoroughly studied (Cherepin, 2002; Levy, 2002). Another approach is Magnetic Induction electrical impedance Tomography (MIT), where the currents are applied by induction as in (Watson, 2003; Korjenevsky, 2000). A set of excitation coils driving a low frequency current surrounds the object to be measured. The electrical fields produce both conductive and displacement currents, depending on the object's electrical properties. Those currents, called eddy currents, result in developing voltages that can be measured on the surface. The main difference in the above approaches is in the depth of current penetration (in MIT the current can be induced in the inner part of the object, while in EIT the current penetrate mainly the layers close to the surface). The current, which can be applied to the body is limited by electrical safety concerns. Most international standards limit the current to 100 μA rms for frequencies up to 1 *kHz* and then increasing with frequency to an absolute limit of 10 *mA* for frequencies above 100 *kHz*.

A major step in developing of an EIT system was made by introducing multi-frequency systems, which enable measurement of tissue impedance at different frequencies. These spectral measurements provide better insight to tissue characterization. It has been shown, that in some cases, pre-malignant changes are associated with large changes in tissue impedance spectra (Brown, 2003).

Usually, technical problems limit the frequency range for spectral measurements. In EIT method the injecting electrodes exhibit some problems: for example, at low frequencies they possess high contact impedance (reducing low frequency currents injection). Thus, some research is devoted to design an efficient current generator (see Ross (2003), for example). The use of very low frequencies also increases the time of measurement such that transient changes, for example, those occurring during the cardiac cycle, cannot be recorded. Almost all current EIT systems operate at the frequency range of 1 *kHz* to 2 *MHz*. It has been shown that even though the dissipative and reactive components are related by the Kramers-Kronig relations (Frohlich, 1958) for a single tissue, the significant information about an ensemble of various tissues can be gained by measuring a complete spectrum of the complex impedance in an appropriate frequency range (Osypka, 1995).

Originally, EIT was developed for medical imaging purposes, such as breast tumor diagnosis, cardiac monitoring, pulmonary disease detection and more. However, many other application, e.g., industrial, can be derived as well.

While unique reconstructions are guaranteed under a variety of assumptions (Isakov, 1998; Isaacson, 2004; Babaeizadeh, 2007), even for the layered structures (Kohn, 1985), studied herein, reconstruction algorithms (Goharian, 2007; Trigo, 2004) for arbitrary conductivity profiles (e.g., piecewise constant, etc.) may lead to unacceptable results, particularly when finite and noisy measurements are involved. In this study efforts are made to gain mathematical-physical understanding to the mechanism of the EIT inverse procedure, particularly to instability of solutions in order to point out potentially **stable** techniques. This is carried out by focusing through the study of piecewise continuous media with planar stratification.

Solution of a full inverse problem, (i.e. reconstruction of the conductivity distribution inside the object) is usually solved via MLS technique (Brown, 2003). For this purpose, the forward electromagnetic problem should be solved in three dimensional (3D) configuration for a prescribed conductivity distribution. The MLS procedures, outlined and discussed in Appendix A, are based on comparison of the data obtained from the forward solution with the potential measured on the boundaries of the body. There are some pitfalls in these procedures that scientists try to deal with (Lionheart, 2004). Firstly, the analytical solution for arbitrary 3D configurations is hard to achieve and there is a need to use numerical solvers repetitively to solve the forward problem. Secondly, the unknowns in a general EIT problem are the conductivities and their locations. The problem is highly non-linear in both the conductivity values and their locations, thus, it is more desirable to assume a specified spatial grid, (i.e. to make the locations known and search only for the conductivities vector). To this end, the reduced inverse schemes utilize standard numerical solvers (e.g., finite element (Soleimani, 2005) and boundary element methods) in conjunction with commonly used MLS procedures (Zlochiver, 2003; Kallman, 1992). Unfortunately, this reduced procedure is highly sensitive to the selection of both the location grid and the initial conductivity values (Borcea, 2003), thus remaining the mls procedure to be nonlinear, which convergence to the global desired minimum is not guaranteed (Dobson, 1992). While the problem of the big time required for forward solvers can be overcome using e.g. (Soleimani, 2005), number of regularization techniques were proposed to obtain **stable** solutions for the nonlinear ill-posed EIT inverse problem, see (Goharian, 2007) for example, and they demand some a priory knowledge or constraints on the reconstructed conductivity distribution, (e.g. [Babaeizadeh, 2007]).

RECONSTRUCTION OF PIECEWISE CONTINOUS LAYERED TISSUES VIA EIT

Problem Definition

The **electromagnetic fields**, induced by a point-source, are governed by Maxwell's equations. At low frequencies and small field strengths the electromagnetic properties of living tissue allow these to be simplified via the potential equation (e.g. Haus & Melcher, 1989)

$$\nabla^2\Phi(\mathbf{r}) + \nabla\Phi(\mathbf{r})\cdot\nabla\ln(\sigma) = -\frac{i(\mathbf{r})}{\sigma}. \quad (1)$$

where $\mathbf{\Phi(r)}$ and $\boldsymbol{i}\mathbf{(r)}$ denote the **electric potential** and the **current** source distribution, respectively, at the point $\mathbf{r}=(\rho,\theta,z)$.. Considering a piecewise continuous **plane stratified** conductivity profile $\boldsymbol{\sigma}\mathbf{(z)}$ and a quasistatic current point-source $\boldsymbol{S}$

$$i(\mathbf{r}) = I\delta(\mathbf{r}-\mathbf{r}'), \quad (2)$$

located at $\mathbf{r}' = (0,0,z')$, we aim to reconstruct $\boldsymbol{\sigma}\mathbf{(z)}$ for $z \geq z_1$ using a noninvasive measurements of the potential $\mathbf{\Phi(r)}$ at the plane $z_1 = 0$, as outlined in Figure 1.

Integral Representation for the Solution of the Forward Problem

The potential $\mathbf{\Phi}$ for the piecewise continuous media described by

$$\sigma(z) = \sigma_i(z), \quad (3)$$

where z belongs to the ***i-th*** layer

Figure 1. Physical configuration and reconstruction setup

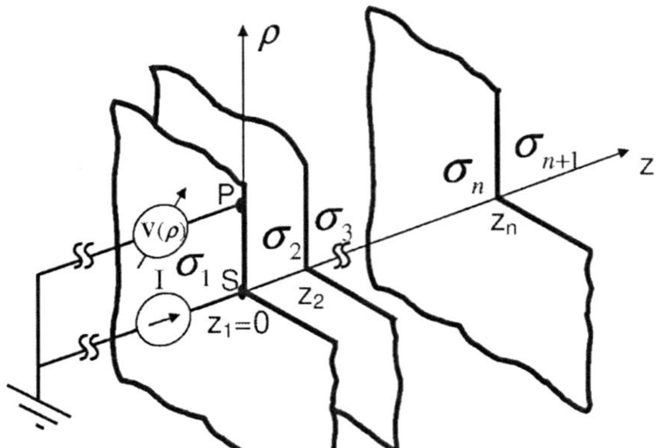

$$z_{i-1} < z < z_i, \qquad i = 1, 2, ..., n+1, \qquad z_0 = -\infty, \qquad z_{n+1} = \infty, \tag{4}$$

can be expressed most effectively by Green's function,

$$\Phi(\mathbf{r}) = \frac{I}{\sigma_1} G(\mathbf{r}, \mathbf{r}'), \tag{5}$$

given via the inverse Bessel transform (Dolgin, 2006; Abramowitz, 1970; Erdelyi, 1954)

$$G(\mathbf{r}, \mathbf{r}') = \frac{1}{2\pi} \int_0^{\infty} \xi g(z, z', \xi) J_0(\xi \rho) d\xi. \tag{6}$$

The differential operators and the associated boundary conditions for both the Green's function $G(\mathbf{r}, \mathbf{r}')$ and the characteristic Green's function $g(z, z', \xi)$ in (6) are specified in Table 1. The characteristic Green's function $g(z, z', \xi)$, for constant σ_1, is given via

$$g_i(z, z', \xi) = \frac{1}{2\xi} \begin{cases} \prod_{p=1}^{i} T_p(\xi) \left[t_i(z, \xi) + R_i(\xi) r_i(z, \xi) \right] e^{\xi z'} & i > 0 \\ \left[e^{-\xi z'} + R_1(\xi) e^{\xi z'} \right] e^{\xi z} & i = 0 \end{cases}, \tag{7}$$

where $t_i(z, \xi)$ and $r_i(z, \xi)$ are the two independent solutions of the ordinary differential equation in Table 1 corresponding to a specified ***i***-th layer, denoting the so-called transmitted and reflected functions, respectively. The functions $t_i(z, \xi)$ and $r_i(z, \xi)$ corresponding to piecewise constant, piecewise linear, and exponential conductivity profiles are given explicitly in Table 2. Both the piecewise constant and the piecewise linear profiles are utilized in subsequent reconstruction calculations.

The global reflection and transmission coefficients, $R_i(\xi)$ and $T_i(\xi)$ are given by the following recursive closed form expressions

$$R_i(\xi) = \frac{R_{i+1}(\xi) + \dfrac{t_{i+1}(z_i,\xi)\sigma_i(z_i)t_i'(z_i,\xi) - t_i(z_i,\xi)\sigma_{i+1}(z_i)t_{i+1}'(z_i,\xi)}{r_{i+1}(z_i,\xi)\sigma_i(z_i)t_i'(z_i,\xi) - t_i(z_i,\xi)\sigma_{i+1}(z_i)r_{i+1}'(z_i,\xi)}}{1 + R_{i+1}(\xi)\dfrac{r_{i+1}(z_i,\xi)\sigma_i(z_i)r_i'(z_i,\xi) - r_i(z_i,\xi)\sigma_{i+1}(z_i)r_{i+1}'(z_i,\xi)}{t_{i+1}(z_i,\xi)\sigma_i(z_i)r_i'(z_i,\xi) - r_i(z_i,\xi)\sigma_{i+1}(z_i)t_{i+1}'(z_i,\xi)}} \times$$

$$\left[-\frac{r_{i+1}(z_i,\xi)\sigma_i(z_i)t_i'(z_i,\xi) - t_i(z_i,\xi)\sigma_{i+1}(z_i)r_{i+1}'(z_i,\xi)}{t_{i+1}(z_i,\xi)\sigma_i(z_i)r_i'(z_i,\xi) - r_i(z_i,\xi)\sigma_{i+1}(z_i)t_{i+1}'(z_i,\xi)} \right],$$

$$R_{n+1}(\xi) = 0 \tag{8}$$

and

$$T_{i+1} = \frac{\dfrac{\sigma_i(z_i)\left(t_i(z_i,\xi)r_i'(z_i,\xi) - r_i(z_i,\xi)t_i'(z_i,\xi)\right)}{t_{i+1}(z_i,\xi)\sigma_i(z_i)r_i'(z_i,\xi) - t_{i+1}'(z_i,\xi)r_i(z_i,\xi)\sigma_{i+1}(z_i)}}{1 + R_{i+1}\dfrac{r_{i+1}(z_i,\xi)\sigma_i(z_i)r_i'(z_i,\xi) - r_{i+1}'(z_i,\xi)r_i(z_i,\xi)\sigma_{i+1}(z_i)}{t_{i+1}(z_i,\xi)\sigma_i(z_i)r_i'(z_i,\xi) - t_{i+1}'(z_i,\xi)r_i(z_i,\xi)\sigma_{i+1}(z_i)}},$$

$$T_1 = 1, \tag{9}$$

respectively. Note that $t'(z, \xi)$, and $r'(z, \xi)$ denote derivatives of $t(z, \xi)$ and $r(z, \xi)$ with respect to z, in Eqs. (8) and (9).

*Table 1. Poisson equations and boundary/continuity conditions for G(**r**,**r**') and g(z, z',ξ)*

	$G(\mathbf{r},\mathbf{r}')$	$g(z,z',\xi)$
Differential equation	$\left(\nabla^2+\nabla\ln(\sigma)\cdot\nabla\right)G(\mathbf{r},\mathbf{r}')=-\delta(\mathbf{r},\mathbf{r}')$	$\left(\frac{d^2}{dz^2}-\xi^2+\frac{d\ln(\sigma(z))}{dz}\cdot\frac{d}{dz}\right)g(z,z',\xi)$ $=-\delta(z-z')$
Source condition at $z=z'$	$\int\limits_{V\to 0}\nabla^2G(\mathbf{r},\mathbf{r}')dV=$ $\oint\limits_{A\to 0}\nabla G(\mathbf{r},\mathbf{r}')\cdot dA=-1$	$\left[\frac{dg(z'+h,z',\xi)}{dz}-\frac{dg(z'-h,z',\xi)}{dz}\right]_{h\to 0}$ $=-1$
Continuity condition at $z=z_i$	$G_i(\mathbf{r},\mathbf{r}')=G_{i+1}(\mathbf{r},\mathbf{r}')$	$g_i(z,z',\xi)=g_{i+1}(z,z',\xi)$
$i>0$	$\sigma_i\frac{G_i(\mathbf{r},\mathbf{r}')}{z}=\sigma_{i+1}\frac{G_{i+1}(\mathbf{r},\mathbf{r}')}{z}$	$\sigma_i\frac{dg_i(z,z',\xi)}{dz}=\sigma_{i+1}\frac{dg_{i+1}(z,z',\xi)}{dz}$
Decay at infinity	$rG_i(\mathbf{r},\mathbf{r}')_{r\to\infty}<\infty$	$(\frac{d}{dz}+\xi)g(z,z',\xi)_{\|z\|\to\infty}=0$

Assuming that the current point-source is located at the origin, i.e., $z'=0$ and the measurements are performed on the plane *z=0*, one obtains explicit representation for the characteristic Green's function $g_1(z,z',\xi)$ on the surface *z=0*,

$$g_1(0,0,\xi)=\frac{1}{2\xi}\left[1+R_1(\xi)\right]. \tag{10}$$

Note however, that $\sigma_1=0$ for air-tissue interface renders $R_1(\xi)=-1$. Thus, **Φ(r)** in (5) should be evaluated by taking the limit of $g_1(0,0,\xi)/\sigma_1$ as $\sigma_1\to 0$ and then performing the integral in (6). Following this sequence, the measured surface potential $V(\rho)$ (Figure 1), defined as

$$V(\rho)=\Phi(\mathbf{r})\,|_{z=z'=0,\sigma_1=0}=\frac{I}{\sigma_1}G(\mathbf{r},\mathbf{r}')\,|_{z=z'=0,\sigma_1=0}, \tag{11}$$

is given explicitly via

$$V(\rho)=\frac{1}{2\pi}\int\limits_0^\infty \xi v(\xi)J_0(\xi\rho)d\xi, \tag{12}$$

where $v(\xi)$ is the Bessel transform of $V(\rho)$

$$v(\xi)=2\pi\int\limits_0^\infty \rho V(\rho)J_0(\xi\rho)d\rho=\frac{I}{\sigma_1}g_1(z,z',\xi)\,|_{z=z'=0,\sigma_1=0}$$

$$=-\frac{I}{\sigma_2(0)}\frac{R_2(\xi)r_2(0,\xi)+t_2(0,\xi)}{t_2'(0,\xi)+R_2(\xi)r_2'(0,\xi)}. \tag{13}$$

Table 2. Canonical form and two independent solutions, $r_i(z,\xi)$ and $t_i(z,\xi)$, corresponding to the ordinary differential equation in Table 1, for three different conductivity profiles. The functions I_0 and K_0 denote the modified Bessel functions of zero order.

$\sigma_i(z)$	Canonical form	y	r_i	t_i
$a_i z + b_i$	$\left(y^2 \dfrac{d^2}{dy^2} + y \dfrac{d}{dy} - y^2\right) f(y) = 0$	$\xi\left(z + \dfrac{b_i}{a_i}\right)$	$I_0(\mid y \mid)$	$K_0(\mid y \mid)$
$e^{a_i z + b_i}$	$\left(\dfrac{d^2}{dy^2} + a_i \dfrac{d}{dy} - \xi^2\right) f(y) = 0$	z	$e^{-\left(a_i - \sqrt{a_i^2 + 4\xi^2}\right) y/2}$	$e^{-\left(a_i + \sqrt{a_i^2 + 4\xi^2}\right) y/2}$
c_i	$\left(\dfrac{d^2}{dy^2} - \xi^2\right) f(y) = 0$	z	$e^{\xi y}$	$e^{-\xi y}$

Novel Reconstruction Procedure for Piecewise Constant Conductivity Profile

Image Series Expansion

The potential $\mathbf{\Phi(r)}$ in (5), for a piecewise constant conductivity profile, has been expended recently into the following rigorous image series representation (Einziger, 2002; Einziger, 2005),

$$\Phi(\mathbf{r},\mathbf{r}') = \frac{I}{4\pi\sigma_1}[\frac{1}{\mid \mathbf{r}-\mathbf{r}' \mid} +$$

$$+\sum_{l_1=0}^{1}\sum_{m_1=0}^{\infty}\cdots\sum_{l_{n-1}=0}^{s_{n-2}}\sum_{m_{n-1}=0}^{\infty}\{\prod_{k=1}^{n-1}\begin{pmatrix} s_{k-1}+1 \\ l_k \end{pmatrix}\begin{pmatrix} s_k \\ m_k \end{pmatrix}$$

$$\times K_k^{l_k}[1-K_k^2]^{s_{k-1}-l_k+1}[-K_k]^{m_k} K_n^{m_k-l_k}\}\frac{K_n}{\mid \mathbf{r}-\tilde{\mathbf{r}}'_k \mid}], \quad (14)$$

where $\mathbf{r}$ and $\tilde{\mathbf{r}}'_k$, denoting the observation and the image points, are given via

$$\mathbf{r} = (x,y,z) \text{ and } \tilde{\mathbf{r}}_k' = \left(0,0,\tilde{z}_k'\right) \quad (15)$$

respectively, and

$$\tilde{z}_k' = 2\sum_{k=1}^{n-1}(s_k+1)(z_{k+1}-z_k) - z', \quad (16)$$

$$s_n = \sum_{k=1}^{n}(m_k - l_k), \quad s_0 = 0. \quad (17)$$

In the WKB limit (Morse, 1953), the intrinsic reflection coefficients K_i, $i = 2,3,\ldots,n,$ given by

$$K_i = \frac{\sigma_i - \sigma_{i+1}}{\sigma_i + \sigma_{i+1}}, \quad K_0 = 0, \quad \sigma_0 = \sigma_1, \quad (18)$$

are assumed to be sufficiently small, i.e.,

$$\left|K_i\right| << 1. \tag{19}$$

Hence, maintaining image terms of $O(|K_i|)$, the expression in (14) is readily reduced into the WKB image series expansion,

$$\Phi_{WKB}(\mathbf{r},\mathbf{r}') = \frac{I}{4\pi\sigma_1}\left[\frac{1}{|\mathbf{r}-\mathbf{r}'|} + \frac{K_1}{|\mathbf{r}-\mathbf{r}'_1|} + \right.$$

$$\left. +(1-K_1^2)\sum_{i=2}^{n}\frac{K_i}{|\mathbf{r}-\mathbf{r}'_i|}\right], \ \mathbf{r}'_i = (0,0,-2z_i - z'). \tag{20}$$

Note that the intrinsic reflection coefficient K_1^2 is contained, however, in (20) as to accommodate the case $\sigma_1 = 0$, leading to a non-WKB coefficient $K_1 = -1$.

Reconstruction Considerations

The voltage probe reading $V(\rho)$ at $\rho = \sqrt{x^2+y^2}$ can be expressed, via Eqs. (10) - (13) and (20), as

$$V_{WKB}(\rho) = \Phi_{WKB}(\mathbf{r},\mathbf{r}')\,|_{z=z'=0,\sigma_1=0} = \frac{I}{2\pi\sigma_2}\left[\frac{1}{\rho} + 2\sum_{i=2}^{n}\frac{K_i}{\sqrt{\rho^2+(2z_i)^2}}\right]. \tag{21}$$

The resultant WKB image series expansion is characterized by an outstanding feature, namely, each image term corresponds analytically and explicitly to a unique layer, leading to a one to one mapping between each image term and the local impedance of the associated layer. This locality feature leads to an effective subsequent linear reconstruction of the electrical impedance profile via **Legendre expansion** in conjunction with Prony's method.

It is readily noted that $\boldsymbol{\rho V(\rho)}$ contains information associated with the image contributions in (21) for a limited $\boldsymbol{\rho}$ range only. Indeed as $\rho/(2z_2) \to 0$, one obtains

$$\rho V_{WKB}(\rho) \approx \frac{I}{2\pi\sigma_2}, \tag{22}$$

whereas the reverse limit $\rho/(2z_n) \to \infty$, leads to

$$\rho V_{WKB}(\rho) \approx \frac{I}{2\pi\sigma_2}\left(1 + 2\sum_{i=2}^{n}K_i\right). \tag{23}$$

Hence, it can be concluded that the effective ρ range, containing independent $\boldsymbol{\rho V(\rho)}$ data, is defined via

$$0 \le \rho \le \rho_{\max}, \quad \rho_{\max}/(2z_n) >> 1 \tag{24}$$

Furthermore, for an intermediate $\boldsymbol{\rho}$ range, $0 \le 2z_q << \rho_q \le \rho \le \rho_p << 2z_{p+1} \le 2z_n << \rho_{\max}$ only the first $\boldsymbol{p}$ images in (21) has to be effectively accounted for, from which the first $\boldsymbol{q}$ are taken collectively, thus, (21) is reduced into a truncated image series expansion

$$\rho V_{WKB}(\rho) \approx \frac{I}{2\pi\sigma_2}\left(1 + 2\sum_{i=2}^{q}K_i + 2\sum_{i=q+1}^{p}\frac{\rho K_i}{\sqrt{\rho^2+(2z_i)^2}}\right). \tag{25}$$

Note that, for $\boldsymbol{q=0}$, the reconstruction resolution is dictated by the maximal number of images $\boldsymbol{p}$ that can be effectively handled by a specific spectral domain reconstruction method.

Furthermore, the window width ρ_p ($\rho_p \leq \rho_n$) defines the effective penetration range, $0 \leq z \leq z_p \leq z_n$.

Linear Transformation: Legendre Expansion

Evidently, Eq. (21) contains all the information required for reconstruction of the layered media. Evaluation of an individual ***i***th image term in (21) leads to reconstruction of K_i and z_i and, consequently, the electrical impedance $\sigma(z)$ of the entire medium (via Eq. (18)). While the standard MLS non-linear optimization procedure seems capable of obtaining the desired information regarding the unknown image terms, its execution for large number of images usually results in a cumbersome global minimum estimation, namely, unacceptable computation time due to the unavoidable local minima identification and elimination, as expected for a non-linear algorithm. Herein, we seek for an alternative linear procedure, which has the potential of accurately reconstructing relatively large number of layers (i.e., distinct image terms) and significantly reducing the execution time (relative to the MLS procedure).

Noting that the geometrical parameters z_i are associated with the singularities of $V(\rho)$ in the complex ρ plane, whereas the electrical parameters K_i are associated with their weights, one is tempted to perform the reconstruction procedure via analytic continuation of $V(\rho)$ into the complex ρ domain. Such approach is always possible for analytic operator (Laplace's equation) relaying on analytic data (Courant, 1989). However, in view of the well-known unstable properties of analytic continuation procedures (i.e., bounded analytic Cauchy boundary data $\Phi_{WKB}|_{z=0}$ and $(\partial\Phi_{WKB} / \partial z)|_{z=0,\rho\neq 0} = 0$, for elliptic operator, does not guarantee bounded solution for $\Phi_{WKB}|_{z>0}$), the focus, herein, is on a real function analysis, namely, determining the radius of convergence for Taylor series expansion associated with each image in the real ρ axis rather than reconstructing its singularity in the complex ρ plane. To this end, standard Taylor series expansion of $V(\rho)$ in (21) is equivalently expressed via orthogonal Legendre polynomial expansion, thereby, effectively evaluating the expansion coefficients by inner products rather than (potentially unstable) matrix inversion. In the radial range $0 \leq \rho < \infty$, shifted Legendre polynomials, $P_l(1-2\rho^2)$ (Abramowitz, 1970), defined on a unit window $0 \leq \rho \leq w, w=1$ [unit length], are most desirable to expand the scaled potential $V(s\rho)$, leading to

$$V(s\rho) = \sum_{l=0}^{\infty} b_l(s) P_l(1-2\rho^2), \tag{26}$$

where the coefficients $b_l(s)$ are given via (Erdelyi, 1954)

$$b_l(s) = 2\left(2l+1\right)\int_0^w \rho V\left(s\rho\right) P_l\left(1-2\rho^2\right) d\rho \tag{27}$$

and s is a positive real scaling factor. Explicitly for WKB,

$$\begin{aligned} b_l(s) &= \frac{2\left(2l+1\right)}{s^2}\int_0^{sw} \rho V_{WKB}\left(\rho\right) P_l\left(1-2(\rho/s)^2\right) d\rho \\ &= \frac{2I}{\pi s \sigma_2}\sum_{i=1}^{n} K_i \left(2z_i / s + \sqrt{1+(2z_i/s)^2}\right)^{-(2l+1)}, \end{aligned} \tag{28}$$

Note that s can also be regarded, via the second equality in Eq. (27), as scaling factor for Legendre's unit window width w=1 [unit length] (with respect to a non-scaled potential $V(\rho)$). Furthermore, while for $i>1, K_i = K_{i,}$, for $i=1$, $K_1=1/2$, and the unknown parameter is σ_2.

Generally, the Legendre polynomial expansion scheme in (26) - (27) represents a discrete linear closed-form transformation of the voltage distribution $V(s\rho)$ into the coefficients $b_l(s)$ space, however there may exist alternative, potentially useful, closed-form linear transformations. Obviously, one such alternative, commonly utilized for separable solution representation of the direct potential problem is given by the Fourier-Bessel transform pair (Dolgin, 2006).

Spectral Domain Estimate - Extended Prony Method

It is readily recognized that the individual n terms contained in the right hand side summation of Eq. (27) may be regarded as n distinct exponentials $\left(2\frac{z_i}{s}+\sqrt{1+\left(2\frac{z_i}{s}\right)^2}\right)^{-2}$ of power l, weighted by $\frac{2IK_i}{\pi\sigma_2 s}\left(2\frac{z_i}{s}+\sqrt{1+\left(2\frac{z_i}{s}\right)^2}\right)^{-1}$. Hence, the PM procedure (Hamming, 1986) exploiting $2n$ data points, i.e., $b_l(s)$, $0 \le l \le 2n-1$, or, equivalently, $2n$ inner products, can be utilized to reconstruct n distinct exponentials and weights characterizing the stratification geometry and electrical parameters, respectively. Also, to avoid dominance of any one of the exponentials contained in the right hand-side of Eq. (27) the scaling factor s should be large enough as to support the entire reconstruction range, i.e.

$$s \ge 2z_i / w, \tag{29}$$

leading to the inclusion of $V(\rho)$ well within the window $0 \le \rho / w \le s$. Note, however, that the selection $s >> 2z_n / w$, results in almost linearly dependant exponentials and, thus, should be avoided.

Following the PM procedure, the n unknown exponentials $\left(2\frac{z_i}{s}+\sqrt{1+\left(2\frac{z_i}{s}\right)^2}\right)^{-2}$ are roots of the n order polynomial equation

$$\sum_{p=0}^{n} c_p(\mu^2)^p = 0, \tag{30}$$

where $c_n = 1$. Let μ_i^2 denote the i th root of (30), then,

$$\mu_i = \left(2z_i / s + \sqrt{1+(2z_i / s)^2}\right)^{-1}, \tag{31}$$

leading to

$$z_i = \frac{\mu_i^2 - 1}{4\mu_i} s. \tag{32}$$

The polynomial coefficients denoted by the vector $\mathbf{C} = \left[c_0, c_1, \ldots, c_{n-1}\right]^T$ are solution of the linear system,

$$\mathbf{AC} = \mathbf{B},\ \mathbf{C} = \mathbf{A}^{-1}\mathbf{B}, \tag{33}$$

where $\mathbf{A}_{j,k} = b_{j+k-1},\ j,k = 0,1,\ldots,n-1$, $\mathbf{B} = -[b_n, b_{n+1}, \ldots, b_{2n-1}]^T$ and ^{T} denotes transpose operation. Finally, the weight coefficients, denoted by the vector

$\mathbf{K} = \frac{2I}{\pi s \sigma_2}[\mu_1 K_1, \mu_2 K_2, \ldots, \mu_n K_n)]^T$, are also solution of the linear system

$$\mathbf{MK} = \mathbf{D}, \quad \mathrm{K} = \mathrm{M}^{-1}\mathbf{D} \tag{34}$$

where $M_{i,j} = (\mu_j^2)^i$ and $\mathbf{D} = [b_0, b_1, \ldots, b_{n-1}]^T$.

Reconstruction Results

The potential promise of the novel EIT reconstruction procedure presented herein is now demonstrated via numerical simulations in the presence of noisy data. The input data is generated using (14), setting $z = z' = 0$ and $\sigma_1 = 0$. Error sources, affecting the reconstruction procedure results, include the WKB approximation, numerical spectral integration, and noisy input data $V(\rho)$ corresponding to inaccurate measurements.

The WKB error is due to approximation (21), which is equivalent to (14) only asymptotically. It can be readily verified that the WKB approximation for oscillating intrinsic reflection coefficients approximates (14) much better than WKB approximation associated with positive intrinsic reflection coefficients. This is due to faster convergence of (14), when consisting of oscillating and monotonically decreasing (WKB and non-WKB) terms, resulting in dominance of the first (WKB) terms in the series representation. Furthermore, in physical terms, while the oscillating reflection coefficients introduce minor deviations of the conductivity profile from its average, large number of monotonically increasing coefficients (layers) may result in an unacceptable difference between the initial and final values of the tissue conductivity, violating the WKB approximation.

The input data bases include both noiseless data sets and noisy sets (Frangi, 2002) characterized by 60 dB signal to noise ratio (SNR), with respect to the signal $V(s\rho)$ at the endpoint $\rho = w$ (Eqs. (27)) and a specified scaling factor s. SNR level of 60 dB can be experimentally maintained utilizing the readily available narrow-band low-frequency active filters. The simulation noise implemented herein is white and gaussian.

The drawback of infinite window extent (poor SNR) is readily avoided for the Legendre's finite extent window by increasing the signal strength $V(s_p\rho)$ well above the noise level, setting $s_p < s_{max}$ $((s_p = \rho_p / w,\ s_{max} = \rho_{max} / w)$, but at the cost of a shallower reconstruction depth, since Eq. (25) leads to $z_p < z_n$ for $s_p < s_{max}$.

To overcome noisy data, we utilize oversampling of the input data. The resultant "ghost" layers, are then eliminated in the Prony procedure by identifying those characterized by complex width or negligibly small intrinsic reflection coefficient. Selection guidelines for the scaling factor s can be inferred via (25) (replacing $2z_i$ by $2z_i / s$).

Finally, the impulse response in (14) and (21), corresponding to the exact potential and its WKB approximation, respectively, is valid as long as the electrodes size (e.g., the diameter of electrodes *S* and *P* in Figure 1) is much smaller than both the layers thickness (Eq. (3)) and the window width *w* (Eqs. (26) - (27)). While the effect of electrodes size is neglected throughout this paper, it can be accounted for (Cheng, 1989), particulary, in conjunction with the image series expansion (Livshitz, 2001).

Reconstruction of Five Layered Media

The reconstructed media parameters, i.e., depths z_i / w and conductivities σ_i / σ_2, for the cases of both oscillating and positive intrinsic reflection coefficients, are given in Table 3. The reconstruction results depicted in Figure 2 reveal that a very

Table 3: Simulation parameters and PM errors for reconstructed parameters z_i / w and σ_{i+1} / σ_2 (Figure 2) relative to the simulation parameters, associated with five layered media, $\sigma_1 = 0[S/m]$, $\sigma_2 = 10[S/m]$, $w = 1[unit\ lenght]$, for oscillating and monotonically decreasing conductivity profiles. Results for noisy data (Frangi, 2002) are contained in the square brackets.

Conductivity profile	layer # i	exact parameters		PM relative error [%]	
		z_i / w	σ_{i+1} / σ_2	z_i / w	σ_{i+1} / σ_2
oscillating	1	0	1	0 [0]	0.007[0.05]
	2	0.1	0.82	0.3 [3.1]	0.1 [1.7]
	3	0.2	1	0.4 [8.2]	0.07 [1.8]
	4	0.5	0.83	0.4 [5.5]	0.005 [0.6]
	5	2	1.13	0.4 [3.2]	0.1 [0.4]
monotonically decreasing	1	0	1	0 [0]	0.0003[0.01]
	2	0.1	0.82	0.1 [0.9]	0.03 [0.8]
	3	0.2	0.67	0.5 [4.2]	0.3 [0.8]
	4	0.5	0.56	0.2 [7]	1.2 [0.01]
	5	2	0.41	3.6 [11]	1.9 [3]

good reconstruction can be obtained via the proposed PM procedure for five layered WKB medium, even for noisy data [Figures 2(b),(d)], i.e., the corresponding maximal relative error in Table 3 is bounded by 5% (SNR $\to \infty$) up to 11% (SNR =60 dB). The successful reconstruction demonstrated in Figures 2(a),(b) and Table 3, for oscillating intrinsic reflection coefficients K_i, is due to the excellent agreement between the WKB potential $V(\rho)$ in (21) and the exact potential $\Phi(\mathbf{r}, \mathbf{r}') |_{z=z'=0, \sigma_1=0}$ in (14). As already noted, this excellent agreement is due to the oscillating reflection coefficients, leading to fast convergence of the image series expansion in (14) and, thus, to minimization of the truncation error caused by non WKB image terms that have been neglected in (21). This, however, is not the case for positive intrinsic reflection coefficients, leading to the somewhat less accurate reconstruction results depicted in Figures 2(c),(d). Note that, a successful reconstruction was demonstrated even for WKB profiles (Table 3) for which $\left|(\sigma_i - \sigma_{i+1}) / \sigma_i\right| \approx 2K_i \leq 0.3,\ \ i = 2,3,4,5$ (Eq. (18)). However, for non-WKB profiles (i.e., when $| (\sigma_i - \sigma_{i+1}) / \sigma_i |$ is much larger than 0.3), the reconstruction schemes have to be modified by replacing the WKB image series expansion in (20) with the rigorous image series representation in (14)-(18), and extending the spectral transformations and estimates accordingly.

Evidently, Table 3 reveals that the Legendre polynomial expansion scheme is preferable over the Fourier-Bessel transforms scheme (Dolgin, 2006), in view of its features, including a build in discretization and a finite extent window (i.e.,

Figure 2. Reconstructed conductivity profiles ($s = 2$): (a),(b) and (c),(d) corresponding to oscillating and monotonically decreasing conductivity profiles, respectively

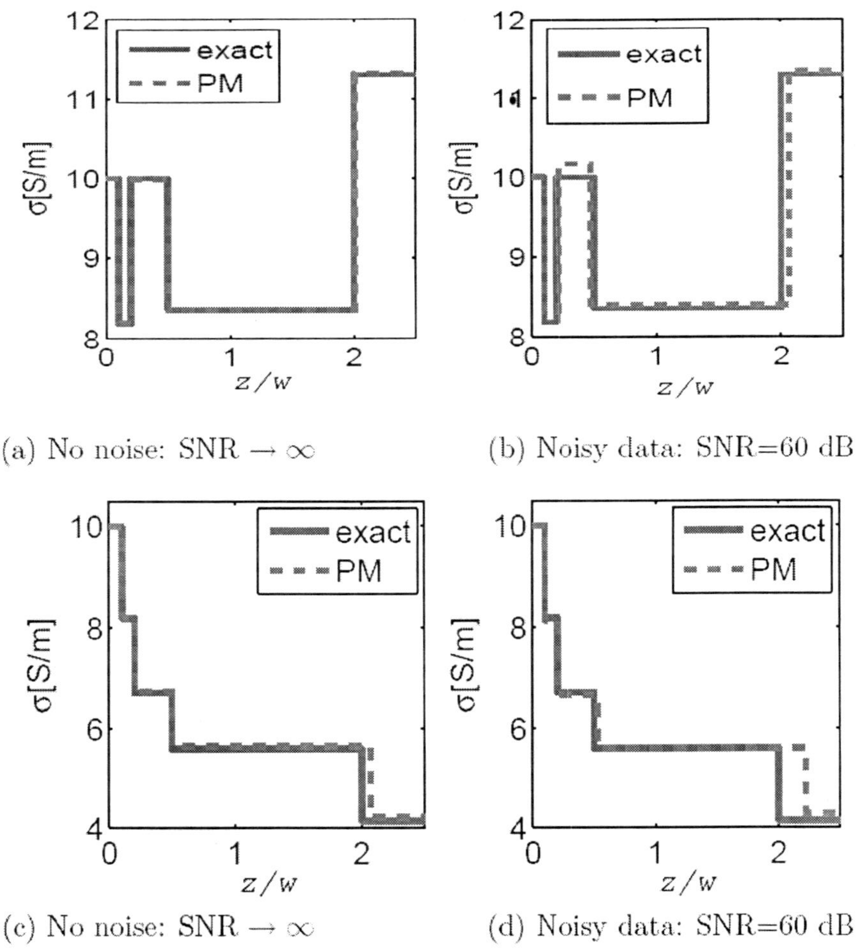

(a) No noise: SNR $\to \infty$

(b) Noisy data: SNR=60 dB

(c) No noise: SNR $\to \infty$

(d) Noisy data: SNR=60 dB

data truncation), leading to a better noise immunity and thus to a more accurate reconstruction.

Stable Reconstruction of Piecewise Continuous Layered Biological Tissues

An efficient reconstruction procedure can be executed through approximating the piecewise continuous profile by a piecewise constant profile, as depicted in Figure 3.

Mathematically, we denote the approximated piecewise constant conductivity by σ_p

$$\sigma(z) = \sigma_p, \quad \bar{z}_{p-1} < z < \bar{z}_p, \tag{35}$$

corresponding to the p-th layer via

$$p = 1, 2, ..., m+1, z_0 = -\infty, z_{m+1} = \infty. \tag{36}$$

It is readily noted that while $\sigma_i(z)$ in (3)-(4) corresponds to the actual piecewise continuous media, σ_p in (35)-(36) corresponds to its discretization via piecewise constant media, as depicted in Figure 3.

Figure 3. Discretization of a piecewise continuous conductivity profile

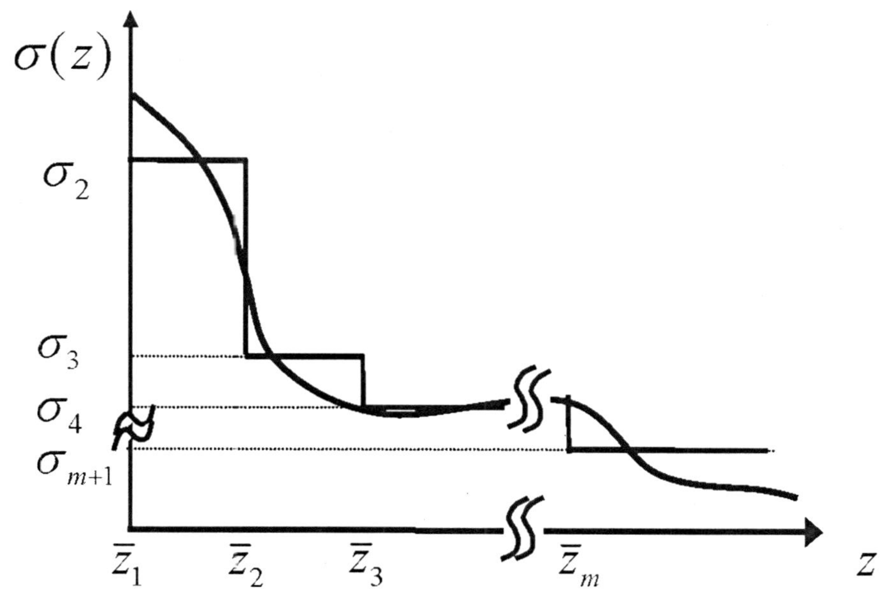

A reconstruction procedure can now be performed by utilizing the previously introduced **Legendre expansion** in conjunction with PM, which is most effective for WKB piecewise constant conductivity profiles (Sec. 3.3). This two-step reconstruction procedure, incorporating WKB image series expansion, are compered to the alternative, widely used, MLS method.

Alternative Reconstruction Procedure: MLS Method

Upon setting prescribed values fcr $\bar{z}_p$, the MLS error function ε, given via

$$\varepsilon = \frac{1}{L}\sum_{l=0}^{L-1}\left(V_{WKB}(\rho_l) - V(\rho_l)\right)^2, \tag{37}$$

is minimized by differentiation with respect to the normalized intrinsic reflection coefficients $\overline{K}_q$, as follows,

$$\frac{\partial \varepsilon}{\partial \overline{K}_q} = 0, \ \overline{K}_1 = \frac{I}{2\pi\sigma_2}, \ \overline{K}_q = \frac{IK_q}{\pi\sigma_2}, \ q = 2,3,\ldots,m. \tag{38}$$

Note that $V_{WKB}(\rho)$ and $V(\rho)$ are given in (21) and (11), respectively. The linear optimization problem, explicitly expressed as

$$\sum_{l=0}^{L-1}\left(\sum_{p=1}^{m}\frac{\overline{K}_p\rho}{\sqrt{\rho_l^2 + (2\bar{z}_p)^2}} - V(\rho_l)\right)\frac{\rho}{\sqrt{\rho_l^2 + (2\bar{z}_q)^2}} = 0,$$

$$q = 1,2,3,\ldots,m, \tag{39}$$

is solved by a matrix inversion. Subsequently, σ_p are reconstructed via Eqs. (18) and (38). Two $\bar{z}_p$ sets are selected for the MLS procedure (39): i) the standard equispaced set, referred as ESMLS, given by

Table 4. Conductivity profiles and corresponding reconstruction procedures parameters. For all three profiles, $b_2 = 10\ S / m$ and $z_3 / w = 2$. For PM procedure, $w = 1$ and $s = 4$.

profile	z_2 / w	b_3 / b_2	l_2	l_3	α	$\bar{z}_2 / w$	$\Delta z / w$
oscillating	1	0.6	$5\ m$	$-3\ m$	2.2	0.2	0.51
decreasing	0.5	0.95	$5\ m$	$9.5\ m$	1.75	0.15	0.54
non-WKB	0.5	0.8	$10 / 6\ m$	$4\ m$	1.76	0.12	0.63

$$\bar{z}_p = (p-1)\Delta z, \quad p = 1,2,\ldots,m, \tag{40}$$

and ii) a non-homogenous set, motivated via PM reconstruction results and referred as PMMLS,

$$\bar{z}_{p+2} - \bar{z}_{p+1} = \alpha(\bar{z}_{p+1} - \bar{z}_p), \quad p = 1,2,\ldots,m-2, \tag{41}$$

where α is a numerically measured constant.

Reconstruction of Four Layered Continuous Media

The simulations performed herein utilize three distinct four layered, $n+1=4$ (Eqs. (3) - (4)), continuous piecewise linear conductivity profiles, given via

$$\sigma_i(z) = \begin{cases} b_2(1 - z / l_2), & z_1 \le z \le z_2, \quad i = 2 \\ b_3(1 - z / l_3), & z_2 \le z \le z_3, \quad i = 3 \\ b_3(1 - z_3 / l_3), & z_3 \le z, \quad i = 4 \end{cases} . \tag{42}$$

and Table 4. Reconstruction results for three distinct conductivity profiles utilizing PM, PMMLS, and ESMLS methods, are depicted in Figure 4. Relative errors associated with the $p-th$ layer reconstruction, defined via

$$Error = 100\left(\int_{\bar{z}_{p-1}}^{\bar{z}_p} \left|\sigma_p - \sigma(z)\right| dz \Big/ \int_{\bar{z}_{p-1}}^{\bar{z}_p} \sigma(z) dz \right)[\%], \tag{43}$$

are specified in Table 5, including noisy data reconstructions.

Figures 4 and Table 5 readily demonstrate the potential promise and the successful implementation of the PM method for reconstruction of continuous conductivity profiles, significant extension of the reconstruction results for piecewise constant layered media outlined in section 3.3 (also, Dolgin, 2004 and Dolgin, 2006). Furthermore, profound analysis of the depths relations, provided by the PM scheme, reveals that there is almost constant ratio between the thickness of the layers (difference between the subsequent depths, Eq. (41)). Incorporating this observation in PMMLS, indeed leads to stable and accurate reconstructions, whereas the selection of a standard equispaced $\bar{z}_p$ set (Eq. (40)), results in poor and unstable reconstructions. It is noted that both PM and PMMLS methods perform very well even for non-WKB conductivity profile (Figures 4(e)-(f) and Table 5, bottom) and noisy measurements (Figures 4(b),(d),(f) and Table 5).

Figure 4. Reconstructed conductivity profiles, specified in Table 4: (a),(b) and (c),(d) correspond to oscillating and monotonically decreasing WKB conductivity profiles, respectively, (e),(f) correspond to non-WKB monotonically decreasing conductivity profile

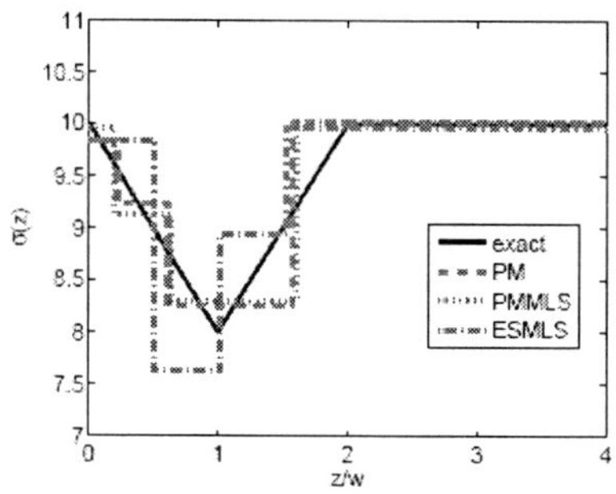

(a) No noise: SNR $\to \infty$

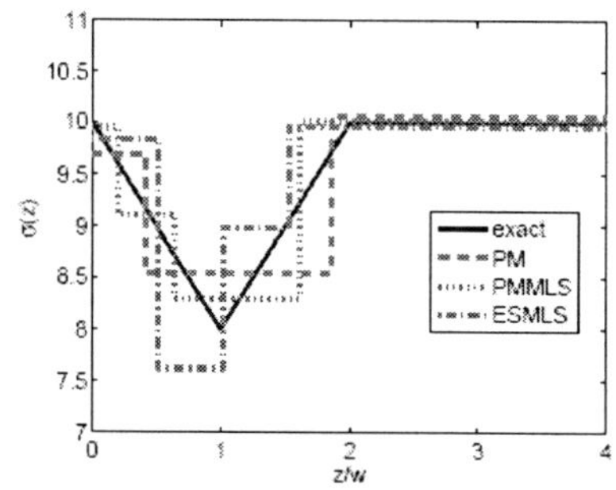

(b) Noisy data: SNR=60 dB

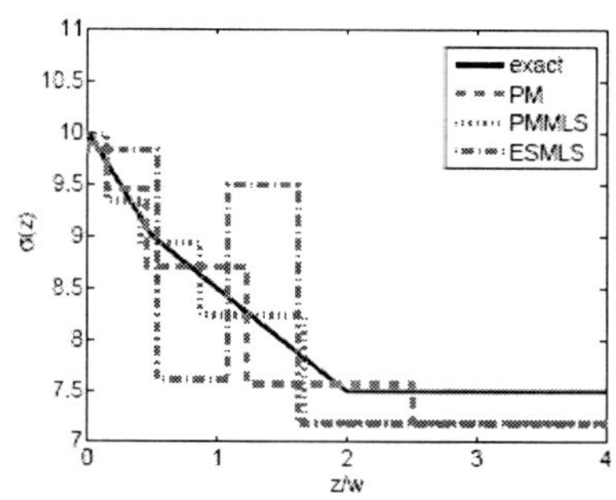

(c) No noise: SNR $\to \infty$

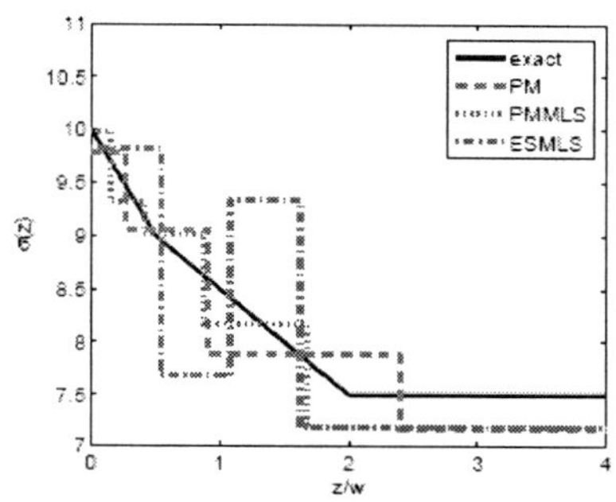

(d) Noisy data: SNR=60 dB

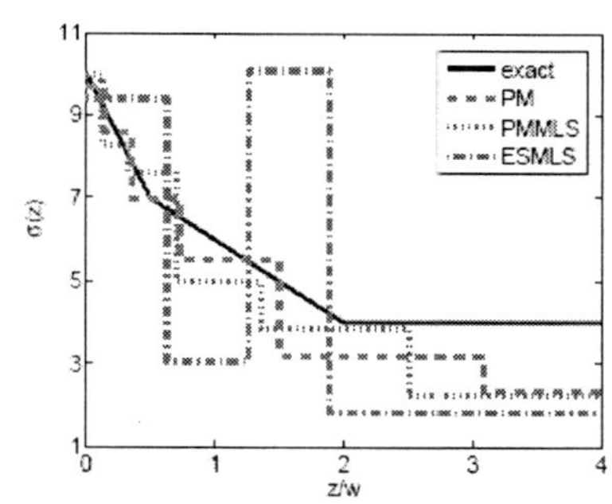

(e) No noise: SNR $\to \infty$

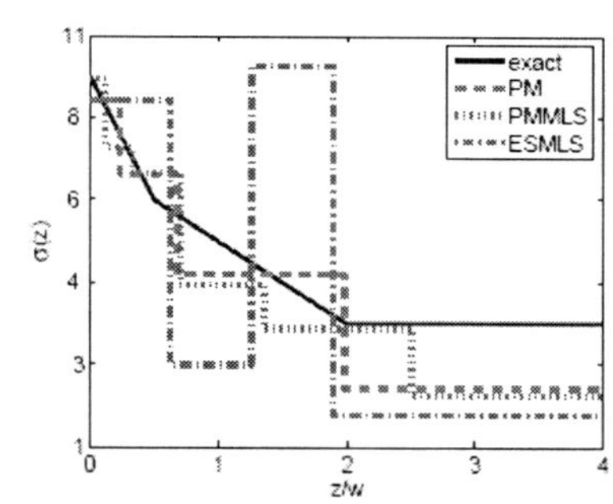

(f) Noisy data: SNR=60 dB

The measurements noise have a lesser effect on the relative error (Eq. (43)) here, than in Figure 2(b),(d) and Table 3, since the noise associated with the discretization of the continuous profile is dominant (Table 5). Finally, the discretization noise can be further reduced in PMMLS by increasing the layers number in Eq. (41).

At all, image theory signifies an appropriate **depth discretization** for EIT inversion, leading to a stable and accurate MLS reconstruction and rendering regularization techniques unnecessary.

FUTURE RESEARCH DIRECTIONS

It will take a while till the EIT will be adopted as a viable medical imaging technique as the additional research should be conducted on both

Table 5. Reconstruction results for the three distinct conductivity profiles, specified in Table 4, utilizing PM, PMMLS, and ESMLS methods. Results for noisy data ($\text{SNR}|_{\rho=sw} = 60\ dB$*, Frangi (2002)) are contained in the square brackets.*

		PM			PMMLS		ESMLS	
Conductivity Profile	Lay-er # i	$\bar{z}_i / w$	$\frac{\sigma_{i+1}}{\sigma_2(0)}$	Error [%]	$\frac{\sigma_{i+1}}{\sigma_2(0)}$	Error [%]	$\frac{\sigma_{i+1}}{\sigma_2(0)}$	Error [%]
oscillating	1	0.0004	0.983	1.2	0.996[0.995]	1.6[1.6]	0.984[0.984]	4[3.9]
	2	0.22[0.0014]	0.923[0.968]	2.2[2.3]	0.912[0.911]	2.4[2.4]	0.762[0.762]	10[10]
	3	0.61[0.41]	0.825[0.854]	3.7[4.7]	0.829[0.83]	3.7[3.6]	0.894[0.898]	4.7[5.1]
	4	1.6[1.86]	1.0014[1.007]	4.6[2.2]	1.002[1.001]	4.2[4.2]	0.997[0.996]	4.6 [4.6]
	5	2[2]	1.0014[1.007]	0.15[0.72]	1.002[1.001]	0.1[0.1]	0.997[0.996]	0.33 [0.38]
monotonically decreasing	1	0.00013	0.99	0.8	0.998[0.998]	1.3[1.3]	0.983[0.982]	4.2[4.1]
	2	0.145[0.0007]	0.946[0.98]	1.7[1.4]	0.934[0.931]	1.6[1.7]	0.762[0.769]	12.3[11.5]
	3	0.458[0.27]	0.87[0.906]	2.3[2.6]	0.893[0.901]	1.5[2]	0.949[0.934]	16.5[14.7]
	4	1.23[0.91]	0.757[0.788]	2.9[4.1]	0.824[0.817]	2.4[2.5]	0.717[0.718]	6.7[6.6]
	5	2.5[2.4]	0.718[0.717]	4.3[4.4]	0.718[0.719]	4.2[4.2]	0.717[0.718]	4.3[4.2]
monotonically decreasing, non-WKB	1	0.0005	0.966	2.2	0.997[0.995]	3.4[3.2]	0.939[0.939]	16[16]
	2	0.14[0.0016]	0.86[0.94]	3.9[4]	0.828[0.829]	4.9[4.8]	0.304[0.304]	50[50]
	3	0.36[0.24]	0.697[0.76]	4.3[7.7]	0.761[0.764]	7.9[8.2]	0.101[0.101]	108[108]
	4	0.73[0.68]	0.55[0.52]	7.5[12.3]	0.499[0.496]	16[16.6]	0.182[0.181]	56[56]
	5	1.5 [1.98]	0.32[0.24]	23.4[40]	0.384[0.388]	12[11]	0.182[0.181]	55[55]
	6	3.1	0.23	42	0.222[0.223]	44[44]		

instrumentation and inverse proceudre subject. In view of the current research, the following three topics can be further investigated:

i) EIT for curved layers, in particular cylindrical and spherical layers. Both the forward and the inverse solutions should be considered.
ii) EIT for three dimensionally varying conductivity profiles.
iii) Reconstruction of non-WKB profiles.

CONCLUSION

It has been readily demonstrated that incorporation of an appropriate forward model, herein, the image series expansion in conjunction with the WKB approximation, results in an effective and informative reconstruction scheme. The reconstruction schemes possess an important locality feature, assigning analytically to each spectral image term a local impedance associated with a unique layer, and thereby leading to efficient and accurate novel reconstruction procedures.

The reconstruction algorithm is preferable for shallow reconstruction, even when a noisy data is involved. It has been demonstrated that the Legendre polynomial expansion performs very well since both the finite extent window and the build-in discretization are its inherent features. Thus, our approach is effective for applications such as breast and skin cancer detection (Assenheimer, 2001) as well as biofilms thickness monitoring (Linderholm, 2007). It should be noted, however, that only inhomogeneous **depth discretization**, dictated by PM, leads to stable and accurate results, including the MLS procedures, and thus rendering regularization techniques unnecessary. Furthermore, the reconstructed media has to be only locally layered, i.e. it can slowly vary laterally as compared with Legendre finite-extent window width. In view of these observations, applying our physically motivated inhomogeneous coordinate discretization in other EIT algorithms may result in an inherent stabilization of these reconstruction algorithms.

The impulse response in (5)-(9) and (21), corresponding to the exact potential and its WKB approximation, respectively, is valid as long as the electrodes size (e.g., the diameter of electrodes S and P in Figure 1 is much smaller than both the layers thickness (Eqs. (3)-(4) and (35)-(36)) and the window width w (Eqs. (26)-(27)). While the effect of electrodes size is neglected throughout this paper, it can be accounted for (Cheng, 1989; Kim, 2007), particulary, in conjunction with the image series expansion [32].

Finally, for non-WKB profiles, the reconstruction schemes have to be modified by replacing the WKB image series expansion in (20) with the rigorous image series representation in (14)-(18), and extending the spectral transformations and estimates accordingly. Further extension of our method is required in order to adopt the findings of the current research for the real-life imaging needs. It can be carried out upon utilizing spherical and cylindrical layered conductive structures, for which closed form image series solutions are also available, thereby accounting for curvature correction.

REFERENCES

Abramowitz, M., & Stegun, I. A. (1970). *Handbook of Mathematical Functions*. New York: Dover Publications.

Assenheimer, M., Laver-Moskovitz, O., Malonek, D., Manor, D., Nahaliel, I., Nitzan, R., & Saad, A. (2001). The T-SCAN™ technology: electrical impedance as a diagnostic tool for brest cancer detection. *Physiological Measurement*, *22*(1), 1–8. doi:10.1088/0967-3334/22/1/301

Babaeizadeh, S., Brooks, D. H., & Isaacson, D. (2007). 3-D Electrical Impedance Tomography for Piecewise Constant Domains With Known Internal Boundaries. *IEEE Transactions on Bio-Medical Engineering*, *54*(1), 2–10. doi:10.1109/TBME.2006.886839

Barber, D. C., & Brown, B. H. (1984). Applied Potential Tomography. *Journal of Physics. E, Scientific Instruments*, *17*, 723–733. doi:10.1088/0022-3735/17/9/002

Barber, D. C., Brown, B. H., & Avis, N. J. (1992). Image Reconstruction in Electrical Impedance Tomography Using Filtered Back-Projection. *Proceedings of the Annual International Conference IEEE EMBS* (Paris, France), *14*, 1691 -1692.

Berryman, J. G., & Kohn, R. V. (1990). Variational Constraints for Electrical Impedance Tomography. *Physical Review Letters*, *65*(3). doi:10.1103/PhysRevLett.65.325

Borcea, L. (2003). Nonlinear multigrid for electrical impedance tomography, In *Proceedings of the SPIE - The International Society for Optical Engineering*: *Vol. 5016*(1), (pp. 49-58). Santa Clara, CA.

Brown, B. H. (2003). Electrical Impedance Tomography (EIT): a review. *Journal of Medical Engineering & Technology*, *27*(3), 97–108. doi:10.1080/0309190021000059687

Cheney, M., & Isaacson, D. (1995). Issues in Electrical Impedance Imaging. *IEEE Computational Science & Engineering*, *2*, 53–62. doi:10.1109/99.476369

Cheng, K. S., Isaacson, D., Newell, J. C., & Gisser, D. G. (1989). Electrode Models for Electric Current Computed Tomography. *IEEE Transactions on Bionedical Engineering*, *36*(9), 918–924. doi:10.1109/10.35300

Cherepin, V. A., Karpov, A. Y., Korjenevsky, A. V., Kornienko, V. N., Kultiasov, Y. S., & Oshapkin, M. B. (2002). Three-Dimensional EIT Imaging of Breast Tissues: System Design and Clinical Testing. *IEEE Transactions on Medical Imaging*, *21*(6), 662–667. doi:10.1109/TMI.2002.800602

Courant, R., & Hilbert, D. (1989). *Methods of mathematical physics*. New York: Wiley.

Dobson, D. C. (1992). Convergence of a reconstruction method for the inverse conductivity problem. *SIAM Journal on Applied Mathematics*, *52*(2), 442–458. doi:10.1137/0152025

Dolgin, M., & Einziger, P. D. (2004). Image series expansion for electrical impedance tomography. *Phyical. Review Letters, 93*(14), 148101/1-4.

Dolgin, M., & Einziger, P. D. (2006). Reconstruction of Layered Biological Tissues via Electrical Impedance Tomography. *IEEE Transactions on Bio-Medical Engineering*, *53*(12), 2464–2471. doi:10.1109/TBME.2006.884638

Dorn, O., Berteta-Aguirre, H., Berryman, J. G., & Papanicolaou, G. (1999). A nonlinear inversion method for 3D-electromagnetic imaging using adjoint fields. *Inverse Problems*, *15*, 1523–1558. doi:10.1088/0266-5611/15/6/309

Einziger, P. D., Livshitz, L. M., & Mizrahi, J. (2002). Rigorous image-series expansions of quasi-static Green's functions for regions with planar stratification. *IEEE Transactions on Antennas and Propagation*, *50*(12), 1813–1823. doi:10.1109/TAP.2002.807365

Einziger, P. D., Livshitz, L. M., & Mizrahi, J. (2006). Image Theory and Applications in Bioelectromagnetics. In Misra, J. C. (Ed.), *Biomathematics: Modeling and Stimulation* (pp. 315–358). Singapore: World Scientific. doi:10.1142/9789812774859_0012

Erdelyi, A. (1954). *Tables of integral transforms* (*Vol. II*). New York: McGraw-Hill.

Frangi, A. R., Riu, P. J., Rosell, J., & Viergever, M. A. (2002). Propagation of measurement noise through backprojection reconstruction in electrical impedance tomography. *IEEE Transactions on Medical Imaging*, *21*(6), 566–578. doi:10.1109/TMI.2002.800612

Frohlich, H. (1958). *Theory of dielectrics: dielectric constant and dielectric loss*. Oxford, UK: Clarendon Press.

Goharian, M., Bruwer, M., Jegatheesan, A., & Moran, G.R., & MacGregor. (2007). A novel approach for EIT regularization via spatial and spectral principal component analysis. *Physiological Measurement*, *28*(9), 1001–1016. doi:10.1088/0967-3334/28/9/003

Hamming, R. W. (1986). *Numerical Methods for Scientists and Engineers*. New York: Dover.

Haus, H. A., & Melcher, J. R. (1989). *Electromagnetic fields and energy*. Englewood Cliffs, NJ: Prentice-Hall.

Henderson, R. P., & Webster, J. G. (1978). An Impedance Camera for Spatially Specific Measurements of the Thorax. *IEEE Transactions on Bio-Medical Engineering*, *25*, 250–254. doi:10.1109/TBME.1978.326329

Holder, D. S. (Ed.). (2005). *Electrical Impedance Tomography, Methods, History and Applications*. Bristol, UK: IOP.

Ingerman, D. V. (2000). Discrete and continuous Dirichlet-to-Neumann maps in the layered case. *SIAM Journal on Mathematical Analysis*, *31*(6), 1214–1234. doi:10.1137/S0036141097326581

Isaacson, D., Mueller, J. L., Newell, J. C., & Siltanen, S. (2004). Reconstruction of Chest Phantoms by the D-Bar Method for Electrical Impedance Tomography. *IEEE Transactions on Medical Imaging*, *23*(7), 821–828. doi:10.1109/TMI.2004.827482

Isakov, V. (1998). *Inverse Problems for Partial Differential Equations*. Wichita, KA: Springer.

Jerbi, K., Lionheart, W. R. B., Vauhkonen, P. J., & Vauhkonen, M. (2000). Sensitivity matrix and reconstruction algorithm for EIT assuming axial uniformity. *Physiological Measurement*, *21*, 61–66. doi:10.1088/0967-3334/21/1/308

Kallman, J. S., & Berryman, J. G. (1992). Weighted least-squares criteria for electrical impedance tomography. *IEEE Transactions on Medical Imaging*, *11*(2), 284–292. doi:10.1109/42.141653

Keller, G. V., & Frischknecht, F. C. (1966). *Electrical Methods in Geophysical Prospecting*. Oxford, UK: Pergamon Press.

Kim, B. S., Boverman, G., Newell, J. C., Saulnier, G. J., & Isaacson, D. (2007). The complete electrode model for EIT in a mammography geometry. *Physiological Measurement*, *8*(7), S57–S69. doi:10.1088/0967-3334/28/7/S05

Kohn, R. V., & Vogelius, M. (1985). Determining conductivity by boundary measurements II. Interior results. *Communications on Pure and Applied Mathematics*, *38*(5), 643–667. doi:10.1002/cpa.3160380513

Kolehmainen, V., Vauhkonen, M., Karjalainen, P. A., & Kaipio, J. P. (1997). Spatial inhomogeneity and regularization in EIT. *Proceedings of the 19th Annual International Conference of the IEEE Engineering in Medicine and Biology SocietY,* (1, pp. 449-452). Chicago.

Korjenevsky, A., Cherepin, V., & Sapetsky, A. (2000). Magnetic Induction Tomography: experimental realisation. *Physiological Measurement*, *21*(1), 89–94. doi:10.1088/0967-3334/21/1/311

Levy, S., Adam, D., & Bresler, Y. (2002). Electromagnetic Impedance Tomography (EMIT): A New Method for Impedance Imaging. *IEEE Transactions on Medical Imaging*, *21*(6), 676–687. doi:10.1109/TMI.2002.800573

Linderholm, P., Vannod, J., Barrandon, Y., & Renaud, P. (2007). Bipolar resistivity profiling of 3D tissue culture. *Biosensors & Bioelectronics*, *22*, 789–796. doi:10.1016/j.bios.2006.02.016

Lionheart, W. R. (2004). EIT reconstruction algorithms: pitfalls, challenges and recent developments. *Physiological Measurement*, *25*(1), 125–142. doi:10.1088/0967-3334/25/1/021

Livshitz, L. M., Einziger, P. D., & Mizrahi, J. (2001). A model of finite electrodes in layered media: a hybrid image series and moment method scheme. *Journal of the Applied Computational Electromagnetics*, *16*(2), 145–154.

Metherall, P. (1998). *Three Dimensional Electrical Impedance Tomography of the Human Thorax*. (Ph.D. Thesis), University of Sheffield, UK.

Morse, P. M., & Feshbach, H. (1953). *Methods of Theoretical Physics*. New York: McGraw-Hill.

Mueller, J. L., Siltanen, S., & Isaacson, D. (2002). A direct reconstruction algorithm for electrical impedance tomography. *IEEE Transactions on Medical Imaging*, *21*(6), 555–559. doi:10.1109/TMI.2002.800574

Nachman, A. I. (1996). Global Uniqueness for a Two-Dimensional Inverse Boundary Value Problem. *The Annals of Mathematics*, *143*(1), 71–96. doi:10.2307/2118653

Osypka, M., & Gersing, E. (1995). Tissue impedance spectra and the appropriate frequencies for EIT. *Physiological Measurement*, *16*(3A), A49–A55. doi:10.1088/0967-3334/16/3A/005

Ross, A. S., Saulnier, G. J., Newell, J. C., & Isaacson, D. (2003). Current Source Design for Electrical Impedance Tomography. *Physiological Measurement*, *24*(2), 509–516. doi:10.1088/0967-3334/24/2/361

Soleimani, M., Powell, C. E., & Polydorides, N. (2005). Improving the Forward Solver for the Complete Electrode Model in EIT Using Algebraic Multigrid. *IEEE Transactions on Medical Imaging*, *24*(5), 577–583. doi:10.1109/TMI.2005.843741

Somersalo, E., Cheney, M., Isaacson, D., & Isaacson, E. (1991). Layer stripping: a direct numerical method for impedance imaging. *Inverse Problems*, *7*, 899–926. doi:10.1088/0266-5611/7/6/011

Sylvester, J. (1992). A convergent layer striping algorithm for the radially symmetric impedance tomography problem. *Communications in Partial Differential Equations*, *17*(11&12), 1955–1994.

Trigo, F. C., Gonzalez-Lima, R., & Amato, M. B. P. (2004). Electrical Impedance Tomography Using the Extended Kalman Filter. *IEEE Transactions on Medical Imaging*, *51*(1), 72–81.

Watson, S., Williams, R. J., Griffiths, H., Gough, W., & Morris, A. (2003). Magnetic induction tomography: phase versus vector-voltmeter measurement techniques. *Physiological Measurement*, *24*(2), 555–564. doi:10.1088/0967-3334/24/2/365

Yorkey, T., Webster, J. G., & Tompkins, W. J. (1987). Comparing reconstruction algorithms for electrical impedance tomography. *IEEE Transactions on Bio-Medical Engineering*, *34*, 843–852. doi:10.1109/TBME.1987.326032

Zlochiver, S., Freimark, D., Arad, M., Adunsky, A., & Abboud, S. (2006). Parametric EIT for monitoring cardiac stroke volume. *Physiological Measurement*, *27*, S139–S146. doi:10.1088/0967-3334/27/5/S12

Zlochiver, S., Rosenfeld, M., & Abboud, S. (2003). Induced-Current Electrical Impedance Tomography: A 2-D Theoretical Simulation. *IEEE Transactions on Medical Imaging*, *22*(12), 1550–1560. doi:10.1109/TMI.2003.820025

ADDITIONAL READING

Hyvönen, N. (2004). Complete electrode model of electrical impedance tomography: Approximation properties and characterization of inclusions. *SIAM Journal on Applied Mathematics*, *64*(3), 902–931. doi:10.1137/S0036139903423303

Jonsson, E. (1999). Electrical conductivity reconstruction using nonlocal boundary conditions. *SIAM Journal on Applied Mathematics*, *59*(5), 1582–1598. doi:10.1137/S0036139997327770

KEY TERMS AND DEFINITIONS

Electrical Impedance Tomography (EIT): is a medical imaging technique in which an image of the conductivity or permittivity of part of the body is inferred from surface electrical measurements. Typically, conducting electrodes are attached to the skin of the subject and small alternating currents are applied to some or all of the electrodes. The resulting electrical potentials are measured, and the process may be repeated for numerous different configurations of applied current. The invention of EIT as a medical imaging technique is usually attributed to John G. Webster and a publication in 1978 (Henderson,1978) although the first practical realisation of a medical EIT system was detailed in 1984 due to the work of David C. Barber and Brian H. Brown (Barber, 1984) (form http://en.wikipedia.org/wiki/Electrical_impedance_tomography).

Inverse Problem: is the task that often occurs in many branches of science and mathematics where the values of some model parameter(s) must be obtained from the observed data. Inverse problems are typically ill posed, as opposed to the well-posed problems more typical when modeling physical situations where the model parameters or material properties are known. Of the three conditions for a well-posed problem suggested by Jacques Hadamard (existence, uniqueness, stability of the solution or solutions) the condition of stability is most often violated. In the sense of functional analysis, the inverse problem is represented by a mapping between metric spaces. While inverse problems are often formulated in infinite dimensional spaces, limitations to a finite number of measurements, and the practical consideration of recovering only a finite number of unknown parameters, may lead to the problems being recast in discrete form. In this case the inverse problem will typically be *ill-conditioned*. In these cases, regularization may be used to introduce mild assumptions on the solution and prevent overfitting. Many instances of regularized inverse problems can be interpreted as special cases of Bayesian inference.

A Forward Problem (direct problem, normal problem): is the problem of calculating what should be observed for a particular model, e.g. calculating the potential that would be measured for a given model. A forward problem is in general a well posed problem in contrast to an inverse problem.

Quasistatic electromagnetic fields: is the fields description in the low frequency (large wavelength) regim. Maxwell's equations are significantly simplifed in this limit enabling an effictive design and implementation in many branches of electrical engineering.

Image Theory (or Image Series Expansion): is a basic problem-solving tool in quasistatics, which enables representation of a point source response (Green's function), associated with generally complex configuration, in terms of elementary point source responses (mirror sources). The name originates from the replacement of certain elements in the original layout with imaginary sources, which replicates the boundary conditions of the problem (i.e., Dirichlet boundary conditions or Neumann boundary conditions).

Poisson's Equation: is a partial differential equation with broad utility in electrostatics, mechanical engineering and theoretical physics. It is named after the French mathematician, geometer and physicist Siméon-Denis Poisson. The Poisson equation is $\Delta\phi = f$ where Δ is the Laplace operator, and *f* and φ are real or complex-valued functions on a manifold. When the manifold is Euclidean space, the Laplace operator is often denoted as ∇^2 and so Poisson's equation is frequently written as $\nabla^2\phi = f$ In three-dimensional Cartesian coordinates, it takes the form $\left(\frac{\partial^2}{\partial x^2} + \frac{\partial^2}{\partial y^2} + \frac{\partial^2}{\partial z^2}\right)\phi\left(x, y, z\right) = f\left(x, y, z\right)$. For vanishing *f*, this equation becomes Laplace's equation $\Delta\phi = 0$ The Poisson equation may be solved using a Green's function (http://en.wikipedia.org/wiki/Poisson's_equation).

Legendre Expansion: expresses an arbitrary (finite extent) function in terms of Legendre functions.

Legendre Functions: are solutions to Legendre's differential equation, $\frac{d}{dx}\left[\left(1 - x^2\right)\frac{d}{dx}P_n(x)\right] + n(n+1)P_n(x) = 0$. They are named after Adrien-Marie Legendre.

This ordinary differential equation is frequently encountered in physics and other technical fields. In particular, it occurs when solving Laplace's equation (and related partial differential equations) in spherical coordinates. The Legendre differential equation may be solved using the standard power series method. The equation has regular singular points at $x = \pm 1$ so, in general, a series solution about the origin will only converge for $|x| < 1$. When n is an integer, the solution $P_n(x)$ that is regular at $x = 1$ is also regular at $x = -1$, and the series for this solution terminates (i.e. is a polynomial). These solutions for $n = 0, 1, 2,...$ (with the normalization $P_n(1) = 1$) form a polynomial sequence of orthogonal polynomials called the Legendre polynomials. Each Legendre polynomial $P_n(x)$ is an nth-degree polynomial. It may be expressed using Rodrigues' formula: $P_n(x) = \frac{1}{2^n n!} \frac{d^n}{dx^n}\left[\left(x^2 - 1\right)^n\right]$. The shifted Legendre polynomials (utilized in this chapter) are defined as $\tilde{P}_n(x) = P_n(2x - 1)$. Here the "shifting" function $x \rightarrow (2x-1)$ (in fact, it is an affine transformation) is chosen such that it bijectively maps the interval [0, 1] to the interval [−1, 1], implying that the polynomials $\tilde{P}_n(x)$ are orthogonal on [0,1]: $\int_0^1 \tilde{P}_m(x)\tilde{P}_n(x)dx = \frac{1}{2n+1}\delta_{mn}$. An explicit expression for the shifted Legendre polynomials is given by $\tilde{P}_n(x) = (-1)^n \sum_{k=0}^{n} \binom{n}{k}\binom{n+k}{k}(-x)^k$, The analogue of Rodrigues' formula for the shifted Legendre polynomials is $\tilde{P}_n(x) = \left(n!\right)^{-1} \frac{d^n}{dx^n}\left[\left(x^2 - x\right)^n\right]$. (from http://en.wikipedia.org/wiki/Legendre_polynomials)

Prony's method (Prony analysis): was developed by Gaspard Riche de Prony in 1795. However, practical use of the method awaited the digital computer. Similar to the Fourier transform, Prony's method extracts valuable information from a uniformly sampled signal and builds a series of damped complex exponentials or sinusoids. This allows for the estimation of frequency, amplitude, phase and damping components of a signal. (from http://en.wikipedia.org/wiki/Prony's_method)

Mean Least Square: method is applied to approximate solutions of overdetermined systems, i.e. systems of equations in which there are more equations than unknowns. Least squares method is often applied in statistical contexts, particularly regression analysis. Least squares may be interpreted as a method of fitting data. The best fit, between modeled data and observed data, in its least-squares sense, is an instance of the model for which the sum of squared residuals has its least value, where a residual is the difference between an observed value and the value provided by the model. The method was first described by Carl Friedrich Gauss around 1794. Least squares corresponds to the maximum likelihood criterion if the experimental errors have a normal distribution and can also be derived as a method of moments estimator. Regression analysis is available in most statistical software packages. (from http://en.wikipedia.org/wiki/Least_squares).

APPENDIX A

Algorithms for Image Reconstruction via EIT

A.1 Problem Definition

The inverse conductivity problem consists of determining an unknown impedance distribution $\gamma(\mathbf{r}) = \sigma(\mathbf{r}) + j\omega\varepsilon(\mathbf{r})$, , where $\mathbf{r}$ denotes the coordinates of the point inside a bounded volume $\Omega \in \mathbf{R}^n$, n=*2* or *3*, from the knowledge of the Dirichlet-to-Neumann, or voltage-to-current, map (see Figure 5).

The inverse impedance problem is modeled by the generalized Laplace equation

$$\nabla \cdot \gamma \nabla \Phi = 0 \quad \text{in} \quad \Omega \tag{44}$$

where $\Phi(\mathbf{r})$ represents the electric potential and $\gamma(\mathbf{r})$ represents the impedance. Applying a known voltage V on the boundary of the region $\Omega \in \mathbf{R}^n$, n=*2*, corresponds to the Dirichlet boundary condition

$$\Phi = V \quad \text{on} \quad \partial\Omega \tag{45}$$

and knowledge of the resulting current density distribution gives rise to the Neumann boundary condition

$$\gamma \frac{\partial \Phi}{\partial \nu} = j \quad \text{on} \quad \partial\Omega \tag{46}$$

Figure 5. Physical configuration of the two dimensional EIT problem. Current I is driven into the region Ω *through electrodes a-b on the surface* $\partial\Omega$*. Surface voltage measurements V are made through electrodes c-d. The internal conductivity of* Ω *is* σ*, while the surrounding region is assumed to have zero conductivity.*

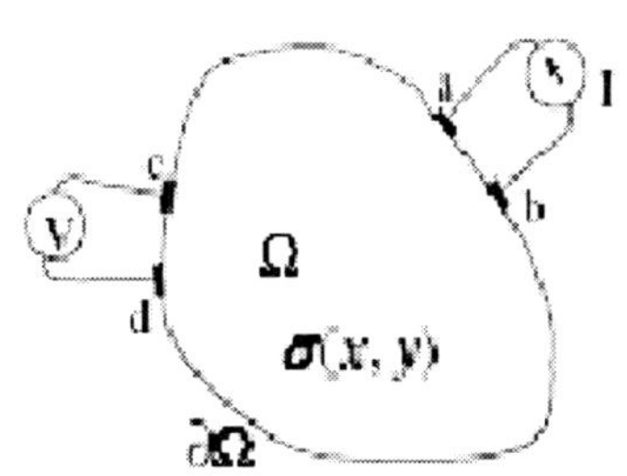

where ν denotes the inward normal to $\partial\Omega$. The mapping, which takes a given voltage distribution on the boundary to the resulting current density distribution on the boundary is referred to as the Dirichlet-to-Neumann or voltage-to-current map and is denoted by Λ_γ (Ingerman, 2000). Since the physical interpretation of Λ_γ is knowledge of the resulting current on the boundary of Ω corresponding to all possible voltage distributions on the boundary, it is taken to be the input data for reconstruction algorithms. Analytical solution of (44) is only possible for simple geometries and boundary conditions.

A.2 Reconstruction Algorithms

The impedance imaging problem is nonlinear and ill-posed (Brown, 2003). Unlike the forward Dirichlet problem, the inverse problem, when considered as Cauchy problem, is expected to be unstable as progressing to the interior from the boundaries. Nevertheless, a huge amount of inverse algorithms have arisen during last two decades. The existing algorithms can be associated with one of the following class: (a) noniterative linearization-based algorithms, (b) iterative algorithms solving the full nonlinear problem, and (c) algorithms using *analytic* derivations, such as layer stripping and $\bar{\partial}$ method.

Examples of linearization algorithms are backprojection method (Barber, 1992), borrowed from computed tomography (CT), sensitivity matrix method (Jerbi, 2000; Metherall, 1998) and one-step NOSER method (Cheney,1995). Linearization algorithms are based on the premise that the conductivity differs only slightly from a known, often constant, conductivity. However, this assumption is often incorrect in physiological applications. Moreover, in many cases the sensitivity matrix is ill-conditioned and methods like singular value decomposition need to be applied or some other feasibility constraints should be involved (Berryman, 1990).

Algorithms solving the full nonlinear problem are iterative in nature. These iterative algorithms are based on output least-squares (Yorkey, 1987; Dorn, 1999; Zlochiver, 2003) in conjunction with modified Newton-Raphson method. While these approaches are promising for obtaining accurate reconstructed conductivity values, they may be slow to converge and often require the computation and inversion of the Hessian matrix which is ill-conditioned, so regularization techniques are usually needed. The representative of these algorithms, the modified Newton-Raphson method, is described in details in the next subsection.

The main disadvantage of the methods mentioned above is the lack of analytical insight of the forward solution. Recently, a new class of algorithms has emerged. The distinguishing feature of the algorithms such as layer stripping (Somersalo, 1991; Sylvester, 1992) and $\bar{\partial}$ (Mueller, 1992) methods is incorporation of some, analytically derived, tools and considerations into the inverse problem solution. So they have a potential to solve the nonlinear problem with satisfactory accuracy. Thus, both algorithms are presented in what follows.

Modified Newton-Raphson Method

The modified Newton-Raphson method uses a FEM solver and a modified Newton-Raphson iterative method (Yorkey, 1987) to compute the conductivity distribution. The region Ω is partitioned into a number of discrete elements, each with assumed uniform conductivity. The forward problem is then solved for each element by ensuring continuity of voltage and current flow between the neighboring elements. A forward transform ***F*** describing the relationship between the boundary voltages ***V*** and the conductivity σ is given by:

$$V = F(\sigma) \tag{46}$$

The quadratic error $e(\sigma)$ between the computed voltages V (see Eq. 46) and the measured voltages V_0 is defined by:

$$e(\sigma) = \frac{1}{2}\left(\mathbf{F}(\sigma) - V_0\right)^T \left(\mathbf{F}(\sigma) - V_0\right) \tag{47}$$

Minimization of this error with respect to the conductivity gives:

$$e'(\sigma) = \left(\mathbf{F}'(\sigma)\right)^T \left(\mathbf{F}(\sigma) - V_0\right) = 0 \tag{48}$$

where $\left[\mathbf{F}'(\sigma)\right]_{ij} = \frac{\partial \mathbf{F}_i}{\partial \sigma_j}$ and is called the Jacobian matrix. Finding the Taylor expansion of equation (48) and ignoring the non-linear terms, a correction factor for the conductivity at the kth iteration is obtained:

$$\Delta\sigma^k = -\left(\left\{\mathbf{F}'(\sigma^k)\right\}^T \left\{\mathbf{F}'(\sigma^k)\right\}\right)^{-1} \left\{\mathbf{F}'(\sigma^k)\right\}^T \left(\mathbf{F}(\sigma^k) - V_0\right) \tag{49}$$

The updated conductivity distribution calculated by:

$$\sigma^{k+1} = \sigma^k + \Delta\sigma^k \tag{50}$$

The process is repeated with the updated conductivity distribution σ^{k+1} till the convergence.

As it was mentioned above, two main problems of this type of algorithms are the rapid use of FEM (or another numerical) solver for the forward problem and inversion of ill-conditioned matrix $\left(\left\{\mathbf{F}'(\sigma^k)\right\}^T \left\{\mathbf{F}'(\sigma^k)\right\}\right)$, both at each iteration step. These result in an unacceptable computational time. Furthermore, the method is prone for many local minima.

Layer Stripping Algorithm

The layer stripping method (Somersalo, 1991) is built of two steps, namely (1) the reconstruction of the conductivity σ at the boundary of a disc or sphere (of radius r_0), and, using this information, (2) the synthesis of the data on an interior surface of radius $r_0 - \Delta$. The algorithm utilizes some analytical properties of the forward operator and the characteristics of high frequency waves. Optimal currents are used to facilitate a direct (non-iterative) solution to the full non-linear reconstruction problem.

Advantages of this method are that it is a direct method of obtaining an approximate solution to the full non linear problem and it is fast comparing to other iterative schemes. However, the quality of images obtained from the reconstruction of real data was rather poor (Cheney, 1995). The authors attribute this to the introduction of further instabilities into the already ill-posed problem.

D-Bar Method

The method, based on the two-dimensional global uniqueness proof of inverse boundary value problem by Nachman (Nachman, 1996), which implements $\bar{\partial}$ method of inverse scattering for EIT problem, consists of two steps:

$$\Lambda_{\sigma} \xrightarrow{1} t \xrightarrow{2} \sigma,$$

where the intermediate object $t : \mathbf{C} \to \mathbf{C}$ is called the *(nonphysical) scattering transform*, σ denotes the conductivity inside the region Ω, and Λ_{σ} is Dirichlet-to-Neumann map. The idea behind the algorithm is to transform the generalized Laplace equation (44) to the Schrodinger equation and use the $\bar{\partial}$ method of inverse scattering to solve the resulting inverse problem.

Chapter 7
Intelligent Decision Support System for Fetal Delivery using Soft Computing Techniques

R. R. Janghel
Indian Institute of Information Technology and Management Gwalior, India

Anupam Shukla
Indian Institute of Information Technology and Management Gwalior, India

Ritu Tiwari
Indian Institute of Information Technology and Management Gwalior, India

ABSTRACT

In the present work an attempt is made to develop an intelligent decision support system (IDSS) using the pathological attributes to predict the fetal delivery to be done normal or by surgical procedure. The pathological tests like Blood Sugar (BR), Blood pressure (BP), Resistivity Index (RI) and systolic / Diastolic (S/P) ratio will be recorded at the time of delivery. All attributes lie within a specific range for normal patient. The database consists of the attributes for cases 2 (i.e. normal and surgical delivery). Soft computing technique namely Artificial Neural Networks (ANN) are used for simulator. The attributes from dataset are used for training & testing of ANN models. Three models of ANN are trained using Back-Propagation Algorithm (BPA), Radial Basis Function Network (RBFN), Learning Vector Quantization Network (LVQN) and one hybrid approach is Adaptive Neuro-Fuzzy Inference System (ANFIS). The designing factors have been changed to get the optimized model, which gives highest recognition score. The optimized models of BPA, RBFN, LVQN and ANFIS gave accuracies of 93.75, 99.00, 87.50 and 99.50% respectively. Hence in our present research the ANFIS is the model whom efficiency and result are best.The ANFIS is the best network for mentioned problem. This system will assist doctor to take decision at the critical time of fetal delivery.

DOI: 10.4018/978-1-61692-004-3.ch007

INTRODUCTION

The motivation behind the present research work is that much less have been contributed so far in literature with regard to fetal delivery. Further the proposed system use intelligent techniques with sound improvement in efficiency.

The present research shall assist the doctor to take right decisions in many complex situations where when a minor mistake can lead to death of the patient. The three ANN architectures, Back-Propagation Network (BPN), Radial Basis Function Networks (RBFN), and Learning Vector Quantization Networks (LVQN) and Adaptive Neuro-Fuzzy Inference System (ANFIS) are used here.

A Back-Propagation Network is a multi-layered feed-forward neural network, making use of Back-propagation algorithm, which involves giving the input vector to the network, comparison of the desired and the network output for the input vector, changing each weight by an amount equal to the derivative of the error with respect to that weight times some learning rate (Shukla Anupam 2009).

RBFN consists of three different layers- an input layer, a hidden layer and an output layer. The hidden units are known as Radial centers and have the same dimensions as that of the input vector. The transformation from the Input space to the hidden space is non-linear whereas the transformation from the hidden unit space to the output space is linear. In the hidden neurons, usually Gaussian activation function is used (Yegnanarayana B. 2003,Orr M.J.L 1996). We use a parameter called spread which controls the network performance. Larger spread means a smoother function approximation.

Learning vector quantization (LVQ) Network consists of an input layer, a competitive layer and a linear layer. For an input, the neurons in the competitive layer compete with each other and the neuron with the most positive output becomes the winning neuron. The weights of the winning neuron (a row of the input weight matrix) are adjusted with the Kohonen learning rule. The only requirement in this network is that the competitive layer must have enough neurons, and each class must be assigned enough competitive neurons (Ghosh, A 2005). Neural Network and fuzzy Toolbox of MATLAB are used (MATLAB, 2000). The ANFIS model can construct an input-output mapping based on both the fuzzy if-then rules and the stipulated input-output data pairs. The if-then rules of SFIM are often applied for obtaining the inference on an imprecise model. A conclusion can be reached in the indefinite system, which is better than human experience. These if-then rules based on stipulated input-output training data pairs suitable membership function (MF) are then produced. The ANFIS model employs the neural network training procedure to adjust the membership function and associated parameter that approaches the desired data sets (Jian-Da Wu 2009).

BACKGROUND

The expert systems are tremendously used in health care involving predicting and diagnosing a particular disease. Medical expert systems are useful in certain situations where either the case is quite complex or there are no medical experts readily available for patients (Zaheeruddin, Garima 2006,Fahad Shahbaz Khan 2008). In past decades, various methods and systems have been proposed to efficiently expertise from domain experts. The time scales into consideration, such that the variant of disease symptoms in different time scales can be precisely expressed (Gwo-Haur Hwang 2006). The use of a fuzzy expert system to predict the need for advanced neonatal resuscitation efforts in the delivery room. This system relates the maternal medical, obstetric and neonatal characteristics to the clinical conditions of the newborn (Braz J Med Biol Res 2004). The diagnosis and management of neonatal birth injuries has been developed for the use of general practitioners and obstetricians handling large number of deliveries (Veena Kumari, C.2002). The blood pressure and heart rate used for early risk assessment, hypertension complications and as a guide to preventive intervention during pregnancy (Ayala, D.E 2002). The hierarchical network where stage networks are radial basis function networks (HRBFN) and using the nearest neighbor method as decision rule instead of the approximation method used (Ky Van Ha, 1998). Success of neural networks in medical diagnosis depends not only on the learning mechanisms and network structure but also on the data quality (Cohen, M.E.2002. Beat-to-beat interval (BBI) and symbolic blood pressure (SP) interactions in pregnant women with chronic hypertension in comparison to those in normotensive pregnant (PRE) and non-pregnant women (Voss, A. 2003).

MAIN FOCUS OF THE CHAPTER

The motivation behind the present research work is that much less have been contributed so far in literature with regard to fetal delivery. Further the proposed system use intelligent techniques with sound improvement in efficiency. This work can assist the doctors for easily diagnosis of the patients. The doctors can also compare their diagnosis with neural networks and reconsider those cases where there is a mismatch between their assessment and diagnosis results obtain from using Artificial Neural Networks models.

Methodology

Figure 1 shows the overall diagram of complete methodology. The collection from blood samples have been done for like Blood Pressure (BP), Blood sugar (BR), Resistivity Index (RI) and Systolic / diastolic (S/P) ratio. Based on the tests results our expert system will predict that the fetal delivery will be done, by normal process or by the surgical operation. If the expert system output will be

Figure 1. Block diagram of complete methodology

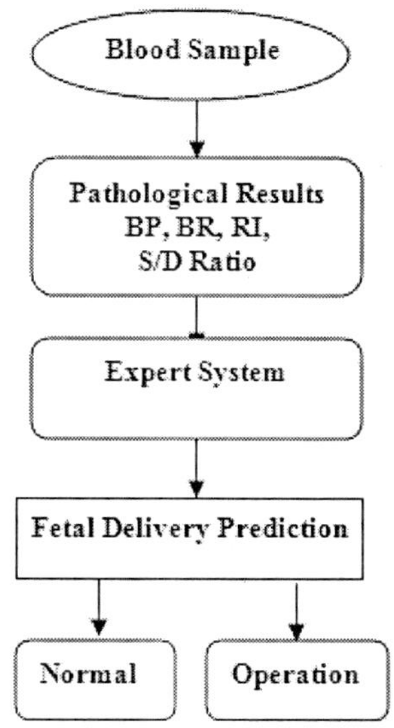

come 0 means fetal delivery done through surgical operation and if 1 delivery through normal process.

Description of Data-Set

The data-set for women pregnancy & delivery was collected and recorded for 640 instances at the time of delivery, which consists of 4 attributes. The attributes are detailed as in the Table 1. In the ANN model the number of instances in training data set is 480 and in testing set are 160.

Simulation Model of ANN using BPA

The BPA normally makes use of the gradient descent to compute the new value of the weight sand biases. It is hence quickly able to adjust the network weights for good performance. The graph or space denoting the error of the system for every combination of weights and biases is called as the error space. The aim of any training algorithm is to find the global optima in this search space. BPA may many a times get trapped in local minima. This is due to the absence of any global guiding strategy or the attempt to cover the

Table 1. Complete attribute documentation

	Goal	Learning Rate	No. of Neurons in Hidden Layer	No. of Epochs	MSE	% Accuracy of Diagnosis
Training Data	0.01	0.001	50	30,000	0.01	95.83
Testing Data	0.01	0.001	50	30,000	0.01	93.75

entire error space which is highly complex and of high dimensionality. The feed- forward neural network architecture used in this experiment consisted of one hidden layers along with input and output layers shown in Figure 2.The transfer function in hidden layer neurons and output layer neurons are sigmoid and purelin respectively. The performance function used was Mean Sum-squared Error (MSE).

Where i, j and k indices referring to the neurons belonging to the output, hidden, and input layers respectively, p, m, and k are the number of neurons in input, hidden and output layer respectively.

- x p X_1 input vector
- h: Weighted sum of input stimuli
- v: m X1 output vector of hidden layer
- g: Weighted sum of v_j
- Y: n X1 output vector of output layer
- $w_{ij:}$ weight connecting i^{th} unit of output layer and j^{th} unit of hidden layer
- $w_{jk:}$ Weight connecting j^{th} unit of hidden layer to k^{th} unit of input layer.
- y: Actual output.
- y^d: Desired output.

All the actual outputs of the network have computed. The computations have done as follows:

$$h_j = \sum_{k=1}^{p} w_{jk} x_k$$

$$v_j = \frac{1}{1 + e^{-h_j}}$$

Figure 2. Model of single hidden feed forward NN

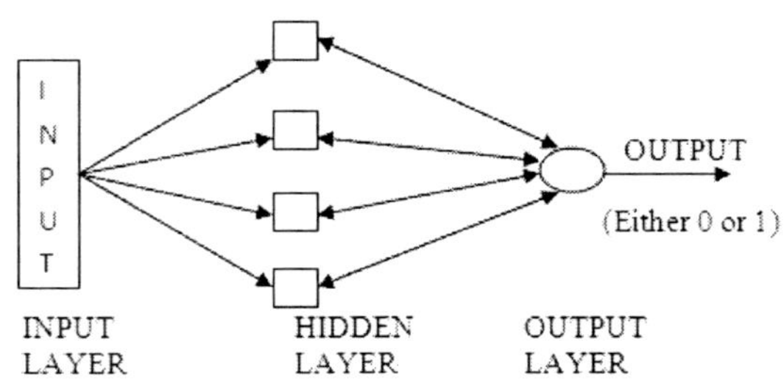

$$g_i = \sum_{j=1}^{m} w_{jk} v_j$$

Backward pass:

1. Compute the error $e=y^d-y$
2. Compute $\delta_i = y \cdot (1 - y) \cdot (y^d - y)$

δ_i is used to distribute the error at the output unit back to the preceding layers. Update the weights connecting hidden layer to output layer using the following updation rule. $w_{ij}(t + 1) = w_{ij}(t) + \eta\delta_i h_j$

3. Compute $\delta_j = v_j(1 - v_j)w_{jk}\delta_j x_k$

It is not necessary to propagate the error back to the input layer. δ_j is used to adapt the weights connecting the input layer to the hidden layer. Update the weights connecting input layer to hidden layer. $w_{ij}(t + 1) = w_{ij}(t) + \eta\delta_i\delta_j x_k$ After all the δ factors have been determined, the weights for all layers adjusted simultaneously.

The experimental results of diagnosis using BP Networks are shown in Table 2. The simulated

Table 2. Best experimental result of BPA NN model

	Goal	Learning Rate	No. of Neurons in Hidden Layer	No. of Epochs	MSE	% Accuracy of Diagnosis
Training Data	0.01	0.001	50	30,000	0.01	95.83
Testing Data	0.01	0.001	50	30,000	0.01	93.75

Figure 3. Training curve of the NN model

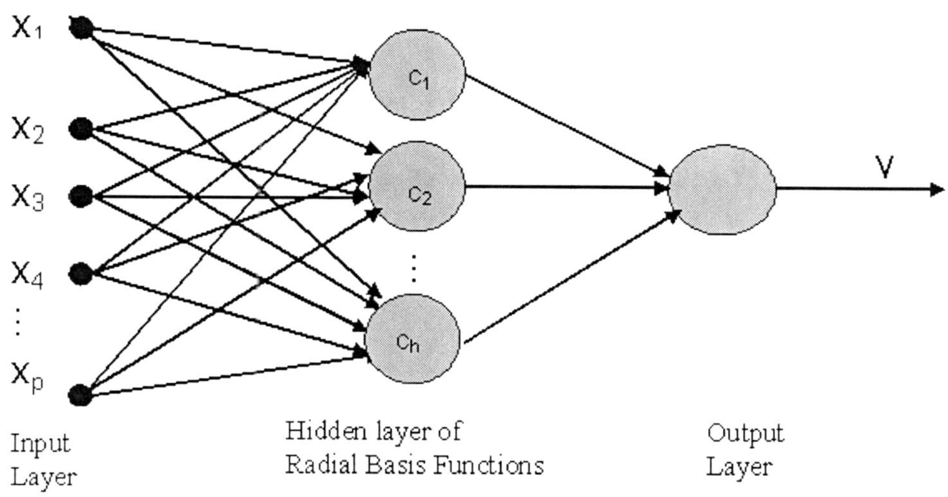

network model consists of 50 hidden neurons and 1 neuron in output layer gains accuracy 93.75%. Figure 3 shows the training curve for this model. Figure 4 and 5 shows the percentage accuracy of diagnosis using the best training and testing for this model respectively. The percentage accuracy of diagnosis was calculated as: % age accuracy = (Correct Results / All Results) * 100.

On the basis of the best possible combination of the parameters (i.e., the %age accuracy of diagnosis and time for training), the best model has been chosen.

Diagnosis using Radial Basis Function (RBF) Networks

In Radial Basis Function Networks, shown in Figure 3, the training is started in the hidden layer with unsupervised learning algorithm. The training is continued in the output layer with supervised algorithm. In the training process weight are set small random values in network. Each input unit $x_{i,}$ for all i= 1 to p, receives input signals and transmits to the next hidden layer which is known as radial center denoted by C. The centers are selects from the set of input vectors. It should be noted that a sufficient number of centers have to be selected to ensure adequate sampling of the input vector space. The number of nodes in hidden layer it should be greater or equal to $2^{p\cdot}$ Calculate the output from the hidden layer unit as follows:

$$v_i(x_i) = \frac{\exp\left[-\sum_{j=1}^{p}(x_{ji} - c_{ji})^2\right]}{\sigma_i^2}$$

Figure 4. Percentage accuracy of diagnosis for the best training BP network

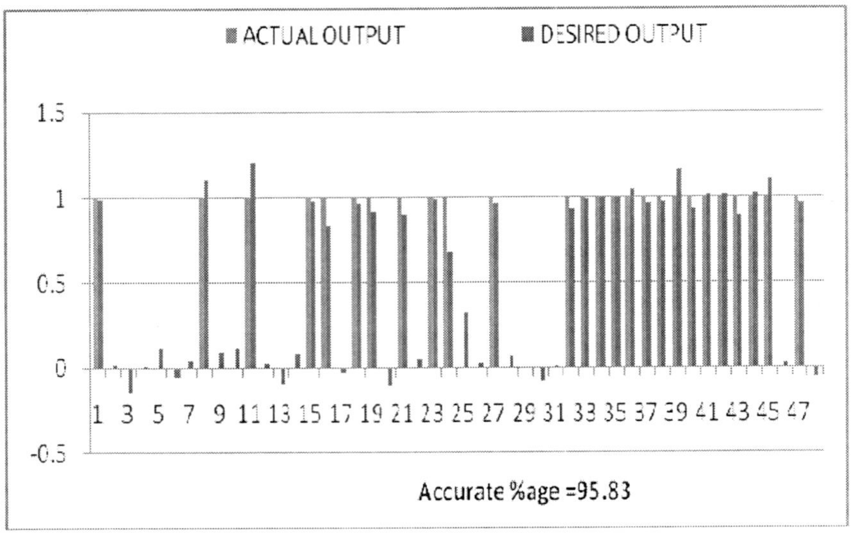

Figure 5. Percentage accuracy of diagnosis for the best testing model

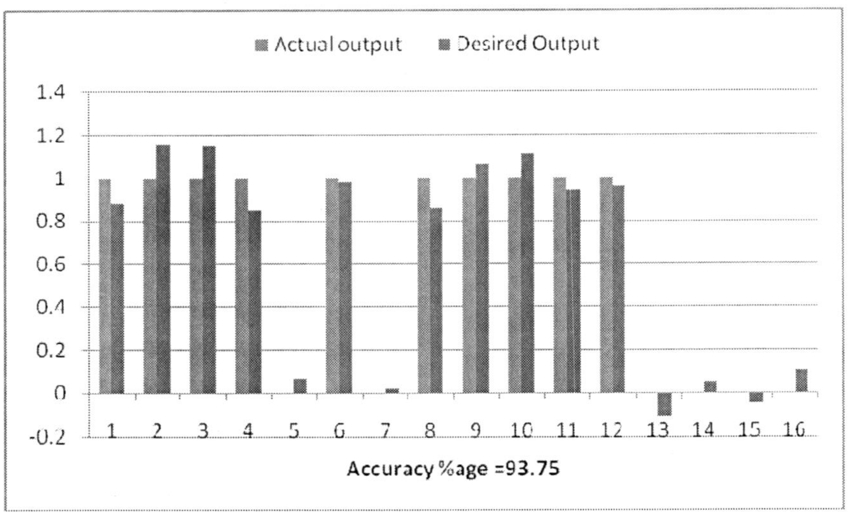

Where

- = center of the RBF unit for input variables.
- = j^{th} variable of input pattern.
- = Width of ith RBF unit.
- p = p is the number of inputs.

Therefore, calculate the output of the neural network.

$$y_{net} = \sum_{i=1}^{k} w_{im} v_i(x_i) + w_0$$

Where

- K = number of hidden layer nodes (RBF function)
- y_{net} = output value of mth node in output layer for the nth incoming pattern.

Figure 6. Architecture of RBF model used in our experiments

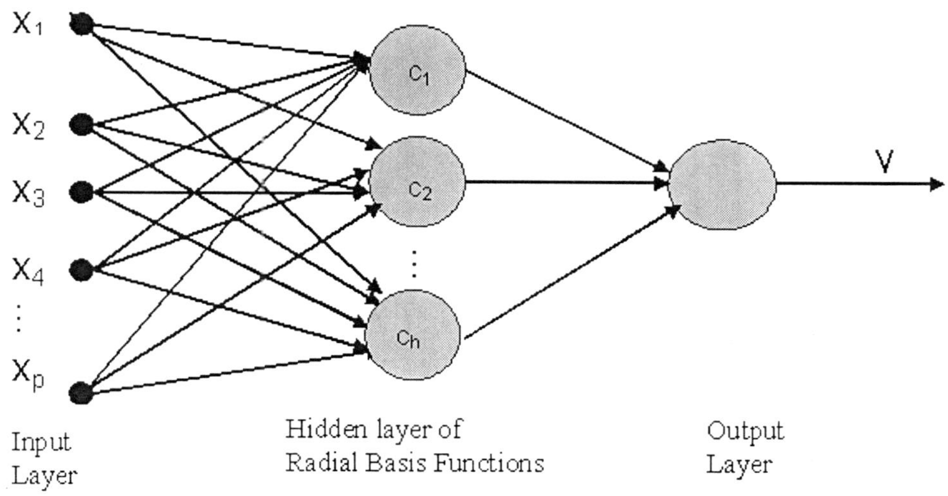

Table 3. Best experimental Result of RBF model

	Goal	Spread	Radial Basis Neurons	No. of Epochs	MSE	% Accuracy of Diagnosis
Training Data	0.01	0.05	50	25	0.01	99
Testing Data	0.01	0.05	50	25	0.01	99

- w_{im}= weight between i^{th} RBF unit and m^{th} output node.
- w_0= biasing term at n^{th} output node.

Calculate the error and to reduce that error we have adjustment weight with the help of number of epochs

In Radial Basis Function Networks, shown in Figure 6, the Gaussian function is used each node produces an identical output for inputs within a fixed radial distance from the center, i.e. they are radially symmetric and an error goal of 0.01 is used. The performance function MSE was used. The value of spread has been modified to get optimized model using RBF. This also resulted into change of number of epochs being used by the network. The experimental results of diagnosis using RBF Networks are shown in Table 3. The RBF network model with spread value 0.05, 50 hidden neurons gives accuracy of 99% is the RBF model for diagnosis and prediction of fetal delivery. Figure 7 shows the training curve for the best RBF Network. The Figure 8 and 9 shows the percentage accuracy of diagnosis and prediction of fetal delivery using the best training and testing RBF network respectively.Provide discussion of the overall coverage of the chapter and concluding remarks.

LVQ: Diagnosis using Learning Vector Quantization Network (LVQN)

It is well known that vector quantization is a data compression method, which encodes a set of data points into a reduced set of reference vectors. In the literature, many vector quantization strategies

Figure 7. Training curve of the best RBF model

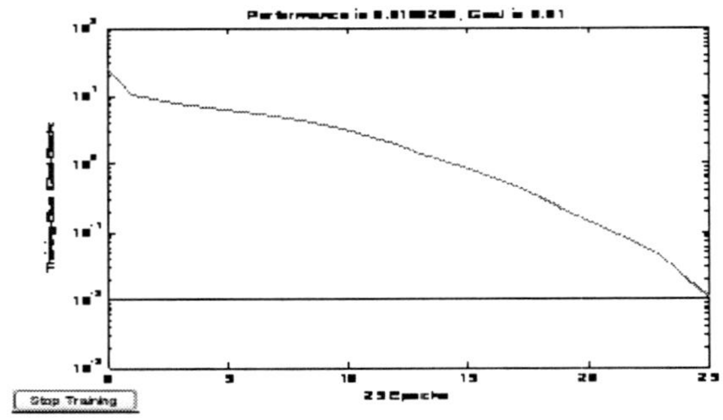

Figure 8. Percentage accuracy of diagnosis for the best training RBF model

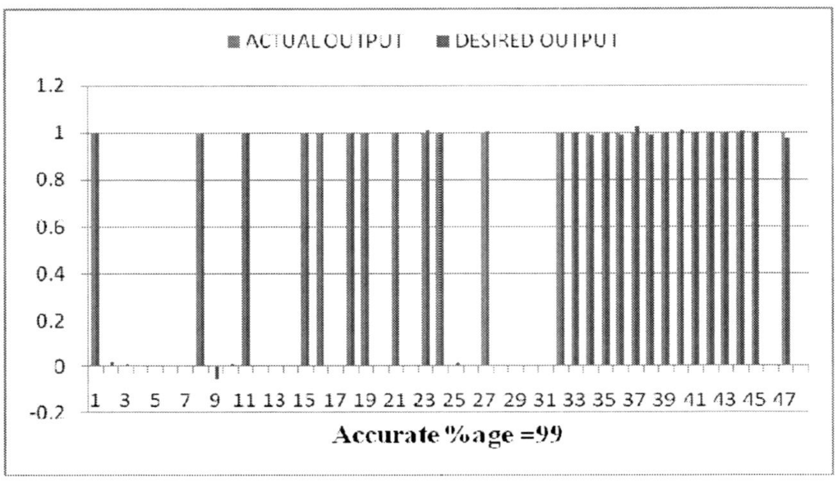

are proposed. One common way to design vector quantizer is based on cluster analysis. It is well known that the number and the centers of radial basis functions play an important role in the performance of RBF neural networks. Similarly, the size of codebook and the reference vectors are the key to vector quantization.

An LVQ network has a first competitive layer and a second linear layer. The competitive layer learns to classify input vectors. Linear layer transforms the competitive layer's classes into target classifications defined by the user. We refer to the classes learned by the competitive layer as *subclasses* and the classes of the linear layer as *target classes*. Original LVQ, however, suffers from several drawbacks such as slow convergence and instable behavior because of which a variety of alternatives have been proposed. there are two major drawbacks of these methods, which have only recently been tackled. On the one hand, LVQ relies on heuristics and a full mathematical investigation of the algorithm is lacking. This problem often leads to unexpected behavior and instabilities of training. Recently, it has rigorously been shown.

Slight variations of the basic LVQ learning scheme yield quite different results. LVQ which can be derived from an explicit cost function are particularly interesting,

Figure 9. Percentage accuracy of diagnosis for the best testing RBF model

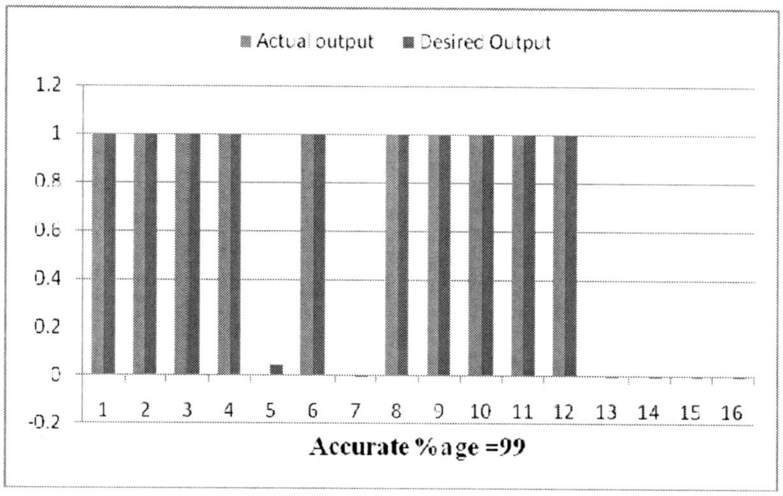

Figure 10. Architecture of LVQ model

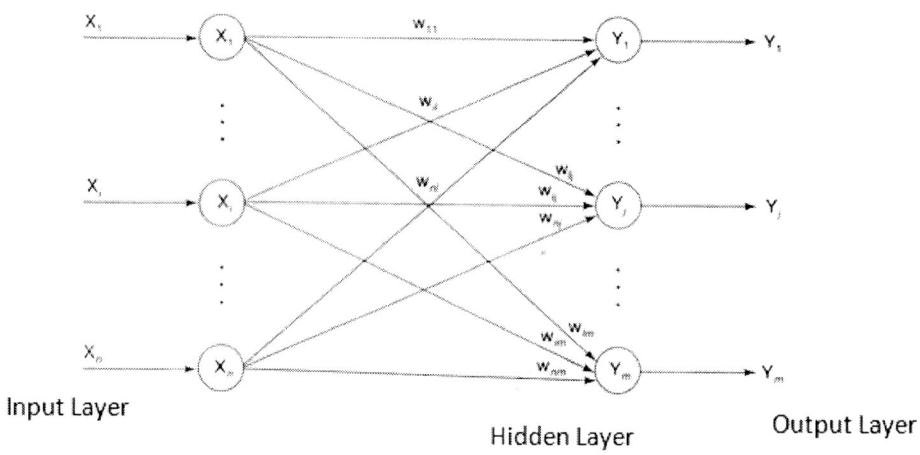

Table 4. The best experimental Result for LVQ model

	Goal	Learning Rate	No. of Neurons in Hidden Layer	No. of Epochs	MSE	% Accuracy of Diagnosis
Training Data	0.01	0.001	50	150	0.01	97.91
Testing Data	0.01	0.001	50	150	0.01	87.50

Figure 11. Training curve of the best LVQ model

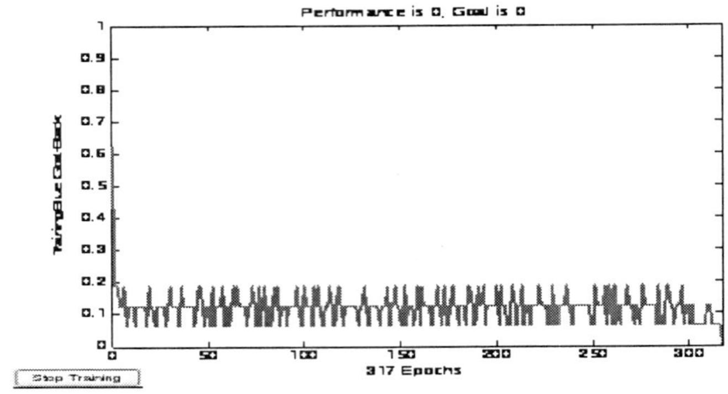

Figure 12. Percentage accuracy of diagnosis for the best training LVQ model

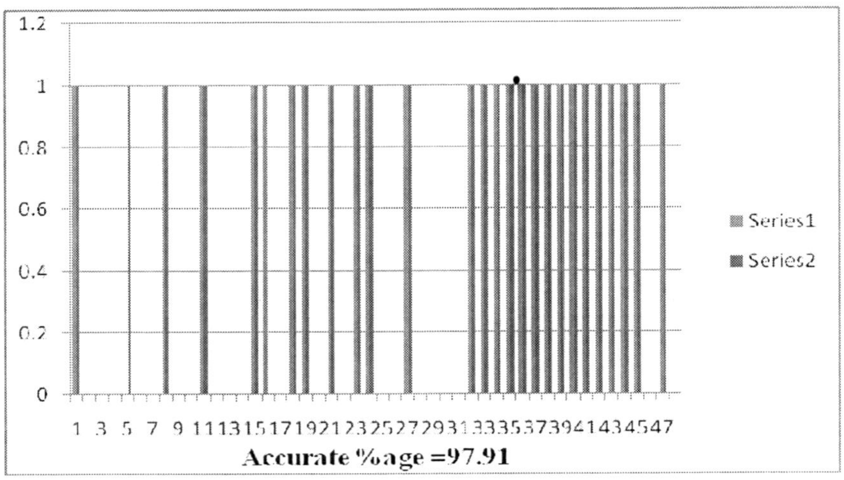

LVQ models are simulated for different neurons in hidden layer (Figure 10). The performance function used is MSE. The Table 4 shows the experimental results for LVQ networks, which differ from each other on the basis of number of hidden neurons used. The network with 50 hidden neurons and an accuracy of 87.5% is the best training LVQ Network. The Figure 11 shows the training curve for the best LVQ Network. The Figures 12 and 13 shows the percentage accuracy of diagnosis using the best training and testing LVQ network. The efficiency is calculated as in section 2.2.

ADAPTIVE NEURO-FUZZY INFERENCE SYSTEM (ANFIS)

Our present model is based on adaptive neuro-fuzzy inference system (ANFIS). An ANFIS is a fuzzy inference system implemented in framework of adaptive neural networks. ANFIS either uses input/output data sets to construct a fuzzy inference system whose membership functions are tuned using a learning algorithm or an expert may specify a fuzzy inference system and then the system is trained with the data pairs by an adaptive network. The ANFIS model for fetal delivery expert system shows in Figure 14.It

Figure 13. Percentage accuracy of diagnosis for the best testing LVQ model

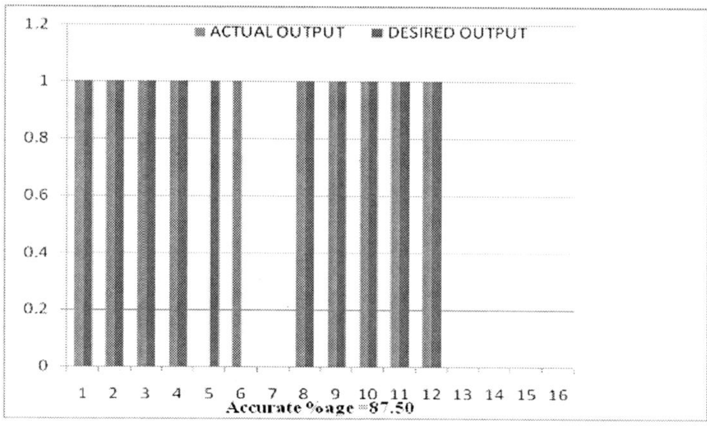

consists of two major components, namely, fuzzy inference system and adaptive neural network (J.S.R. Jang, 1993).

A fuzzy inference system has six functional layers.

- **Input layer**: This layer simply transmits these input variables to the fuzzification layer.
- **Fuzzification layer**: The fuzzification layer describes the membership function of each input fuzzy set. Membership functions are used to characterize fuzziness in the fuzzy sets (Abraham and B. Nath, 2001).
- **Inference layer**: An inference engine performs the inference operations on the rules to infer the output by a fuzzy reasoning method. It is perform interpretation of connective "AND" and connective "OR" rule (Kribeche, A 2004 and Kam, A.2000).
- **Normalization layer:** The node of this layer is also a fixed node and calculates the ratio of the rule's firing strength in inference layer to the sum of all the rules' firing strength (G.J. Klir 1995).
- **Output layer**: This layer represents the THEN part (i.e., the consequent) of the fuzzy rule. The operation performed by the nodes in this layer is to generate the qualified consequent (either fuzzy or crisp) of each rule depending on firing strength (G.J. Klir 1995).

Figure 14. ANFIS system architecture for fetal delivery system

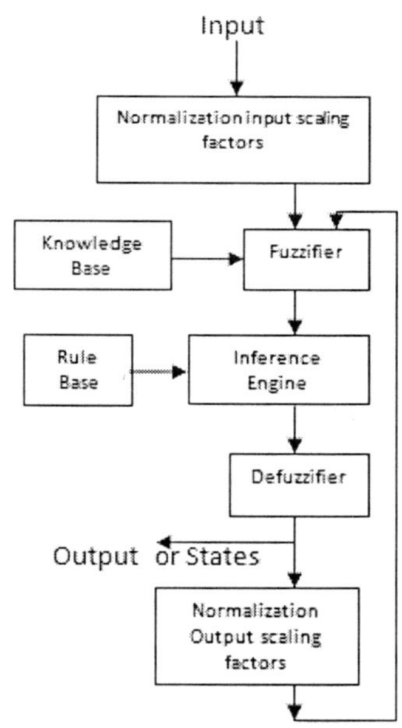

- **Defuzzification layer:** Defuzzifier converts the fuzzy outputs obtained by inference engine into a non-fuzzy output real number domain (D. Kukolj 2002 and J. R. Harding, 1996).

Figure 15. Input membership function

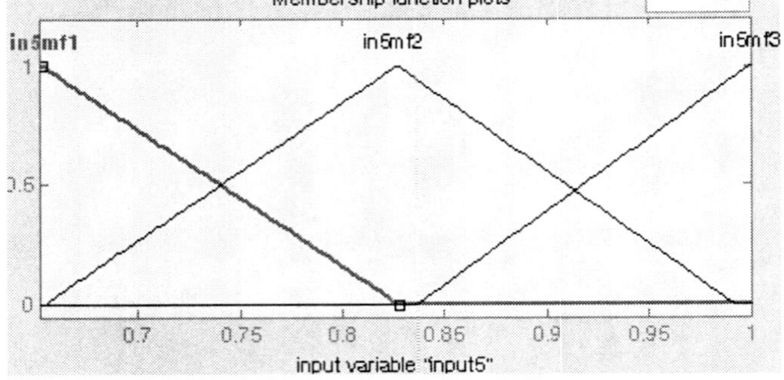

Figure 16. Outcome of testing the training data sets

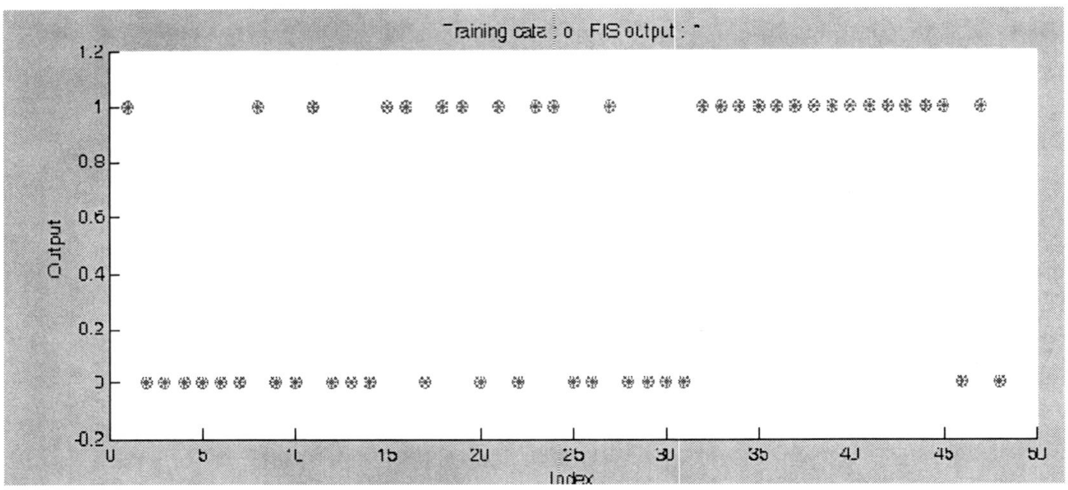

Specimen Rule Base sets:

ANFIS contains 244 rules some of them are given below.

- If (BP Upper is high) or (BP Lower is Low) and (R-R is high) and (R--I is high) and (S/D-Ratio is high) then Fetal-Delivery-Expert-System out Put is 1 mean Surgical.
- If (BP Upper is Normal) and (BP Lower is Normal) and (R-R is Normal) and (R-I is Normal) normal (S/D-Ratio is Normal) then Fetal-Delivery-Expert-System Output is 0 means Normal process.

We have simulated our model using ANFIS (Fuzzy Logic Tool box) of MATLAB. The system is first designed using Sugeno Fuzzy Inference System. It is a five input–one output system. The input is blood tests; type of task, and exposure time and the reduction in work efficiency is taken as the output variable. The input parameters are represented by fuzzy sets (or linguistic variables). We have chosen gbell shaped membership functions to characterize these fuzzy sets. The membership functions for input variables are shown in Figure 15. Training result is shown in Figure 16. Blue circle (o) represents desired output while pink asterisk (*) represents actual output.

Figure 17. ANFIS model structure

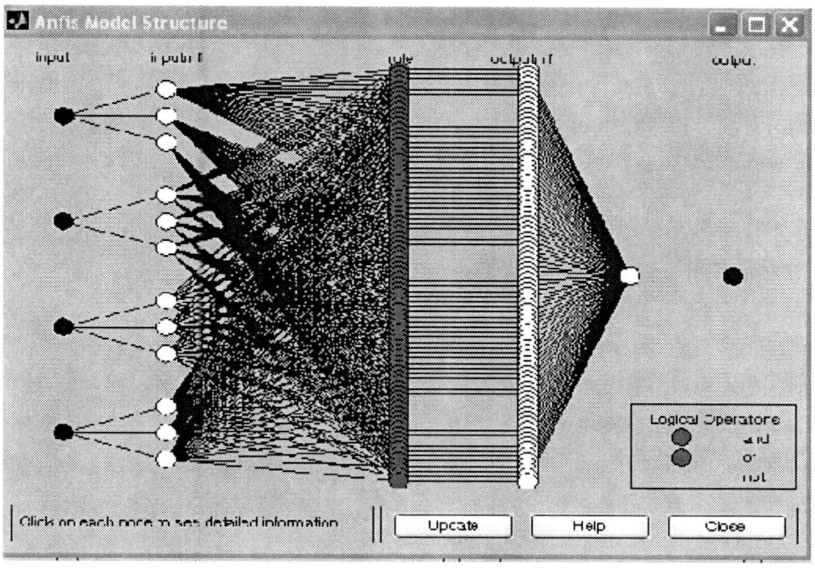

Figure 18. Real time fetal delivery expert system model

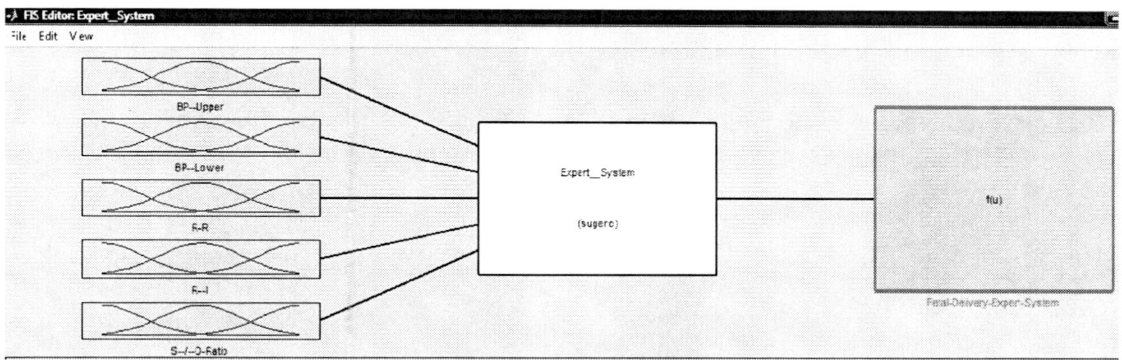

ANFIS model used Sugeno type fuzzy inference system, training optimization method is hybrid, error tolerance is 0%, number of epochs is 3,no of member function in each input (feature) is 3,no of inputs (features)is 5, no of output is 1, data set for training is 480 and data set for training is 160. ANFIS model and real time fetal delivery expert system model are shown in Figures 17 and 18 respectively.

FUTURE RESEARCH DIRECTION

The presented work and comparisons talk about the application of Artificial Neural network for the detection of fetal delivery mode. On the basis of the experimental observations of four neural networks based system and ANFIS, ANFIS gives the highest accuracy of 99.50% for diagnosis of fetal delivery system. Further the results obtained in case of RBFN gives the midway results i.e., efficiency of 99%.Further more the performance of each of the diagnostic system is basically application dependent, and depends a lot on the kind of data set being used for training and testing. The work can assist the doctors for easily diagnosis of the patients. The doctors can also compare their diagnosis with neural networks and reconsider those cases where there is a mismatch between their assessment and diagnosis results obtain from using Artificial Neural Networks models.

The completely multi-disciplinary nature of the field puts a serious limitation over its growth and development. A lot many diseases are yet to come under the hood of computational intelligence. The iterative nature of correcting the model at various stages to achieve greater prediction efficiency is a major task. This may be another focus for the readers for contribution and work in this field. This work can be extended using other algorithm of neural networks to improve efficiency. These techniques may be used for other problems like blood pressure identification, heart attack prediction, and fetal health prediction, fetal delivery time structure prediction and blood follow control between pre-natal fetus and maternity abdomen.

CONCLUSION

In this chapter we saw the working of four different ANN methods for the problem of detection of fetal delivery mode. In all the cases we were able to solve the problem with fine accuracies using the intelligent approaches. The first experiment done was of the use of ANN with LVQ. These systems used the generalizing capabilities of the ANN for problem solving. We were able to get sufficient accuracies using these systems. Various limitations of the LVQ motivated the use of another system for solving the same problem. The next implementation was using BPA and RBF. These systems removed the shortcomings of ANN with LVQ. This resulted in a rise in accuracy of the systems. The results reveal that the system performed very well on the training data set but did not do that well on the testing data set. The last approach was using the ANFIS. These systems gave good performances. This would prove to be a very useful system considering the present scenario where diseases are on a hike and there is a lack of availability of specialized doctors.

REFERENCES

Abraham, & Nath, B. (2001). A Neuro-fuzzy approach for modelling electricity demand in Victoria, *Appl. Soft Comput. 1*, 127–138.

Ayala, D. E., Hermida, R. C., Mojon, A., Fernandez, J. R., Alonso, I., Silva, I., et al. (2002). Blood pressure and heart rate variability during gestation in healthy and hypertensive pregnant women, In *Proceedings of the Engineering in Medicine and Biology Society, Ann. Int. Conf. IEEE,* (vol.1., pp 367 – 370).

Ayala, D. E., Hermida, R. C., Mojon, A., & Iglesias, M. (2002). Circadian blood pressure variability in healthy human pregnancy. Comparison with gestational hypertension. In *Proceedings of Engineering in Medicine and Biology Society, IEEE Annual Conference,* (vol. 1., pp. 639 – 640).

Braz, J. (2004, May). Med Biol Res Fuzzy expert system in the prediction of neonatal resuscitation. *Brazilian Journal of Medical and Biological Research*, *37*(5), 755–764.

Cohen, M. E., & Hudson, D. L. (2002). Meta neural networks as intelligent agents for diagnosis. *Neural Networks*, *1*, 233–238.

Gilleard, W., Lai, D. T. H., Levinger, P., & Begg, R. K. (2008, August 20-24). Detecting trunk motion changes due to pregnancy using pattern, recognition techniques. In *Proceedings of the 30th Annual International IEEE EMBS Conference*, British Columbia, Canada.

Harding, J. R., & Wright, A. M. (1996). Non-invasive imaging in the investigation of deep vein. In *Proceedings of the 18th Annual International Conference of the IEEE Engineering in Medicine and Biology Society*. Amsterdam. IR Imaging in Medicine II - Quantitative Clinical Applications.

Hwang, G. H., Chen, J. M., Hwang, G. J., & Chu, J. C. (2006). A time scale-oriented approach for building medical expert systems. *Expert Systems with Applications*, 299–308. doi:10.1016/j.eswa.2005.09.050

Jang, J.-S. R. (1993). ANFIS: adaptive-network-based fuzzy inference system. *IEEE Transactions on Systems, Man, and Cybernetics*, *23*, 665–685. doi:10.1109/21.256541

Kam, A., & Cohen, A. (April, 2000). Separation of twins fetal ECG by means of blind source separation (BSS). In *Proceedings of the 21st IEEE Electrical and Electronic Engineers in Israel.* (pp. 342 – 345).

Khan, F. S., Maqbool, F., Razzaq, S., Irfan, K., & Zia, T. (2008, February). The Role of Medical Expert Systems in Pakistan. In *Proceedings of world academy of science, engineering and technology* (volume 27).

Ibrahim, F., Taib, M. N., Saadiah, S., Abu Bakar, W., & Abas, W. (2001). Dengue fever and dengue haemorrhagic fever symptoms analysis from an expert system respective. In *Proceedings of the IEEE Int. Conf. 2001.*

Ghosh, A., Biehl, M., & Hammer, B. (2005). Dynamical analysis of LVQ type learning rules. In *Proceedings of the Workshop on the Self-Organizing-Map WSOM'05*, Univ. de Paris (I).

Klir, G. J., & Yuan, B. (1995). *Fuzzy Sets and Fuzzy Logic: Theory and Applications*. Englewood Cliffs, NJ: Prentice-Hall.

Kribeche, A., Benderbous, S., Tranquart, F., Kouame, D., & Pourcelot, L. (2004). Detection and analysis of fetal movements by ultrasonic multi-sensor Doppler (ACTIFOETUS). In *Proceedings of the 2004 IEEE Ultrasonics Symposium,* (Vol. 2, pp. 1457 – 1460).

Kukolj, D. (2002). Design of adaptive Takagi–Sugeno–Kang fuzzy models. *Applied Soft Computing*, *2*, 89–103. doi:10.1016/S1568-4946(02)00032-7

Orr, M. J. L. (1996). *Introduction to Radial Basis Function Networks (Technical report)*. Edinburgh, Scotland: Center for Cognitive Science, University of Edinburgh.

Peng, C., Xiao, S., Nie, Z., & Wang, Z. (1996). Application of Bayes Theorem in medical expert system. In *Proceedings of the IEEE Engineering in medicine and Biology*.

Pereira, M. A., Schaefer, M. B., & Marques, J. L. B. (2004, Septmeber 1-5). Remote Expert System of Support the Prostate Cancer Diagnosis. In *Proceedings of the 26th Annual International Conference of the IEEE EMBS*. San Francisco, CA.

Shukla, A., Tiwari, R., Janghel, R. R., & Kaur, P. (2009, March 6-7). Diagnosis of Thyroid Disorders using Artificial Neural Networks on (2009). IEEE International Advance Computing Conference. Patiala, India, (pp. 2722-2726).

Shukla, A., Tiwari, R., & Kaur, P. (2009, March 6-7). Knowledge Based Approach for Diagnosis of Breast Cancer. In *Proceedings of the IEEE International Advance Computing Conference*. Patiala, India. (pp. 6-12).

Tsumoto, S. (2001). *Rule Induction System based on Characterization of Medical Diagnosis using Rough Sets*. Washington, DC: IEEE Press.

Van Ha, K. (1998). Hierarchical radial basis function networks. *Neural Networks Proceedings*, *3*, 1893–1898.

Veena Kumari, C., Sndara Rao, G., Madhusudhana Rao, G., & Reddy, K. V. V. S. (2002). *Expert system on neonatal birth injuries*, (vol. 6, pp. 1999 – 2000).

Voss, A. Baumert, M. Baier, V. Stepan, H. Walther, T. Faber, R., (2003). Analysis of interactions between heart rate and blood pressure in chronic hypertensive pregnancy, Engineering in Medicine and Biology. In *Proceedings of the Ann.Conf. of Biomedical Engineering Society*. (Vol. 2 pp. 1615-1616).

Wu, J. D., Hsu, C.-C., & Chen, H.-C. (2009, May). An expert system of price forecasting for used cars using adaptive neuro-fuzzy inference. *Expert Systems with Applications*, *36*(4), 7809–7817. doi:10.1016/j.eswa.2008.11.019

Yegnanarayana, B. (2003). *Artificial Neural Networks*. New Delhi, India: Prentice Hall of India Pvt. Ltd.

Zaheeruddin, G. (2006, March). A neuro-fuzzy approach for prediction of human work efficiency in noisy environment. *Computing Volume, 283-294.*

KEY TERMS AND DEFINITIONS

Blood Pressure (BP): Arterial pressure is most commonly measured via a sphygmomanometer, which historically used the height of a column of mercury to reflect the circulating pressure. Today BP values are still reported in millimeters of mercury (mmHg), though aneroid and electronic devices do not use mercury.

Systolic Pressure: Systolic pressure is peak pressure in the arteries, which occurs near the end of the cardiac cycle when the ventricles are contracting.

Diastolic Pressure: Diastolic pressure is minimum pressure in the arteries, which occurs near the beginning of the cardiac cycle when the ventricles are filled with blood.

Blood Sugar (RR): A blood glucose test measures the amount of a type of sugar, called glucose, in your blood. Glucose comes from carbohydrate foods. It is the main source of energy used by the body.

Artificial Neural Networks: Networks consisting of a number of artificial neurons arranged in a layered manner, where each neurons takes input, processes it and gives it to the out neuron for further processing, or as system output. They are excellent agents for problem solving where some inputs are mapped to outputs in an unknown manner.

Classification: Problems consisting of a number of inputs or attributed which need to be mapped to a set of predefined classes. Each input is said to be belonging to some output class out of all the available classes.

Fetal: fetal include the fetus genome, nutrient production and hormone output.

Intelligence System: It is a system which learns during its existence. It senses its environment and learns, for each situation, which action permits it to reach its objectives. It continually acts, mentally and externally and by acting reaches its objectives more often than pure chance indicates.

APPENDIX A: SIMULATION RESULTS

Table 5. The experimental result for ANFIS model with linear output

Output Type: Linear					
	Epoch 3	**Training Data**		**Testing Data**	
MF Type	**Error**	**Avg Testing Error**	**%**	**Avg Testing Error**	**%**
Triangular	1.34E-05	1.34E-05	100	0.53093	93.75
Trapezoidal	**2.30E-05**	**2.00E-05**	**100**	**0.48412**	**99.50**
Generalized Bell	3.03E-05	2.66E-05	100	0.79057	62.5
Gaussmf	1.85E-05	1.85E-05	100	0.79057	62.5
Gauss2mf	2.16E-05	2.16E-05	100	0.79057	62.5
Pimf	**2.10E-05**	**2.10E-05**	**100**	**0.48412**	**99.50**
Dsigmf	2.13E-05	2.13E-05	100	0.79057	62.5
Psigmf	2.13E-05	2.13E-05	100	0.79057	62.5

Table 6. Performance comparison of our work

Neural Network Algorithm	**Accuracy %**
LVQ	87.5
BPA	93.75
RBF	99
ANFIS	99.50

Table 7. The results comparison of the previous models

Methods/Techniques	**Accuracy in %**
Support Vector Machine (SVM) [31]	71.43
Linear Discriminant Analysis (LDA) [31]	28.57
Thermal Imaging Technique [26]	97.00
Fuzzy Logic [27]	70-80
Rule Chaining [28]	90.00
Baye's Formula [29]	73.00
Rough Set Approach [30]	86.20

Chapter 8
Handling Large Medical Data Sets for Disease Detection

Rahul Kala
Indian Institute of Information Technology and Management Gwalior, India

Anupam Shukla
Indian Institute of Information Technology and Management Gwalior, India

Ritu Tiwari
Indian Institute of Information Technology and Management Gwalior, India

ABSTRACT

The breakthrough in the field of intelligent systems has spread its fruits to the field of biomedical engineering as well; where a series of models are being applied to automatically detect diseases based on some parameters or inputs. The continuous research in this field has resulted in a large amount of database being created for many diseases which becomes very difficult to train. Also the number of attributes is under constant rise. This increases the dimensionality of the problem and ultimately leads to poor performance. In this chapter we deal with the methods to handle these situations. We discuss the mechanism to divide data between different sub-systems. We also discuss the method of division of the attributes to reduce the training time and complexity. The resultant systems are able to train better due to low computational cost and hence give better performance. We validated this with the Breast Cancer database from the UCI Machine Learning repository and found our algorithm optimal.

INTRODUCTION

Computational Intelligence has given rise to automation in numerous spheres. Bio-medical engineering is one of these spheres where the computationally intelligent systems have automated the task of detection of diseases. These systems are able to affectively detect the presence or absence of any disease. These systems take the various parameters as inputs that can potentially affect the decision regarding the presence or absence of disease. The system analyzes these inputs and then makes its decision. Every input or parameter affects the decision of the system to some extent. Some parameters are very important whereas the others may behave rather passive in nature. Ideally the larger the number of parameters, the more is the chance of detection of the disease. This is

DOI: 10.4018/978-1-61692-004-3.ch008

because of the fact that the system is given more information that may be consulted for decision making.

The detection system usually makes use of historic data to formulate rules regarding the analysis. The historic data is a collection of large amount of information regarding the presence or absence of disease in multiple scenarios. The system tries to extract valuable information or rules from this database by the process of machine learning. It then tries to generalize the extracted information or rules to the unknown data. The entire knowledge of the system to detect the disease is based on the learning of the historical data. Hence it can effectively only effectively predict the presence or absence of some disease if the behavior was recorded by the system sometimes earlier and presented at the time of learning as the historical database. In case the same does not hold, the system might not behave as desired and it may give any random or abrupt output. Hence ideally a larger historical database is preferred that can capture as much diversity as possible. The aim is that in the future any unknown input is related to one of the inputs in the historical database.

The large number of attributes in the system as well as the large number of training data size in the historical database seems to be a big boon for the system. However, this may have a negative impact on the system in terms of computational time. The larger number of attributes or data set instances has a multiplicative impact on the time of training. It may hence be possible that the system is unable to train itself in finite time. This would drop the efficiency of the system and the entire system would become sub-optimal. Further, the larger number of attributes makes the system very flexible. The entire system can now assume more behavior by different values of outputs for different inputs. In other words there is an increase in the number of parameters of the systems that require more data and time for training. There is always an associated risk of sub-optimal training as a result of the added attributes. Hence an increase in attributes or the number of inputs is not always desirable.

The larger number of instances of training data in the training data set also has negative affects apart from the time complexity being increased. More data added to the system may add unique characteristics to the system which is to be modeled. This may be an exception to the present state and behavior of the system. As a result the system would have to formulate new rules or learning to accommodate the input that acts as an exception. This would add to the complexity of the system. Further the complex systems are more computationally expensive and difficult to train due to the large system parameters. Also the training may be sub-optimal. This puts a serious limitation to the increase of data.

It may not always be the case that adding attributes or training instances is poor for the system. Some added attributes showing behavior of correlation to one or more of the already existing attributes may not make the system that sensitive. Similarly if all of the added inputs show normal behavior as the rest of the inputs in the database, there would not be much adverse affect on the system performance. In such cases we may consider the addition to play role in time only. It may at the same time help in optimal system tuning.

Modular Neural Networks (MNNs) (Shadabi, Sharma and Cox, 2006) are neural networks that exploit the modularity in the problem. The whole problem is divided into a set of modules which are Artificial Neural Networks (ANNs) in themselves. All the modules behave independent of each other. Each module tries to solve its part of the problem independently. After all the modules have solved the problem, the results are communicated to the integrator. The integrator is responsible for combining the results of the individual modules to form the result of the entire problem. In such a manner the problem is solved by the combined effect of the various modules. Each module is ultimately a neural network that has to undergo training before it can be put to use. The training of the various modules is independent of each other and is carried out by their part of the problem. Modular neural networks are effective means to solve problem where the conventional system is unable to solve the problem due to its complex size or other limitations. These networks give a good performance boost to the system with a very little loss of generality.

Large number of attributes or data instances is not always desirable. However not considering any of them would make the system miss out valuable piece of information, which might be needed for optimal training. Hence in this chapter we study the manner in which we can make the system perform well in computationally feasible time, at the same instance not delete any valuable piece of information. We study both the problems independently one by one. First we would be discussing the problems of a large number of attributes in the training data set. For this we would distribute the attributes among different modules of a modular neural network. All these compute their result and the same are used by the integrator to compute the final result.

The second problem is one large training data size. For this problem also we make use of modular neural network. The first step is to cluster the training data into clusters. Each cluster has a separate neural network of its own. The training data set is divided into cluster and each cluster is trained by the inputs that belong to that cluster. For unknown input we first compute the cluster to which it belongs. We then use the neural network of the same cluster to compute the final output. This is the output of the system.

This chapter is organized as follows. In section 2 we present some of the works from literature. Section 3 discusses the problem of division of attributes. In section 4 we discuss about the clustering based division of training data set. The results to solve the problem of Breast Cancer are given in Section 5. We give the directions for future research in section 6 and the conclusions in section 7.

BACKGROUND

Modular Neural Networks are hybrid systems that effectively solve the problem. A lot of work is being done in use of hybrid systems for problem solving. Rutwoski (2004) did a major work to build flexible neuro fuzzy systems. Here he presented various models build of neuro fuzzy systems. Kuo et al (2008) proposed a hybrid model for learning fuzzy if-then rules. These have been applied to variety of problems (Grigore and Gavat 1998; Lee et al 1999, Taur and Tao, 2000). A lot of work is going on in the various parts of these algorithms like clustering, genetic optimizations, rule forming, parameter updating etc (Er and Zhou 2008; Mu et al 2006; Sandhu, Salaria and Singh, 2008). The algorithms try to optimize the performance in clustering by designing various models based on the architecture of neuro-fuzzy systems (Chaudhuri and Bhattacharya, 2000; Lin, Chun and Cheng 2007, Lin and Hong, 2007; Pinero et al 2007, Vieira and Barradas, 2003). Adams (2009) proposed the use of Genetic Algorithms to decide the connectivity of associative memory that can be generalized to artificial neural networks. Maravall et al (2009) also proposed a hybrid model of Genetic Algorithms with reinforcement learning for robotic controllers.

The problem of detection of disease is classificatory in nature where we need to classify the inputs to either of the two output classes that stand for the presence or absence of disease. Classification is a major problem of study in literature. People are trying to better adapt the present algorithms to make them more suitable for classificatory problems. Amin et al. (2009) presented a model of single layered complex valued artificial neural network for classificatory problem. Here they had made use of new activation functions. Hu (2008) used Choquet Integral with neural network and genetic algorithms for pattern classification. Estudillo et al (2008) proposed multiplicative nodes instead of additive in neural networks to build neural network classifiers. Ang, Tan and

Al-Mamum (2008) used probability to genetically evolve a neural network from smallest size to larger sizes. They proposed variable probabilities.

Genetic Algorithms are being constantly studied and modified for better performances at various situations. One of the major landmark here is the evolution of Particle Swarm Optimizations. Nani (2009) used the Nearest Neighbor approach for prototype reduction using Particle Swarm Optimization and the found the Nearest Neighbor approach to be good. Grammatical Evolution is another area of work. Tsoulus et al (2008) proposed grammatical evolution for neural network construction and training. O'Neill et al (2001 and 2005) has highlighted various developments in these fields in terms of representation and working of the algorithm. Ryann, Collins and O'Neil (2005) proposed these algorithms for program generation in arbitrary language.

A lot of work is being done in the field of neural network for validating, generalizing and better training of the neural network (Daghici, 1997; Gerlot, Flink and Thomas 2006; Graves et al 2008; Shadabi, Sharma and Cox, 2006). The problems also employ the concept of Hidden Markov Models (Hewavitharana, Fernando and Kodikara 2002; Sandhu, Salaria and Singh, 2008; Shi, Shu and Liu 1998). These are statistical models that can be used to predict the consequence of the unknown input. These models have found a variety of use in handwriting recognition, speech recognition etc. Instantaneously trained neural networks (Kak 1998; Rajagopal 2003) are a good approach for faster training with a smaller generalization capability. These networks require very less training time as the weights are decided just by seeing the inputs. Self organizing maps have also been used extensively for the problem solving. Various other mathematical models have been proposed. These employ mathematical techniques like point to point matching for solving the problem.

DIVISION OF ATTRIBUTES

The first problem of study is where we have a large number of attributes on which the decision regarding the presence or absence of disease depends upon. Consider the case of skin diseases it has 34 attributes that are considered for deciding the presence or absence of the disease (Ilter, Guvenir and Altey, 1998). Such a large number of attributes need to be computed which has its own advantages and disadvantages as discussed. We hence build a modular neural network over this system that helps in solving the problem.

In this problem, we first divide the problem into modules. Here the attributes are divided into modules. Every module gets a set of attributes. It is possible that an attribute is given to more than one module. Similarly it is possible that an attribute is not given to any of the attributes at all. This however must be avoided as it leads to a loss of valuable information.

Then each module independently calculates the output. These use ANNs for the task. At the end each ANN returns the probabilities of the occurrence of each of the class. These probabilities lie in the range of -1 to 1. A '-1' means that the given class is definitely absent. Similarly a '1' means that the class is present for sure. The numbers denote the certainty of the ANN in the occurrences of the class as the final output class.

At the end the integrator does the task of combining the individual solutions to give the final output. This is in the form of 1st averaging the various probabilities returned by the individual systems. Here the performance of the systems at the time of training is used as weights. Then the summation takes place to return the final class that is declared as the final output. The basic working of the system is shown in Figure 1. We discuss each of the steps in the next section.

Figure 1. The general structure of the algorithm

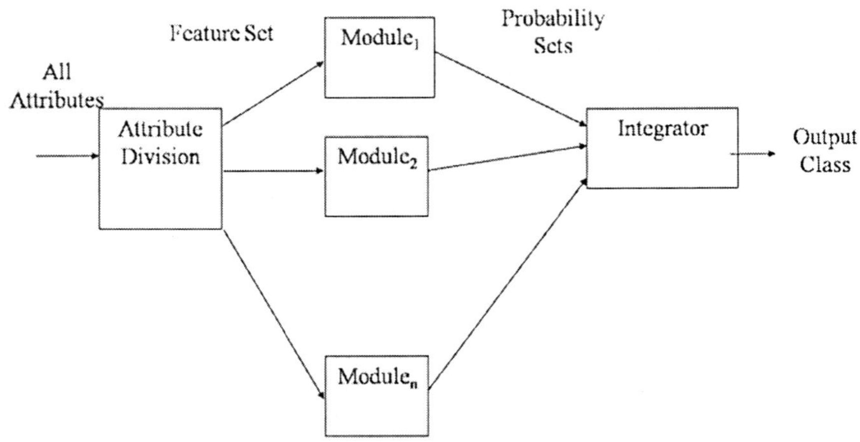

Figure 2. The division of inputs between modules

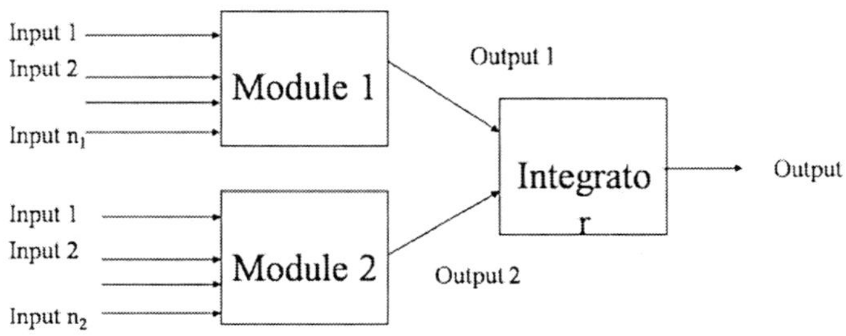

Modules

Here we are supposed to exploit the modularity in the features. We would be dividing the entire feature set into the various modules. The basic motive is to ensure that each module after getting its feature set must be in a condition to appreciably solve the problem. It must have the related attributes to enable it to do so. Hence the attributes given to any module must be diverse and must collectively supply the entire information. Redundancy in features may be removed. The redundant features would unnecessary increase computation. Also loading too many features to an ANN would be not desirable. This would also increase the computation on it unnecessarily. Here we also try to ensure that all attributes collectively get the complete feature set. This would avoid the loss of information from the system.

Consider that the disease being considered had 'a' attributes $X<X_1, X_2, X_3, \ldots, X_a>$. Let us say we are to divide this attribute set X into b modules. In such a case we form b new modules each consisting of a set of X_is such that each attribute X_i belongs to some or the other module Y_j. It must be additionally kept in mind that the distribution must be such that each module Y_j must be able to give a decent performance even by its own. There must be a very high correlation between attributes of different modules and a very low correlation between the attributes of same module.

The structure in general related to the division of the features among modules is shown in Figure 2. Here the input comes to the system and is divided among these modules. Each module calculates its output and gives it to the integrator to decide the final output.

Artificial Neural Networks

The job of classification of the inputs is carried out with the help of ANNs with Back Propagation Algorithm as the training algorithm. The ANNs are a natural choice because of their ability to learn from the historical data and to generalize the results. The ANNs map any input to some class or person here. We use a classificatory model of ANN here. This has as many output neurons as the number of classes. Each output neuron stands for some person or class. The output at this neuron for any input *i* is the probability of occurrence of this person or class according to the ANN. Hence the ANN gives as its output c number of probabilities in the output vector. Let this output vector for any input *i* be represented by $<v_{i1}, v_{i2}, v_{i3}, \ldots v_{ic}>$.

The probabilities here are measured in the range of -1 to 1. A probability of 1 means that according to the ANN this is the output class with full confidence. On the other hand a probability of -1 means that according to the ANN this class is not the output with full confidence. Hence the ideal output for any input for the ANN should be a 1 for any one element of the output vector and a -1 for all the other elements. However due to practical reasons, the output lies anywhere in the complete region. Figure 3 shows the system inputs and outputs with the ANN as a black box.

Integrator

The last part to implement according to the entire algorithm is the integrator. This is the major part of the whole system that does the task of finding the final output class after getting inputs from the individual modules. The integrator analyzes all the outputs by the various modules and then decides the final output class that according to the system is the output.

Figure 3. The ANN inputs and outputs

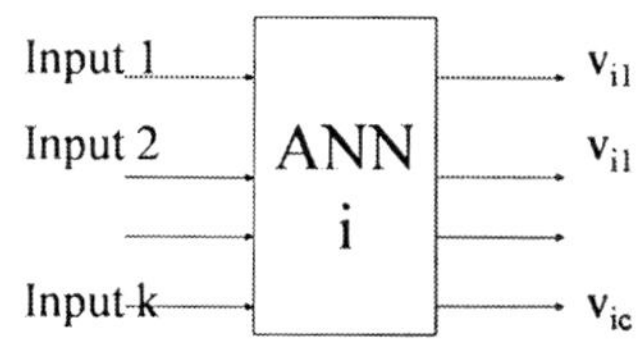

The input given to the integrator is the solution vector of every module of ANN. Let the vector of the module *i* be $<v_{i1}, v_{i2}, v_{i3}, \ldots v_{ic}>$ where each v_{ik} is the probability of the occurrence of the class *k* measured on a scale of -1 to 1. The integrator decides the output by first taking the weighted averages of the probabilities given to it and then selecting the class with the maximum probability. This class is declared as the winner. This is shown in Figure 4.

The weighted average is calculated for each and every class in the system on which the output can map to. The weights of the various modules or ANNs here are their performances on the training data. Each ANN was given the same data set for the training purposes with a different feature set. The performance here is calculated as a ratio between the numbers of elements the ANN correctly classifies in the validation data set by the total number of elements in the validation data set. The higher the performance of the ANN in the validation data set, the more would be its weight and more dominant it would be to decide the final output at the time of integration.

Using these calculated weights, the integrator calculates the weighted average for all the classes. This gives the final probability vector comprising of c probabilities with each probability associated with some class. These probabilities again lie in the range of -1 to 1 with the same meaning of the probabilities.

The next task of the integrator is to find out the final output class. For this the integrator selects the output class with the largest value of the probability out of all the available classes. The class or the person corresponding to this largest

Figure 4. The Integrator

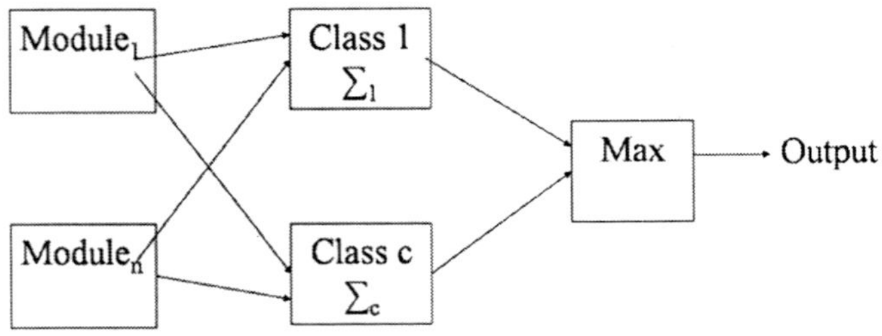

Figure 5. The hierarchical training algorithm

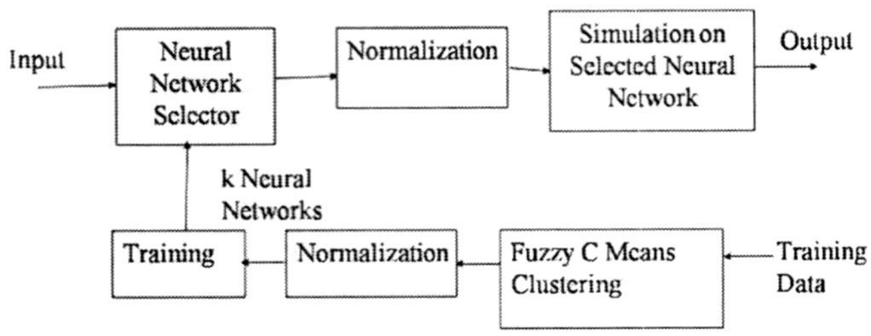

probability is declared as the winner and this is the output that the system gives.

DIVISION OF TRAINING DATA

The other problem that we have considered is of division of the training data into a set of modules. We know that a large amount of training data has an adverse affect on training. Besides it exhibits a complex relation between the inputs and the outputs which is difficult to model. In this approach we try to divide the entire problem into independent modules that can be independently trained and tested. Here each module is a cluster in the input space. In other words we may say that we divide the entire multi-dimensional input space into a set of clusters. Each cluster has a vague boundary which demarcates it from the other clusters. Further, each cluster has a separate neural network of itself through which it is trained.

A conventional Artificial Neural Network (ANN) gives the inputs to the system and the output is calculated by the processing by the various nodes of the system. Every time an input is given from the input nodes and the output is collected after processing from the output nodes. The system consists of a number of parallel processing nodes that work on the input to generate the output.

In this approach we first cluster the input training data into *k* number of clusters. Each of the *k* clusters is a module of the modular neural network. It represents an ANN. This module or ANN caters to the needs of inputs that lie within its cluster range. Hence every neural network or cluster has a boundary. Any input that lies within this boundary is processed by this neural network and the corresponding output is generated solely by this network. This is decided by the clustering of the input test data.

The major steps of the algorithm are given in Figure 5. As it can be seen from figure, the algorithm has two phases, training and testing. The purpose of training is to make the *k* modules and decide their clusters. The training data is clustered using Fuzzy C Means clustering. This gives us the center of every cluster. We also get the members of every cluster. Every cluster has

Figure 6. The hierarchical structure of the algorithm

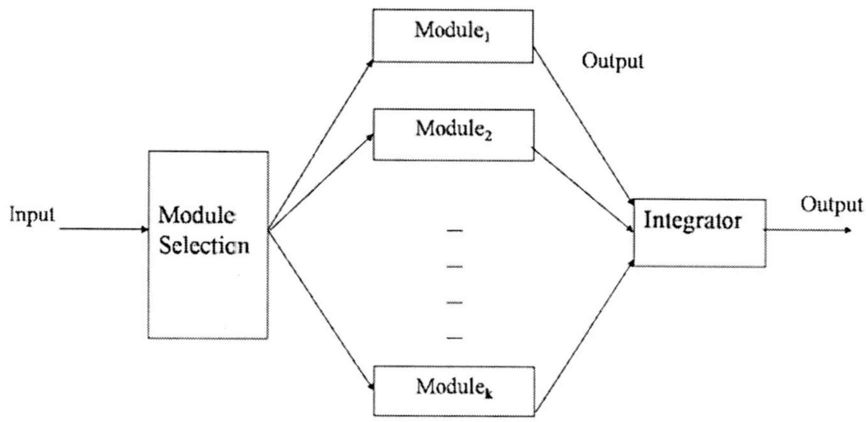

its own ANN. This ANN is trained independently of all other networks using the members of this cluster. When this process is over for all the *k* ANNs, we have the networks ready for the testing. In testing phase, whenever an input is given, we select the best cluster or module that is closest to the input. We then process the input by this ANN or module. The general architecture of the system is given in Figure 6.

We discuss more about the various phases of the algorithm in detail in the next few subsections. We discuss the two phases of training and testing, one by one.

Training

The purpose of this stage is to form the *k* ANNs or modules, each trained by its set of inputs. Each module has its own range in which it operates. Fuzzy C Means Clustering is a clustering algorithm that is extensively used for clustering of input data in various applications. In this algorithm, we need to specify the number of clusters in advance. The algorithm clusters the input data into these many clusters. We get the centers of the clusters at the end. This clustering algorithm is called a fuzzy algorithm, as any data element is not a member of just one cluster, rather it is associated with more than one clusters each with a different membership degree. This clustering algorithm also gives us the membership degrees of the various inputs.

In our algorithm, we first of all need to decide the number of clusters. This value depends of the level of modularity of the problem. The higher value of *k* would result in larger number of ANNs. The inputs would be distributed over a larger number of modules. This would improve the training time but result in a loss of generalization. By analyzing the training data set and the system requirements, we decide the value of *k*. The other parameters that we need to fix in this algorithm are Maximum number of iterations, Minimum improvement and exponent. Once we run the algorithm, the data is analyzed and the various clusters are formed. At the end of the algorithm, we get to know the centers of the *k* clusters that we had intended to find.

Suppose that our training data is $<I_{11}, I_{12}, I_{13}, I_{14}....I_{1n}>$, $<I_{21}, I_{22}, I_{23}, I_{24}....I_{2n}>$ ..... $<I_{m1}, I_{m2}, I_{m3}, I_{m4}....I_{mn}>$ Using Fuzzy C Means Clustering we get the *k* centers as $<C_{11}, C_{12}, C_{13}, C_{14}....C_{1n}>$, $<C_{21}, C_{22}, C_{23}, C_{24}....C_{2n}>$ ..... $<C_{k1}, C_{k2}, C_{k3}, C_{k4}....C_{kn}>$.

Now we allocate every input to a corresponding cluster. This is decided based on the distance between the input and the cluster. We select the cluster with the least distance from the given input. The distance between any two points $X<x_1,$

$x_2, x_3, x_4 \ldots x_n>$ and $Y<y_1, y_2, y_3, y_4 \ldots y_n>$ is given in equation (1).

$$d(X,Y) = \sum_{i-1}^{n} (x_i - y_i)^2 \qquad (1)$$

The cluster p to which any given input I belongs is given by equation (2). We select only one value of p.

Cluster(I) = { p: d(I, C_p) ≤ d(I, C_i) for all 1≤ i ≤ k } (2)

We look at all the training data and decide the cluster to which they belong. We group up data and hence at the end each cluster has some input training data associated with it. Through this step, we have clustered the input data into various clusters.

The input data may be having very high ranges. Since we are using back propagation algorithm, we need to make sure that data in every step lies within workable ranges. If the input data is very high, it is possible that it may overshoot the workable range in any step of internal processing. This is a common observation while working with the ANN toolkit of MATLAB. If the input data sizes are even slightly higher, the results are badly affected. Hence it is usually preferred to keep all inputs between -1 to 1. This improves the performance. In order to make sure that the inputs are within range, we apply a step of normalization. In this step every input is divided by the maximum value that the input can take. Usually we take this maximum value as the maximum value that is present in the training input. This is given by equation (3).

$$I_{new} = \frac{I_{old}}{\prod_{i=1}^{cluster\ size} Max\left(\left|I_i\right|\right)} \qquad (3)$$

If the outputs are also quite large, then we need to normalize them as well. This can be done by dividing them with the maximum output, as we did for the input. This would ensure that the output is within the range of –1 to 1, under which the artificial neural network would be able to perform well.

These maximum values need to be preserved, as we would need them in the testing phase as well. While testing also, whenever an input is applied, we first find out the cluster to which it belongs. Then we divide the input by the same value as we did for all the training data of that cluster.

The most commonly used method for training is the Back Propagation Algorithm (BPA). In this algorithm, the inputs are applied one after the other and the outputs are calculated. The actual results to each of these inputs are known. The difference is calculated between the actual and the observed outputs. This error is back propagated to all the layers. The layers uses the concepts of steepest descend to calculate the new weights. The weights are changed to the new weights. Next time when same inputs are applied, the errors are smaller. This process is repeated for a few iterations or epochs.

We have the k clusters ready, each with a set of normalized data sets from the previous step. We use the back propagation algorithm in all these k ANNs and train them independently. The limited inputs are given and hence training is a lot better and faster.

Testing

Once the k modules are ready, we need to test them for unknown inputs. This is done in the testing phase of the algorithm. We need to select one of the k modules. This selection is done by finding the cluster that is closest to the given input. This selection is the same as given in equations (1) and (2). We need to normalize the input as we did for the training data. Every cluster had a maximum value per input which we used to divide the input to make it lie within the range of -1 to 1. We divide the input by the same value as we did for all the training data of that cluster. This value is given in equation (3).

Once we have selected the module and the normalized input to be processed. We now apply the input to this module or ANN using the forward pass of the artificial neural network. The various nodes process the inputs and pass the results to the subsequent layers. The final answer is given by the output node. This is the output to the given input that may be interpreted as per the requirements of the system. It may be noted that the integrator always gets a response from a single module in the presented approach. The integrator simply outputs this value as the final system output.

RESULTS

In this section we present an experimental framework for the problems discussed. The problem that we choose for the experimental purposes is the detection of Breast Cancer. Here we are given a set of attributes and these needs to be classified into malignant or benign. We take the breast cancer data from the UCI Machine Learning Repository for this purpose (Wolberg, Mangasarian and Aha, 1992). This database consists of 29 real valued inputs. These correspond to the following features for each cell nucleus: radius (mean of distances from center to points on the perimeter), texture (standard deviation of gray-scale values), perimeter, area, smoothness (local variation in radius lengths), compactness (perimeter2 / area - 1.0), concavity (severity of concave portions of the contour), concave points (number of concave portions of the contour), symmetry, fractal dimension ("coastline approximation" - 1). The entire data set consists of a total of 357 benign and 212 malignant cases, totaling to 569 instances in the database.

The basic methodology consists of first division of the database into training and testing data sets. We keep a total of approximately 70% data for the training purpose and the rest 30% for the testing purpose. The entire algorithm is applied as per sections 3 and 4 on the training and the testing data sets. The final performance for both of these is noted. We discuss the results to both the experiments of division of attributes and division of training data sets one by one in the next sub-sections.

Attribute Division

First we took the data from the data set and divided it into 2 separate modules. There were a total of 30 attributes in the data set. We took the first 15 attributes for the first module and the next 15 attributes for the second part. There was no repetition or sharing of attributes between these two modules. The whole data set comprising of training and testing data set was hence partitioned vertically into separate parts. Each of these was trained separately. The integrator was made that carried forward the task of combining the results of these two modules.

Each of the two ANNs used in the problem had the same architecture. They were separately trained using Back Propagation Algorithm. There was 1 hidden layer consisting of 4 neurons. The hidden layer had an activation function of '*tansig*' and the output layer had an activation function of '*purelin*'. The learning rate was fixed to be 0.05. Momentum was kept as 0.8. The maximum number of epochs were 3500.

The system so formed with two ANNs and an integrator, making a complete modular neural network gave a performance of 98.21% in the training data where it could identify 385 of the 392 cases. The efficiency of the testing data was 94.35% with the identification of 167 out of 177 cases presented. The system hence gave a good performance.

Training Data Division

The next problem that we have is where we need to divide the training data set into clusters and assign each ANN a different cluster. We make 3 clusters where the data would be clustered into.

Figure 7. Fuzzy C means clustering of training input data

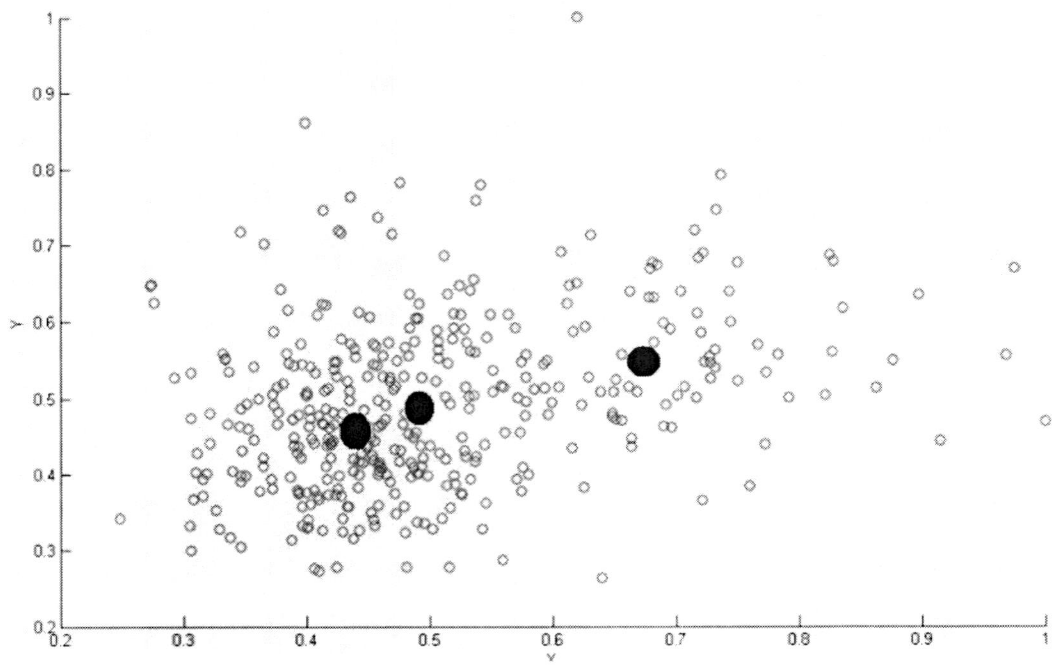

Fuzzy C means clustering was used for the clustering purposes. 100 iterations were used with a minimum improvement of 10^{-5} and exponent of 2. The clustered plot of two of the axis from the input space is shown in Figure 7. Here the black dots denote the cluster center.

From this we get the training centers for further processing. 3 different ANNs are made based on these clusters. Each of them is given its share of the training input to train with. Later the testing is performed. Here also we first select the cluster or the ANN and then find the output corresponding to the input.

All the three ANNs used in the problem had the same architecture. They were separately trained using Back Propagation Algorithm. There was 1 hidden layer consisting of 6 neurons. The hidden layer had an activation function of '*tansig*' and the output layer had an activation function of '*purelin*'. The learning rate was fixed to be 0.05. Momentum was kept as 0.8. The maximum number of epochs were 3500.

The entire system in the stated configuration gave an accuracy of 91.3% in the training data set and 90.5% in the testing data set. Again it may be seen that the system was able to effectively solve the problem of diagnosis of the breast cancer.

FUTURE RESEARCH DIRECTIONS

In this chapter we presented solutions to the common problems of handling large data sizes. The solutions proposed were effective in diagnosis of breast cancer where we achieved large computational speedup with a minute loss of generality. The data set chosen for this problem was itself quite small in nature. For future, work may be carried out on data sets which are massively large in nature and fail to train by a single method. This would be the ideal testing of the proposed algorithm. These data sets may be large horizontally or vertically. The small computational availability has been the reason for low pace of research in numerous fields. The proposed methods promise an effective solution where the data can be easily partitioned to solve the problem. The algorithm may be used over newly built large datasets of large sizes.

We have proposed two independent solutions to the problem of large data sizes. The former divides the data vertically by division of the attributes. At the same time the other divides the data horizontally by the division of instances. These methods may be combined in an intelligent manner to solve complex problems. The design, training and testing of this combined approach may be carried out in future. This would effectively solve the problem of data sets which are very vast in nature. As more and more problems are coming under automation, there is a growth in the number of attributes as well as the entire data set size. The combined method would prove to be very beneficial in such scenarios.

In the proposed algorithm we made use of ANN with Back Propagation Algorithm. Various other models may be tried like Self Organizing Maps, Learning vector Quantization, etc. Also the application of Hybrid Systems including Neuro-Fuzzy Systems, Genetic Training and Evolution of the System may be studied in the future.

CONCLUSION

In this chapter we discussed the problem and solution of having large data set. The size could either be large due to a high number of input attributes that caused a problem in the system training and testing. The size could also be large due to the size of the training data instances. These problems were solved by the use of modular neural networks. For the first problem we divided the input attributes in different modules. This division resulted in a reduced workload as well as reduced the problem complexity. For the second problem we made the division horizontally where the data set was divided by clustering into different data segments or clusters. Each cluster was trained by a separate ANN.

The algorithm was validated by executing it against the breast cancer database. The database contained 30 attributes and 569 instances. The attributes were divided into two sets for the first part of the problem. For the second part of the problem, the data was divided into three clusters using Fuzzy C Means clustering. This made the problem less complex that could easily be solved.

We divided the data set available into training and testing data sets. The training data set was used for training the system with the designed algorithm. The testing was performed by the testing data set. The efficiency of the algorithm to correctly identify the disease from the testing dataset is given as the final diagnostic efficiency. Using this system we could get a sufficiently large efficiency of diagnosis of the disease. The computational time was much less. As a result the system could optimally train itself. This solved the problem of training and testing of large data sets that is becoming an issue of concern for many problems.

ACKNOWLEDGMENT

This work has been supported and sponsored by Indian Institute of Information Technology and Management Gwalior.

REFERENCES

Adams, R., Calcraft, L., & Davey, N. (2009). Using a genetic algorithm to investigate efficient connectivity in associative memories. *Neurocomputing*, *72*(4-6), 732–742. doi:10.1016/j.neucom.2008.05.017

Amin, M. F., & Murase, K. (2009). Single-layered complex-valued neural network for real-valued classification problems. *Neurocomputing*, *72*(4-6), 945–955. doi:10.1016/j.neucom.2008.04.006

Ang, J. H., Tan, K. C., & Al-Mamun, A. (2008). Training neural networks for classification using growth probability-based evolution. *Neurocomputing*, *71*(16-18), 3493–3508. doi:10.1016/j.neucom.2007.10.011

Chaudhuri, B. B., & Bhattacharya, U. (2000). Efficient training and improved performance of multilayer perceptron in pattern classification. *Neurocomputing*, *34*, 11–27. doi:10.1016/S0925-2312(00)00305-2

Conor, R., Collins, J. J., & Neill, M. O. (n.d.). *Grammatical Evolution - Evolving Programs for an Arbitrary Language*

Draghici, S. (1997). A neural network based artificial vision system for license plate recognition, International Journal of Network Security. *International Journal of Neural Systems*, *8*(1). doi:10.1142/S0129065797000148

Er, M. J., & Zhou, Y. (2008). A novel framework for automatic generation of fuzzy neural networks. *Neurocomputing*, *21*(4-6), 584–591. doi:10.1016/j.neucom.2007.03.015

Estudillo, F. J., Martinez, C. H., Gutierrez, P. A., & Estudillo, A. C. (2008). Evolutionary product-unit neural networks classifiers. *Neurocomputing*, *72*(1-3), 548–561. doi:10.1016/j.neucom.2007.11.019

Gernot, A., & Fink, P. & Thomas (2006). Unsupervised Estimation of Writing Style Models for Improved Unconstrained Off-line Handwriting Recognition. In *Proceedings of the Tenth International Workshop on Frontiers in Handwriting Recognition.*

Graves, A., Fernandez, S., Liwicki, M., Bunke, H., & Schmidhuber, J. (2008). Unconstrained Online Handwriting Recognition with Recurrent Neural Networks, In Proceedings of Advances in Neural Information Processing Systems.

Grigore, O., & Gavat, I. (1998). Neuro-fuzzy Models for Speech Pattern Recognition in Romanian Language. In *Proceedings of European Symposium on Intelligent Techniques* (CONTI'98). Timisoara, Romania, (pp. 165–172).

Hewavitharana, S., Fernando, H. C., & Kodikara, N. D. (2002). Off-line Sinhala Handwriting Recognition using Hidden Markov Models

Hu, Y.-C. (2008). Nonadditive grey single-layer perceptron with Choquet integral for pattern classification problems using genetic algorithms. *Neurocomputing*, *72*(1-3), 331–340. doi:10.1016/j.neucom.2008.01.008

Ilter, N., Guvenir, H., & Altay (1998). *UCI Machine Learning Repository*. Rerieved from http://www.ics.uci.edu/~mlearn/MLRepository.html

Kak, S. C. (1998). On generalization by neural networks. *Information Sciences*, *111*, 293–302. doi:10.1016/S0020-0255(98)10009-9

Kala, R., Shukla, A., & Tiwari, R. (2009). Fuzzy Neuro Systems for Machine Learning for Large Data Sets. In *Proceedings of the IEEE International Advance Computing Conference*, (pp. 541-545) Patiala, India.

Kuo, R. J., Hong, S. M., Lin, Y., & Huang, Y. C. (2008). Continuous genetic algorithm-based fuzzy neural network for learning fuzzy IF–THEN rules. *Neurocomputing*, *71*(13-15), 2893–2907. doi:10.1016/j.neucom.2007.07.013

Lee, S. G., et al. (1999). A Neuro-Fuzzy Classifier for Land Cover Classification. In *Proceedings of the 1999 IEEE International Fuzzy Systems Conference Proceedings*, Seoul, Korea.

Lin, C. J., Chung, I. F., & Chen, C. H. (2007). An entropy-based quantum neuro-fuzzy inference system for classification applications. *Neurocomputing*, *70*(13-15), 2502–2516. doi:10.1016/j.neucom.2006.08.008

Lin, C. J., & Hong, S. J. (2007). The design of neuro-fuzzy networks using particle swarm optimization and recursive singular value decomposition. *Neurocomputing*, *71*(1-3), 297–310. doi:10.1016/j.neucom.2006.12.016

Maravall, D., Lope, de, Martin, J., & Antonio, J. (2009). Hybridizing evolutionary computation and reinforcement learning for the design of almost universal controllers for autonomous robots. *Neurocomputing*, *72*(4-6), 887–894. doi:10.1016/j.neucom.2008.04.058

Mu, C. S., Chien, H. C., Eugene, L., & Jonathan, L. (2006). A new approach to fuzzy classifier systems and its application in self-generating neuro-fuzzy systems. *Neurocomputing*, *69*(4-6), 586–614. doi:10.1016/j.neucom.2004.11.033

Nani, L., & Lumini, A. (2009). Particle swarm optimization for prototype reduction. *Neurocomputing*, *72*(4-6), 1092–1097. doi:10.1016/j.neucom.2008.03.008

O' Neill, M., & Brabazon, A. (2005). Recent Adventures in Grammatical Evolution. In *Proceedings of CMS 2005 Computer Methods and Systems*. (Vol. 1, pp. 245-253).

O' Neill, M., & Ryan, C. (2001). Grammatical Evolution. *IEEE Transactions on Evolutionary Computation*, *5*(4).

Pinero, P. (2004). Sleep stage classification using fuzzy sets and machine learning techniques. *Neurocomputing*, *58–60*, 1137–1143. doi:10.1016/j.neucom.2004.01.178

Rajagopal, P. (2003). *The Basic Kak Neural Network with Complex Inputs* (Master of Science in Electrical Engineering Thesis). Tamil Nadu, India: University of Madras

Rutkowski, L. (2004). *Flexible Neuro-Fuzzy Systems, Structures, Learning and Performance Evaluation*. Amsterdam: Kluwer Academic Publishers.

Sandhu, P. S., Salaria, D. S., & Singh, H. (2008). A Comparative Analysis of Fuzzy, Neuro-Fuzzy and Fuzzy-GA Based Approaches for Software Reusability Evaluation. In *Proceedings of Worlds Academy of Science* (*Vol. 29*). Engineering and Technology.

Shadabi, F., Sharma, D., & Cox, R. (2006). Learning from Ensembles: Using Artificial Neural Network Ensemble for Medical Outcomes Prediction, *Innovations in Information Technology*, 1-5.

Shi, D., Shu, W., & Liu, H. (1998). Feature Selection for Handwritten Chinese Character Recognition Based on Genetic Algorithms. In *Proceedings of the Intl' Conf. on Systems, man and Cybernetics*, (Vol. 5, No 5, pp. 4201-4206).

Som, T., & Saha, S. (2008). Handwritten character recognition by using Neural-network and Euclidean distance metric. *Social Science Research Network*. Retrieved from http://ssrn.com/abstract=1118755

Soryani, M., & Rafat, N. (2006). Application of Genetic Algorithms to Feature Subset Selection in a Farsi OCR. In *Proceedings of World Academy of Science* (*Vol. 18*). Engineering and Technology.

Taur, J. S., & Tao, C. W. (2000). A New Neuro-Fuzzy Classifier with Application to On-Line Face Detection and Recognition. *The Journal of VLSI Signal Processing*, *26*, 397–409. doi:10.1023/A:1026515819538

Tsoulos, I., Dimitris, G., & Glavas, E. (2008). Neural network construction and training using grammatical evolution. *Neurocomputing*, *72*(1-3), 269–277. doi:10.1016/j.neucom.2008.01.017

Vieira, A., & Barradas, N. (2003). A training algorithm for classification of high-dimensional data. *Neurocomputing*, *50*, 461–472. doi:10.1016/S0925-2312(02)00635-5

Wolberg, W. H., Mangasarian, O. L., & Aha, D. W. (1992). UCI Machine Learning Repository, University of Wisconsin Hospitals. Retrieved from http://www.ics.uci.edu/~mlearn/MLRepository.html

KEY TERMS AND DEFINITIONS

Artificial Neural Networks: Mathematical model consisting of parallel processing neurons that perform information processing in a layered manner. They are excellent agents for regression, functional prediction or classification.

Classification: Problems in which the input always lies in one of the available classes based on the input attributes.

Fuzzy C Means Clustering: A clustering algorithm that forms fuzzy cluster where each member is associated to every cluster by some degree of membership that lies in a scale of 0 to 1.

Generalization: Ability of a system to give correct outputs to unknown inputs.

Hybrid Systems: Systems made by a combination of soft computing systems (Artificial neural Networks, Evolutionary Algorithms or Fuzzy Logic) along with heuristics.

Input Space: A multi-dimensional space plotting the output values of the Artificial Neural Network (or any other system) for every combination of inputs for a specific system state.

Integrator: Part of the Modular Neural Network that carries forward the task of division of problem into modules and the computation of the final output by the individual module output.

Machine Learning: Forming rules, trends or patterns in the historical database, so that the correct outputs may be computed whenever this data is presented again to the systems.

Modular Neural Networks: Neural Networks that work on the modularity in the problem. The problem is divided into modules and given to various sub-systems that independently solve part of the problem. The overall result is communicated to an integrator and the final output is computed.

Modules: Independent Neural Networks that solve a part of the whole problem in a Modular Neural Network and communicate their results to the integrator.

Chapter 9

Breast Cancer: Advancement in Diagnostic and Treatment

Yos S Morsi
Swinburne University of Technology, Australia

Pujiang Shi
Swinburne University of Technology, Australia

Amal Ahmed Owida
Swinburne University of Technology, Australia

Rafiul Hassan
University of Melbourne, Australia

Rezaul Karim Begg
Victoria University, Australia.

ABSTRACT

Breast cancer is the second most common cancer in the world and is difficult to accurately identify and treat. Diagnostic computational tools can be used effectively, with high degree of accuracy, to recognize and differentiate between the two known types of breast lesion, namely benign and malignant. These modelling tools include artificial intelligence techniques such as Artificial Neural Networks (ANNs), Fuzzy Logic (FL), Hidden Markov Model (HMM) and Support Vector Machines (SVMs). These tools can identify the important features that play pivotal roles in the classification task, and can aid physicians to diagnose and prognosticate breast cancer. Moreover, recent advancement in nanotechnology indicates that with the aid of nanoparticles, nanowires, nanorobots and nanotubes, the disease of breast cancer can be potentially eradicated totally. The chapter highlights the limitations of the current therapies used in breast cancer and discusses the concept of nanotechnology as a possible future therapy.

INTRODUCTION

Breast cancer is the most common type of cancer amongst women in the developed world, with approximately 1 in 12 having the disease sometime during their life, with the incidence in Australia being slightly higher at 1 in 11 women (Breast Screen Australia, 2000-2001). While most breast cancer patients fall within the age group of 35-

DOI: 10.4018/978-1-61692-004-3.ch009

54, it is not uncommon to find malignant breast lesion at a much earlier age. Moreover, men have also been diagnosed with breast cancer as breast tissue is identical for male and female. Because of the prolonged, complicated and intensive treatment procedure, early detection of breast cancer is crucial for effective treatment. Although, there have been many different methods for identifying breast cancer (mammography, MRI, and biopsy), all of them produce results which can be interpreted differently depending on the consultant physician's knowledge and experience. This underscores the need for a reliable and imperial automated method to assist the physician to identify breast cancer accurately. There exist a number of automated tools for the diagnosis of this disease. However, these tools are very complex and suffer from poor performance. This suggests there is a need for the development of new effective diagnostic tools. Now-a-days various computer aided diagnostic methods, including Artificial Neural Networks (ANNs), Fuzzy Logic (FL), Hidden Markov Model (HMM) and Support Vector Machines (SVMs) have been proposed to identify and distinguish between the benign and malignant breast lesion with a high degree of precision. Modern microarray technologies produce high dimensional read outs of molecular activities in patient specimens that can describe the characteristic features of the cancer types. A major challenge of these technologies is to identify the most influential gene set from a large number of genes that are responsible for the occurrence of the disease and can be used as predictors for the cancer. However, the advancement of nanotechnology aided with **nanowires, nanotubes,** and **nanorobots** for cancer treatment appears to be the most successful choice of option which has the potential to eradicate the cancerous cells and prove to be the future treatment therapy.

DIAGNOSIS AND MODELING TECHNIQUES

It is well recognized that in treatment and diagnostic of breast cancer, clinicians are often presented with identical clinical information. However, unfortunately clinicians can act in different ways depending on their knowledge and experience which highlighted the need to introduce diagnostic tools to support the scientific homogeneity and accountability of healthcare decisions and actions. The benefits expected from such actions include an overall reduction in cost, improved quality of care as well as patient and public opinion satisfaction. Recently, computer-based medical data processing research has yielded methods and tools for managing the task away from the hospital management level and closer to the desired disease and patient management level.

In search of an accurate tool for distinguish and diagnostic cancer lesions various techniques have been proposed. Recent research focuses primarily on the application of computer vision and for early lesion identification in mammograms and breast-imaging volumes through computer-aided diagnostics (CAD) tools with particular emphasis on computational diagnostics methodology for the analysis of molecular disease mechanisms in cancer. To this end, advanced applications of information and disease process modeling technologies have already demonstrated an ability to significantly augment clinical decision making. One of the main obstacles that need to be overcome is the development of systems that treat both information and knowledge as clinical objects with same modeling requirements. Here we briefly describe some of the existing computational models used for classification of the types of breast lesion in brief here.

Artificial Neural Networks: There are a number of studies where ANNs have been proposed to diagnose and prognosticate the two known types of breast cancers: Benign and Malignant. Among these, Fogel et al. (Fogel, Wasson Iii et al., 1995) who applied ANNs to classify the types of breast cancer while they evolved the structure of the ANN by employing evolutionary programming. They validated their approach using the Wisconsin breast cancer dataset (WBCD) that was first introduced by Wolberg and Mangasarian (Wolberg and Mangasarian, 1990). Abbas achieved a better classification performance compared to that of Fogel Fogel et al. (Fogel, Wasson Iii et al., 1995). by using an evolutionary artificial neural network approach based on the pareto differential evolution algorithm for the same dataset.

Fuzzy Logic: Fuzzy Logic (FL) uses a number of rules to define the data structure and combine the output of all these rules to obtain an aggregated result. Although FL is popular where it is difficult to classify an object in which group it belongs to (i.e., the degree of membership of a specific object is overlapped among two or more groups/classes) due to the fuzziness involved in the system, there are studies where researchers have proposed FL approaches to classify the types of breast cancer with varying success. Nauck et al. (1995) used FL to classify the WBCD dataset. In their approach, they modified the state of art neuro-fuzzy model through introducing shared weights between the connections of two neurons in the neuro-fuzzy structure. This approach has been referred as NEFCLASS. In another study, Setioni et al. used FL where the fuzzy rules were generated using a trained ANN. This system called Neuro rules has been applied to classify breast cancer using the WBCD. Hassan et al. (2006) proposed a method by combining HMM and FL to classify the two types of breast cancer. HMM log-likelihood value for each data vector was used to rank the data vector and the ranked data vectors were partitioned to generate fuzzy rules. To obtain a better classification performance, in another study Hassan et al. (2010) used the area under the ROC curves (AUC) to select the influential features from the dataset. Then the hybrid of HMM and FL was used to classify the dataset with the selected features.

Support Vector Machine (SVM): SVM is a popular computational tool for classifying binary class problem. Fung et al.(2002) proposed knowledge-based SVM classifiers to classify types of breast cancer, where prior knowledge from the dataset was used to reformulate a linear support vector machine.

Now a days, a number of **Artificial Intelligence (AI) tools** based on Artificial Neural Network (ANN) have been proposed to diagnose and prognosticate the dataset for the two known types of breast cancers: Benign and Malignant (Fogel, Wasson Iii et al., 1995). Recently, a hybrid computational model has been developed (e.g. Hidden Markov Model (HMM), Fuzzy Logic (FL) and ANN) for the diagnosis and prognosis of a number of human diseases such as breast cancer, balanced impairment problem and malignant lymphoid tissue identification (Kamruzzaman, Lim et al., 2005) It is claimed that this tool can successfully identify and distinguish the two types of breast cancer, with higher accuracy than the existing ones. Furthermore, tools such as ANN and FL have been applied on WBCD dataset to diagnose and prognosticate the two known types of breast cancers. Others researchers such as Fung et al. (Mangasarian et al., 2005) have used Support Vector Machine (SVM) with the same dataset to analyze breast cancer.

In addition to the tissue or breast fluid data, the application of gene expression level information is widely used for diagnosis and prognosis of general diseases. For instance, (Vijver et al., 2002) found that the **gene expression profile** is a more powerful predictor of the outcome of the disease in younger patients with breast cancer than standard systems based on clinical and histological criteria. These authors evaluated the predictive power of the profile using both uni-variate and multi-variants statistical analysis to prognosticate breast cancer.

Recently, Hassan et al. (2009) proposed a multi-classifier voting approach to classify the Vijver et al.s, 2002) gene expression dataset into two classes: poor prognosis and good prognosis. In a study, (Lim et al., 2007) achieved an improved performance in classifying cancerous lymphoid tissue from Lymphochip gene expression data by using SVM followed by a gene selection technique. Huang et al., Cheng et al., (2003) analyzed DNA microarray data from samples of primary breast tumors, using nonlinear statistical analyses to assess multiple patterns of interactions of groups of genes that have predictive values for the individual patient, with respect to lymph node metastasis and cancer recurrence. They further introduced a computer-based system for cancer diagnosis using microarray data and found that the **Multi-category SVMs (MC-SVMs)** were the most effective classifier for accurate cancer diagnosis from gene expression data. Alexe et al. (2006) applied Logical Analysis of Data (LAD) tool to analyze the microarray data for diagnosis and prognosis of the breast cancer dataset. They identified that 17 genes out of the 25,000 genes are capable of distinguishing patients with poor or good prognosis.

In addition to breast cancer related data, researchers have focused on the use of the best classifier to optimize the recognition model. The most common classifiers used are: (ANN; Gruvberger, Ringner et al., 2001), (SVM; Alizadeh, Elsen et al., 2000), (FL; Kuznetsov, Ivshina et al., 1996), (k-Nearest Neighbor clustering (k-NN); Yang, Haddad et al., 2003) and hierarchical clustering (Bittner, Meltzer et al., 2000). Based on the micro-array data expression, these classifiers have been widely used to diagnose and classify several cancers (e.g. lung, ovarian, leukemia and breast). Moreover, to reduce the redundant and less significant genes in identifying the cancerous tumor, a number of data reduction methods have also been proposed. The widely used data reduction methods are: t-test, f-test, significant analysis of micro-arrays (SAM), principal component analysis (PCA) and clustering.

FUTURE RESEARCH DIRECTIONS

There are still many important and challenging issues in developing and optimizing a breast cancer diagnostic tool. One approach is that, by totally analyzing the cancerous gene expression data and incorporating improved AI technique, the resulting software would have greater influences on physicians' decisions for early diagnosis and classification of cancer. However, it is a challenging task to generate the best HMM to capture the fluctuations among the data features, Moreover, it is difficult to find the exact relationship among the initial parameters and the performances of the HMM. Genetic algorithm (GA) is well known for solving such problems where the exact mathematical relationship is hard to identify.

Investigating the less important fuzzy rules (Figure 1) and condense them will further optimize the method of HMM-based rule generation. To examine the less important fuzzy rules, an approach to identify the redundant rules, namely a new 'subset hood-based" rule identification need to be developed. No tools perform universally for all dataset, several alternative approaches e.g. ANN. SVM and Bayesian network are being investigated worldwide along with the FL for the same dataset, which will result in generating the best ANN model to diagnose and prognosticate the same dataset. Similar tests can be performed with SVM by varying the kernel functions. On presentation of a test data, the outcome predicted by each model are then combined using a weighted decision system to generate a single output indicating the status of the patient.

Nanotechnology and Treatment of Cancer

Recently the use of nanotechnology for the treatment of cancer has received a lot of attention and now various possible techniques have been proposed for treatment. Cancer hyperthermia treatment where the heat is used at various depths

Figure 1. Fuzzy rule generation based on HMM log likelihood values

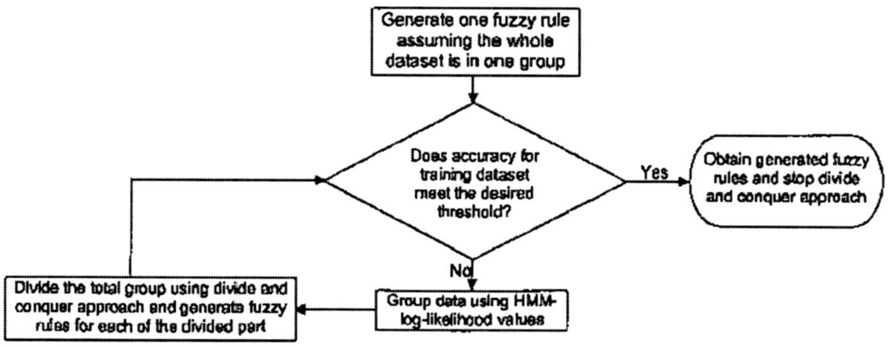

in human cancer tissue to target the cancerous cells and eradicate or neutralize them has been widely accepted. Another technique is the use of the magnetic nano-particles that being subjected to a magnetic AC field which has shown remarkable heating effects related to loss during the magnetization reversal process of the particles. The literature suggests that such effect can be used for the eradication of cancerous cells including breast cancer. Although these techniques are promising there are still a number of challenges to overcome before bringing this treatment to clinical implementation. Currently an extensive research on the use of radio frequency and microwave hyperthermia systems as non-invasive instruments to produce sufficient and accurate temperature gradients within the biological tissues for efficient and effective treatment of breast cancer is being investigated worldwide with various degree of success.

In line with this other innovative techniques have been recently proposed for the treatment of cancer such as nanoscale devices like nanowire and nanotube. These devices at least in theory can diagnose and treat the cancer directly and effectively. This concept ignited a lot of excitement among researchers and as a result there are various nano-devices that have been searched and developed for the treatments of cancer. These devices (having at least one dimension less than 100 nanometers) can penetrate the cells and interact with DNA and proteins present inside. Moreover, theoretically speaking miniaturization will allow the development of various tools for the treatment of various diseases and could make it possible to run various diagnostic tests simultaneously with high degree of sensitivity and accuracy and enter and control and encapsulate cells within a human body..

The combined drug delivery research with nanotechnology is now one of the most widely proposed methods which have the potential to create opportunity in developing targeted drug delivery strategies for cancer treatments in general and breast cancer in particular. The theory behind this concept is that when drug device is inserted in the body, it finds the required target, such as tumour, and releasing the required dose of drug on target effectively with precious timing and minimum if any adverse effect. As stated by Goldberg and Langer, the main purpose of these devices and particles is to deliver nanoscale drugs and various classes of biomacromolecules, such as peptides, proteins, plasmid DNA and synthetic oligodeoxynucleotides (Goldberg, Langer et al., 2007).

However, for drug delivery nanomaterials there are still a number of challenges to over come, such as controlled composition, shape, size and morphology. Nanomaterials and their surface properties and shapes can be optimised to control solubility, immune-compatibility and cellular uptake. To date identified limitations of developments and designs of drug delivery system are still suffering from factors such as potential cytotoxicity suboptimal bioavailability and very limited effective drug targeting. However, the literature now suggest that improved delivery of inefficient water-soluble drugs, with specific targeted delivery of drugs in a cell or tissue-, delivery of large macromolecule drugs to intra-cellular sites of action as well as co-delivery of two or more drugs or therapeutic modality for combination therapy. Visualization of target sites of drug delivery by combining therapeutic agents with imaging modalities with real-time is also possible in the future. (Ferrari, 2005).

However, a among such an excitement it should be noted that the short and long terms side effects of nanoscale treatments are still unknown and in a controversial stage, as the exact mechanics and the physical properties of various nanoparticles materials are not fully understood..

Nanotube in Drug Delivery

Carbon nanotubes is one of the promising choice of cancer therapies among all the various conceptual ideas that have been proposed for the treatment of drugs, (Ikai, Smith et al., 2007). These future devices are well researched as possible drug delivery vehicles, and they possess good precision and, biocompatibility with minium adverse effects. In fact researcher in the field suggest that there are several clear advantages associated with the use of carbon nanotube such as;, the inner diameter of the nanotubes is lager, hence more larger volume for the encapsulation of the drugs, the inner volume could be easily manipulated by simply removing the end cap of nanotubes, the inner and outer walls of the nanotubes are easily recognized which is an advantage in drug delivery applications, finally these tubes have the capability in penetrating into cell nuclei, which are useful in handling genes (Ikai, Smith et al., 2007).

As suggested by Kai, Smith et al delivering of the drugs using carbon nanotubes can be illustrated in (Figure 2) and follow the below basic steps:

- the carbon nanotube is coated by chemical receptor such as folate-targeting and the open end is used to insert drug molecules.
- the open end made from biodegradable cap, hence degradation is controlled by the environmental factors such as pH, temperature and external supply,
- the nanotube after injection will find their defined targets by use of chemical receptors, such as folate receptors on cancer cells. The nanotube will penetrate the tumour walls and timely release the drug.

Moreover, recently the combination of nanoparticles and hyperthermia method has been widely proposed in the past few decades to potentially provide cancer clinics with more effective and advanced cancer treatment. However, it should be noted that despite the enormous research efforts, all the proposed hyperthermia techniques to date are found to be not effective and have various adverse effects. For example the low heating temperature generated owing to the heat loss through a relatively big gap between targeted cells and hyperthermia agents caused by the hard to control agent transport. Moreover, killing healthy cells attributed to the difficulties of cell differentiations by hyperthermia agents, are considered as the main reasons for the undesirable outcomes which make such proposed treatment unattractive. The introduction of the use of nanoparticles to address some of above drawbacks to fill the following requirements: (i) non-toxicity; (ii) a sufficient chemical stability in bio-environment; (iii) an appropriate circulation time in the blood; and (iv) in addition a harmless biocompatible, biodegradable nanoparticles have been proposed in literature.

Figure 2. Process of drug delivering using carbon nanotubes (Ikai, Smith et al. 2007 [12])

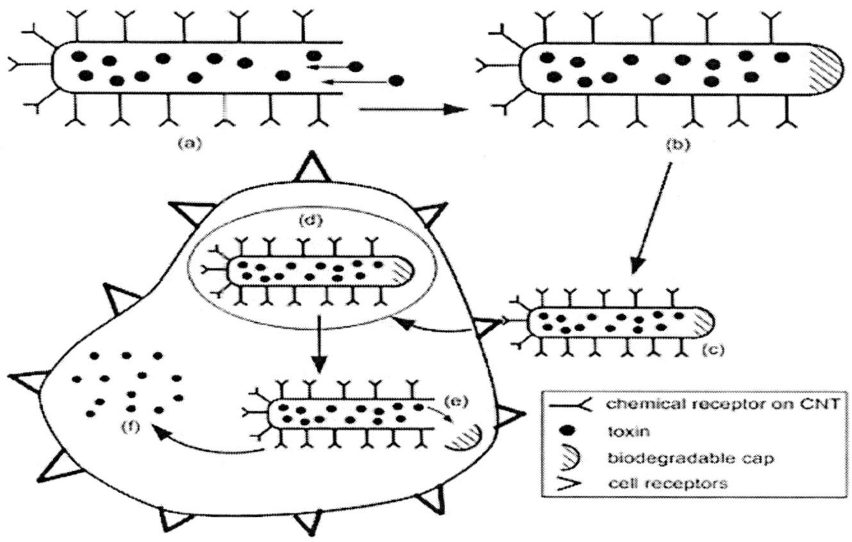

Furthermore, it should be noted that cancer cells are temperature sensitive compared with the other cells and therefore, relative higher temperature could be used to treat cancer. This method is called photo induced hyperthermia where heat is generated by light energy. The idea is that gold nanoparticles are first subjected to infrared light and then transferred it to heat the sight where the cancer cells are located. The theory behind that when heat is generated through UV infrared light or other sources such as microwave, cancerous cells which bound to gold nanoparticles are eliminated. Alexander HR Jr.et al (2008) Conversely the literature also suggest that in the process of converting light to heat energy, rod shape gold nanoparticles are more effective than normal spherical gold particles as the shape of the gold nanoparticles can influence their responding infrared frequency. Furthermore, in this process the drugs are attached to the surface of the nanoparticles which are exposed to sensitive frequency of infrared light, and then the nanoparticles will melt and release the drugs effectively. Moreover, the melting time of the nanoparticles can be controlled by their shape and the energy input and tremendous amount of research are currently being carried out on the optimisation of the melting time using various type of materials and time realise.

The use of polymer nanoparticles has been proposed due to the fact that polymer nanoparticles could be coated with biomolecules which can be made to act as special signals to recognize cancer cells among patient tissues. Therefore, the side effects such as killing healthy cells could be minimized or eliminated, as the nanoparticles are only accumulating around the cancer cells. On the other hand, not like the inorganic nanoparticles, the polymer will degrade and only stay in the body for a short time, therefore, the possible adverse effects of gold particles such as calculus and mutation can be totally eliminated. Hence the choice of the biodegradable polymers and the optimization of the degradation time and geometry of the particles are issues of ongoing concern to the researchers in the field. **Q A Pankhurst et al (2003)**

Conversely, the special characteristics of DNA have been proposed as suitable to serve as a construction material in nanosciences (Seeman, 1999). This because, the DNA on the nanoparticles can only connect to the cancer gene and get into the cancer cells and has a relatively high physicochemical stability. The idea of using DNA on the nanoparticles is based on the fact the one can enhance the power of DNA as a molecular tool by synthesize its sequence using automated methods and use, polymerase chain reaction (PCR) and to amplify such DNA sequence from microscopic to macroscopic forms (PCR). Moreover, DNA offers a great mechanical rigidity of short double helices as they can be considered as a rigid rod spacer between two tethered functional molecular components on both ends. Moreover, it should be noted that nature provides a complete toolbox of highly specific biomolecular reagents, such as endonucleases, ligases, and other DNA-modifying enzymes, which can process DNA material with atomic precision and accuracy on the Angström level.

Similarly nanorobots have been proposed as a diagnostic tool in the therapy of cancer or as a targeted drug delivery agent to eradicate cancer cells.

CONCLUSION

Breast cancer is a major cause of deaths and predominantly affects women over the age of 40. Cancer diagnosis and prognosis have become one of the major National Health Service issues attracting various federal and state government initiatives worldwide. Dealing with the increasing cost of health care delivery and the detrimental consequences on the quality and effectiveness of clinical outcomes requires supportive and corrective actions to be taken much closer to the source of the problem. The disease can be most efficiently treated if detected at an early stage.

To detect the breast cancer accurately and quickly, computational models are currently being developed. Some notable ones are based on techniques such as Hidden Markov Model (HMM), Fuzzy Logic (FL) and ANN, and these have demonstrated promise for the detection and future treatments of breast cancer as well as assisting clinicians with the updated knowledge for treatment. On the other hand, nanotechnology is currently being researched for effective treatment of cancer. It can be stated that the use of nanotechnology in breast cancer treatment is a revolutionary approach instead of surgery, chemotherapy, radiation therapy and hormonal therapy whose side effects can be considered significant. This is particularly the case for drug delivery system research, including nano particles, nanowires, nanorobots and nanotubes. All the advanced diagnostic and therapeutical techniques discussed in this chapter are promising but are still in experimental stage Therefore, the research and the development of this technology is the key to the success to the development of an accurate diagnostic and effective treatment of such a disease.

REFERENCES

Alexander, H. R. Jr. (2008). Isolation Perfusion. In DeVita, V. T., Lawrence, T. S., & Rosenberg, S. A. (Eds.), *Cancer Principles and Practice of Oncology* (8th ed., pp. 701–710). Philadelphia: Lippincott, Williams, & Wilkins.

Alexe, G. (2006). Breast cancer prognosis by combinatorial analysis of gene expression data. *Breast Cancer Research*, *8*(4). doi:10.1186/bcr1512

Alizadeh, A. A. (2000). Distinct types of diffuse large B-cell lymphoma identified by gene expression profiling. *Nature*, *403*(6769), 503–511. doi:10.1038/35000501

Bittner, M. (2000). Molecular classification of cutaneous malignant melanoma by gene expression profiling. *Nature*, *406*(6795), 536–540. doi:10.1038/35020115

Ferrari, M. (2005). Cancer nanotechnology: Opportunities and challenges. *Nature Reviews. Cancer*, *5*(3), 161–171. doi:10.1038/nrc1566

Fogel, D. B., Wasson Iii, E. C., & Boughton, E. M. (1995). Evolving neural networks for detecting breast cancer. *Cancer Letters*, *96*(1), 49–53. doi:10.1016/0304-3835(95)03916-K

Fung, G., Mangasarian, O. L., & Shavlik, J. (2005). Knowledge-based support vector machine classifiers. In *Proceedings of NIPS 2002*.

Goldberg, M., Langer, R., & Jia, X. (2007). Nanostructured materials for applications in drug delivery and tissue engineering. *Journal of Biomaterials Science. Polymer Edition*, *18*(3), 241–268. doi:10.1163/156856207779996931

Gruvberger, S. (2001). Estrogen receptor status in breast cancer is associated with remarkably distinct gene expression patterns. *Cancer Research*, *61*(16), 5979–5984.

Hassan, R. Begg,Y.Morsi,K.Lynch,HMM-fuzzy model forbreast cancer diagnosis, in: Proceedings of the 15th International Conference on Machines in Medicineand Biology,2006.

Hassan, R., Hossain, M. M., Bailey, J., Macintyre, G., Ho, J., & Ramamohanarao, K. (2009). A voting approach to identify a small number of highly predictive genes using multiple classifiers. *BMC Bioinformatics*, *10*(Suppl I), S19. doi:10.1186/1471-2105-10-S1-S19

Hassan, R., Hossain, M. M., Begg, R. K., Ramamohanarao, K., & Morsi, Y. (2010). Breast-Cancer identification using HMM-fuzzy approach. *Computers in Biology and Medicine*, *40*(Issue 3), 240–251. doi:10.1016/j.compbiomed.2009.11.003

Huang, E. (2003). Gene expression predictors of breast cancer outcomes. *Lancet*, *361*(9369), 1590–1596. doi:10.1016/S0140-6736(03)13308-9

Ikai, A., Smith, A., & Tsukada, M. (1999). Nanomechanics. *Current Nanoscience*, *3*(1), 1. doi:10.2174/157341307779940517

Kamruzzaman, J., et al. (2005). Gene selection and classification of human lymphoma from microarray data, In Lecture Notes in Computer Science (including subseries Lecture Notes in Artificial Intelligence and Lecture Notes in Bioinformatics (pp. 379-390).

Kamruzzaman, J., et al. (2007). Gene selection and classification of human lymphoma from microarray data. In *Proceedings of TENCON: The IEEE Region 10 Annual International Conference*.

Kuznetsov, V. A. (1996). Syndrome approach for computer recognition of fuzzy systems and its application to immunological diagnostics and prognosis of human cancer. *Mathematical and Computer Modelling*, *23*(6), 95–119. doi:10.1016/0895-7177(96)00021-0

Lacroix, M. (2006). Significance, detection and markers of disseminated breast cancer cells. *Endocrine-Related Cancer*, *13*(4), 1033–1067. doi:10.1677/ERC-06-0001

Merck Manual Home Edition. (2007). *Introduction: Breast Disorders. Whitehouse Station*. NJ: Merck.

Nauck. D., Nauck, U. and Kruse, R. (1996). 'Generating Classification rules with the Neuro Fuzzy system NEFCLASS', Proceedings of IEEE Conference, pp. 466-470.

Pankhurst, Q. A., Connolly, J., Jones, S. K., & Dobson, J. (2003). Applications of magnetic nanoparticles in biomedicine, J. Phys. D: Appl. Phys. **36** R167–R181 PII: S0022-3727(03)40035-1.

Seeman, N. C. (1999). DNA engineering and its application to nanotechnology. *Trends in Biotechnology*, *17*(11), 437–443. doi:10.1016/S0167-7799(99)01360-8

Vijver, Van De., He, M. J., et al. (2002). A gene-expression signature as a predictor of survival in breast cancer. *The New England Journal of Medicine*, *347*(25), 1999–2009. doi:10.1056/NEJMoa021967

Wolberg, W. H., & Mangasarian O. L., (1990). Multisurface method of pattern separation for medical diagnosis applied to breast cytology. *National Academy of Sciences, 87*(23), 9193-9196.

Yang, H., et al. (2003). A segmental nearest neighbor normalization and gene identification method gives superior results for DNA-array analysis. *National Academy of Sciences, 100*(3), 1122-1127.

KEY TERMS AND DEFINITIONS

Breast Cancer: A disease in which the cells in the breast show abnormal behaviour in their growth and multiply in uncontrolled manner and spread to other parts of the body through lymphatic system.

Hidden Markov Model (HMM): HMM is a statistical model which is widely used for cancer applications to identify regions of genes with abnormal expression levels from microarray gene expression data.

Fuzzy Logic (FL): Fuzzy Logic model is a combination of accuracy and interpretability. By applying these two objectives on cancer, Fuzzy Logic Model can precisely describes the different kind of lesions in breast cancer patients.

Artificial Neural Network (ANN): It is one of the signal processing technology based on the operation of biological neuron networks and is used to recognize the medical image patterns associated with breast cancer.

Nanotechnology: Nanotechnology is the science of building functional systems at the molecular scale. This technology may be very useful for developing ways to eradicate cancer cells without causing any damage to the healthy, neighbouring cells.

Drug Delivery System: It is a type of method of administrating a pharmaceutical drug to achieve a biological effect at the targeted site in humans or animals.

Chapter 10
Techniques for Decomposition of EMG Signals

Arun Kumar Wadhwani
MITS, India

Sulochana Wadhwani
MITS, India

ABSTRACT

The information extracted from the EMG recordings is of great clinical importance and is used for the diagnosis and treatment of neuromuscular disorders and to study muscle fatigue and neuromuscular control mechanism. Thus there is a necessity of efficient and effective techniques, which can clearly separate individual MUAPs from the complex EMG without loss of diagnostic information. This chapter deals with the techniques of decomposition based on statistical pattern recognition, cross-correlation, Kohonen self-organizing map and wavelet transform.

INTRODUCTION

The electrical signals produced by the muscles and nerves are analyzed to assess the state of neuromuscular function in subjects with suspected neuromuscular disorders. The repetitive activation of several individual motor units (MUs) results in a superposed pulse train and constitutes the electromyogram (EMG) signal. The analysis of the EMG is based on its basic constituent i.e. motor-unit action potentials (MUAPs). The motor unit is the smallest functional unit of a muscle, which can be activated voluntarily. It consists of a group of muscle fibers, which are innervated from the same motor nerve. The shape of MUAP reflects the pathological and functional states of the motor unit. With increasing muscle force, the EMG signal shows an increase in the number of activated MUAPs recruited at increasing firing rate, making it difficult for the neurophysiologist to distinguish individual MUAP waveforms. In most of the clinical EMG examinations, it is the shape of the action potential that is analyzed for diagnostics

The shape and amplitude of MUAP waveform generally differ from motor unit to motor unit due to unique geometric arrangement of the muscle fibers in each motor unit. However, the MUAP

DOI: 10.4018/978-1-61692-004-3.ch010

waveforms from different motor units may also be nearly similar in amplitude and shape when the muscle fibers of two or more motor units have a similar spatial arrangement in detectable vicinity of electrode. The variations in the MUAP waveform are greater when the MUAP waveform actually arises from two or more of the motor units fibers at approximately same distance from the electrode and thus of similar amplitude. The variable latencies in the onset of individual muscle fiber action potentials may produce large uncorrelated changes in compound MUAP waveform from one firing to the next. When few (less than three) motor unit action potential train (MUAPTs) are present in the EMG signal, much of the noise actually results from variations in an MUAP waveform from one firing to the next. When a greater number of MUAPTs is present, the additional noise is also produced by many low amplitude MUAP waveforms.

Number of different factors attribute for noise in MUAPs, namely, increase in degree of severity, instrument noise, neuromuscular junction jitter, detection electrode movement, and interference from the MUAPs of nearby motor units [2]. The shape of the MUAP waveforms within a MUAPT remains constant, if (i) all the initial relationships between the electrode and the active muscle fibers remain constant (i.e. there is no variation in geometrical arrangement between the recording electrode and active muscle fibers), (ii) the relative time difference between the initiation of each constituent fiber action potential, and (iii) the properties of the recording electrode remain constant, and (iv) there are no significant biochemical changes in the muscle tissues. The presence of noise in the EMG signal is a major problem to obtain clean MUAPs after decomposition.

Due to overlapping of MUAPs in the EMG signal, physicians have great difficulty in classifying superimposed waveforms and have no valid reason for their conclusions. With the help of decomposition technique, it is possible to provide more accurate information w.r.t. the EMG signal and MUAPs to know the state of a subject's peripheral neuromuscular system.

DECOMPOSITION OF EMG

The parameters of the MUAPs have proven to be of major importance for the clinical diagnosis of myopathies and neuropathies [1]. For perfect diagnosis, accurate decomposition of EMG signal is needed. The success of EMG signal decomposition is decided by the accurate classification of the MUAPs. There is a long list of limiting factors, which hamper the process of successful decomposition. Some of them arise from the characteristics of the MUAPs. The MUAPs have different durations (finite) and overlap in time and frequency domains. They occur at different time instants are time varying in nature and contaminated by noise and background activity produced by non detectable MUAPs. The repetition frequencies are so high that individual MUAPs rarely appear as isolated potentials [1].

The major challenge in decomposition is to break down the waveforms and analyze them accurately as these are the outcome of a complicated activity and require complete understanding of the electrical fields generated within and around the muscle fibers. Manual decomposition of EMG signal has been successfully done for a long time for clinical diagnosis. It has been shown that the relevant MUAP parameters such as shape, amplitude, duration, and number of phases and turns can be identified manually. However, manual analysis is tedious, time-consuming and inaccurate, and therefore, the investigators have worked for long time to automate the process of decomposition. Significant features and other details of various techniques for automatic decomposition of an EMG signals. are given in (Figure 1).

It has been found that most automatic detection schemes cannot accommodate slow changes in shape or amplitude in MUAPs.

Figure 1. Comparison of various decomposition techniques

S N	Decomposition Techniques	Workers	Features
1.	Template matching & Firing statistics	R S Lefever & C J De Luca, March 1982 R S Lefever A P Xenakis & C J De Luca, March 1982	For generation of synthetic EMG; precise knowledge of MUAPs is required. Firing of MUAPs is decided by the operator.
2.	Tumbling algorithm	R M Studer, R J P de Figueiredo & G S Moschytz, March 1984	Maximum 3 number of overlapping MUAPs can be separated.
3.	Multiple decision approach	A Gerber, R M Studer, R J P de Figueiredo & G S Moschytz, December 1984	Maximum 3 number of overlapping MUAPs can be separated. Reference signal is shortened.
4.	Template matching	K C Mc Gill, K L Cummins & L J Dorfman, July 1985	8 to 15 MUAPs are detected. Suppresses the MUAP sharp peaks.
5.	Statistically pattern recognition technique	D Stashuk & H D Bruin, January 1983	Power spectrum feature & firing time criteria. 3 to 5 MUAPs are detected. For stability of data and initialization of templates, help of the operator is required.
6.	Median average & split sweep median averaging	S D Nandedkar & D B Sanders, November 1989	Signal to noise ratio is improved. Suppresses the large -amplitude noise spikes. Split sweep median averaging is fast technique.
7.	IBC & TBC	D W Stashuk & R K Naphan, April 1992	IBC neglects the errors and missing data in the training set.
8.	Template matching	G H Loudon, N B Jone & A S Sehmi, November 1992	Fuzzy firing statistics.
9.	Statistically & Kohonen Pattern recognition technique	I. Christodoulos & Constantinos S. Pattichis, February 1999	Euclidean distance criteria. 5 to 6 MUAPs are detected.
10.	Wavelets	J Fang, G C Agarwal & B T Shahani, June 1999	1 to 8 MUAPs are detected. Spikes, which are less sensitive to waveform variation, can be classified easily.
11.	Modeling	D Farina, A Crosetti & R Merletti, January 2001	Euclidean distance criteria. Fuzzy firing statistics.

SEGMENTATION

The segmentation (scan the EMG signal) is done to determine the number and shape of different MUAPs present, to know the approximate location of each peak and to know the amount of change in the MUAP waveforms throughout the EMG signal. In segmentation phase, the EMG signal is cut into the segments of possible MUAP waveform and the low activity signal is eliminated. The segmentation technique algorithm calculates threshold depending on maximum value of the complete signal. Peaks over the calculated threshold are considered as the candidate MUAPs. This selected threshold is dependent upon level of background noise in the data. Determination of this threshold is very critical. Generally speaking, lower value of threshold may generate extra number of peaks and tend to increase the error, which mistakenly classifies the spikes belonging to the same motor unit into different groups. On the other hand, if threshold is higher, it may generate less number of groups and increase the error, which fails to distinguish the spikes of different motor units.

CLASSIFICATION TECHNIQUES

As per literature survey, it has been found that to obtain clean MUAPs, the statistical pattern recognition, cross correlation coefficients, Kohonen self-organizing feature map, and Wavelet transform methods can be used. Therefore these methods have been described here in detail.

Statistical Pattern Recognition Technique

The statistical pattern recognition approach is based on the Euclidean distance [2]. Euclidean distance is determined to identify and group similar waveforms(segment) using a constant threshold. The MUAP waveform, which is having minimum distance (having greatest similarity) from the reference waveform and is above the threshold, is considered belonging to the same class. The steps of the decomposition technique are as follows:

STEP 1.

Start with the first segment, x, as the reference waveform; being the first member of the class.

STEP 2.

a. Calculate the Euclidean distance, l_x of the reference waveform as follows:

$$l_x = \sum_{i=1}^{N} x_i^2$$ where N is number of samples,

x_i is the ith sample of waveform x.

b. Calculate the Euclidean distance, d_{xy}, between the x and all the other segmented waveforms

$$d_{xy} = \sum_{i=1}^{N} \left(x_i - y_i\right)^2$$ where, y_i is the ith sample of waveform y.

STEP 3.

Find those waveforms which have $d_{xy} \leq 0.125 * l_x$ (set threshold)

If number of identified waveforms > 2, then form a new MUAP class and calculate its average waveform and store; else class members are superimposed

STEP 4.

Take the new reference from the remaining segments and go to step 2(b) and determine the Euclidean distance. If it satisfies the threshold criteria, then MUAP class is determined accordingly.

Threshold values are chosen after extensive testing. It was found that there are no widely applicable threshold criteria for assigning a MUAP a class. This threshold is critical because a very low value may spilt a MUAP class with high waveform variability in two or more subclasses, whereas, a greater value may merge the resembling classes of MUAPs.

Cross-Correlation Coefficient Technique

This cross-correlation coefficient technique is widely used for detecting the individual wave shapes from a complex signal. This technique is also suitable for the MUAP detection. The principle of this technique is based on template matching. The cross -correlation coefficient indicates the degree of similarity between templates. In this method, from the recorded EMG signals, the individual segments having high correlation coefficients in a template matching are recognized as the MUAP. All possible combinations of predetermined templates are determined by searching for the best match. In case of clustering, feature analysis criteria show that the clusters can be better separated and boundaries can be better detected by using cross-correlation coefficients. And finally, in case of the supervised classification of active segments, cross-correlation coefficients analysis achieves a higher recognition rate compared to other techniques. Following steps are used to calculate the cross-correlation coefficient between the segments obtained after segmentation of the EMG signal:

STEP 1. Start with the first waveform, x, as reference, being the first member of the class.
STEP 2. Calculate the cross -correlation coefficient, C(r), of this reference waveform with all the other segmented waveforms.
STEP 3. Find those waveform for which, C (r) ≥ 0.82, (a set threshold), if the number of the waveform satisfying the above relation is > 2, then form a new MUAP class and calculate its average and store; else class members are superimposed.
STEP 4. Take the new reference from the remaining segments and go to 'STEP 2' and determine the cross-correlation coefficient C(r) in a similar manner; if it satisfies the threshold criteria, then MUAP class is determined accordingly.

For determination of other classes, any one of remaining segments is taken as the reference and its cross-correlation coefficients with the segments is calculated. This procedure is repeated till all segments are classified.

Kohonen Self-Organizing Feature Map Technique

The unsupervised, Kohonen self-organizing neural network (NN) is considered a potential technique for the decomposition of EMG signal. The classification of the MUAPs into groups of similar shapes is a typical case of an unsupervised learning pattern recognition problem. The identified MUAPs are classified by an unsupervised NN. The term unsupervised identifies a structure able to recognize the presence of different classes in the input set, without any priori knowledge. When an input pattern is presented, each unit in the first layer takes a value of the corresponding entry in the input pattern. The output layer then sums up inputs and completes it to find a single winning unit. Each interconnection in the Kohonen feature map has an associated weight value. The initial state of the network has randomized values for the weights. The weight values are updated during training of the network.

In this technique, there is no prior knowledge of correctly labeled (classified) inputs, but the system is expected to discover statistically salient features of the input population. With this algorithm, the training process involves the presentation of pattern vectors from the training set one at a time. A winning neuron (node) is selected in a systematic manner after all input vectors are presented. A weight adjustment process takes place by using the neighborhood concept that shrinks over time. After several input vectors are presented, weights form clusters or vector centers that sample the input space such that the point density function of the vector centers tend to approximate the probability density function of the input vectors. The weights are also organized such that topologically close output nodes are sensitive to inputs that are physically similar. Thus, the output nodes are ordered in a natural way.

The Kohonen network provides advantages over classical pattern-recognition techniques because it utilizes the parallel architecture of a neural-network and provides a graphical organization of pattern relationships. It is found from literature that the maximum number of MUAPs that can be identified for needle EMG at low to moderate force level is at most 6 [2,3]. Therefore 8 output nodes are sufficient in the map. Following are the steps for training the Kohonen-NN:

STEP 1. Initialize the weights.
STEP 2. Create a competitive layer of eight nodes.
STEP 3. Train the neural network.
STEP 4. The training stops when number of epochs (replications) is reached to its maximum set value.

STEP 5. After training, the competitive layer is used as classifier with each neuron in the competitive layer as a class.
STEP 6. All the segmented MUAPs are given to this trained competitive layer and the output is obtained in the form of sparse matrix, then it contains the winner neuron for each candidate MUAP.

Wavelet Based Technique

Wavelet Transform (WT) is a powerful alternative to Fourier Transform, Discrete Fourier Transform and Fast Fourier Transform for the analysis of EMG signal. Wavelet transforms (WT) have become powerful alternative to Fourier transforms in medical applications, where the signals are non-stationary in nature like EMG. Wavelet algorithms process data at different scales and resolutions. If we look at a signal with a large 'window', we should notice gross features. Similarly, if we look at a signal with a small window, we should notice detail features. In addition to helping in recognition and detection of key diagnostic features, they provide a powerful tool for the disease diagnostics.

In order to select a suitable WT, that matches the physics of the problem, due weightage be given to some important properties of the wavelets such as smoothness, spatial localization, frequency localization, and ability to represent local polynomial function, orthogonality, and symmetry.

A good wavelet is the one which results in a small number of non negligible WT coefficients or a best approximation of a given signal up to a given scale. Thus, the scaling function associated with a good wavelet usually has a shape similar to the shape of the given signal. WT is a very promising technique for time-frequency analysis. By decomposing signals into elementary building blocks that are well localized both in time and frequency, WT can characterize the local regularity of the signal. This feature can be used to distinguish EMG signal from serious noise, artifacts and baseline drift.

In the present technique, the second order Daubechies wavelet has been used as its waveform is biphasic similar to most of the spikes of the MUAPs. This is also orthogonal and compactly supported. The 1st, 2nd and 3rd decompositions, namely w1, w2 and w3, of each waveform using db-2 wavelet have not give the considerable difference therefore these decompositions are not taken into account. The decomposition steps are as follows:

STEP 1. Calculate 4th, 5th and 6th decompositions, namely w_4, w_5 and w_6, of each waveform using db-2 wavelet and save all the decompositions.
STEP 2. Take first waveform, x, as reference waveform being first member of the class.
STEP 3. Determine distances of all the decompositions separately. Calculate three Euclidean distances (d_4, d_5 and d_6) between the waveform, x, and all the other segmented waveforms y_i as

$$d_4 = \sum_{i=1}^{\text{Length}(w_4)} \left(x_{4i} - y_{4i}\right)^2$$

where, i = ith sample in 4th decomposed signal.

$$d_5 = \sum_{j=1}^{\text{Length}(w_5)} \left(x_{5j} - y_{5j}\right)^2$$

where, j = jth sample in 5th decomposed signal.

$$d_6 = \sum_{k=1}^{\text{Length}(w_6)} \left(x_{6k} - y_{6k}\right)^2$$

where, k = kth sample in 6th decomposed signal.

STEP 4. Find the similarity measure, D = max (d_4, d_5 and d_6)
STEP 5. Find all those waveforms having $D \leq 0.9$ (a set threshold).

The maximum values of all three calculated distances are compared to the threshold for classification of MUAPs. If the maximum value of the distance is less than or equal to the threshold, then detected MUAP belongs to the class of reference MUAP; if not, then it belongs to some other class.

STEP 6. If number of waveforms (satisfying above condition) > 2, form a new class and take the average of all and store.
STEP 7. Take the new reference from the remaining segments and go to step (ii) and determine the Euclidean distance in a similar manner; if it satisfies the threshold criteria, then MUAP class is determined accordingly.

It is observed that db-2 wavelets has proved to be the best suitable for MUAP separation. There is one advantage of this technique as the classification procedure is based on spectrum matching. The spectrum matching technique is considered to be more effective than the waveform matching technique in the time domain, especially when the interference is induced by baseline drift or by high-frequency noise. In both the cases, interference affects two small portions of the frequency spectrum.

DECOMPOSITION OF SUPERIMPOSED WAVEFORMS

It was found after classification phase that superimposed waveform were also present in the segmented waveform. Therefore it is necessary to separate out these MUAPs from the superimposed waveform. The following steps are implemented for the decomposition of superimposed MUAP waveforms:

a. Take average MUAP of class 1. Reduce its length in such away that its start and end points have magnitude less than 10μV. Take this waveform as a reference.
b. Take any superimposed waveform x.
c. Slide the reference waveform (reduced MUAP waveform) on superimposed waveform and find the best matching value, where Cross correlation coefficient has its maximum value. This value indicates the best matching point.
d. For each matching point, calculate the normalized Euclidean distance (N_d), with the reference waveform.

$$N_d = \sum_{i=1}^{M}\left(x_i - y_i\right)^2 / \sum_{i=1}^{M} y_i \quad N_d < Th = 0.2$$

PERFORMANCE COMPARISION AND DISCUSSIONS

The general expected accuracy of the decomposition is dependent on the quality of data. The quality of the data is determined by its signal to noise ratio, stability, and actual separation of the motor unit class templates. If any one of these aspects of the data is degraded, accuracy of the process suffers. When there is increased recruitment or noise, one must acquire a large number of MUAP discharges for all above methods except wavelet technique and to identify a modest number of similar templates. Statistical pattern recognition and cross-correlation techniques require recordings of the EMG signal that are more free of noise. Kohonen self-organizing feature technique is a fast method for extracting MUAPs that requires recordings of the EMG signal relatively free of noise. Overall Wavelet technique has the best performance. This study demonstrates the versatility of Kohonen technique. When the recordings are relatively free of background activity, the decomposition of EMG signal by this method are similar to those obtained by the statistical pattern recognition and cross-correlation techniques. When background activity is increased and statistical pattern recognition and cross-correlation techniques fail, decomposition of EMG signal are similar to Wavelet technique. Cross-correlation technique examines all possible combinations of templates and their waveforms shifts in each possible time location (exhaustive search scheme performed in the time domain) to determine the best template match. Obviously, any exhaustive search technique is usually time consuming and is normally applicable only when the number of available templates is small. The final task in MUAP classification is the selection of reference template. Identification of MUAP templates mainly relies on the number of MUAPs present in one set of data, which indicates the number of repetitions of a MUAP. Therefore, a group containing more MUAPs has a higher chance to be selected as a reference template.

Training effort for the wavelet technique and Kohonen self-organizing feature map were significantly less as compared to the cross-correlation and statistical pattern recognition techniques. Decomposition performances of correlation approach and statistical technique were found to be similar. Statistical technique has the disadvantages of using a constant threshold for classification that make it less flexible, especially when the signal is noisy and with high variability. It is observed that number of classes which can be detected by the statistical technique is unlimited depending only on the number of actual MUAP classes existing in the signal. The Kohonen-NN performed better than the statistical pattern recognition technique and yielded a higher success rate. Wavelet spectrum of a spike describes not only frequency components of the spike but also their time locations. Thus, waveform matching in the wavelet preserves the best properties of matched filter techniques in both the time and frequency domains. The excitability and variability of MUAPs are easily evaluated with the help of Kohonen map and wavelet based techniques. The success-rate of classification for NOR, MYO and MND cases is found to be highest using wavelet technique.

When decomposition and clustering were performed on the acquired myoelectric signal, it was found that the number of action potentials were missing due to unresolved superpositions which occur at times when many neurons fire almost simultaneously. When the myoelectric signal is recorded, it is initially decomposed into individual action potentials. The decomposed signals are then clustered, using physical characteristics, into classes representing single motor neuron sources and the lumping of more than one neuron's firings into a single class. The clustering step, however, is never fully successful due to unresolved signal superpositions and, less frequently, missed detection by the electrode. Number of action potential firings are therefore missed resulting in an incomplete data set. This often manifests itself in the data as an inter pulse interval (IPI) that is too large. It was also observed that in statistical pattern recognition and cross-correlation techniques, due to waveform variability, the MUAP classes coming from the same motor unit, although looked similar, were not grouped together. Merging of these classes can be achieved by using higher constant threshold.

It is seen visually from the MUAPs of NOR, MYO and MND cases that there is a wide variation in some of the clinically important parameters. The duration measure is the key parameter being used in the clinical practice. Myopathy patients usually have MUAPs with short durations, low amplitudes and a small number of phases; whereas the MND patients have MUAPs with long durations, high amplitudes and a large number of phases. Sometimes waveform are more complex and have as many as six-phase reversal even in normal muscles. In complex EMG signals, where more active motor units were present, the physician was not able to confidently classify MUAPs based on a visual analysis of the data. The physician could only suggest how many motor units were active in a signal. The decomposition techniques were able to confidently classify motor units in a complex EMG signal. The decision of reference MUAP is very important, because sometimes, it happens that when we are taking any one MUAP as a reference and find the members of the class and second time when we are taking the reference MUAP from this obtained class then the number

Figure 2. Performance comparison of techniques

S. N.	Conditions	Statistical Pattern Recognition technique	Cross Correlation Coefficient technique	Kohonen Self-Organizing NN technique	Wavelet technique
1.	If there is need of base-line correction?	Yes	Yes	Yes	No
2.	For large amount of data	-	-	Best	-
3.	Is their need to give reference signal?	Yes	Yes	No	Yes
4.	Computational time	Highest	Less than Statistical technique but greater than Kohonen and Wavelet techniques	Lowest	Higher than Kohon but less th Statistical and Correlation techniques
5.	Accuracy	Lowest	Lowest	Less than wavelet technique but higher than Statistical and Correlation techniques	Highest

of members change for the same class. This is due to location of the peak in the given MUAPs. In all above techniques, which are fully automatic, the data processing permits analysis without any loss or distortion of information.

CONCLUSION

The following major conclusions are drawn on the basis of present work:

1. The performance of decomposition by Cross-Correlation approach is comparable to statistical pattern recognition technique. The main problem of both the techniques is the large amount of computational time to process all the possible combinations of time shifted templates by taking different template as the reference.
2. The Kohonen-NN require smaller architecture and thus less computational effort and is found more appropriate for the classification of MUAPs because of their ability to adapt and to create complex classification boundaries. When Cross-Correlation approach is combined with the Kohonen-NN, then it results in an integrated approach for decomposition, which is fast, efficient, accurate and requires less computational time.
3. Wavelet technique is easily implementable and has better performance in respect of speed and accuracy. In the wavelet technique, it is observed that in all above five

decompositions
4. 3rd, 4th and 5th decompositions show significant difference for MUAPs classification.
5. If number of templates is small, then statistical pattern recognition technique and Cross-Correlation approach are good; and if number of templates is high, then Kohonen-NN and wavelet decomposition technique are very good.
6. Wavelet-based analysis provides the MUAP morphology in the time-frequency plane. It allows fast extraction of localized frequency components and there is no need of correction for baseline drift or high-frequency noise. Therefore, wavelet technique has proved to be the best for decomposition and classification of MUAPs.

The outcome of this work will be very useful for diagnosing the neuromuscular disorders in planning aspects of curative and rehabilitation therapy and for evaluating response to treatment.

REFERENCES

Chauvet, E., Fokapu, O., Hogrel, J.-Y., Gamet, D., & Duchene, J. (2003, November). Automatic Identification of Motor Unit Action Potential Trains from Electromyographic signals Using Fuzzy Techniques. *Journal of Medical and Biological Engineering and Computing. SpringerLink, 41*(6), 646–653.

Christodoulos, I., & Pattichis, C. S. (1999, February). Unsupervided pattern recognition for the classification of EMG signals. *IEEE Trans. on BME, 46*(2), 169–178. doi:10.1109/10.740879

De Luca, C. J., Alexander, A., Wotiz, R., Gilmore, L. D., & Nawab, S. H. (2006). Decomposition of Surface EMG Signal. *Journal of Neurophysiology, 96*, 1646–1657. doi:10.1152/jn.00009.2006

Fever, R. S., & Luca, C. J. (1982, March). A procedure for decomposing the myoelectric signal into its constituent action potentials-part 1: Technique, Theory and Implementation. *IEEE Trans. on BME, 29*(3), 149–157. doi:10.1109/TBME.1982.324881

Fever, R. S., Xenakis, A. P., & Luca, C. J. (1982, March). A procedure for decomposing the myoelectric signal into its constituent action potentials-part 2: Execution and Test for Accuracy. *IEEE Trans. on BME, 29*(3), 158–164. doi:10.1109/TBME.1982.324882

Gerber, A., Studer, R. M., Figueiredo, R. J. P., & Moschytz, G. S. (1984, December). A new framework and computer program for quantitative EMG signal analysis. *IEEE Trans. on BME, 31*(12), 857–863. doi:10.1109/TBME.1984.325248

Gill, K. C. M., Cummins, K. L., & Dorfman, L. J. (1985, July). Automatic decomposition of the clinical Electromyogram. *IEEE Trans. on BME, 32*(7), 470–477. doi:10.1109/TBME.1985.325562

Holobar, A., & Zazula, D. (2004). Correlation-based decomposition of surface electromyograms at low contraction forces. *Journal of Medical and Biological Engineering and Computing. SpringerLink, 42*(4), 487–495.

Khandpur, R. S. (1987). *Hand book of biomedical instrumentation*. New York: McGraw-Hill Publishing Company Limited.

Kleine, B. J., vanDijk, B., Lapatki, M., & Zwarts, D., Stegeman. (2007). Using two-dimensional spatial information in decomposition of surface EMG signals. *Journal of Electromyography and Kinesiology, Elsevier, 17*(5), 535–548. doi:10.1016/j.jelekin.2006.05.003

Loudon, G. H., Jone, N. B., & Sehmi, A. S. (1992, November). New signal processing techniques for the decomposition of EMG signals. *Medical & Biological Engineering & Computing, 30*(6), 591–599. doi:10.1007/BF02446790

Mallet, Y., Coomans, D., Kautsky, J., & Olivier, D. V. (1997, October). Classification using adaptive wavelets for feature extraction. *IEEE Trans. on PAMI*, *19*(10), 1058–1066.

Nandedkar, S. D., & Sanders, D. B. (1989, November). Median averaging of electromyographic motor unit action potentials: comparison with other techniques. *Medical & Biological Engineering & Computing*, *27*(6), 566–572. doi:10.1007/BF02441637

Stashuk, D., & Bruin, H. D. (1988, January). Automatic decomposition of selective needle detected myoelectric signals. *IEEE Trans. on BME*, *35*(1), 1–10. doi:10.1109/10.1330

Chapter 11
Regional and Community Health Information Exchange in the United States

Adi V. Gundlapalli
University of Utah School of Medicine, USA

Jonathan H. Reid
University of Utah School of Medicine, USA & Utah Department of Health, USA

Jan Root
Utah Health Information Network, USA

Wu Xu
Utah Department of Health, USA

ABSTRACT

A fundamental premise of continuity in patient care and safety suggests timely sharing of health information among different providers at the point of care and after the visit. In most healthcare systems, this is achieved through exchange of written medical information, phone calls and conversations. In an ideal world, this exchange of health information between disparate providers, healthcare systems, laboratories, pharmacies and payers would be achieved electronically and seamlessly. The potential benefits of electronic health exchange are improved patient care, increased efficiency of the healthcare system and decreased costs. The reality is that health information is electronically exchanged only to a limited extent within local communities and regions, much less nationally and internationally. One main challenge has been the inability of health information exchange organizations to develop a solid business case. Other challenges have been socio-political in that data ownership and stewardship have not been clearly resolved. Technological improvements over the past 20 years have provided significant advances towards safe and secure information exchange. This chapter provides a general overview of community health information exchange in the United States of America, its history and details of challenges faced by stakeholders. The lessons learned from successes and failures, research and knowledge

DOI: 10.4018/978-1-61692-004-3.ch011

gaps and future prospects are also discussed. Current and future technologies to facilitate and invigorate health information exchange are highlighted. Two examples of successful regional health information exchanges in the US states of Utah and Indiana are highlighted.

"Things do not happen. Things are made to happen."

—John F. Kennedy

INTRODUCTION

Imagine a situation where a patient is sitting in a medical office for a visit. The doctor arrives, greets the patient, logs in to the electronic medical record and accesses the patient's medical chart on a computer in the room. After verifying the full name and date of birth with the patient, the doctor proceeds to a screen that provides a historical view of the patient's medical visits. "I see that you live in the neighboring town, and you have been seen by a medical group there for the past 5 years. I also see that you have transferred your care to my practice today, and your doctors have provided a summary of your condition for me to review. You have a history of high blood pressure, diabetes and high cholesterol. Looks like you have had laboratory testing performed in the past 3 months and all your numbers look great! Your recent chest x-ray and echocardiogram show no abnormalities. You are on several medications for your medical conditions and have been regular in picking up and refilling your medications. I also note that you experienced chest pain while visiting your daughter in another state last year and, fortunately, the hospital admission and testing there revealed no damage to your heart. According to your personal health record that you maintain and have given me access to, you have been feeling well and are quite active. Your local public health department identifies you as an early recipient of the new H1N1 swine flu vaccine. Let's pick up from here. Please tell me how you are feeling today…"

This elaborate introduction signals the start of an excellent medical visit that is both satisfying and time well spent for the patient as well as the doctor. If you look carefully at this visit, the patient's medical history, detailed medical records, laboratory testing, diagnostic imaging and pharmacy records from several different unaffiliated providers and healthcare systems were available to the doctor instantaneously at the point of care. This held true whether the prior visit was in the neighboring town or another state. The new doctor would not need to repeat any of the testing recently performed nor would he/she have to "reinvent the wheel" in caring for this patient. The personal health record was a bonus feature that provided information on current and ongoing health issues as reported by the patient. The result is increased patient satisfaction, preserved patient safety, improved efficiency of the healthcare system and overall decreased expenditures.

All of this was made possible by an efficient and seamless exchange of electronic health information between providers, most likely linked by a master patient index and a record locator service. The exchange was facilitated by cooperative agreements between healthcare systems and providers and the use of robust health information technology (HIT). These represent the quintessential "meaningful use" and "meaningful users" concepts that have been proposed by the US federal government to encourage the adoption of HIT across the highly fragmented health case system in the US to improve quality of care using health information exchange (HIE). Does such an ideal health information exchange exist anywhere in the United States? In a few settings and to a limited extent, this is possible within integrated healthcare systems such as the US Department of Defense, US Veteran's Administration (VA) (Dayhoff and Maloney 1992; Lloyd 1992; Martin 1992; Lau, Banning et al. 2005; Warnekar, Bouhaddou et al. 2007; Bouhaddou, Warnekar et al. 2008), Kaiser Permanente in California (Kaiser Permanente 2009) and Intermountain Healthcare in Utah (Intermountain Healthcare 2009). There are examples of regional HIE among healthcare providers that have achieved some meaningful exchange of information. A state-by-state directory is listed by the eHealth Initiative (eHealth Initiative 2009) that includes successful ventures in Indiana and Pennsylvania. There are also examples of opportunities for HIE with public health departments; these have mainly focused on immunization records and other data relevant to public health emergencies (Public Health Informatics Institute 2005; Shapiro 2007; Hessler, Soper et al. 2009; Hinman and Davidson 2009). For the most part though, this scenario and vision of seamless HIE remains utopian.

Communication and exchange of information are central themes of healthcare and form the basis of relationships between patients and their providers (Weiner, Barnet et al. 2005). Furthermore, the various unaffiliated providers involved in healthcare such as clinicians, laboratories, imaging facilities, healthcare systems and payers such as insurance companies have to exchange health information to ensure continuity of care for patients and payments for services rendered. At the present time, for the most part, patient-provider interactions are in person, by phone and/or by written communication. Electronic means of communication are slowly increasing between patients and their providers (Gagnon, Legare et al. 2009). These include email communications (Gagnon, Legare et al. 2009), patient-centered medical homes (American Association of Family Physicians 2009), personally controlled health records (PCHR) (Ball and Gold 2006; Einbinder and Bates 2007; Mandl, Simons et al. 2007; Ozkaynak, Marquard et al. 2007; Montelius, Astrand et al. 2008) and web-based consumer health solutions such as Google Health (Google 2009) and Microsoft HealthVault (Microsoft 2009). Electronic exchange of information is more advanced in certain areas that have government mandates and standards such as coding and billing, where the majority of the exchange is electronic. Other patient-provider and provider-provider exchanges remain largely paper-based.

The basic premise of HIE is to improve patient care, contribute to patient safety increase efficiency and decrease overall healthcare expenditures (Kaelber and Bates 2007; Adler-Milstein, McAfee et al. 2008; Adler-Milstein, Bates et al. 2009). In an ideal world, all patient encounters with the healthcare system would be electronic. Data generated from these encounters would be available for exchange between all parties that had legitimate need to see and use these data. The access to these data would be with appropriate security restrictions to protect patient privacy. To elaborate on these themes, the remainder of this chapter will review arguments and use cases to support HIE, the barriers to large scale implementation of HIE, lessons learned from current successful efforts and from failures. There will be a focus on technology and informatics related to HIE. We will also identify current and future areas of research that ultimately should form the evidence base for policy and funding for HIE. In this chapter, we use the term health information exchange (HIE) to broadly refer to electronic exchange of health information between two or more parties.

BACKGROUND

Electronic health information exchange traces its roots to the advent of modem technology that allowed transmission of information over local telephone lines. Released in 1981, the Hayes SmartModem was the first modem that allowed computer aided dialing and answering of calls. This meant that users no longer had to manually initiate or receive calls. This was achieved automatically by placing the telephone handset onto a modem coupler. As a result, unmanned computers could host services that were accessible anytime. This led to the explosion of the computerized Bulletin Board System (BBS). A BBS is a system that allows users to connect and share information, files, electronic mail or real-time chat with other users. As more users starting using modems to communicate, small community networks started to appear among individual users and organizations. These networks were the forerunners of the modern internet with early innovators being the US Government and academic universities. As the technology adoption increased, the bulletin board systems offered a way for public users to connect to community networks and use the services being offered through the internet. A community network consists of one or more computers providing services to people using computers and terminals to gain access to those services and to each other (Cisler 1994). In 1986 Dr. T.M. Grunder at Case Western Reserve University in Cleveland, Ohio, created a free community computing network known as Free-Net (Sievers 1992). Free-Net was envisioned to be a completely free, open-access community computer system that allowed anyone to call in 24 hours a day and access a wide range of electronic services and features. Free-Net offered users the ability to exchange health information between patients and clinical staff, and even hospital to hospital for the first time. Early HIE was referred to as electronic data interchange.

With the ability to share information electronically demonstrated and validated, a new health information sharing experiment started. This was referred to as the Community Health Information Network (CHIN) and can be considered the precursor to current day regional HIE (Noss and Zall 2002). While there were many types, generally, a CHIN could be defined as an inter-organizational system using information technologies and telecommunications to store, transmit and transform clinical and financial information. This information can be shared among cooperative as well as competitive participants, such as payers, hospitals, alternative delivery systems, clinics, physicians and home health agencies (Payton and Brennan 1999). A CHIN comprised three main components: key stakeholders from the health community, a network to transmit data between the CHINs trading partners and a central data repository of clinical data (Rubin 2003). At that time, CHIN supporters were focused on improving care and reducing operating costs. The essential concept behind the CHINs was to "connect the dots" for providers. In other words, the idea was to allow complete patient-level information to be available to authorized clinicians at the point of care.

An early example of a CHIN was a system called ComputerLink. This was a network-delivered, computer-based utility that provided health services to homebound persons. This network represented the first effort to systematically replicate functions provided by formal support services such as peer support, professional advice, education, and counseling for vulnerable populations (Brennan 1995; Payton, Brennan et al. 1995; Brennan 1999).

The concept and hope for CHINs was laudable; however, they faced tremendous challenges, and by the year 2000 most CHINs had failed (Appleby 1995; Furukawa 1997; Lassila, Pemble et al. 1997; Noss and Zall 2002; Lorenzi 2003). One main reason was lack of evidence to show benefits such as increased efficiency or effectiveness. Another reason was the perceived loss of control over the data. The ownership issues related to patient data were never resolved between the participating organizations, and this led to a lack of trust. Another reason was financial. There were no sustainable business models, and there was constant disagreement on how a CHIN should be financed. The information technology was not advanced enough to create a federated data model, so, out of necessity; a centralized data repository was created. This increased the lack of trust and brought data ownership and stewardship issues to the forefront again.

CHINs served to highlight the basic premise and potential benefits of health information exchange. Their failure forced stakeholders and supporters to regroup and rethink data stewardship and business models.

The business case for exchanging data electronically was sound and provided the market to exchange claims electronically between payers and providers through the use of proprietary clearinghouses. However, the essential problem of how to create a single "virtual" health record that would be available to appropriate providers remained largely unsolved. In addition, healthcare costs continued to rise far above inflation. The failure of CHINS may have, in part, contributed to the high costs of healthcare in the US. The current healthcare crisis has fueled a renewed sense of urgency in achieving the fundamental CHIN goal.

This led to the birth of Regional Health Information Organizations (RHIO) that promoted heath information exchange in the region (McDonald, Overhage et al. 2005) (Brennan, Ferris et al. 2005; Conn 2005; Koval 2005; Orlova, Dunnagan et al. 2005; Rollins 2005; Blair 2006; Raths 2006; Scalise 2006; Stein 2006; Lawrence 2007; Martin 2007; McGowan, Jordan et al. 2007). The business case or funding model proposed was a mix of federal grants, private funding and user fees. The data stewardship was more federated and less restrictive. Several RHIOs have been formed in the past two decades, and many have survived using these funding models. It is important to highlight the failure of one of the most famous RHIOs, the Santa Barbara County Care Data Exchange. Despite good intentions, fairly advanced technology and adequate funding, this RHIO failed after only a few months of data exchange. The main reason cited is the lack of value for the data exchange as perceived by the stakeholders (Holmquest 2007; Miller and Miller 2007). This is a significant concern that needs to be addressed for the future of HIE to be secure in terms of financial models, stakeholder participation and perception of benefit (Adler-Milstein, McAfee et al. 2008, Rudin, 2009 #186; Grossman, Kushner et al. 2008; Hurd 2008; Maffei 2008; Nocella, Horowitz et al. 2008; Adler-Milstein, Bates et al. 2009).

From RHIOs, the next iteration of the theme is health information exchange (HIE), the term that is in vogue today.

HEALTH INFORMATION EXCHANGE

Stakeholders

In general, patients in the US receive their healthcare from disparate medical providers that are not affiliated with each other. Most practice as small businesses with less than 10 physicians or providers. Regardless of their affiliation or financial ties, intuitively it would appear that all parties involved in healthcare are natural stakeholders in supporting HIE. Starting with patients and providers, this would include various healthcare systems, clinical laboratories, imaging facilities and insurance companies. Though the common goal should be to share information electronically to improve the quality of healthcare for their mutual patients, in reality, this is not the case. There are market forces and competing theories among individual providers and healthcare systems who consider patient data to be owned assets that should not or cannot be shared (Grossman, Bodenheimer et al. 2006; Malepati, Kushner et al. 2007). Reasons for not sharing patient data range from competitive interests in provided services to financial constraints as small outpatient clinics rarely have the resources to invest heavily in health information technology. For the larger healthcare systems, a long-held marketing strategy that seeks to tie patients and physicians to a particular system by using exclusive HIE mechanisms has also kept information from being shared.

Table 1. Key concepts of Regional and Community Health Information Exchange

Regional and Community Health Information Exchange	
Stakeholders	• Patients • Providers • Healthcare systems • Hospitals • Clinical laboratories • Diagnostic imaging facilities • Insurance companies • Public health agencies • Consumer health groups
Models	• Private • Public • Federated • Centralized • Blended
Challenges and Barriers	• Access to electronic medical systems • Financial support • Legal and regulatory issues involving privacy of patient data • Technology • Trust across institutions • Data stewardship
Lessons Learned and Potential Solutions	• Develop workable business model • Establish trust • Reward use of HIE • Prove usefulness, efficiency and security • Newer technologies to address data stewardship, security and privacy issues
Future Research Directions	• Outcomes research to demonstrate benefits • Research from other fields on sustainable business models

Key stakeholders in HIE vary based on the type of information being exchanged (Table). The most common types of information exchanged are laboratory and diagnostic imaging study results (eHealth Initiative 2009). For this type of HIE, the stakeholders are medical providers, hospitals, clinical laboratories and providers of diagnostic imaging. Hospital and independent pharmacies provide prescription medication data. If information on outpatient visits and emergency department visits are included, the stakeholders include hospital and healthcare systems that own outpatient practices and emergency departments. These groups of stakeholders also facilitate other functions of HIE such as the ability to provide alerts to medical providers regarding specific topics and electronic prescribing of medications. Health insurers who are the payers for healthcare also have a need to receive clinical information. Insurers need clinical information for utilization management, for prior authorizations and for claim adjudication.

Connectivity to electronic medical records and exchange of these records forms the next major functions of HIE. For these functions, the stakeholders are hospitals and practices with their disparate electronic medical record systems.

A more recent function of HIE has been to provide and electronically exchange information of relevance to public health such as immunizations, notifiable and reportable infectious diseases and deaths (Shapiro 2007; Hessler, Soper et al. 2009; Hinman and Davidson 2009). For these HIE efforts, public health agencies such as local and state/provincial health departments become key stakeholders along with medical providers, hospitals and clinical laboratories.

From a patient perspective, consumer health groups are engaged in safeguarding the interests of the patients amidst all the exchange that is or could take place. These groups are key stakeholders that could advocate for and facilitate HIE. Even though HIE is rarely profitable, additional stakeholders include health information technology vendors that provide infrastructure, software and support services for HIE. Finally, standards organizations that provide expertise on interoperability and messaging standards for effective sharing of health information should be considered important stakeholders.

Models

There are several models of HIE currently in the US. A common type is a *private* HIE that is formed when affiliated organizations exchange information. An example of this (and a likely forerunner of HIE) is the electronic transmission of laboratory results from laboratory information systems to ordering providers. This type of direct exchange of information may be considered *domain-specific* HIE. Other domains in which private HIE is routinely seen is administrative functions such as insurance verification, pre-authorization of services by the payer and provider's billing office.

A *public* HIE is formed when a third-party organization, usually a non-profit, brokers the exchange of information between stakeholders. A common version of this is seen in regional health information organizations (RHIOs) where entities facilitate the exchange between medical providers and hospitals or laboratories. They provide the means of exchanging information to increase efficiency and patient care in the system while maintaining privacy and confidentiality. These "honest brokers" typically do not have access to the information and function much like a post office—they deliver the letter without ever looking inside.

Logistically and functionally, HIEs can be *federated, centralized* or *blended.* The federated model appeals to many stakeholders as each participating organization retains control of its information. The organization then responds to specific queries for information and provides information conforming to strict privacy and confidentiality laws. This usually requires pre-determined levels of access to information and business agreements to exchange legitimate health information.

In the centralized model, the coordinating organization collects, collates and stores information in a centralized location. Here, too, the access is carefully controlled when providing information across organizations. This system works well within large integrated or affiliated healthcare providers. When there are no organizational, financial or other strong affiliations, it is unlikely that entities will part with large amounts of information for storage in a centralized location.

Usually, HIE follows a blended model, whereby data, such as a master patient index or record locator service, are centrally stored and stakeholders are queried for other information in a federated manner.

Challenges and Barriers

There are several challenges and barriers to the large scale adoption of HIE in the US. Broadly, these fall into the categories of access to electronic medical systems, financial, socio-political and, to an extent, technological.

One major barrier to the adoption of HIE between key stakeholders such as private physicians and hospitals appears to be the surprisingly low penetration of electronic medical records in both the outpatient and hospital setting. A recent survey of ambulatory care practices in the US has revealed that 13% of physicians reported having a basic system in their outpatient offices, and only 4% had a fully functional system (DesRoches,

Campbell et al. 2008). A survey of hospitals in the US revealed that only 8% had a basic electronic medical record in at least one unit of the hospital, and an astonishingly low 1.5% of them had a comprehensive electronic records system (Jha, DesRoches et al. 2009).

Major arguments against investing in HIE by private stakeholders are financial investment and lack of a solid business model. As noted above, with CHINs, there still exists a perception that HIE fails to improve efficiency or be otherwise useful. The HIE concept also challenges a long-held marketing strategy of tying providers and patients to a particular system (usually a hospital or a laboratory information system) through a private HIE.

An additional challenge has been the current healthcare reimbursement system. The United States uses a fee-for-service payment model for healthcare. Essentially, providers are paid only when they perform a service; therefore, more services and procedures equal more income. Hence, there is no financial incentive for providing more efficient and effective care, particularly if it involves fewer procedures.

Apart from the initial set-up cost of infrastructure, time and personnel, there are operational costs involved in maintaining and supporting HIE. Many entities charge fees for facilitating exchange of information, either a flat fee or a per transaction fee. It is not encouraging that a recent survey of HIE in the US found only 55 active RHIOs. Of these, only 41% reported receiving enough revenue from participating organizations to cover their annual operating costs (Adler-Milstein, Bates et al. 2009). Most of the exchange was for laboratory test results and pharmacy data. Of those who had been surveyed in the prior year (2007), most had made no progress in expanding exchange capabilities. The failure rate over the past year was a very significant 20%. The authors concluded that the scope of RHIOs remains limited and their viability remains uncertain. The business model for HIE remains a challenge from inception to operation to viability (Adler-Milstein, McAfee et al. 2008).

Even if financial concerns were overcome, there still remain key concerns about data stewardship and the feeling that patient data are proprietary and not to be shared with other competitor entities in the same market place (Grossman, Bodenheimer et al. 2006; Malepati, Kushner et al. 2007).

Other barriers often mentioned are the legal and regulatory issues involved in exchange of patient data. Most countries, including the US, have enacted strict privacy and confidentiality laws governing the exchange of patient health information. Many of these regulations vary by state creating a quagmire of conflicting rules about who may exchange what information. Electronic exchange of patient information between entities without appropriate safeguards, business agreements and patient authorizations is perceived to increase risk, and has dampened the large scale adoption of HIE, particularly across state lines.

As noted above, data stewardship and ownership issues contributed to the failure of CHINs. These concerns were not overcome with existing technology in the 1990s. With advances in technology and the notion of "federated" data, technology is not considered a major barrier to HIE. The availability of high-level security that meets federal standards further bolsters the argument that current technologies will support HIE to the satisfaction of all stakeholders involved.

In summary, financial concerns, lack of tangible benefits given the current reimbursement system, competitive pressures and regulatory concerns have limited the large scale adoption of HIE in the US. It appears that the notion of "common good" is not incentive enough to initiate and sustain HIE.

Lessons Learned and Potential Solutions

The barriers facing HIE are not easy to overcome but inform the lessons learned. From the failures, we have learned that the business model for HIE needs to be revamped. It may not be possible for all HIEs to have an identical business model; very likely the "successful" model will vary according to the local or state healthcare market landscape. A fee-for-service or subscription model are options that should be considered by all HIE, with adequate safety nets of federal grants and private funding for initial start-up and maintenance. The culture must evolve to allow stakeholders to believe that investing their time and money in return for effective HIE will result in tangible benefits such as improved reimbursement. Widespread HIE will fundamentally shift market forces in ways that are probably not well appreciated at this time.

The importance of data ownership and trust issues have been difficult lessons learned from both failures and successes. Here again, trust between competitors and with patients must be built slowly between stakeholders. In reviewing the success of regional HIE, it is evident that stakeholder buy-in is key. The HIE must develop a defensible business plan that offers significant return on investment for the various stakeholder groups in the market. In addition, it is crucial that the HIE include the right stakeholders and utilize technology that is widely available. Patience is an important virtue.

The impetus to receive and exchange records electronically across disparate healthcare systems will increase as the adoption of electronic medical records and information systems increases in the US. This is a slow and tedious process that will be driven by government and private funding, increased awareness and, ultimately, reimbursement systems that reward or even mandate the use of electronic records and HIE. The recent push for increasing the use and adoption of electronic medical records by the US government, through the American Recovery and Reinvestment Act (ARRA) of 2009 Title XIII – Health Information Technology (HITECH), will provide a much needed boost to this field. Similarly, federal funding to initiate and sustain HIE through regional partnerships will also provide an impetus to HIE financing in general.

The perception that HIE is not useful or that it may not improve efficiency can only be solved with continued research into the field. There are examples of limited success of HIE in specific areas (Hayward, Warren et al. 2007; Kuhn, Giuse et al. 2007; Phillips and Welch 2007; Frisse, King et al. 2008; Nocella, Horowitz et al. 2008). However, there are no large scale successes reported in the literature. On the other hand, there are studies that show a high failure rate and fears regarding sustainability among entities engaged in HIE (Adler-Milstein, McAfee et al. 2008; Adler-Milstein, Bates et al. 2009). A consensus needs to be reached among different stakeholders regarding the common goals, benefits and risks, especially for large scale HIE (Kuhn, Giuse et al. 2007).

The perception that HIE may fundamentally change market strategies for the large systems—hospitals and clinical laboratories—inevitably increases resistance to the adoption of HIE in markets dominated by large for-profit systems. These markets will require significant changes in the reimbursement system to change, and even then the change will be strongly resisted.

Barriers such as trust among stakeholders in the HIE, who are usually competitors, will only be overcome on a broad geographic scale when the financial incentives are compelling enough to require (in a financial sense) a change to their current business practices of using patient data as a competitive advantage. A recent push has been to actively involve the patient in HIE. It is the patient's data that is exchanged, and if patients are convinced of the benefits, they may be advocates for increased adoption of HIE (Diamond and Ricciardi 2006; Tripathi, Delano et al. 2009). However, without adequate education, patients could also kill the HIE effort if they are not convinced that this is a change that directly benefits them.

Closely aligned with trust issues are issues associated with privacy and confidentiality of patient information and the law. While these issues have been used as an excuse to not encourage HIE, with greater involvement from stakeholders, including patients, and with greater safeguards, the situation will change in favor of HIE (McGraw, Dempsey et al. 2009). This will involve changes to both state and federal laws in the US.

In areas where HIEs have been successful, they have largely been driven by health insurers. It could be argued that the benefits of making the healthcare system more efficient and effective through an HIE largely accrue to health insurers. Private and government insurers in states such as Florida, Michigan, Colorado and Delaware have funded HIEs that have brought significant return on investments. This approach is limited by the structure of the various healthcare markets across the country and is most successful in markets that are dominated by a single insurer. In the majority of the country where there is active competition, it has been a significant challenge to bring competing payers together to support an HIE.

To resolve the issues raised above, it is hoped that "disruptive technology" will enable and foster HIE. For example, privacy and security issues of access to patient data are solved with greater security and controlled access built in to current HIE systems (Carter, Lemery et al. 2006; Gravely and Whaley 2009; Marshall, Gillespie et al. 2009). The current "paper" system is extremely insecure and has essentially no "audit" functionality. Technology could also enable more cost-effective solutions to exchange of information as has been shown in every industry that has adopted information exchange to date. Adoption of national messaging standards such as HL7 will also translate to improved HIE and interoperability that may in turn lead to increased adoption of HIE (Orlova, Dunnagan et al. 2005; Walker, Pan et al. 2005; Donnelly, Mussi et al. 2006; Zafar and Dixon 2007; Hammond 2008; Raths 2008; Rogoski 2008).

Technology may contribute to HIE with regard to software and architecture. Open source technologies may have the benefit of a cost-effective solution for HIE (Open Source Health Records Exchange 2009). Service-oriented architecture (Wright and Sittig 2008) and grid-based systems have the potential of transforming HIE both regionally and nationally by creating federated databases and offering solutions to data stewardship. An example of grid-based exchange of data that could be emulated for the HIE world is the widely used and accepted cancer Biomedical Informatics Grid, caBIG (Manion, Robbins et al. 2009). This concept may also benefit exchange of information with public health agencies (Staes, Xu et al. 2009).

AN EXAMPLE HEALTH INFORMATION EXCHANGE SET UP AND ARCHITECTURE

HIE: Health Information Exchange, **HIS:** Health Information System, **CA:** Certificate Authority.

HIE between stakeholders can be set up using various systems and architectures. In general, HIE consists of data sources, an intermediary HIE services layer and a portal to access data. (Figure 1) provides a simplified example of a HIE architecture that could be established within a region.

In this example, a hospital and a clinical laboratory are the data sources that provide authorized access to patient data through secured communication. They each set up a resource server that resides outside the entity firewall so that no breach of internal security occurs. The hospital and laboratory identify the data that they would like to provide to the HIE; this could be negotiated by prior agreement based on stakeholder views and needs.

The middle layer is the HIE services layer that provides the basic functionality of identifying patients uniquely, identifying and authorizing users and exchanging data. The most common elements in an HIE are the record locater service (RLS) or

Figure 1. A simplified system architecture for health information exchange between stakeholders

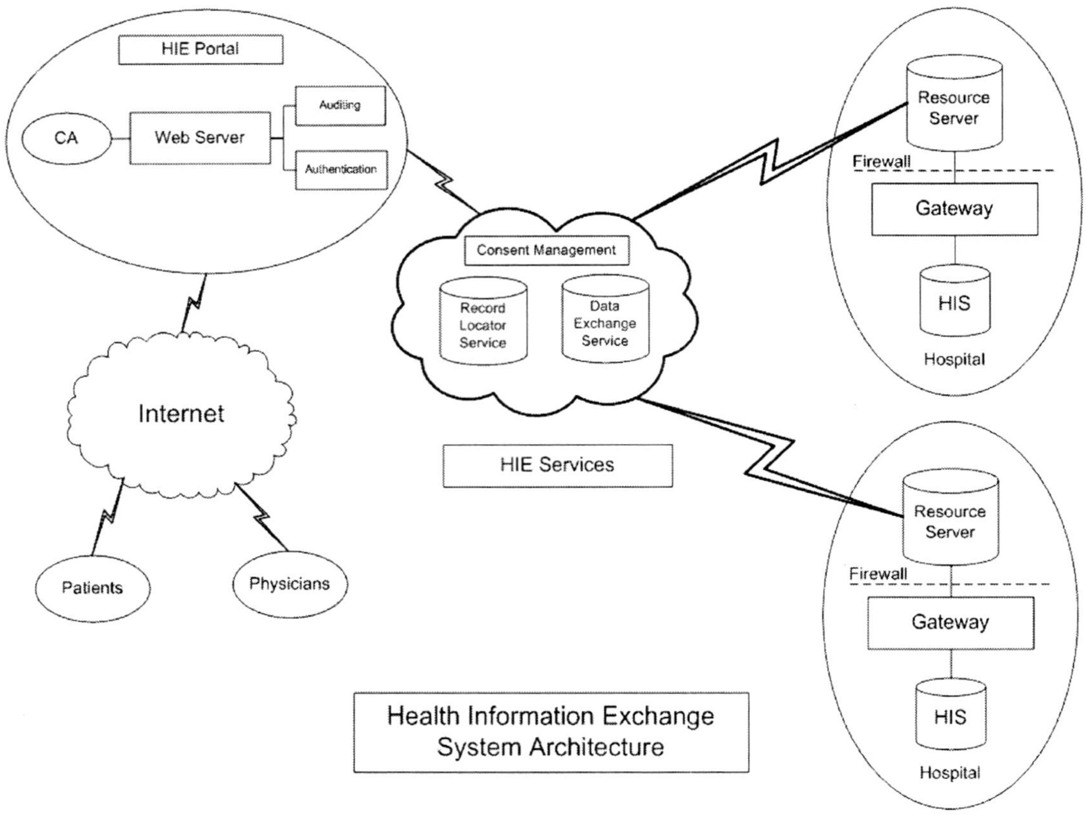

master patient index (MPI), data exchange service (DES), consent management service, the data repository, user authentication and auditing server.

The RLS is an electronic index of identifying information that allows the system to uniquely identify a patient and locate associated data. This index directs providers to the data source location of the patient health records. The core responsibilities of the RLS are to 1) identify a patient within an HIE or in a remote community and 2) identify the electronic location of a patient's clinical data. HIE users search for a patient with full or partial demographic information including first name, last name, date of birth, gender, zip code or other parameters. An RLS improves the efficiency of the HIE by allowing it to send the data request to the correct data source.

The DES provides HIPAA-compliant clinical data exchange in standard data formats, including HL7 2.x, CCS, CCR, XML, CSV, DICOM, other text files, images, scans, etc.. Security is usually achieved used PKI and Web Services (SOAP, XML-RPC) technologies.

The second part of HIE services consists of a HIE portal that includes a web server with auditing and authentication capability. This is the component that directly interacts with the end-users, which, in this example, are patients and physicians. Each user is authenticated to a level of access that has been pre-determined by a business agreement with the HIE after discussions with the stakeholders.

When a provider wishes to access records on a particular patient, he or she would log on to the system using a secure web portal and be presented with a menu of options. The provider must first attest that he or she has a treatment relationship with the patient prior to accessing records. The provider could then search for records using patient identifiers and, in this case, the RLS would locate records associated uniquely with that patient. The data would then be retrieved on demand from the resource servers of the hospital or laboratory and displayed for the provider. While retaining these basic components and architecture, HIE could incorporate data from pharmacies, outpatient clinics, public health agencies and any other entity with an interest and need for HIE.

UTAH HEALTH INFORMATION NETWORK

Utah has long been a national leader in HIE. The Utah Health Information Network (UHIN) was founded in 1993 as a public-private partnership in response to a community problem: how could a state with a (relatively) small population, where the healthcare market was dominated by local group health insurers and local healthcare providers create an efficient system for exchanging health information, specifically claims? Blue Cross Blue Shield of Utah, as the Medicare contractor, had been successfully receiving electronic claims for many years, but most of the other Utah payers were just beginning to implement systems. At the time, Utah was such a small market that it was of no interest to the then-major clearinghouses. Rather than each payer implementing its own proprietary system, which would have resulted in chaos for the Utah provider community, the entire community, payers and providers alike, came together to create a single commonly held utility, UHIN, that would benefit the *entire* community. Thus, all stakeholders were represented and claimed ownership of UHIN.

Because UHIN was serving members who were competitors, it was decided that UHIN would not function as a clearinghouse; instead, it would act as a Value Added Network (VAN). That is, it would not "open the envelope" and edit or format data; it would essentially be a post office picking up and delivering electronic mail. UHIN utilizes a single electronic commerce agreement (ECA) that all members must sign. The ECA is available on the UHIN web site (www.uhin.org). The ECA covers HIPAA privacy and security issues and allows the members to avoid signing HIPAA Business Associate Agreements with everyone else on the network.

This forced the fledging UHIN into using electronic data interchange standards. In 1993 the Utah Legislature adopted a law that gave the Utah Insurance Department (UID) the authority to adopt standards for administrative exchanges. The UID gave UHIN the responsibility of convening the community to create the administrative standards that UID would subsequently adopt, and UHIN's long-standing career as a Standards Development Organization for the State of Utah began. Since that time, the Utah healthcare community, through the UHIN Standards process, has created over 80 standards and has adopted available national standards as well.

The business case for UHIN is based on the premise that all the parties on the exchange (payers and providers) benefit from exchanging patient claim/billing data. Although both parties must make a significant initial investment to enable this exchange, the return on investment occurs very quickly. UHIN started its operations with the exchange of administrative data.

Since its inception, UHIN has operated by collecting membership fees. The basic UHIN formula for determining membership fees is to first determine who receives value for the transaction. In the case of a claim, the UHIN board decided that payers received 70% of the value and providers received 30% of the value. The basic idea is that the "price" of each claim exchanged through UHIN is divided 70-30: each stakeholder group pays for its share of the value received by exchanging that claim. UHIN payers pay a click fee for claims, and UHIN providers pay an annual membership fee. Currently more than 90% of all insurers' administrative claims, remittance and eligibility data in Utah are exchanged through the UHIN electronic communication system

The business model and pricing strategy for UHIN stakeholders involves a "click charge" for payers to receive and send claims and remittances. Providers using the services pay an annual membership fee. As the number of stakeholders and the volume of transactions increases, the average price per claim and the average cost of each transaction goes down. This savings is passed on directly to the payers and providers in the form of lower charges and annual fees.

After 16 years of service to the community, it is clear that UHIN is one of the successful regional HIE entities (Rubin 2003). One of the reasons for the success is that its governing board required that it be operated first and foremost as a *business*: a non-profit business, but nonetheless a business. It had to bring value to its members (reduce the cost of care). Second, the board decided to move in *small increments*. UHIN began operations by exchanging healthcare claims. Claims, from a business perspective, are a win-win: payers and providers alike benefit from moving from paper into electronic data interchange. UHIN has spent many years solidifying their position with regard to exchange of claim data before even considering the next step in HIE. And third, the board decided to be *inclusive*. From its beginning, UHIN's business strategy was to offer electronic data interchange to any Utah entity that wanted to participate. This helped develop trust among the stakeholders and set the stage for a successful venture.

UHIN is currently moving into its next phase by expanding its portfolio beyond administrative data. Since early 2009, UHIN has initiated pilot testing of exchange of clinical data between partners in two communities of Utah.

INDIANA HEALTH INFORMATION EXCHANGE

Indiana Health Information Exchange (IHIE) is another example of a successful statewide venture with advances in clinical information exchange. Its history can be traced back to Indiana University Medical Center's adoption of the Regenstrief Medical Record System (RMRS) in 1973. The RMRS evolved into a comprehensive clinical data repository used extensively by three hospitals and 30 clinics in Indianapolis (McDonald, Overhage et al. 1999). In 1994, Regenstrief Institute of Medical Informatics expanded the RMRS into the Indiana Network for Patient Care (INPC) with funding from the National Institutes of Health and the National Library of Medicine. The INPC is a citywide electronic medical record system exchanging information among 5 health systems (McDonald, Overhage et al. 2005). The INPC's success led to the formation of the Indiana Health Information Exchange, Inc. (IHIE) in 2004 as a not-for-profit umbrella organization for the region's HIE projects.

The IHIE provides clinical data to clinicians at the point of care and serves more than half of the population in the state of Indiana. The IHIE's clinical data include laboratory results, radiology reports and images, pathology reports, dictated reports, admission discharge and transfer (ADT) data, electrocardiograms, vital signs, etc. Since 2004, over 50 million test results and other clinical information have been exchanged among clinicians, hospitals, emergency departments, laboratories, imaging centers, pharmacies, public health, payers, researchers and patients (www.ihie.com).

The IHIE technical architecture consists of federated data repositories, centralized Concept Dictionary, Global Patient Index, and Global Provider Index. Patient registration records from all participating providers are linked in the Global Patient Index. The data received from a wide variety of sources are converted to standard representations such as HL7 and LOINC. These standardized data are then used to deliver a variety of HIE services for stakeholders (McDonald, Overhage et al. 2005).

Health informatics research plays an instrumental role in the formation and development of IHIE. The Director for Medical Informatics at Regenstrief Institute is also IHIE's President and Chief Executive Officer. The IHIE's technical architecture and applications were developed by researchers at the Regenstrief Institute. The Institute continuously provides clinical information repository services to IHIE and operates the INPC. IHIE's Vice President for Marketing described this collaboration as:

The functions, services, and technogolgy of IHIE and Regenstrief are intertwined. ... Regenstrief does informatics research and "invents" and proves really cool HIE technology; IHIE uses the really cool HIE technology and "sells" HIE services to the healthcare stakeholders in Indiana. (Kansky 2008).

Besides HIE application development, Regenstrief researchers have solved several major technical challenges for effectively managing and improving the operational system over the years. For example, studies by Grannis and Overhage compared the linkage quality of deterministic vs. probabilistic linkage algorithm and supported decision-making for operational efficiency (Grannis, Overhage et al. 2002; Grannis, Overhage et al. 2003). Vreeman developed automated tools to reduce manual efforts to keep up with changing source system terms among disparate systems which contribute data for the ongoing health information exchange (Vreeman 2007). To some degree, IHIE becomes a HIE translational research laboratory for the Regenstrief Institute.

Though research-based innovation is one of IHIE's strengths, grant-based research projects usually have a limited life span. For example, the INPC has largely been funded by various federal grants and its sustainability was a concern. Having been integrated into IHIE, INPC has finally found a fiscal/business home for its long-term success. The collaboration between Indiana Health Information Exchange and Regenstrief Insitute is a powerful demonstration of mutual values of HIE translational research for stakeholders, academic researchers and health practitioners.

FUTURE RESEARCH DIRECTIONS

Many reports of failures and successes of HIE have been reported in the US. (See references and additional reading.) These are mainly descriptive reports of regional HIE with regard to successes and failures, perspectives and surveys of entities engaged in HIE. There are also a limited number of published articles on the technology and standards involved. Several research areas need to be addressed in the field of HIE.

A major research need is outcomes research to show the benefits of HIE. These studies are difficult to conduct as not all benefits of HIE are tangible and can be measured using traditional metrics. In some instances, simply the availability of key patient information that affects patient care is a benefit. Tangible benefits such as reduced costs, increased efficiency and positive patient outcomes are difficult to ascertain. Even more difficult is to show a meaningful difference in patient care. In many instances, it is appropriate to postpone these "outcome studies" (McDonald, Overhage et al. 2005; Vest 2009).

Outcomes research may have to wait for research on sustainable business models. It may be appropriate to have researchers from other fields such as traditional business economics assist in these evaluations in an inter-disciplinary manner. A similar approach may be necessary to further research on technologies related to HIE, bringing in professionals from other fields such as standards, computer science, grid, etc.

CONCLUSION

HIE is a key component of healthcare. Effective exchange of information between stakeholders is necessary for patient care and for the business of healthcare in the US. Regional and community HIE has evolved from humble beginnings and is still in its infancy with regard to wide-scale adoption. From the community health information networks in the early 1990s to the robust health information networks of today, technology has been a key factor in advancing HIE and offering solutions to barriers such as security, privacy and controlled access to patient data.

Stakeholders have learned many valuable lessons from the large number of failures and few successful ventures. The basic premise of HIE is intuitive and should be universally accepted for the "common good." However, major issues such as financial viability, sustainability, marketing strategies, reimbursement, data stewardship and perception of usefulness of HIE remain. The result is that there are only a limited number of regional and community HIE entities that are providing any meaningful exchange of patient information today. Increased funding from government and private sources, more outcomes research and increased stakeholder buy-in combined with further advances in health information technology are necessary to secure the future of HIE in the US. The increased adoption of electronic medical records and information systems is also a key pre-requisite for furthering HIE. The full potential of HIE is yet to be realized.

ACKNOWLEDGMENT

The authors wish to gratefully acknowledge funding and support from the CDC-funded Rocky Mountain Center for Translational Research in Public Health Informatics; Division of Epidemiology, University of Utah School of Medicine; Utah Health Information Network and Utah Department of Health. We would also like to thank our colleagues in our parent institutions for providing references and description of various HIE efforts in Utah and elsewhere. We also acknowledge technical assistance from Ms. Marianne Madsen of the University of Utah.

REFERENCES

Adler-Milstein, J., & Bates, D. W. (2009). U.S. Regional health information organizations: progress and challenges. *Health Affairs (Project Hope)*, *28*(2), 483–492. doi:10.1377/hlthaff.28.2.483

Adler-Milstein, J., & McAfee, A. P. (2008). The state of regional health information organizations: current activities and financing. *Health Affairs (Project Hope)*, *27*(1), 60–69. doi:10.1377/hlthaff.27.1.w60

American Association of Family Physicians. (2009). *Patient-Centered Medical Home*. Retrieved from http://www.aafp.org/online/en/home/membership/initiatives/pcmh.html.

Appleby, C. (1995). The trouble with CHINS (community health information networks). *Hospitals & Health Networks*, *69*(9), 42–44.

Ball, M. J., & Gold, J. (2006). Banking on health: Personal records and information exchange. *Journal of Healthcare Information Management*, *20*(2), 71–83.

Blair, R. (2006). RHIO nation. *Health Management Technology*, *27*(2), 56–62.

Bouhaddou, O., & Warnekar, P. (2008). Exchange of computable patient data between the Department of Veterans Affairs (VA) and the Department of Defense (DoD): Terminology Mediation Strategy. *Journal of the American Medical Informatics Association*, *15*(2), 174–183. doi:10.1197/jamia.M2498

Brennan, C. P. (1995). Managed care and health information networks. *Journal of Health Care Finance, 21*(4), 1–5.

Brennan, P. F. (1999). Health informatics and community health: support for patients as collaborators in care. *Methods of Information in Medicine, 38*(4-5), 274–278.

Brennan, P. F., Ferris, M., et al. (2005). Modeling participation in the NHII: operations research approach. In *Proceedings of the AMIA Annu. Symp.* (pp. 76-80).

Carter, P., & Lemery, C. (2006). Privacy and security in health information exchange. *Journal of American Health Information Management Association, 77*(10), 64A–64C.

Cisler, S. (1994). Community computer networks: building electronic greenbelts. In Bishop, A. P. (Ed.), *Emerging Communities: Integrating Networked Information into Library Services: Clinic on Library Applications of Data Processing* (pp. 16–31).

Conn, J. (2005). Destination RHIO. As regional data networks continue to grow in number, some find financial strength. *Mod Healthc, 35*(42), 28, 32.

Dayhoff, R. E., & Maloney, D. L. (1992). Exchange of Veterans Affairs medical data using national and local networks. *Annals of the New York Academy of Sciences, 670*, 50–66. doi:10.1111/j.1749-6632.1992.tb26074.x

DesRoches, C. M., & Campbell, E. G. (2008). Electronic health records in ambulatory care--a national survey of physicians. *The New England Journal of Medicine, 359*(1), 50–60. doi:10.1056/NEJMsa0802005

Diamond, C., & Ricciardi, L. (2006). Building consumer trust into health information exchange. *J. AHIMA, 77*(10),36, 38.

Donnelly, J., & Mussi, J. (2006). Building an interoperable regional health information network today with IHE integration profiles. *Journal of Healthcare Information Management, 20*(3), 29–38.

eHealth Initiative. (2009). *HIE Directory*. Retrieved from http://www.ehealthinitiative.org/directory-health-information-exchange-initiatives.html

eHealth Initiative. (2009, October 1). *Migrating Toward Meaningful Use: The State of Health Information Exchange. Retrieved from*http://www.ehealthinitiative.org/sites/default/files/file/2009%20Survey%20Report%20FINAL.pdf

Einbinder, J. S., & Bates, D. W. (2007). Leveraging information technology to improve quality and safety. *Yearbook of Medical Informatics*, 22–29.

Frisse, M. E., King, J. K., et al. (2008). A regional health information exchange: architecture and implementation. In *Proceedings of AMIA Annu. Symp.*, 212-216.

Furukawa, M. (1997). Models for evolving community health information networks. *Topics in Health Information Management, 17*(4), 11–29.

Gagnon, M. P., & Legare, F. (2009). Interventions for promoting information and communication technologies adoption in healthcare professionals. *Cochrane Database of Systematic Reviews*, (1): CD006093.

Google. (2009). *Google Health*. Retrieved from https://www.google.com/health

Grannis, S. J., Overhage, J. M., et al. (2002). Analysis of identifier performance using a deterministic linkage algorithm. In Proceedings of AMIA Symp., (pp. 305-309).

Grannis, S. J., Overhage, J. M., et al. (2003). Analysis of a probabilistic record linkage technique without human review. In *Proceedings of AMIA Annu. Symp.*, (pp. 259-263).

Gravely, S. D., & Whaley, E. S. (2009). The next step in health data exchanges: trust and privacy in exchange networks. *Journal of Healthcare Information Management, 23*(2), 33–37.

Grossman, J. M., & Bodenheimer, T. S. (2006). Hospital-physician portals: the role of competition in driving clinical data exchange. *Health Affairs (Project Hope), 25*(6), 1629–1636. doi:10.1377/hlthaff.25.6.1629

Grossman, J. M., Kushner, K. L., et al. (2008). Creating sustainable local health information exchanges: can barriers to stakeholder participation be overcome? *Res Briefs,* (2), 1-12.

Hammond, W. E. (2008). eHealth interoperability. *Studies in Health Technology and Informatics, 134*, 245–253.

Hayward, M. K., & Warren, R. D. (2007). Jackson Community Medical Record: a model for provider collaboration in a RHIO. *Journal of Healthcare Information Management, 21*(3), 31–36.

Hessler, B. J., & Soper, P. (2009). Assessing the relationship between health information exchanges and public health agencies. *Journal of Public Health Management and Practice, 15*(5), 416–424.

Hinman, A. R., & Davidson, A. J. (2009). Linking children's health information systems: clinical care, public health, emergency medical systems, and schools. *Pediatrics, 123*(2), S67–S73. doi:10.1542/peds.2008-1755D

Holmquest, D. L. (2007). Another lesson from Santa Barbara. *Health Affairs (Project Hope), 26*(5), 592–594. doi:10.1377/hlthaff.26.5.w592

Hurd, A. (2008). The federated advantage. Data exchange between healthcare organizations in RHIOs is a hot topic. Can federated models end the debate? *Health Manag, Technol., 29*(4), 14, 16.

Intermountain Healthcare. (2009). Intermountain Healthcare. Retrieved from http://intermountainhealthcare.org/Pages/home.aspx

Jha, A. K., & DesRoches, C. M. (2009). Use of electronic health records in U.S. hospitals. *The New England Journal of Medicine, 360*(16), 1628–1638. doi:10.1056/NEJMsa0900592

Kaelber, D. C., & Bates, D. W. (2007). Health information exchange and patient safety. *Journal of Biomedical Informatics, 40*(6), 40–45. doi:10.1016/j.jbi.2007.08.011

Kaiser Permanente. (2009). *Kaiser Permanente.* Retrieved from https://www.kaiserpermanente.org/

Kansky, J. (2008). Indiana Health Information Exchange: HIE success in the Heartland - Indiana Network for Patient Care. In *Proceedings of the 2008 HIMSS Conference.*

Koval, D. (2005). Real-world RHIO. A regional health information organization blazes a trail in Upstate New York. *Journal of American Health Information Management Association, 76*(3), 44–48.

Kuhn, K. A., & Giuse, D. A. (2007). Expanding the scope of health information systems - from hospitals to regional networks, to national infrastructures, and beyond. *Methods of Information in Medicine, 46*(4), 500–502.

Lassila, K. S., & Pemble, K. R. (1997). Assessing the impact of community health information networks: a multisite field study of the Wisconsin Health Information Network. *Topics in Health Information Management, 18*(2), 64–76.

Lau, L. M., Banning, P. D., et al. (2005). Mapping Department of Defense laboratory results to Logical Observation Identifiers Names and Codes (LOINC). In *Proceedings of the AMIA Annu. Symp.*, (pp. 430-434).

Lawrence, D. (2007). "Doing it right. While the key to the perfect RHIO may still be a mystery, a number of them are off and running." Healthc Inform**24**(9): 38, 40.

Lloyd, S. S. (1992). Automated information systems provide health information management support to veterans' healthcare. *Journal of American Health Information Management Association*, *63*(6), 63–67.

Lorenzi, N. (2003). *Strategies for Creating Successful Local Health Information Infrastructure Initiatives*. Nashville, TN: Vanderbilt University.

Maffei, R. (2008). Determining Business Models for Financial Sustainability in Regional Health Information Organizations: A Literature Review. In *Proceedings of the AMIA Annu. Symp.*, (pg.1038).

Malepati, S., & Kushner, K. (2007). RHIOs and the value proposition. Value is in the eye of the beholder. *Journal of American Health Information Management Association*, *78*(3), 24–29, quiz 31–32.

Mandl, K. D., & Simons, W. W. (2007). Indivo: a personally controlled health record for health information exchange and communication. *BMC Medical Informatics and Decision Making*, *7*, 25. doi:10.1186/1472-6947-7-25

Manion, F. J., & Robbins, R. J. (2009). Security and privacy requirements for a multi-institutional cancer research data grid: an interview-based study. *BMC Medical Informatics and Decision Making*, *9*, 31. doi:10.1186/1472-6947-9-31

Marshall, G. F., & Gillespie, W. (2009). Privacy and security in Pennsylvania: ensuring privacy and security of health information exchange in Pennsylvania. *Journal of Healthcare Information Management*, *23*(2), 38–44.

Martin, D. K. (1992). Making the connection: the VA-Regenstrief project. *M.D. Computing*, *9*(2), 91–96.

Martin, Z. (2007). Virginia RHIO taking baby steps. *Health Data Manag.*, *15*(2), 120, 122.

McDonald, C. J., & Overhage, J. M. (1999). The Regenstrief Medical Record System: a quarter century experience. *International Journal of Medical Informatics*, *54*(3), 225–253. doi:10.1016/S1386-5056(99)00009-X

McDonald, C. J., & Overhage, J. M. (2005). The Indiana network for patient care: a working local health information infrastructure. An example of a working infrastructure collaboration that links data from five health systems and hundreds of millions of entries. *Health Affairs (Project Hope)*, *24*(5), 1214–1220. doi:10.1377/hlthaff.24.5.1214

McGowan, J. J., Jordan, C., et al. (2007). Rural RHIOs: common issues in the development of two state-wide health information networks. In *Proceedings of the AMIA Annu. Symp.*, (pp. 528-532).

McGraw, D., & Dempsey, J. X. (2009). Privacy as an enabler, not an impediment: building trust into health information exchange. *Health Affairs (Project Hope)*, *28*(2), 416–427. doi:10.1377/hlthaff.28.2.416

Microsoft. (2009). *Microsoft HealthVault*. Retrieved from http://www.healthvault.com/

Miller, R. H., & Miller, B. S. (2007). The Santa Barbara County Care Data Exchange: what happened? *Health Affairs (Project Hope)*, *26*(5), 568–580. doi:10.1377/hlthaff.26.5.w568

Montelius, E., & Astrand, B. (2008). Individuals appreciate having their medication record on the web: a survey of attitudes to a national pharmacy register. *Journal of Medical Internet Research*, *10*(4), e35. doi:10.2196/jmir.1022

Nocella, K. C., & Horowitz, K. J. (2008). Against all odds: designing and implementing a grassroots, community-designed RHIO in a rural region. *Journal of Healthcare Information Management*, *22*(2), 34–41.

Noss, B., & Zall, R. J. (2002). A review of CHIN initiatives: what works and why. *Journal of Healthcare Information Management*, *16*(2), 35–39.

Open Source Health Records Exchange. (2009). *Open Source Health Records Exchange*. Retrieved from http://www.openhre.org/

Orlova, A. O., Dunnagan, M., et al. (2005). Electronic health record - public health (EHR-PH) system prototype for interoperability in 21st century healthcare systems. In Proceedings of the AMIA Annu. Symp., (pp, 575-579).

Ozkaynak, M., Marquard, J., et al. (2007). Are lay people ready for health information exchange? In *Proceedings of the AMIA Annu. Symp.,* 1065.

Payton, F. C., & Brennan, C. P. (1999). How a community health information network is really used. *Communications of the ACM*, *42*(12), 85–89. doi:10.1145/322796.322814

Payton, F. C., & Brennan, P. F. (1995). Cost justification of a community health information network: the ComputerLink for AD caregivers. In *Proceedings of Annu* (pp. 566–570). Symp. Comput. Appl. Med. Care.

Phillips, B. O., & Welch, E. E. (2007). Challenges for developing RHIOs in rural America: a study in Appalachian Ohio. *Journal of Healthcare Information Management*, *21*(3), 37–43.

Public Health Informatics Institute. (2005). *Public Health Opportunities in Health Information Exchange*. Retrieved from http://www.phii.org/resources/doc/Opportunities_0605.pdf

Raths, D. (2006). Real solutions for RHIO problems. Pioneering data exchange groups seek sustainability by solving business problems for members. *Healthcare Informatics*, *23*(8), 26–29.

Raths, D. (2008). Setting the standards stage. If health information exchange is to get to the next level, formulating standards will be an absolute key. *Healthcare Informatics*, *25*(3), 34–35.

Rogoski, R. (2008). A lack of data standards & sets will hamper information exchange. Healthcare CIOs must pressure government bodies and industry organizations to make true data standards a reality. *Healthc. Inform., 25*(2), 58, 60.

Rollins, G. (2005). Finding RHIOs. HIM professionals seek, fill roles in emerging health data networks. *Journal of American Health Information Management Association*, *76*(8), 32–34, 36.

Rubin, R. (2003). The Community Health Information Movement: Where It's Been, Where It's Going. In O'Carroll, P. W., Yasnoff, W., Ward, M., Ripp, L., & Martin, E. (Eds.), *Public Health Informatics and Information Systems* (pp. 595–616). New York: Springer. doi:10.1007/0-387-22745-8_27

Scalise, D. (2006). Technology. Which way RHIO? *Hosp. Health. Netw., 80*(6), 20, 22.

Shapiro, J. S. (2007). Evaluating public health uses of health information exchange. *Journal of Biomedical Informatics*, *40*(6), 46–49. doi:10.1016/j.jbi.2007.08.003

Sievers, A. (1992). Free-Net in Cleveland and Case Western Reserve University Library: Linking Community and University. (pp. 187-203). Clinic for Library Applications of Data Processing. Urbana, IL: Graduate School of Library and Information Science.

Staes, C. J., & Xu, W. (2009). A case for using grid architecture for state public health informatics: the Utah perspective. *BMC Medical Informatics and Decision Making*, *9*, 32. doi:10.1186/1472-6947-9-32

Stein, T. (2006). Writing the RHIO fine print. Model policies and specifications speed data exchange start-ups. *Journal of American Health Information Management Association*, *77*(2), 38–40, 42.

Tripathi, M., & Delano, D. (2009). Engaging patients for health information exchange. *Health Affairs (Project Hope)*, *28*(2), 435–443. doi:10.1377/hlthaff.28.2.435

Vest, J. R. (2009). Health information exchange and healthcare utilization. *Journal of Medical Systems*, *33*(3), 223–231. doi:10.1007/s10916-008-9183-3

Vreeman, D. J. (2007). Keeping up with changing source system terms in a local health information infrastructure: running to stand still. *Studies in Health Technology and Informatics*, *129*(Pt 1), 775–779.

Walker, J., & Pan, E. (2005). The value of health care information exchange and interoperability. *Health Affairs (Project Hope)*, (Suppl Web Exclusives), W5-10–W5-18.

Warnekar, P. P., Bouhaddou, O., et al. (2007). Use of RxNorm to exchange codified drug allergy information between Department of Veterans Affairs (VA) and Department of Defense (DoD). In Proceedings of AMIA Annu. Symp., (pp. 781-785).

Weiner, S. J., & Barnet, B. (2005). Processes for effective communication in primary care. *Annals of Internal Medicine*, *142*(8), 709–714.

Wright, A., & Sittig, D. F. (2008). SANDS: a service-oriented architecture for clinical decision support in a National Health Information Network. *Journal of Biomedical Informatics*, *41*(6), 962–981. doi:10.1016/j.jbi.2008.03.001

Zafar, A., & Dixon, B. E. (2007). Pulling back the covers: technical lessons of a real-world health information exchange. *Studies in Health Technology and Informatics*, *129*(Pt 1), 488–492.

ADDITIONAL READING

http://healthit.ahrq.gov/portal/server.pt/gateway/PTARGS_0_3882_874953_0_0_18/09-0071-EF.pdf: A US Government-sponsored report on liability coverage for regional health information organizations

http://healthit.ahrq.gov/portal/server.pt?open=514&objID=5554&mode=2&holderDisplayURL=http://prodportallb.ahrq.gov:7087/publishedcontent/publish/communities/k_o/knowledge_library/key_topics/health_briefing_01232006093812/health_information_exchange.html: The official website of the US Agency for Healthcare Research and Quality (AHRQ) with information on current projects and reports on HIE

http://healthit.hhs.gov/portal/server.pt?open=512&objID=1142&parentname=CommunityPage&parentid=2&mode=2&in_hi_userid=10741&cached=true: The official website of the US Government initiative National Health Information Network (NHIN)

http://health.utah.gov/phi/publications/Utah-ClinicalInfoExchange2008.pdf: Progress report of clinical health information exchange in the state of Utah, 2008

http://www.ahima.org/hie/index.asp: The official website of the The American Health Information Management Association (AHIMA) and information on HIE toolkit

http://www.cdc.gov/phin/: The official website of the US Government sponsored Public Health Information Network (PHIN) http://www.ehealthinitiative.org/: The official website of non-profit organizations eHealth Initiative and Foundation for eHealth Initiative whose mission is to engage multiple and diverse stakeholders to define and implement actions to address quality, safety and efficiency challenges through the use of interoperable information technology.

http://www.ehealthinitiative.org/ehealth-initiative-releases-results-2009-survey-health-information-exchange.html: A current listing of HIE initiatives in the US

http://www.ehealthinitiative.org/ehealth-initiative-releases-results-2009-survey-health-information-exchange.html: The eHealth Initiative 2009 Annual Survey on National Health Information Exchange

http://www.himss.org/asp/topics_rhio.asp: A portal for information on regional health information exchange in the US

http://www.nhinwatch.com/index.cms: A portal to US health information exchanges with channels for federal and regional initiatives

http://www.uhin.org/: The official website of the Utah Health Information Network

KEY TERMS AND DEFINITIONS

Health Information Exchange (HIE): The electronic movement of health-related information among organizations within a hospital system, community, region or nation. In its broadest sense, this refers to electronic exchange of health information between two or more parties.

Community Health Information Network (CHIN): Information network linking providers, insurers, patients and suppliers throughout a community. A CHIN could be defined as an inter-organizational system using information technologies and telecommunications to store, transmit, and transform clinical and financial information.

Regional Health Information Organization (RHIO): A nongovernmental, multi-stakeholder organization that enables or oversees the business and legal issues involved in the exchange and use of health information in a secure manner for the purpose of promoting the improvement of health quality, safety and efficiency.

Electronic Health Records (EHR): A digital form of an individual's longitudinal health record. EHR is often used interchangeable with Electronic Medical Records (EMR). Health care providers with electronic health records can participate in health information exchange (HIE).

Master Patient Index (MPI): A database that maintains a unique index for every patient in the network of Health Information Exchange. To assure the uniqueness of linked patient records from diverse sources is a major technical challenge for all HIE.

Indiana Health Information Exchange (IHIE): A non-profit HIE organization established in 2004. IHIE is the most successful RHIO for clinical health information exchange in the United States.

Utah Health Information Network (UHIN): A non-profit HIE organization established in 1993. UHIN is the most successful RHIO for administrative health information exchange in the United States.

Chapter 12
E-Medical Education: An Overview

D. John Doyle
Case Western Reserve University, USA & Cleveland Clinic Foundation, USA

ABSTRACT

The World Wide Web has made available a large variety of medical information and education resources only dreamed of two decades ago. This review discusses a number of Web-based e-Medical education concepts and resources likely to be of interest to the medical education community as well as a number of other groups. The resources described focus especially on those that are free and those that have an interactive component. The importance of interactivity and its role in the "constructivist" approach to education is emphasized. Problem-based learning in medical education is also discussed. In addition, the importance of "Web 2.0" and related developments is discussed, along with an overview of Web-based medical simulation software that can complement medical education programs. The importance of podcasts and videocasts as an educational resource are also emphasized. Other concepts such as mash-ups and the semantic Web are briefly described. Intellectual property issues are also discussed, such as Creative Commons license arrangements, as well as the concept of "information philanthropy". Finally, the importance of peer-review and technology evaluation for online educational materials is discussed.

DOI: 10.4018/978-1-61692-004-3.ch012

INTRODUCTION

The Rise of Web-Based Educational Systems

"The student begins with the patient, continues with the patient, and ends his studies with the patient, using books and lectures as tools, as means to an end."

—Sir William Osler, Aequanimitas, 1905

Since the coming of age of the World Wide Web a little over a decade ago, a true revolution in access to information of all kinds has taken place. In particular, recent years have witnessed a quasi-revolution in conventional and distance education as a result. Web-based educational technologies now allow for new approaches to education not previously dreamed of. While this is especially true in the field of distance education generally, it has also had a tremendous impact on medical education in particular (Gallagher, Dobrosielski-Vergona, Wingard, and Williams, 2005; Glinkowski and Ciszek, 2007; Jang, Hwang, Park, Kim and Kim, 2005; McKimm, Jollie and Cantillon, 2003; Sajeva, 2006; Schilling, Wiecha, Polineni and Khalil, 2006; Smith, Roberts and Partridge, 2007; Zary, Johnson, Boberg and Fors, 2006). Clinicians and medical students now have available to them a countless array of online medical journals, CME educational sites, discussion forums, medical search engines, podcasts, wikis, and blogs that they can use to enhance their ongoing learning. A great number of these resources are entirely free.

WEB-SITE DEVELOPMENT SOFTWARE

Web pages are a particularly useful means of providing information of almost any kind. They are easily accessed and are updated relatively easily, at least with some development systems. Links to related documents can be provided, while support for tables, graphics and multimedia objects like audio and video clips can usually be managed with minimal difficulty. As a result, Web pages have proven to be very popular for medical education.

Web pages are primarily built using the HTML language or one of its successors (Katzman, 2001; Lynch and Horton, 1998; Ryan, Louis and Yee, 2005; Wiggins, Davidson, Harnsberger, Lauman and Goede, 2001). There are many advantages to using HTML for Web site development, one of which is that one does not need to buy any special software in order to use it - one can write Web pages directly in HTML using almost any text editor. Still, most Web developers prefer to use a specialized Web page editor, and there are a number of inexpensive or free HTML editors available (as a simple Google search will quickly reveal). Professionals usually use packages such as Macromedia's *Dreamweaver or* Microsoft's *Expression Web.* While these are excellent, comprehensive, general-purpose Web page editors, they are not especially friendly to beginners, and for a number of small projects I have used a less well-known but very easy-to-use system known as *Homestead* (www.homestead.com).

Regardless of the system chosen, consideration must also be given to the use of appropriate design principles in Web page construction (Cook and Dupras, 2004; Gotthardt et al, 2006; Wong, Greenhalgh, Russell, Boynton, and Toon, 2003). In this respect, Where possible, consideration should also be given to adding some degree of interactivity to the process (Coiera, 2003; Despont-Gros, Mueller, and Lovis, 2005; Reynolds, Mason and Harper, 2008; Ridley, 2007; Stout, Villegas, and Kim 2001). Web-based interactivity, discussed in more detail later in this article, can be implemented in various ways. For instance, a section of a Web page may ask the student a question, and offer four possible answers the student may select from. Depending on the student's response, the Web page can provide a different commentary. Other forms of Web-based interactivity may involve the use of discussion forums or online surveys and polls. Providing e-mail addresses (and "mailto" links) for authors or instructors can also help make material more interactive. Advanced interactivity may also be achieved using JavaScript, a popular and relatively easy to learn programming language for Web pages, as well as via a number of other specialized languages.

Another concern is with Web site maintenance. All good web sites need periodic updating – otherwise the content becomes dated, hyperlinks become broken and other problems arise. You should plan for quarterly maintenance updates to your site to keep it topical and respectable.

A final point concerns Intellectual Property (IP) issues. It is not uncommon for individuals involved in the development of educational materials to utilize in their work useful material (especially images) found on the Web. However, if done without permission, this practice is potentially problematic, even with appropriate attribution, as the use of the Intellectual Property belonging to others – whether commercial or otherwise - generally requires that permission be granted.

It should be noted, however, that a number of excellent educational resources such as Wikipedia operate under a "Creative Commons" license arrangement. Creative Commons is "a nonprofit corporation dedicated to making it easier for people to share and build upon the work of others, consistent with the rules of copyright." Creative Commons works "to increase the amount of creativity (cultural, educational, and scientific content) in "the commons" — the body of work that is available to the public for free and legal sharing, use, repurposing, and remixing." This arrangement often greatly facilitates the legal reuse of valuable educational materials. The interested reader is directed to http://creativecommons.org for further details.

As an example of such an arrangement, an individual seeking to freely use an illustration of a sugammadex molecule encapsulating a rocuronium molecule can get one that the creator has generously released into the public domain at http://en.wikipedia.org/wiki/Image:Sugammadex_encaps_rocuronium.jpg).

WHAT IS WEB 2.0 AND WHY IS IT IMPORTANT?

The original launch of the World Wide Web circa 1994 soon developed into a series of offerings that took the online world by storm and quickly created no small number of multi-millionaires. Such early offerings soon included corporate and personal Web sites, Web-based mail, Internet commerce, Internet radio, etc. For convenience, some authors describe this "original" version of the Web as Web 1.0.

Since that time, however, the Web has advanced and developed so much that some authors now use the term "Web 2.0" to describe the many recent developments that stress openness, sharing, cooperation and collaboration among Web users (Atreja, Messinger-Rapport, Jain, and Mehta, 2006; Boulos, Maramba, and Wheeler 2006; Kamel Boulos, and Wheeler, 2007; McGee, and Begg, 2008; McLean, Richards, and Wardman 2007). Such developments include Wikis, blogs, podcasts, mashups, and RSS feeds (*vide infra*).

While a formal definition of Web 2.0 that everyone agrees on would be hard to find, one way of understanding it would be to point out its emphasis on participation through open applications and services, rather than define it (as others might) in terms of newer languages such as AJAX or XML, or advanced online applications such as Google Maps or Wikipedia. The emphasis in Web 2.0 is thus on developing applications and systems so that they get smarter and more comprehensive the more people use them (leveraging collective efforts and intelligence), rather than emphasizing any technical properties or specifications. It is this special 'collaborationware' focus of many Web

2.0 applications as well as their simplicity of use and speed of deployment, that has lead their enthusiastic adoption in many medical educational arenas. Another emphasis in Web 2.0 is on the automatic granting of permission to use existing content in new and exciting ways ("information philanthropy") (Doyle, Ruskin and Engel, 1996), discussed later. Yet another focus is that of services over software. Finally, as Web 2.0 continues to develop, it is expected to embrace new modes of communication and interaction such as the use of communication via cell phones, the use of instant messaging, learning via virtual reality techniques, and even learning via online social gaming. In some cases the connections between these technologies and clinical practice may be surprising. For instance, in a study by Rosser, Lynch, Cuddihy, Gentile, Klonsky and Merrell (2007) the authors discovered that surgical trainees who had played video games more than 3 hours per week worked faster and made fewer errors when performing laparoscopic surgical tasks. Let us now look at some of these tools in more detail.

Wikis

A Wiki is a collaborative informational Web site whose content is open (freely accessible) and can be edited by anyone who is duly authorized. The name comes from the Hawaiian word *wiki*, meaning *to hurry* or *swift*. The best known Wiki is ***Wikipedia*** (www.wikipedia.org), which as of this writing has over 2.6 million articles in English. It is sometimes held out as a one of the best examples of Web 2.0, with its openness in both access and in its participation model.

However, Wikipedia's openness in allowing virtually anyone to participate has lead to criticism (Taylor-Mendes, 2007), even though there is evidence that it may be just as accurate as commercial encyclopedias (Giles, 2005). Still, such concerns have lead to the launching of more rigorously edited free online encyclopedias such as ***Scholarpedia*** (http://www.scholarpedia.org) and ***Citizendium*** (http://citizendium.org). For instance, the approach of Scholarpedia is to avoid competing with Wikipedia, but rather to complement it, covering a few narrow fields (such as computational neuroscience) in an exhaustive manner.

It should also be pointed out that some of the "alternatives" to Wikipedia that have been developed may be seriously flawed. As an example, ***Conservapedia*** (http://www.conservapedia.com) is a Web-based encyclopedia written from a Conservative Christian point of view. As a result, it contains articles that support the "Young Earth" creationist model (the earth being a mere 6000 years old) or that present evolution as a discredited scientific theory in conflict with the fossil record.

Medical Education Wikis

One challenge with Wikipedia is that its entries dealing with medical topics tend to vary greatly in quality. While blatant technical inaccuracies are unusual, many of Wikipedia's medical entries lack the perspective and balance usually found in well-established medical textbooks. This situation exists in part because no special training or clinical experience is required to contribute to any Wikipedia article. While it is true that clinicians unhappy with any Wikipedia medical article can take it upon themselves to edit it to their satisfaction, this seems not to be done frequently. In all likelihood, this is at least partly because academics generally get no credit towards tenure or promotion for contributions of this kind.

Because Wikipedia is often weak and incomplete in their treatment of medical subjects, efforts to develop medical Wikis have been launched. ***Ganfyd*** (http://ganfyd.org) is an online collaborative medical reference that is edited by medical professionals and other experts. ***Sermo*** (http://sermo.com) is a wiki-like medical resource that is only accessible by physicians practicing in the USA who can prove their medical credentials by providing their "DEA number". A more specialized medical wiki example is ***Flu Wiki*** (http://www.fluwikie.com), which was launched to assist in the planning for possible avian influenza pandemics. ***Wikisurgery*** (http://www.wikisurgery.com) is a free collaborative surgical encyclopaedia "with over 1,300 articles for surgeons and patients, including news, articles, operation scripts, biographies and images." Yet another example is the ***Diabetes Wiki*** (http://diabetes.wikia.com/wiki/Diabetes_Wiki). A fairly comprehensive list of medical Wikis is available at http://www.davidrothman.net/ list-of-medical-wikis. For more information on Wikis in a medical context see a review by Johnson, Freeman and Dellavalle (2007).

Blogs

Blogs (short for "Web logs") are Web sites intended for online audiences containing a diary-like account of events and personal insights. While a great many blogs are social, political or technical in nature, a number focus on medical issues. Often written by doctors, these blogs regularly discuss the latest developments in diagnosis, treatment or basic science. Some give the authors a chance to rant at "Big Pharma" and their expensive drugs, to complain about HMOs and their "unreasonable" policies, or to complain about malpractice lawyers and the ever rising cost of medical liability insurance. Others are more focused on providing up-to-date clinical information or in telling interesting clinical anecdotes. For an excellent example of a medical blog, see http://www.kevinmd.com. For more general information in a medical context see a review by Sethi (2007).

Finally, loosely related to blogging is ***Twitter*** (http://twitter.com), a microblogging technology where users can send and receive concise, text-based information. While it has not yet seen deep penetration in the medical field, this may be only a matter of time as this and other social media services, such as YouTube, Facebook, MySpace, and Second Life emerge as popular sources of health information, especially for young adults.

Critique of Wikis and Blogs

One concern with both wikis and blogs is the quality of their content, an issue identified earlier. However, there is hope that, at least for some popular resources, the collaborative nature or the resource will lead to self-correction. For instance, the openness of many wikis has given rise to the concept of "Darwikinism" where "unfit" wiki material content is zealously edited by other users (McLean, Richards, and Wardman, 2007).

One interesting question that arises in relation to medical blogging is: "What ethical standards should medical bloggers be held to in their postings?" I would argue that where these individuals are health professionals, ideally at least, they should be ethically bound to the same rules and standards of professionalism as professional journalists: any specific medical information posted should be accurate, should come from a trusted, authoritative source, and a citation to that source should be provided. This is not always the case, as exemplified by some blogs that promote the view that HIV does not cause AIDS (e.g., http://www.aids-science.blogspot.com)

When medical bloggers write about situations or cases encountered in their own clinical practice, specific attention should be given to protecting patient confidentiality. Ideally, medical bloggers may wish to have their blog or medical Web site accredited by the Health on the Net Foundation, which provides endorsement to websites which adhere to the foundation's guidelines. (More information is available at the foundation's Web site (http://www.hon.ch), which outlines the eight principles that the Health on the Net Foundation requires for endorsement.)

Podcasts / Videocasts

A podcast is a downloadable audio or video presentation for replay on a personal media player such as Apple's iPod. A rich variety of medical podcasts are available to interested individual (e.g., itunes.com, podcast.com), although many require a subscription or payment While podcasts are sometimes used for undergraduate medical education, they are most commonly used in post-graduate medical education. A great many medical education podcasts consist of edited recordings of lectures at major medical conferences. In the case of lecture podcasts offered by Audio Digest and some other suppliers, it is possible to get formal CME credit upon completion of a quiz. This is important to many physicians who must obtain a particular number of CME credits to maintain their medical license. Users wishing free medical podcasts may wish to take advantage of those offered by the New England Journal of Medicine (http://content.nejm.org/misc/podcast.dtl). For more information on podcasts see a review by Abbasi (2006).

Mashups

A mashup is a web application that presents information integrated from two or more data sources. An example of a health mashup is ***HealthMap*** (http://healthmap.org), which uses information from Google Maps (http://maps.google.com) or other sources to add cartographic context to epidemiological data so as to create a new service not originally provided by either source.

RSS (Really Simple Syndication)

An RSS document is a Web resource known as a "feed" or "channel" that scans the Web to provide links to updated content (blog entries, news headlines, podcasts, etc.) in which one has previously indicated an interest. RSS documents also include "metadata" such as publication dates and authorship information in a standardized file format ("XML") allows the information to be viewed by many different programs. For more information on RSS services in a medical context see a review by Wu and Li (2007).

Semantic Web

A member of individuals such as Tim Berners-Lee, the inventor of Web 1.0, have expressed concerns about a number of aspects of Web 2.0 and have proposed as an alternative the concept of the "**Semantic Web**", an ambitious undertaking where information would be automatically exchanged and acted upon on our behalf by the Web itself. While humans are capable of using the Web to carry out tasks such as ordering merchandise on eBay or searching for a good price on a cruise vacation, because web pages are designed to be read by people and not machines it is exceedingly hard for a computer to accomplish the same tasks without human direction. However, the vision offered by the Semantic Web is that the information it carried would be formatted so that it is "understandable" by computers, thereby reducing much of the tedious work involved in information-related web activities. Tim Berners-Lee originally expressed the vision of the semantic web as follows (Berners-Lee and Fischetti, 1999):

"I have a dream for the Web [in which computers] become capable of analyzing all the data on the Web – the content, links, and transactions between people and computers. A 'Semantic Web', which should make this possible, has yet to emerge, but when it does, the day-to-day mechanisms of trade, bureaucracy and our daily lives will be handled by machines talking to machines. The 'intelligent agents' people have touted for ages will finally materialize." In the domain of biomedicine, the Semantic Web has now begun to be explored in earnest (Mukherjea, 2005; Good and Wilkinson, 2006; Antezana, Kuiper and Mironov, 2009).

Related to the Semantic Web is the notion of "**Semantic Publishing**", where information and documents are published with explicit "semantic markups" intended to allow computers to comprehend the structure and meaning of published information. While the Semantic Web and Semantic Publishing is expected to eventually change the face of web publishing in dramatic ways, there is much progress to be made before it becomes commonplace. For more information the reader is directed to discussions by Berners-Lee and Hendler (Berners-Lee and Hendler, 2001) and Shadbolt and -Lee (Shadbolt and Berners-Lee, 2008).

INFORMATION PHILANTHROPY

Recent years have seen the growth of a movement I have called "Information Philanthropy" (Doyle, Ruskin and Engel, 1996), which has as its goal making quality intellectual property available for free, usually as an Internet download. This material might be textbooks, graphic illustrations, photographs, videos, musical compositions, blueprints, schematics, DNA and amino acid sequences, computer programs, mathematical algorithms, poetry, chemical synthesis procedures, detective novels, simulation procedures, and even raw scientific data. In all such cases, the creator/owner of the material makes this material available without charge subject to possible restrictions—such as not allowing the material to be used for commercial or military purposes, or perhaps not permitting the material to be reworked (edited, remixed, etc.) into a derivative product. In a great many cases such materials are governed by a Creative Commons license, as discussed earlier.

Interactivity and the "Constructivist" Approach to Education

Constructivism is the view that knowledge is "constructed" by the learner by testing ideas, concepts and approaches based on existing knowledge and one's actively acquired experiences and those of others. Constructivist theory holds that knowledge is not merely acquired passively and that students learn best when they actively (often collaboratively) participate in problem-solving and critical thinking while involved in a well-formulated learning activity.

Many experts in adult learning argue that traditional lecture-based didactic teaching all-too-often encourages passive learning instead of the development of the higher order cognitive skills needed for "true" education. Arguing that active involvement is essential for effective learning, they suggest that adults learn best when drawing on previous experiences, using techniques such as group discussion, simulation exercises, and problem solving. That is, going beyond mere looking and listening motivates people to learn on their own, gives students the motivation to try out new ideas, and encourages them to critically examine issues that were once simple accepted passively.

One educational element that has been advocated as a means to achieve active learning is "interactivity" (Table 1) since it is well-matched to the constructivist model of learning (ConCeição and Taylor, 2007). The *Oxford English Dictionary* defines interactivity as reciprocally active, allowing a two-way flow of information between source and user, responding to the user's input. In recent years interactivity has been viewed as a particularly important component to educational undertakings, although the nature of the "interaction" will naturally vary with factors such as the subject domain (e.g., philosophy versus physics), and format (e.g., conventional versus distance education). Well-designed interactivity in educational systems can, at least in principle, help capture the learner's interest, has the potential to speed learning, and even allows for continuous assessment of the degree to which the material is mastered. These goals are met by providing frequent and relevant user feedback, by recognizing when students misunderstand a concept, and

Table 1. Types of Interactivity in teaching and education, with examples focusing on medical Education

Person-to-person (student / teacher) interaction with both persons in direct verbal communication ("same place interaction")
formal classroom or auditorium teaching (such as a question and answer period at the end of a lecture)
informal hallway or bedside discussions
Person-to-person interaction (student / teacher) using remote communication technology ("different place interaction")
telephone and audio conferencing
writing (paper, e-mail)
video conferencing
telemedicine (e.g., clinical discussion centering around a radiographic image)
Paper-based interactivity [can also be made into a computer model]
interactive paper scenarios (If X is true then go to page Y otherwise go to page Z)
Example 1: Patient with chest pain presents to the ER where X= "admit patient to hospital"
Example 2: Patient with abdominal pain presents to the ER where X= "operate on patient [laparotomy]"
Paper-based interactivity based on "developer pen" technology [can also be made into to a computer model]
developer pen technology allows the student to see the result of a study or laboratory test once it has been "ordered"; based on the result of the selected investigation the student selects other clinical options (e.g., asks more questions, attempts to elicit a particular clinical finding, orders another test)
Computer based interactivity not using the World Wide Web. This usually involves using programming languages such as C++ or various older authoring platforms.
Web-based interactivity. This usually involves using programming languages such as JavaScript or authoring platforms with Web support.

Note: further distinctions can to be made between immediate ("synchronous", "real time") and delayed ("asynchronous") interaction.

by providing learning aids such as animations or graphs that vary depending on user input. However, badly designed interactivity can also impede student progress (*vide infra*).

The importance of interactivity in learning is perhaps best illustrated by the fact that a number of journals either directly or peripherally address this topic. For instance, the Journal of Interactive Learning Research (JILR), available online at http://www.aace.org/pubs/jilr/default.htm, publishes manuscripts having to do with "the underlying theory, design, implementation, effectiveness, and impact on education and training of the following interactive learning environments."

Stevan Harnard (1992) has pointed out that electronic publication (and especially electronic publication via the Internet) provides a dimension of interactivity in document publication that is radically new. He notes:

No other medium can offer an author the possibility of virtually instantaneous and ubiquitous interaction with his intended audience. Electronic publication is not just a more efficient implementation of paper publishing, it offers the possibility of a phase transition in the form (and hence also the content) of scholarly inquiry. Not only are the boundaries between "informal" and "formal" literature blurred, but scholarly inquiry has always been a continuum, from the inchoate birth of new ideas and findings to their (in principle) endless evolution as inquiry carries on.

Interactivity is also important in distance education. One simple definition of "distance education" is that it is the delivery of instruction that does not require the learner to be present in the same physical location as the instructor. Students in such learning environments are thus said to interact variously with the instructor, the content, the technology, and with other students. In addition to these four forms of interaction, further distinctions must to be made between instantaneous ("real time", "synchronous") and delayed ("asynchronous") interaction, as well as between "same-place" and "different-place" interaction. Generally speaking, delayed and different-place interaction offer the student more flexibility and opportunities for thought and reflection, while immediate and same-place interaction, some would say, allow for a greater sense of spontaneity, impulsiveness and even exhilaration.

By contrast, with conventional classroom-based teaching, the focus is predominantly on student-teacher interaction, with student-content interaction also taking place, especially when out-of-classroom reading takes place. In the distance education setting, with the heavy use of self-study materials, the focus is usually on student-content interaction although interaction with technology is also frequently important.

Various learners and instructors will have preferences regarding interactivity, and some forms of education will rely on some forms of interactivity more than others. Regardless, the wise use of interactivity will help "engage" students and help ensure an enduring learning experience. One particularly engaging form of interactivity in educational materials is the use of multiple choice questions (MCQs) (Collins, 2006; Moss, 2001). The use of MCQs not only make the material more engaging but also help detect learning gaps. In recent years the most popular format for MCQ's is the "pick the best single answer" format (e.g., Which one of the following drugs would be the most likely to increase heart rate in a normal adult?). If the question has been answered correctly, the student is given an encouraging note with more details. If answered incorrectly, a different note is shown to the student.

Until recent years, educational technology was not especially capable of maintaining a high degree of interactivity with a learner, in contrast, say, to the very high level of possible interaction between a teacher and a student discussing a complex philosophical matter, where a series of verbal exchanges may occur that involves a cognitive effort much more advanced than mere memorization or rote repetition. This matter is expected to change favorably as software technology continues to become more sophisticated and as computer hardware advances in speed and power. In particular, advances in Artificial Intelligence (AI), and educational authoring systems will likely have a direct impact on the evolution of computer-based interactivity. Still, computer-based learning is much more complex than working through a textbook, and many students who are uncomfortable with computers see no reason to deviate from a curriculum based on well-written textbooks, particularly well-polished classics that are current and are accompanied by study guides and solutions manuals.

Many advocates of computer-mediated distance education draw attention to the helpful aspects offered by computer-based methods and understate the kinds of communicative and technical difficulties learners may experience. When students use complicated equipment in their learning environment, it is important to ensure the technologies used help rather than hinder the learning experience. Students using unfamiliar technologies may experience frustration, anxiety and confusion and students involved in distance education using computer technologies may face numerous stumbling blocks unrelated to the material to be learned. These include computer hardware problems, software problems at the level of the operating system or the various software applications, as well as difficulties with Internet access. Files may mysteriously "disappear". Attachments sent by e-mail may be "lost" in transit. Random "disconnects" from the Internet may frustrate the user. Unless students are moderately familiar with computers, substantial effort may be expended on technology-related issues rather than learning the intended materials.

Thus technologies that are awkward, unintuitive or present the learner with a steep learning curve may hinder interaction and even impede learning. Various means by which technology can impede interactivity include: haphazard, unintuitive or disorganized user interfaces; poor screen layout; poor use of fonts and icons; systems that respond too slowly to user inputs; or systems that crash frequently. While a detailed discussion of this matter is beyond the scope of this review, books by design gurus Jakob Nielsen (1994) and Donald Norman (1999) are recommended as a good place to explore the nature of good and bad user-interface design.

Studies show that technical problems can occasionally render the educational undertaking to be a substantially negative experience. For instance, Hara and Kling (1999) carried out a study of a web-based distance education course at an American university and commented that distance learners may experience problems and frustrations that are not well documented in the distance education literature. They noted that three interrelated sources accounted for most of the problems: "lack of prompt feedback, ambiguous instructions on the web, and technical problems". They concluded that the frustrations the students experienced "inhibited their educational opportunity". In a related paper (Hara and Kling, 2000) similar concerns were voiced.

The importance of interactivity in medical education is supported by a landmark meta-analysis of the effectiveness of formal CME by Davis, O'Brien, Freemantle, Wolf, Mazmanian and Taylor-Vaisey (1999) who showed that traditional didactic methods do not generally lead to a change of clinical practice, or to an improvement in patients' health outcomes, whereas interactive techniques are more likely to. As result, some regulatory bodies, such as the Royal College of Physicians and Surgeons of Canada (RCPSC) specifically mandate that at least 25 per cent of the time of an approved educational event should be allocated for interactive learning, such as in the form of a question and discussion period. This serves to further engage the listener as well as to clarify some of the issues that may remain unanswered at the end of the formal part of the presentation.

PROBLEM-BASED LEARNING

Traditional education practices from kindergarten through professional school often produce students who are disenchanted and bored with their education. All too often students are faced with a vast amount of information to memorize, a good deal of which is of little apparent relevance to future career goals. In particular, in the field of medical education, medical students have been traditionally provided with a series of lectures, laboratories and clinical sessions for four years (six years in Europe), and then released into internship and clinical practice with little in the way of actual skills in real-world clinical problem solving, the prevailing view being that these skills will emerge quickly enough in the hustle-bustle of the busy clinical world (Barrows, 1983).

Studies in classical medical education have often been critical of this approach. What students learn, despite intense efforts on the part of both students and teachers, often fades quickly (Levine & Forman, 1973) and there is even evidence that natural problem solving skills may be impaired by this process (Barrows & Bennett, 1982). It also seems that many physicians are not able to continue their education after completion of their training (Ramsey & Carline, 1991). Problem-based learning (PBL) has been advocated as one means to get around these difficulties (Albanese & Mitchell, 1993).

Traditional education involves the delivery of information to students by means of lectures and demonstrations, usually supported by tutorials and laboratory sessions. In this model the instructor provides students with the information that they need. In Problem-based Learning (PBL) the students work in small groups under the guidance of an instructor or tutor to find for themselves the knowledge they need to solve real world problems. The tutors are usually not experts in the subject matter of the tutorial, but rather are facilitators who help the students find the answers for themselves. At the conclusion of a PBL module, the students should have encountered the information necessary to solve the problem and, in so doing, should have gained knowledge and skills that in a traditional medical curriculum would have been circulated by lecture. PBL emphasizes group problem-analysis and independent self-directed study over teacher- or examination-driven education. As a consequence, it is believed that PBL may encourage students to become thoughtful problem-solvers and life-long learners (Barrows, 1983).

The introduction of a PBL-based medical curriculum began in 1969 at McMaster University in Hamilton, Ontario, Canada (Schmidt et al., 1991). From the school's outset, McMaster medical school structured the curriculum around actual clinical cases instead of teaching based on the traditional subjects of anatomy, biochemistry, physiology, pharmacology and so on. The introduction of PBL was based on a concern that many medical schools put too much emphasis on memorization of facts and little weight on developing problem solving skills or the self-directed study skills necessary for the life-long practice of medicine.

Following its introduction at McMaster University, the PBL teaching model was later adopted by a significant number of other medical schools, as well as by schools teaching other professional disciplines such as business. PBL is now the instructional method of choice in an increasing number of medical schools around the globe (Schmidt et al., 1991).

Problem-based learning is a ground-breaking and demanding approach to medical education - ground-breaking because it involves a new way of using clinical material to help students learn, and demanding because it requires the instructor to play a facilitating and supporting role rather than a didactic one. For the student, problem-based learning emphasizes the application of knowledge and skills to the solution of problems (clinical cases) rather than the mere recall of facts.

Since the quantity of direct teaching is substantially reduced in a PBL curriculum, students are expected to assume greater responsibility for their own education, and the instructor's role becomes variously one of coach, group facilitator, subject matter expert, instructional resource guide, and group consultant, where the instructor is expected to promote and support student involvement, to provide guidance to help keep students on track, to help prevent anyone giving inappropriate negative criticism, and even to assume the role of fellow learner. This arrangement is intended to promote group acquisition of information rather than the mere imparting of information to passive students by faculty (Vernon & Blake, 1993).

In a PBL class, students are given a problem to work on. They then proceed through a number of stages as they move towards their solution: exploring the nature of the problem; making a clear statement of the problem; identifying the information needed to understand the problem; identifying resources needed to gather this information; generating possible solutions to the problem; scrutinizing the various solutions for strengths and weaknesses; identifying the best solution among the various possible solutions; and presenting the solution. These stages usually take place over several class discussion sessions along with students working individually on assigned tasks related to the problem outside of class time.

Problem-based learning has now entered the realm of eMedical education. For example, Table 2 lists some sample medical PBL problems that may be viewed from the Internet.

Table 2. Some sample medical problem-based learning (PBL) cases available on the internet

Bad Reaction - A Case Study in Immunology
http://ublib.buffalo.edu/libraries/projects/cases/immunology/immunology1.html
Pediatric Infection Case
http://medicalpblukm.blogspot.com/2009/08/case-files-3-peds-im-hot-and-drooling.html
Into Thin Air - A Case Study in Physiology
http://ublib.buffalo.edu/libraries/projects/cases/Denali1.html
A Series of Cases in the Field of Obstetrics and Gynecology
http://www.healthsystem.virginia.edu/internet/obgyn-**clerkship/PBLCases.cfm**
A Series of Biology Cases
http://capewest.ca/pbl.html

WEB-BASED MEDICAL SIMULATION SYSTEMS

In many respects, simulators offer the ultimate in interactivity and appear to have an excellent future in medical education. Computer-based simulators used in medical education fall into four general categories: (1) Screen-based text simulators, (2) Screen-based graphical simulators, (3) Manikin-based simulators, and (4) Virtual reality trainers. We briefly discuss the first two of these here, since both can be Web-based.

Screen-based text simulators create verbal scenarios in which the user picks one of several responses and, based on the chosen response, a new text scenario is produced. For instance, in a scenario involving a patient presenting with a severe headache, the user may be offered options such as prescribing an analgesic or getting a CT-scan of the head. Based on the user's choice, a new narrative is then generated and more management choices are offered. Being purely text-based, screen-based text simulators are relatively simple to construct and require little memory, making them popular in early medical simulation efforts. However, since they are lacking in graphical elements, they are rarely used today.

Screen-based graphical simulators such as 'Gasman' (Philip, 1986) and 'Body' (Smith and Davidson, 1999) aim to recreate elements of reality in graphic form on a computer screen, often to elucidate the pharmacokinetic and pharmacodynamic processes associated with drug administration. Usually, only a mouse interface is involved. While these simulations help one understand the conceptual theory underlying clinical practice, they usually do not confer actual practical skills. Their strength lies in an ability to help one understand abstract concepts while remaining portable and relatively inexpensive.

For individuals interested in respiratory medicine, ThoracicAnesthesia.com offers a free "education, information, and reference service" which include a series of didactic pieces and teaching slide sets, a series of journal article synopses, a bronchial anatomy quiz, and a bronchoscopy simulator. The bronchoscopy simulator is unquestionably the best part of the site. Here, using real time video based on an Adobe Flash platform one can navigate through the tracheobronchial tree with controls for moving your virtual bronchoscope forward, backwards, and in diagonal directions. This process is aided by a "macro" view on the left panel (called a "bronchial tree navigational map view") and a "micro" view on the right panel ("bronchoscope view"). If desired, zooming in and out and adding or removing labels on the displayed material can be controlled simply by clicking on the appropriate controls. Most importantly, clicking on various labels in the bronchoscope view will launch further information in the map view, making the experience intuitive and even enjoyable.

PEER-REVIEW OF ONLINE EDUCATIONAL MATERIALS

When an instructor selects teaching resources - especially in the case of medical teaching resources - he or she wants some assurance that the material is timely, accurate, well-written, and developed using sound pedagogical principles. Such assurances, some would argue, can be best obtained via a process of peer-review. While the peer-review process in scientific publishing is as old as scientific publishing itself, the idea of peer-review procedures for educational resources in relatively new. However, it is clearly an idea whose time has come.

Typically, scientific materials submitted for publication are reviewed by two or more expert referees who are particularly knowledgeable in the subject matter being discussed. Their comments and opinions form the basis upon which an editor will decide whether or not to publish the submitted material, and with what changes, if any. By contrast, formal peer-review of educational materials remains relatively uncommon. Historically, this was because until recently, publishing educational resources like books was usually always done in conjunction with a publishing house with its own internal quality control system. For instance, some book companies employ a pre-publication internal and external reviews to establish whether a manuscript is worthy of publication and to determine how it might be enhanced.

With the rise of the Internet, however, the landscape has changed, and publishing no longer requires enormous expense and the cooperation of a publishing house. The prevalence of electronic scholarly publishing has thus increased dramatically in recent years due, largely as a consequence of the reach and immediacy of the Internet and its ability to handle varied forms of electronic media.

The idea of establishing a peer-review process for educational resources is not entirely new. For instance, Project Merlot, located at http://merlot.org, seeks to provide high-quality teaching materials in a number of disciplines of higher education. It conducts reviews along three dimensions: 1) quality of the content, 2) usefulness as a teaching tool, and 3) ease of use.

For peer-reviewed medical education materials, MedEdPORTAL, an offering from the Association of American Medical Colleges (AAMC) maintains an online presence at http://www.aamc.org/mededportal. According to its Web site MedEdPORTAL "is a Web-based tool that promotes collaboration across disciplines and institutions by facilitating the exchange of peer-reviewed educational materials, knowledge, and solutions" and serves "as a central repository of high quality educational materials such as PowerPoint presentations, assessment materials, virtual patient cases, and faculty development materials". Any medical educator may submit materials for possible publication on MedEdPORTAL. The material is then screened by an AAMC staff member to ensure that it meets the minimal requirements for inclusion and does not violate patient privacy. Suitable material is then assigned to three reviewers, at least one who will have expertise in the content area, and at least one who will have expertise in the educational format of the material.

Another peer-reviewed medical resource is The Health Education Assets Library (HEAL), which maintains an online presence at http://www.healcentral.org. Established in 2000, HEAL has grown over time to provide over 22,000 resources such as images, video clips, audio clips, PowerPoint slidesets, documents in PDF format, etc.

HEAL, MERLOT and MedEdPORTAL all make use of the well-known Creative Commons copyright system with their works. In general, all resources in these collections are licensed for free use, reproduction, and modification by users according to the specific terms of the Creative Commons license associated with that resource.

Despite these encouraging developments, formal peer-review of educational resources remains uncommon. However, with academic credit now starting to be granted to individuals who produce freely downloadable peer-reviewed educational material such as that offered by HEAL and MedEdPORTAL, the volume and quality of such resources is bound to increase over time.

EDUCATIONAL TECHNOLOGY EVALUATION

As new educational technologies (ETs) become available there is a need to evaluate them in some systematic way. Ideally any new ET would be compared to an existing standard ET using a randomized trial design, such as in randomly assigning students to one of two teaching systems and testing for differences in outcome. In reality these kinds of studies are relatively rare because of high resource requirements and for other reasons, and we may be thus forced to use less perfect instruments to gauge the value of a new ET, using measures such as user preference scores, as a surrogate for rigorous outcome data. Thus, for instance, when some educators declare that interactive teaching provides better educational outcomes than the mere non-interactive display of information, they generally do not argue on the basis of randomized clinical trials (as one would generally do, for instance, in evaluating a new drug) but instead support their position on the basis of general principles. Thus the notion that adding interactivity to a teaching event such as a lecture improves learning retention has not been proven to be true on the basis of randomized trials such as those done in domains like oncology, but is held to be true on the basis of a collective wisdom in the medical education community via a process driven primarily by thought leaders in education, where these leaders periodically explore, review and comment on this and other issues on a regular basis.

CONCLUSION

In the past, medical education relied predominantly on classic methods of instruction such as formal lectures, laboratory demonstrations, and examining patients in clinics or at the bedside. Even today, these methods of instruction remain important, and in particular, contact with patients as a learning experience remains paramount. However, the use of electronic and Web-based teaching methods has now become an important additional modality in medical education. When properly designed so as to be engaging and interactive, such methods can have a particularly favorable impact on the way medical education is carried out. As these methods continue to be developed and refined it is expected that they will continue to impact favorably on medical education in the future.

As compared to medical education from two decades ago that relied heavily on textbooks and lectures, medical education today utilizes a large number of web-based resources that make learning more engaging, more pleasant, and easier. For example, no longer is a trip to the library required to obtain up-to-date information on an unusual condition that a medical student may encounter in a clinical encounter. Instead, the student can get reliable clinical information virtually instantly from an increasingly rich number of trustworthy online clinical sources. The future of medical education is indeed very promising.

REFERENCES

Abbasi, K. (2006). Journals join the podcast revolution. *Journal of the Royal Society of Medicine*, *99*, 329. doi:10.1258/jrsm.99.7.329

Albanese, M., & Mitchell, S. (1993). Problem-based learning: A review of the literature on its outcomes and implementation issues. *Academic Medicine*, *68*, 52–81. doi:10.1097/00001888-199301000-00012

Antezana, E., Kuiper, M., & Mironov, V. (2009). Biological knowledge management: the emerging role of the Semantic Web technologies. *Briefings in Bioinformatics*, *10*, 392–407. doi:10.1093/bib/bbp024

Atreja, A., Messinger-Rapport, B., Jain, A., & Mehta, N. (2006). Using Web 2.0 technologies to develop a resource for evidence based medicine. In *Proceedings of the AMIA Annu. Symp.*, (pg. 847).

Barrows, H. S. (1983). Problem-based, self-directed learning. *Journal of the American Medical Association*, *250*, 3077–3080. doi:10.1001/jama.250.22.3077

Barrows, H. S., & Bennett, K. (1982). Experimental studies on the diagnostic (problem-solving) skill of the neurologist, their implications for neurological training. *Archives of Neurology*, *26*, 273–277.

Berners-Lee, T., & Fischetti, M. (1999). *Weaving the Web: the original design and ultimate destiny of the world wide web by its inventor*. San Francisco: Harper San Francisco.

Berners-Lee, T., & Hendler, J. (2001). Publishing on the semantic web. *Nature*, *26*, 1023–1024. doi:10.1038/35074206

Boulos, M. N., Maramba, I., & Wheeler, S. (2006). Wikis, blogs and podcasts: a new generation of Web-based tools for virtual collaborative clinical practice and education. *BMC Medical Education*, *15*, 41. doi:10.1186/1472-6920-6-41

Coiera, E. (2003). Interaction design theory. *International Journal of Medical Informatics*, *69*, 205–222. doi:10.1016/S1386-5056(02)00106-5

Collins, J. (2006). Education techniques for lifelong learning: writing multiple-choice questions for continuing medical education activities and self-assessment modules. *Radiographics*, *26*, 543–551. doi:10.1148/rg.262055145

Conceição, S. C., & Taylor, L. D. (2007). Using a constructivist approach with online concept maps: relationship between theory and nursing education. *Nursing Education Perspectives*, *28*, 268–275.

Cook, D. A., & Dupras, D. M. (2004). A practical guide to developing effective web-based learning. *Journal of General Internal Medicine*, *19*, 698–707. doi:10.1111/j.1525-1497.2004.30029.x

Davis, D., O'Brien, M. A., Freemantle, N., Wolf, F. M., Mazmanian, P., & Taylor-Vaisey, A. (1999). Impact of formal continuing medical education: do conferences, workshops, rounds, and other traditional continuing education activities change physician behaviour or health outcomes? *Journal of the American Medical Association*, *282*, 867–874. doi:10.1001/jama.282.9.867

Despont-Gros, C., Mueller, H., & Lovis, C. (2005). Evaluating user interactions with clinical information systems: a model based on human-computer interaction models. *Journal of Biomedical Informatics*, *38*, 244–255. doi:10.1016/j.jbi.2004.12.004

Doyle, D. J., Ruskin, K. J., & Engel, T. P. (1996). The Internet and medicine: past, present, and future. *The Yale Journal of Biology and Medicine*, *69*, 429–437.

Gallagher, J. E., Dobrosielski-Vergona, K. A., Wingard, R. G., & Williams, T. M. (2005). Web-based vs. traditional classroom instruction in gerontology: a pilot study. *Journal of Dental Hygiene*, *79*, 7.

Giles, J. (2005). Internet encyclopaedias go head to head. *Nature*, *15*, 900–901. doi:10.1038/438900a

Glinkowski, W., & Ciszek, B. (2007). WWW-based e-teaching of normal anatomy as an introduction to telemedicine and e-health. *Telemedicine Journal and e-Health*, *13*, 535–544. doi:10.1089/tmj.2006.0077

Good, B. M., & Wilkinson, M. D. (2006). The Life Sciences Semantic Web is full of creeps! *Briefings in Bioinformatics*, *7*, 275–286. doi:10.1093/bib/bbl025

Gotthardt, M., Siegert, M. J., Schlieck, A., Schneider, S., Kohnert, A., & Gross, M. W. (2006). How to successfully implement E-learning for both students and teachers. *Academic Radiology*, *13*, 379–390. doi:10.1016/j.acra.2005.12.006

Hara, N., & Kling, R. (1999). *Students' frustrations with a web-based distance education course: A taboo topic in the discourse*. Indiana University, Rob Kling Center for Social Informatics. Retrieved June 15, 2009, from http://rkcsi.indiana.edu/archive/CSI/WP/wp99_01-octoberB.html

Hara, N., & Kling, R. (2000). *Students' distress with a web-based distance education course: An ethnographic study of participants' experiences*. Indiana University, Rob Kling Center for Social Informatics. Retrieved June 15, 2009, from http://rkcsi.indiana.edu/archive/CSI/WP/wp00-01B.html

Harnad, S. (1992). *Interactive Publication: Extending American Physical Society's Discipline-Specific Model for Electronic Publishing*. Serials Review, Special Issue on Economics Models for Electronic Publishing, pp. 58–61. Retrieved from http://users.ecs.soton.ac.uk/harnad/ Papers/Harnad/harnad92.interactivpub.html

Jang, K. S., Hwang, S. Y., Park, S. J., Kim, Y. M., & Kim, M. J. (2005). Effects of a Web-based teaching method on undergraduate nursing students' learning of electrocardiography. *The Journal of Nursing Education*, *44*, 35–39.

Johnson, K. R., Freeman, S. R., & Dellavalle, R. P. (2007). Wikis: the application of Web 2.0. *Archives of Dermatology*, *143*, 1065–1066. doi:10.1001/archderm.143.8.1065

Kamel Boulos, M. N., & Wheeler, S. (2007). The emerging Web 2.0 social software: an enabling suite of sociable technologies in health and health care education. *Health Information and Libraries Journal*, *24*, 2–23. doi:10.1111/j.1471-1842.2007.00701.x

Katzman, G. L. (2001). Adobe acrobat: an alternative electronic teaching file construction methodology independent of HTML restrictions. *Journal of Digital Imaging*, *14*, 9–13. doi:10.1007/s10278-001-0018-8

Levine, H. G., & Forman, P. B. (1973). A study of retention of knowledge of neurosciences information. *Journal of Medical Education*, *48*, 867–869.

Lynch, P. J., & Horton, S. (1998). Hypertext markup language as an authoring tool for CD-ROM production. *The Journal of Biocommunication*, *25*, 20–25.

McGee, J. B., & Begg, M. (2008). What medical educators need to know about "Web 2.0". *Medical Teacher*, *30*, 164–169. doi:10.1080/01421590701881673

McKimm, J., Jollie, C., & Cantillon, P. (2003). ABC of learning and teaching: Web based learning. *BMJ (Clinical Research Ed.)*, *19*, 870–873. doi:10.1136/bmj.326.7394.870

McLean, R., Richards, B. H., & Wardman, J. I. (2007). The effect of Web 2.0 on the future of medical practice and education: Darwikinian evolution or folksonomic revolution? *The Medical Journal of Australia*, *6*, 174–177.

Moss, E. (2001). Multiple choice questions: their value as an assessment tool. *Current Opinion in Anaesthesiology*, *14*, 661–666. doi:10.1097/00001503-200112000-00011

Mukherjea, S. (2005). Information retrieval and knowledge discovery utilising a biomedical Semantic Web. *Briefings in Bioinformatics*, *6*, 252–262. doi:10.1093/bib/6.3.252

Nielsen, J. (1994). *Usability Engineering*. San Francisco: Morgan Kaufmann Publishers.

Norman, D. A. (1999). *The Invisible Computer: why good products can fail, the personal computer is so complex, and information appliances are the solution*. Cambridge, MA: MIT Press.

Philip, J. H. (•••). (No date.). 'Gasman' - Understanding Anesthesia Uptake & Distribution. [Computer software]. Chestnut Hill, MA: Med Man Simulations. *International Journal of Clinical Monitoring and Computing*, *3*, 165–173. doi:10.1007/BF01716358

Ramsey, P. G., & Carline, J. D. (1991). Changes over time in the knowledge base of practicing internists. *Journal of the American Medical Association*, *266*, 1103–1107. doi:10.1001/jama.266.8.1103

Reynolds, P. A., Mason, R., & Harper, J. (2008). The many faces of interaction. *British Dental Journal*, *24*, 565–570. doi:10.1038/sj.bdj.2008.409

Ridley, R. T. (2007). Interactive teaching: a concept analysis. *The Journal of Nursing Education*, *46*, 203–209.

Rosser, J. C., Lynch, P. J., Cuddihy, L., Gentile, D. A., Klonsky, J., & Merrell, R. (2007). The impact of video games on training surgeons in the 21st century. *Archives of Surgery (Chicago, Ill.)*, *142*, 181–186. doi:10.1001/archsurg.142.2.181

Ryan, A. G., Louis, L. J., & Yee, W. C. (2005). Informatics in radiology (infoRAD): HTML and Web site design for the radiologist: a primer. *Radiographics*, *25*, 1101–1118. doi:10.1148/rg.254045119

Sajeva, M. (2006). E-learning: Web-based education. *Current Opinion in Anaesthesiology*, *19*, 645–649. doi:10.1097/ACO.0b013e328010bec8

Schilling, K., Wiecha, J., Polineni, D., & Khalil, S. (2006). An interactive web-based curriculum on evidence-based medicine: design and effectiveness. *Family Medicine*, *38*, 126–132.

Schmidt, H. G. (1993). Foundations of problem-based learning: some explanatory notes. *Medical Education*, *27*, 422–432. doi:10.1111/j.1365-2923.1993.tb00296.x

Sethi, S. K. (2007). Blog/web log - a new easy and interactive website building tool for a non-net savvy radiologist. *Journal of Thoracic Imaging*, *22*, 115–119. doi:10.1097/01.rti.0000213578.47398.aa

Shadbolt, N., & Berners-Lee, T. (2008). Web science emerges. *Scientific American*, *299*, 76–81. doi:10.1038/scientificamerican1008-76

Smith, N. T., & Davidson, T. M. (1999). *'Body' simulation - Anesthesia, physiology and pharmacology simulation* [Computer software]. Point Roberts, WA: Advanced Simulation Corporation.

Smith, S. F., Roberts, N. J., & Partridge, M. R. (2007). Comparison of a web-based package with tutor-based methods of teaching respiratory medicine: subjective and objective evaluations. *BMC Medical Education*, *1*, 41. doi:10.1186/1472-6920-7-41

Stout, P. A., Villegas, J., & Kim, H. (2001). Enhancing learning through use of interactive tools on health-related websites. *Health Education Research*, *16*, 721–733. doi:10.1093/her/16.6.721

Taylor-Mendes, C. (2007). Proceed with caution: using Wikipedia as a reference. *Neonatal Network*, *26*, 140–141.

Vernon, D. T., & Blake, R. L. (1993). Does problem-based learning work? A meta-analysis of evaluative research. *Academic Medicine*, *68*, 550–563. doi:10.1097/00001888-199307000-00015

Wiggins, R. H. III, Davidson, H. C., Harnsberger, H. R., Lauman, J. R., & Goede, P. A. (2001). Image file formats: past, present, and future. *Radiographics*, *21*, 789–798.

Wong, G., Greenhalgh, T., Russell, J., Boynton, P., & Toon, P. (2003). Putting your course on the Web: lessons from a case study and systematic literature review. *Medical Education*, *37*, 1020–1023. doi:10.1046/j.1365-2923.2003.01673.x

Wu, W. G., & Li, J. (2007). RSS made easy: a basic guide for librarians. *Medical Reference Services Quarterly*, *26*, 37–50. doi:10.1300/J115v26n01_04

Zary, N., Johnson, G., Boberg, J., & Fors, U. G. (2006). Development, implementation and pilot evaluation of a Web-based Virtual Patient Case Simulation environment--Web-SP. *BMC Medical Education*, *21*, 10. doi:10.1186/1472-6920-6-10

ADDITIONAL READING

Atienza, A. A., Hesse, B. W., Baker, T. B., Abrams, D. B., Rimer, B. K., Croyle, R. T., & Volckmann, L. N. (2007). Critical issues in eHealth research. *American Journal of Preventive Medicine*, *32*, S71–S74. doi:10.1016/j.amepre.2007.02.013

Atreja, A., Messinger-Rapport, B., Jain, A., & Mehta, N. (2006). Using Web 2.0 technologies to develop a resource for evidence based medicine. In *Proceedings of AMIA Annu. Symp.*, (pg. 847).

Beard, L., Wilson, K., Morra, D., & Keelan, J. (2009). A survey of health-related activities on second life. *Journal of Medical Internet Research*, *11*, e17. doi:10.2196/jmir.1192

Boulos, M. N., Maramba, I., & Wheeler, S. (2006). Wikis, blogs and podcasts: a new generation of Web-based tools for virtual collaborative clinical practice and education. *BMC Medical Education*, *6*, 41. doi:10.1186/1472-6920-6-41

Catwell, L., & Sheikh, A. (2009). Evaluating eHealth interventions: the need for continuous systemic evaluation. *PLoS Medicine*, *6*, e1000126. doi:10.1371/journal.pmed.1000126

Cook, D. A., Beckman, T. J., Thomas, K. G., & Thompson, W. G. (2008). Adapting web-based instruction to residents' knowledge improves learning efficiency: a randomized controlled trial. *Journal of General Internal Medicine*, *23*, 985–990. doi:10.1007/s11606-008-0541-0

Costin, D. L., Mackinnon, A. J., Griffiths, K. M., Batterham, P. J., Bennett, A. J., Bennett, K., & Christensen, H. (2009). Health e-cards as a means of encouraging help seeking for depression among young adults: randomized controlled trial. *Journal of Medical Internet Research*, *11*, e42. doi:10.2196/jmir.1294

Donnelly, L. S., Shaw, R. L., & van den Akker, O. B. (2008). eHealth as a challenge to 'expert' power: a focus group study of internet use for health information and management. *Journal of the Royal Society of Medicine*, *101*, 501–506. doi:10.1258/jrsm.2008.080156

Eysenbach, G. (2008). Medicine 2.0: social networking, collaboration, participation, apomediation, and openness. *Journal of Medical Internet Research*, *10*, 22. doi:10.2196/jmir.1030

Frame, I., Austen, K. F., Calleja, M., Dove, M. T., White, T. O., & Wilson, D. J. (2009). New tools to support collaboration and virtual organizations. *Philosophical Transactions. Series A, Mathematical, Physical, and Engineering Sciences*, *367*, 1051–1056. doi:10.1098/rsta.2008.0193

Gerard, J. M., Scalzo, A. J., Laffey, S. P., Sinks, G., Fendya, D., & Seratti, P. (2006). Evaluation of a novel Web-based pediatric advanced life support course. *Archives of Pediatrics & Adolescent Medicine*, *160*, 649–655. doi:10.1001/archpedi.160.6.649

Gorini, A., Gaggioli, A., Vigna, C., & Riva, G. (2008). A second life for eHealth: prospects for the use of 3-D virtual worlds in clinical psychology. *Journal of Medical Internet Research*, *10*, e21. doi:10.2196/jmir.1029

Hall, W., De Roure, D., & Shadbolt, N. (2009). The evolution of the Web and implications for eResearch. *Philosophical Transactions. Series A, Mathematical, Physical, and Engineering Sciences*, *367*, 991–1001. doi:10.1098/rsta.2008.0252

Hellström, L., Waern, K., Montelius, E., Astrand, B., Rydberg, T., & Petersson, G. (2009). Physicians' attitudes towards ePrescribing-evaluation of a Swedish full-scale implementation. *BMC Medical Informatics and Decision Making*, *9*, 37. doi:10.1186/1472-6947-9-37

Hughes, B., Joshi, I., & Wareham, J. (2008). Health 2.0 and Medicine 2.0: tensions and controversies in the field. *Journal of Medical Internet Research*, *10*, e23. doi:10.2196/jmir.1056

Lemley, T., & Burnham, J. F. (2009). Web 2.0 tools in medical and nursing school curricula. *Journal of the Medical Library Association*, *97*, 50–52. doi:10.3163/1536-5050.97.1.010

McLean, R., Richards, B. H., & Wardman, J. I. (2007). The effect of Web 2.0 on the future of medical practice and education: Darwikinian evolution or folksonomic revolution? *The Medical Journal of Australia*, *187*, 174–177.

Mohammed, S., Orabi, A., Fiaidhi, J., Orabi, M., & Benlamri, R. (2008). Developing a Web 2.0 telemedical education system: the AJAX-Cocoon portal. *International Journal of Electronic Healthcare*, *4*, 24–42. doi:10.1504/IJEH.2008.018919

Nordqvist, C., Hanberger, L., Timpka, T., & Nordfeldt, S. (2009). Health professionals' attitudes towards using a Web 2.0 portal for child and adolescent diabetes care: qualitative study. *Journal of Medical Internet Research*, *11*, e12. doi:10.2196/jmir.1152

Norman, G. J., Zabinski, M. F., Adams, M. A., Rosenberg, D. E., Yaroch, A. L., & Atienza, A. A. (2007). A review of eHealth interventions for physical activity and dietary behavior change. *American Journal of Preventive Medicine*, *33*, 336–345. doi:10.1016/j.amepre.2007.05.007

Rethlefsen, M. L., Piorun, M., & Prince, J. D. (2009). Teaching Web 2.0 technologies using Web 2.0 technologies. *Journal of the Medical Library Association*, *97*, 253–259. doi:10.3163/1536-5050.97.4.008

Somal, K., Lam, W. C., & Tam, E. (2009). Computer and internet use by ophthalmologists and trainees in an academic centre. *Canadian Journal of Ophthalmology*, *44*, 265–268. doi:10.3129/i09-057

Timpka, T., Eriksson, H., Ludvigsson, J., Ekberg, J., Nordfeldt, S., & Hanberger, L. (2008). Web 2.0 systems supporting childhood chronic disease management: a pattern language representation of a general architecture. *BMC Medical Informatics and Decision Making*, *8*, 54. doi:10.1186/1472-6947-8-54

van Straten, A., Cuijpers, P., & Smits, N. (2008). Effectiveness of a web-based self-help intervention for symptoms of depression, anxiety, and stress: randomized controlled trial. *Journal of Medical Internet Research*, *10*, e7. doi:10.2196/jmir.954

van Zutphen, M., Milder, I. E., & Bemelmans, W. J. (2009). Integrating an eHealth program for pregnant women in midwifery care: a feasibility study among midwives and program users. *Journal of Medical Internet Research*, *11*, e7. doi:10.2196/jmir.988

KEY TERMS AND DEFINITIONS

Blogs: Web sites intended for online audiences containing a diary-like account of events and personal insights.

Information Philanthropy: A movement which has as its goal making quality intellectual property available for free, usually as an Internet download.

Problem-based Learning (PBL): An educational modality where students work in small groups under the guidance of an instructor to find for themselves the knowledge they need to solve real world problems.

Podcasts: A podcast is a downloadable audio or video presentation for replay on a personal media player such as Apple's iPod.

Web 2.0: A term used to describe the recent technical developments (e.g., Wikis, blogs, podcasts, mashups, and RSS feeds) that stress openness, sharing, cooperation and collaboration among Web users

Wikis: A collaborative informational Web site whose content is open (freely accessible) and can be edited by anyone who is duly authorized.

Semantic Publishing: A technology where information and documents are published with explicit "semantic markups" intended to allow computers to comprehend the structure and meaning of published information.

Semantic Web: A vision of the future where information is automatically exchanged and acted upon on our behalf by the Web itself by virtue of formatting to make it readily "understandable" by computers.

Chapter 13
Medical Transcription a Pioneer in the Healthcare Informatics

Shilpi Srivastava
DMC Management Consultants Ltd., India

ABSTRACT

Despite the importance of medical records, relatively little is known about medical transcription, a process through which voice files are transformed into healthcare documentation. This lack of knowledge is evident in academic research with no previous studies of medical transcriptionists (MTs) or the medical transcription service organizations (MTSOs) in existence despite the central role of the industry in the creation of healthcare documentation. The proposed chapter is a detailed ethnographic study of the medical transcription process. While its general aim is to document the impact of technology on the process of medical transcription, the topic resides in a broader array of issues that include the impact of technology on the workplace, and how assumptions of work drive technological design. The central issue being examined is what is the extent to which technology can replace workers and how design decisions impact practice by either facilitating or impeding it. Given the thing being produced is vital for medical treatment, resolving this question is not only of academic interest, but important to everyone who has a medical record.

INTRODUCTION

Quality medical care often depends on a quality medical record. For most doctors, one of the most time consuming functions are having to go through a patient's medical history. This could include the patient's pre-visits, family and social history, recommended medication, the follow up check up, and so on. What if all these functions could be taken care of with an Electronic Medical Record (EMR) system that would not only speed up the doctor's interaction with the patient chart, but ensures better care for the patients. Electronic Medical Record software does exactly this. More than just medical practice management software, it is a HIPAA compliant physician software ap-

DOI: 10.4018/978-1-61692-004-3.ch013

plication that simplifies the way patient charts are managed in the doctor's office. Our experience in **medical transcription** field helps us to do this in a most fruitful way.

Medical transcription (MT) is one of the most sophisticated medical language specialty allied healthcare profession, which has become an indispensable element in the modern healthcare industry. The main challenge that medical transcription business face in an increasingly competitive marketplace is the ability to offer high quality and cost effective customer support to all customers all the time. This is only possible with the automation of as many parts of the customer support process as possible in order to handle large workload on a regular basis while maintaining the human aspect of the experience. Since its inception, emerging technologies focused on the research and development of software solutions based on the speech recognition technology is going on. This chapter incorporate various aspects of medical transcription from the process, issues, controversies, problems, hardwares and software's used, future research directions, etc. (en.wikipedia.org/wiki/Medical_transcription, 2008)

BACKGROUND

The evolution of transcription dates back to the 1960s. The method was designed to assist in the manufacturing process. The first transcription that was developed in this process was MRP, which is the acronym for Manufacturing Resource Planning, in 1975. This was followed by another advanced version namely MRP2, but none of them yielded the benefit of medical transcription.

However, transcription equipment has changed from manual typewriters to electric typewriters to word processors to computers and from plastic disks and magnetic belts to cassettes and endless loops and digital recordings. Today, speech recognition (SR), also known as continuous speech recognition (CSR), is increasingly being used, with medical transcriptionists and/or "editors" providing supplemental editorial services, although there are occasional instances where SR fully replaces the MT. Natural-language processing takes "automatic" transcription a step further, providing an interpretive function that speech recognition alone does not provide (although MTs do).

In recent years, medical records have changed considerably. Although many physicians and hospitals still maintain paper records, there is a drive for electronic records. Filing cabinets are giving way to desktop computers connected to powerful servers, where patient records are processed and archived digitally. This digital format allows for immediate remote access by any physician who is authorized to review the patient information. Reports are stored electronically and printed selectively as the need arises. Many MTs now utilize personal computers with electronic references and use the internet not only for web resources, but also as a working platform. Technology has gotten so sophisticated that MT services and MT departments work closely with programmers and information systems (IS) staff to stream in voice and accomplish seamless data transfers through network interfaces. In fact, many healthcare providers today are enjoying the benefits of handheld PCs or personal data assistants (PDAs) and are now utilizing software on them for dictation. Also, a software named Computer Aided Medical Transcription (CAMT) software is exclusively designed for medical transcription industry. The CAMT software change spoken words to texts. Using this software you can easily increase your editing speed. In this software, editing is done as fast as keyboard stokes and shortcuts.

As with most industry, **medical transcription service organization** is also experiencing expanded distribution and globalization of its work. This is resulting in questions regarding which technologies will evolve to increase efficiency & accuracy, decrease turnaround time, and support data capture. While many of these technologies such as digital dictation and electronic signature exist today, several technologies are still on the horizon. (en.wikipedia.org/wiki/Medical_transcription, 2008)

OVERVIEW

Pertinent, up-to-date, confidential patient information is converted to a written text document by a medical transcriptionist (MT). This text may be printed and placed in the patient's record and/or retained only in its electronic format. Medical transcription can be performed by MTs who are employees in a hospital or who work at home as telecommuting employees for the hospital; by MTs working as telecommuting employees or independent contractors for an outsourced service that performs the work offsite under contract to a hospital, clinic, physician group or other healthcare provider; or by MTs working directly for the providers of service (doctors or their group practices) either onsite or telecommuting as employees or contractors. Hospital facilities often prefer electronic storage of medical records due to the sheer volume of hospital patients and the accompanying paperwork. The electronic storage in their database gives immediate access to subsequent departments or providers regarding the patient's care to date, notation of previous or present medications, notification of allergies, and establishes a history on the patient to facilitate healthcare delivery regardless of geographical distance or location.

The term transcript or "report" as it is more commonly called, is used as the name of the document (electronic or physical hard copy) which results from the medical transcription process, normally in reference to the healthcare professional's specific encounter with a patient on a specific date of service. This report is referred to by many as a "**medical record**". Each specific transcribed record or report with its own specific date of service is then merged and becomes part of the larger patient record commonly known as the patient's medical history. This record is often called the patient's chart in a hospital setting.

Medical transcription encompasses the MT, performing document typing and formatting functions according to an established criteria or format, transcribing the spoken word of the patient's care information into a written, easily readable form. MT requires correct spelling of all terms and words, (occasionally) correcting medical terminology or dictation errors. MTs also edit the transcribed documents, print or return the completed documents in a timely fashion. All transcription reports must comply with medico-legal concerns, policies and procedures, and laws under patient confidentiality.

In transcribing directly for a doctor or a group of physicians, there are specific formats and report types used, dependent on that doctor's speciality of practice, although history and physical exams or consults are mainly utilized. In most of the off-hospital sites, independent medical practices perform consultations as a second opinion, pre-surgical exams, and as **IMEs (Independent Medical Examinations)** for liability insurance or disability claims. Some private practice family doctors choose not to utilize a medical transcriptionist, preferring to keep their patient's records in a handwritten format, although this is not true of all family practitioners.

Currently, a growing number of medical providers send their dictation by digital voice files, utilizing a method of transcription called speech or voice recognition. Speech recognition is still a nascent technology that loses much in translation. For dictators to utilize the software, they must first train the program to recognize their spoken words. Dictation is read into the database and the program continuously "learns" the spoken words and phrases.

Poor speech habits and other problems such as heavy foreign accents and mumbling complicate the process for both the MT and the recognition software. An MT can "flag" such a report as unintelligible, but the recognition software will transcribe the unintelligible word(s) from the existing database of "learned" language. The result is often a "word salad" or missing text. Thresholds can be set to reject a bad report and return it for standard dictation, but these settings are arbitrary. Below a set percentage rate, the word salad passes for actual dictation. The MT simultaneously listens, reads, and "edits" the correct version. Every word must be confirmed in this process. The downside of the technology is when the time spent in this process cancels out the benefits. The quality of recognition can range from excellent to poor, with whole words and sentences missing from the report. Not infrequently, negative contractions and the word "not" is dropped all together. Voice recognition is similar to the voice prompts one hears on dialing "411", when information provides the wrong number and charges for the "411" call. These flaws trigger concerns that the present technology could have adverse effects on patient care. Control over quality can also be reduced when providers choose a server-based program from a vendor Application Service Provider (ASP).

Downward adjustments in MT pay rates for voice recognition are controversial. Understandably, a client will seek optimum savings to offset any net costs. Yet vendors that overstate the gains in productivity do harm to MTs paid by the line. Despite the new editing skills required of MTs, significant reductions in compensation for voice recognition have been reported. Reputable industry sources put the field average for increased productivity in the range of 30%-50%; yet this is still dependent on several other factors involved in the methodology. Metrics supplied by vendors that can be "used" in compensation decisions should be scientifically supported.

Another unresolved issue is high-maintenance headers that replace simple interfaces to become the "platform" of choice. Pay rates should reflect this lost-opportunity cost for the MT.

Operationally, speech recognition technology (SRT) is an interdependent, collaborative effort. It is a mistake to treat it as compatible with the same organizational paradigm as standard dictation, a largely "standalone" system. The new software supplants an MT's former ability to realize immediate time-savings from programming tools such as macros and other word/format expanders. Requests for client/vendor format corrections delay those savings. If remote MTs cancel each other out with disparate style choices, they and the recognition engine may be trapped in a seesaw battle over control. Voice recognition managers should take care to ensure that the impositions on MT autonomy are not so onerous as to outweigh its benefits.

Medical transcription is still the primary mechanism for a physician to clearly communicate with other healthcare providers who access the patient record, to advise them on the state of the patient's health and past/current treatment, and to assure continuity of care. More recently, following Federal and State Disability Act changes, a written report (IME) became a requirement for documentation of a medical bill or an application for Workers' Compensation (or continuation thereof) insurance benefits based on requirements of Federal and State agencies. (en.wikipedia.org/wiki/Medical_transcription, 2008)

AS A PROFESSION

Medical Transcription is one of the fastest growing fields in health care. Medical Transcriptionists are in demand in Western countries especially in the US where the entire healthcare industry is based on insurance and detailed medical records are needed for processing insurance claims. Medical transcription could be one of the speedy growing IT enabled service in India also, with the rapid change in the outlook in Indian healthcare and privatization of the insurance sector. India provides an ideal location for conducting medical transcription with the large population of educated English speaking people and the comparative low cost, which encourages companies abroad to outsource their work to the Indian Medical Transcription field.

Medical transcription is an interesting and challenging career. It is the process whereby one accurately and swiftly transcribes medical records dictated by doctors and others, including history and physical reports, clinic notes, office notes, operative reports, consultation notes, discharge summaries, letters, psychiatric evaluations, laboratory reports, x-ray reports and pathology reports. An individual who performs medical transcription is known as a medical transcriptionist or an MT. The equipment the MT uses is called a **medical transcriber**. The individual who performs medical transcription should always be called a "medical transcriptionist." A medical transcriptionist is the person responsible for converting the patient's medical records into typewritten format rather than handwritten, the latter more prone to misinterpretation by other healthcare providers. The term transcriber describes the electronic equipment used in performing medical transcription, e.g., a cassette player with foot controls operated by the MT for report playback and transcription. In the late 1990s, medical transcriptionists were also given the title of Medical Language Specialist or Health Information Management (HIM) paraprofessional.

Transcription services range from small, one-person home-based businesses to sophisticated, high-tech corporations which employ transcriptionists. Some medical transcription services now employ both 'on-site' and home-based medical transcriptionists.

There are no "formal" educational requirements to be a medical transcriptionist. Education and training can be obtained through traditional schooling, certificate or diploma programs, distance learning, and/or on-the-job training offered in some hospitals, although there are countries currently employing transcriptionists that require 18 months to 2 years of specialized MT training. Working in medical transcription leads to a mastery in medical terminology and editing, MT ability to listen and type simultaneously, utilization of playback controls on the transcriber (machine), and use of foot pedal to play and adjust dictations - all while maintaining a steady rhythm of execution.

While medical transcription does not mandate registration or certification, individual MTs may seek out registration/certification for personal or professional reasons. Obtaining a certificate from a medical transcription training program does not entitle an MT to use the title of Certified Medical Transcriptionist (CMT). The CMT credential is earned by passing a certification examination conducted solely by the Association for Healthcare Documentation Integrity (AHDI), formerly the **American Association for Medical Transcription (AAMT),** as the credentialing designation they created. AHDI also offers the credential of Registered Medical Transcriptionist (RMT). According to AHDI, the RMT is an entry-level credential while the CMT is an advanced level. AHDI maintains a list of approved medical transcription schools.

There is a great degree of internal debate about which training program best prepares a MT for industry work. Yet, whether one has learned medical transcription from an online course, community college, high school night course, or on-the-job training in a doctor's office or hospital, a knowledgeable MT is highly valued. In lieu of these AHDI certification credentials, MTs who can consistently and accurately transcribe multiple document work-types and return reports within a reasonable turnaround-time (TAT) are sought after. TATs set by the service provider or agreed to by the transcriptionist should be reasonable, but consistent with the need to return the document to the patient's record in a timely manner.

As of March 7, 2006, the MT occupation became an eligible U.S. Department of Labor Apprenticeship, a 2-year program focusing on acute care facility (hospital) work. In May 2004, a pilot program for Vermont residents was initiated, with 737 applicants for only 20 classroom pilot-program openings. The objective was to train the applicants as MTs in a shorter time period. (See Vermont HITECH for pilot program established by the Federal Government Health and Human Services Commission).

Curricular Requirements, Skills, and Abilities

Experience that is directly related to the duties and responsibilities specified, and dependent on the employer (working directly for a physician or in hospital facility).

- Knowledge of medical terminology.
- Above-average spelling, grammar, communication and memory skills.
- Ability to sort, check, count, and verify numbers with accuracy.
- Skill in the use and operation of basic office equipment/computer; eye/hand/foot coordination.
- Ability to follow verbal and written instructions.
- Records maintenance skills or ability.
- Good to above-average typing skills.

Basic Mt Knowledge, Skills, and Abilities

- Knowledge of basic to advanced medical terminology is essential.
- Knowledge of Anatomy and Physiology.
- Knowledge of disease processes.
- Knowledge of Medical Style and Grammar.
- Average verbal communication skills.
- Above-average memory skills.
- Ability to sort, check, count, and verify numbers with accuracy.
- Demonstrated skill in the use and operation of basic office equipment/computer.
- Ability to follow verbal and written instructions.
- Records maintenance skills or ability.
- Above-average typing skills.
- Knowledge and experience transcribing (from training or real report work) in the Basic Four work types.
- Knowledge of and proper application of grammar.
- Knowledge of and use of correct punctuation and capitalization rules.
- Demonstrated MT proficiencies in multiple report types and multiple specialties.

Duties and Responsibilities

- Accurately transcribes the patient-identifying information such as name and Medical Record or Social Security Number.
- Transcribes accurately utilizing correct punctuation, grammar and spelling, and edits for inconsistencies.
- Maintains/consults references for medical procedures and terminology.
- Keeps a transcription log.
- Foreign MTs may sort, copy, prepare, assemble, and file records and charts (though in the United States (US) the filing of charts and records are most often assigned to Medical Records Techs in Hospitals or Secretaries in Doctor offices).
- Distributes transcribed reports and collects dictation tapes.
- Follows up on physicians' missing and/or late dictation, returns printed or electronic report in a timely fashion (in US Hospital, MT Supervisor performs).
- Performs quality assurance check.
- May maintain disk and disk backup system (in US Hospital, MT Supervisor performs).
- May order supplies and report equipment operational problems (In US, this task is most often done by Unit Secretaries, Office Secretaries, or Tech Support personnel).
- May collect, tabulate, and generate reports on statistical data, as appropriate (in US, generally performed by MT Supervisor).

(en.wikipedia.org/wiki/Medical_transcription, 2008)

COURSE MODULE OF MEDICAL TRANSCRIPTION

Unit I: Introduction, Ethics and Medical Documents

Module 1: Introduction

This first module provides an overall review of the practice of medical transcription. Students learn about the role of a medical transcriptionist and are introduced to medical documents and reports. They also receive instruction in the particular code of ethics all transcriptionists must adhere to.

Unit II: Keyboarding, Grammar and Style

Module 2: Punctuation

In this module, students receive instruction in grammatically correct punctuation. Proper punctuation is required to ensure accuracy in medical records.

Module 3: Capitalization

The third module covers the proper use of capitalization in medical transcription. Students learn how to capitalize medical terms, as well as general capitalization rules for standard correspondence.

Module 4: Transcribing Numbers, Figures, and Abbreviations

Module 4 provides instruction in the correct transcription of numbers and abbreviations. Transcription of roman numerals, numeric measurements, military time and medical abbreviations is covered.

Module 5: Letter Transcription

This module provides a full overview proper letter format, and addresses the specific concerns MTs must take into account when transcribing a letter. Several professional letter formats are described.

Module 6: Proofreading and Making Corrections

Accuracy is essential when transcribing for medical records. In this module, students are presented with examples of common errors. They are provided with tips that allow them to accurately review their own work.

Module 7: References

In module 7, students learn to make best use of the reference books that come with the course. Medical dictionaries and word books are described, as well as techniques of cross referencing.

Module 8: Word Endings, Antonyms, Eponyms, and Homonyms

In this module, students expand their vocabulary skills. They learn how to deal with common word endings, identify eponyms, and distinguish sound alike medical words based on context.

Module 9: Business Letters and More

Module nine is geared towards transcriptionists who are also responsible for a range of medical office duties. The module covers general letter writing skills, as well as the particular filing and mail routing needs of a healthcare office.

Unit III: Terminology

Module 10: Word Recognition

Module 10 provides an introduction to Word Building, an essential skill for any medical transcriptionist. Students learn to break medical words into their basic elements in order to discover their definition.

Module 11: Suffixes and Prefixes

The basic skill of Word Building is expanded upon in this module. Specialized medical suffixes and prefixes are defined, and their usage described. Knowledge of these allows students to expand their word recognition and building skills.

Module 12: Medical Specialties and the Body

In this module, students continue to build upon their word recognition skills. Medical specialties are introduced, along with general anatomical terms. The module also provides a basic introduction to human anatomy.

Module 13: Appendix B Combining Forms

This module contains an extensive list of medical combining forms, an essential study tool for student transcriptionists, and a useful reference for professionals.

Module 14: Appendix C – Prefixes and Suffixes, Appendix D – Frequently Misspelled Words

Module 14 serves as a transcription reference tool. Students may check their knowledge of prefixes and suffixes, and check the proper spelling of commonly misspelled words.

Module 15: Appendix E – State and Provincial Abbreviations, Appendix F – Common Abbreviations

Module 15 contains lists of additional commonly used abbreviations. State and Province short-forms are listed, along with a number of abbreviations specific to the medical industry.

Module 16: Appendix G – Homonyms, Appendix H Short Forms, Brief Forms, and Medical Slang

Lists of commonly mistaken words are presented in this module, as well as a glossary of short forms often used by health-care staff.

Unit IV: Anatomy

Module 17: Digestive System, Urinary System, Reproductive System

In this module, students receive an introduction to the human digestive, urinary, and reproductive systems. The module presents a basic guide to the organs and elements that make up these respective systems, and a list of specialized terminology and facts related to those systems.

Module 18: Nervous System, Cardiovascular and Lymphatic Systems, Respiratory System

Module 18 continues the overview of the body systems. The module contains a complete glossary and description of the nervous, cardiovascular, lymphatic and respiratory system, as well as valuable information links.

Module 19: Musculoskeletal System, Integumentary Systems, Sense Organs, Endocrine Systems

In module 19, students are provided with more information about the internal and external structure of the body. Sense organs, glands, and the skeletal structure are covered, and a glossary of terms for all systems is provided.

Module 20: Body Systems

Module 20 provides an overall review of the body systems, and the terms and combining forms related to them.

Module 21: Diagnostic Tests and Procedures

This module contains an introduction and description to many of the diagnostic tests transcriptionists may record in their work. Tests and procedures such as angiographies and White Blood Cell counts are detailed and described.

Module 22: Medical Abbreviations and Symbols

An extensive list of medical abbreviations is presented in module 22, along with definitions for each. Module 22 serves as a study tool for other modules.

Module 23: Medical Terms

In Module 23 students have access to an A to Z list of medical terms, and to a glossary of medical suffixes and prefixes.

Unit V: Pharmacology

Module 24: Introduction of Pharmacology, Dermatologic Drugs, Urinary Tract Drugs, Musculoskeletal Drugs

This module presents a basic history of pharmacology and clinical drug use. It then details the specific drugs used for a variety ailments affecting various systems of the body.

Module 25: Cardiovascular Drugs, Endocrine Drugs, Pulmonary Drugs, ENT Drugs, Ophthalmic Drugs

Module 25 continues the list of drugs used for specific body systems, detailing possible prescriptions for heart conditions, glandular conditions, and ear, nose and throat diseases.

Module 26: Obstetrtic-Gynecological Drugs, Neurologic Drugs, Gastrointestinal Drugs, A Quick Refrence to Pharmacology

Module 26 concludes the listing and descriptions of prescriptions specific to various body systems. It also contains a brief overview of the pharmacology industry.

Module 27: Disease Listing

This module contains an alphabetical listing of hundreds of the most commonly diagnosed diseases. Module 27 is a useful adjunct to the reference books used by practicing transcriptionists.

Module 28: Drug Listing – Part 1

Module 28 contains part one of an extensive and current list of prescription and over-the-counter drugs. Generic names are included along with brand-name drugs.

Module 29: Drug Listing – Part 2

Module 29 concludes the alphabetical listing of the most commonly encountered drugs.

Unit VI: Transcription

Module 30: Tips for Medical Transcriptionists, Challenging Medical Words, Phrases, and Prefixes, Difficult Words for New MTs

In this module, students are presented with a concluding overview of the practice of medical transcription. Career tips are presented, along with a final list of challenging or difficult words.

Unit VII: Review, Resume

Module 31: Apply for a Position

This final module contains valuable direction on finding work as a medical transcriptionist. Tips on resume preparation and submission are included, as well as an initial contact list of potential employers.

Depending on the course edition, advanced surgical, pathology and radiology modules may also be offered. (http://transcription.thevlc.com/information/course_outline.html, 2009)

MEDICAL TRANSCRIPTION PROCESS

Medical transcription service providers adhere to stringent processes to ensure 100 percent precision in their service delivery. The medical transcription processes have been standardized based on HIPAA stipulations to avoid risks associated with poor transcription quality. In a simple way, the process of medical transcription works in the manner given below.

Figure 1.

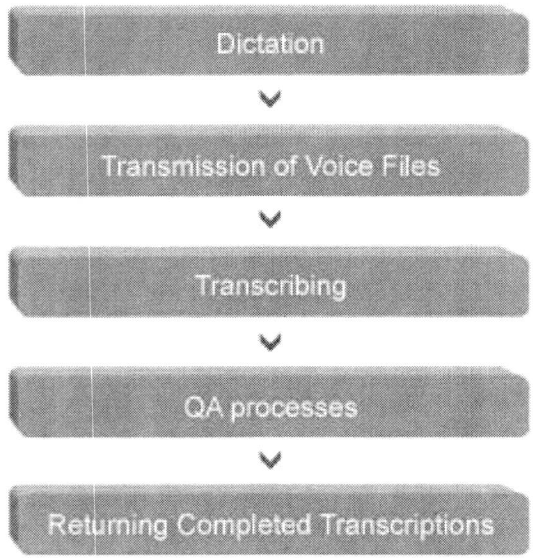

1. Dictation

Medical practitioners record patient information into recording devices such as hand-held digital or analog recording devices, phone-in recorders, personal computers, or other state-of-the-art recording equipment. The choice of recording equipment has direct bearing on the voice quality of the dictation and consequently on the quality and accuracy of the transcription.

Digital recording devices give superior voice quality and clarity to dictations. Sophisticated software modules are also installed into PCs of medical practitioners and doctors allowing them ease of use in dictating and transmitting the voice file to hospital servers thereby enhancing the medical transcription process.

2. Transmission of Voice Files

The digitally recorded dictations are transmitted from the doctors' PCs to the hospital's central server by using a memory card from where they are accessed by the medical transcription service provider for transcribing. Alternatively, with outsourcing of medical transcription processes becoming an increasingly common practice, voice files are often directly routed to the transcription vendor's secure, encrypted server in real-time via the internet from where they are accessed by transcriptionists for immediate typing. This allows 24x7 access to dictations and faster turnaround in the outsourced medical transcription process.

3. Transcribing

The voice files once downloaded from the central server of the medical transcription vendor are allotted to the transcription team. Individual files have distinct job IDs and a centralized allocation system is put in place to avoid duplication of the same files by different transcriptionists.

This is the actual production stage in the medical transcription process where voice files are converted into text format. Transcriptionists use the following tools:

- Foot-pedals: This is used to run the dictations and is useful to editors as well, as it allows the voice file to be replayed for purposes of retyping and correcting where required.
- Headphones: The dictations are accessed using these.
- PCs
- Word processing packages: The files are typed in text format using these packages.
  4. QA processes

There are multiple levels of QA (Quality Assurance) in medical transcription services with the larger players offering as many as 2 levels of quality assurance.

A. Editing

Experienced transcriptionists are moved up as editors in the medical transcription process and undertake:

- Proofreading.
- Electronic spell-check.
- Check for accuracy of data.
- Check formatting, standardization, dates etc.

Stringent quality control processes are necessary at the medical transcription service provider's end to ensure that medical records are error-free and 100 percent accurate. Strong QA measures ensure that patients do not face the risks associated with the entry of incorrect medical records. It also raises the medical fraternity's confidence in outsourced medical transcription processes.

B. Reviewing

Completed transcripts are reviewed by the doctor concerned or a designated member of the medical staff of the healthcare facility. This ensures that all comments are seen by the designated doctor and all transcripts that are flagged off can be checked. Reviewing also ensures that the medical transcription outsourcing process is 100 percent accurate.

5. Returning Completed Transcriptions

The medical records are returned to the hospital servers in real-time, ready to be accessed. The entire medical transcription outsourcing process is designed to be performed seamlessly and within stringent turnaround time. The completed transcripts are uploaded to the client in any of the following ways:

- Zipped e-mail attachment.
- Uploaded into the client hospital's server storage to be accessesed by their staff.
- Send to specialized service providers for automated downloading and saving for in-house batch processing, printing and filing at the hospital.

- All transcriptions sent back to the clients' servers are available for download at the medical transcription service provider's server for 2 years. (www.outsource2india.com. 2009)

MEDICAL TRANSCRIPTION SOFTWARE

Medical transcription software is used to convert voice-recorded reports dictated by physicians or healthcare professionals into text format automatically. It is a universal, user-friendly, abbreviation expander program for the Windows operating system. MT software is most powerful & easy to use shortcut typing, even your e-mail and instant message boxes. This program can save 60% of your typing time. There are many types of MT software's available in the market like **Speed Type**, Spectra Medi. etc. These software's are also used for medical billing and coding for healthcare organizations.

Medical transcription software is based on three types of modules:

1. Input Modules
2. Core Modules
3. Output Modules

Input Modules: Input modules are designed to improve dictation services for high- and low-volume. These modules are easy-to-implement and easy-to-use.

Output Modules: Output modules provide a full-set of extended transcription management features.

Core Modules: Core modules are used to extend dictation and transcription services. They provide easy flow of data between input & output modules.

Features of medical transcription software:

1. A medical transcription software should have capability of easy voice capture & speech re-organization. With this, medical transcriptionist can easily get doctor's dictation with accuracy.
2. It should have ability of medical spell checking & dictionaries so that any coding specialist who doesn't have knowledge of medical terminology can easily do transcription accurately & save the time.
3. It should have easy document distribution. Medical transcription software provides documents available in a variety of formats and doctors can choose any of them.
4. It should provide variety of audio-video format which facilitates doctors to use different types of technology.
5. It should have features of editing any interface quickly & accurately. This will reduce turnaround time.
6. It should be integrated with many healthcare systems & programs. This will help doctors & physicians to access data in readable form easily without wasting time.
7. Medical transcription software should have ability to work with medical billing & coding for healthcare organizations. (www.webraydian.com/content/view/1009/32/, 2009)

MEDICAL TRANSCRIPTION TOOLS AND EQUIPMENTS

Medical transcription has evolved over the years and has always made use of the cutting edge technologies. Many different tools/equipments are used during the medical transcription process. Here is a list of the different tools/softwares, and equipments that are used either during home-based medical transcription or at a bigger work unit that may consist of transcriptionists, editors, quality assurance leaders, etc. This list of equipment and tools is not exhaustive.

1. MP3 playback software.
2. Document processor software (like LYX).
3. Version Control software.
4. Time markers.
5. Bud microphone.
6. Digital voice recorder.
7. Headphone.
8. Computer with Internet/PrinterDesk and comfortable chair.
9. AAMT Book of StyleEncryption software.
10. File/Documents management software.
11. Blue Cross/ Blue Shield Directory.
12. Electronic Medical Dictionary.
13. Fax machine.
14. Document shredder.
15. Word processing program.
16. Audio playback software.
17. Anti virus program.
18. Thesaurus/dictionary for windows.
19. System recovery software.
20. Drug/pharmaceutical reference guide.
21. Foot pedal.
22. Ad blocker.
23. Medical specialty books.
24. Google toolbar.
25. Spyware removal utility.
26. Monthly newsletter.
27. Telephone line.
28. Editing software.
29. Conference recorder.
30. Voice recognition software.
31. Dictation recording equipment.
32. Text counting software (for home-based work). (http://www.outsourcestrategies.com/blog/medical-transcription/2008/02/medical-transcription-tools-and.html, 2009)

MEDICAL TRANSCRIPTION PRODUCTION HARDWARE DETAILS

The production unit workspace is spacious open area holding a network of 80 computers, which includes 3 servers in a separate room for network management and 80 workstations. Additional network equipment includes three 16-port Ethernet hubs, which leave ample scope for immediate expansion if necessary.

Servers

Two Primary Domain Server which handles file distribution and internal mail, and one Backup Domain Server which handles the Internet file transfers and backup system of the entire network are in the specific configuration.

HOME-BASED MEDICAL TRANSCRIPTION

A home based medical transcription office requires a computer, Internet access, speakers, and a quiet work space. There are multiple formats that medical transcripts can be provided as, including electronic or traditional tape recording. The files are sent either physically or electronically to the home based medical transcription office. Upon receipt of the files, the transcriptionist can begin the process.

The role of the medical transcriptions is to listen to the recording and create clean, logical, accurate, medical notes. This information is added to the patient's electronic file, or submitted to the appropriate party on behalf of the doctor. A clear understanding of medical terms, definitions, common short forms, and phrases of speech are all very important. These records are usually spot checked by the physician for accuracy, but it is the responsibility of the transcriptionist to ensure that they are accurate and complete.

Table 1. (www.escubestechnologies.com/facilities.htm, 2009)

NO. OF SERVERS	3
MAKE	ASSEMBLED / AMD & PENTIUN IV
CPU	ATHLON 600 MHz & 2.6 GHz / 80 GB HDD / 1GB DDR
CACHE -	L1 Data Cache 128 Kb/L1 inst. Cache 128 Kb/L2 cache 512 Kb
RAM	1GB DDR
HDD	80 GB
FDD	1.44 MB
CDROM	52x
VDU	17" Color
CABINET	ATX & AT Super tower with 230W SMPS.
WORKSTATIONS	37
	ASSEMBLED/AMD & PENTIUM III
NO. OF WORKSTATIONS	667 MHz /20GB HDD/ 256 MB SD RAM
MAKE	WINDOWS 98/ME/XP STAR.
CPU	
OPERATING SYSTEM	
NETWORKING DETAILS	3
	E LINK UTP CAT – 5
No. OF SWITCHES/HUBS	WINDOWS NT
MAKE OF CABLES	MAIN BACKUP GENERATOR(10KVA); UPS FOR INDIVIDUAL SYSTEMS.
PLATFORM	UPS: 3.5 KVA (ZENITH)
BACKUP POWER DETAILS	CENTRALIZED NETWORK DISTRIBUTION & TRACKING.
MAKE OF BACKUPS	WAVE PEDAL (9 PINS) AND JOYSCRIBE.
TRACKING OF FILES	LICENSED QUICKHEAL ANTIVIRUS.
FOOT PEDAL	WINZIP 9.
ANTIVIRUS	NO SPACE IS REQUIRED AS WE UPLOAD THE WORK DIRECTLY ON CLIENTS FTP SPACE.
ZIPPING	HOWEVER, AS A BACK UP WE HAVE 50 MB SPACE.
FTP	(accessibility details will be provided on request)
CONVERTER	GOLDWAVE.
	EASYWAVE.
	AUDIO CONVERTER.

There are two sets of skills that are very important as a medical transcriptionist: listening and data entry. Accurate recording of the exact words used is a skill that takes time and effort to learn. Many people begin the process with a high degree of accuracy, but quickly begin to translate, adding in their own words, grammar, and edits as they deem appropriate to the document.

Technology has completely revolutionized the operation of a home-based medical transcription business. Voice recognition software is now easily accessible and quite affordable. Many physicians use this type of software to transcribe the vast majority of their notes and rely on a transcriptionist to simply edit and correct the text as needed. The drawback of home based of medical transcription is that this type of service does not pay as well as a full medical transcriptionist service.

The first step in setting up this type of business is to register with the government. Running a business requires some basic overhead activities, such as bookkeeping, tax filing, and keeping track of expenses and revenue. However, business owners operating from a home office can deduct various costs related to the business. This includes space in the home, car, supplies, and Internet costs. It is important for a home-based medical transcription business to invest in computer backup system, so that doctor's files and work in progress is not lost, should there be a computer hardware failure.

(http://www.wisegeek.com/what-is-home-based-medical-transcription.htm, 2009)

OUTSOURCING OF MEDICAL TRANSCRIPTION

Due to the increasing demand to document medical records, countries started to outsource the services of medical transcription. In the United States, the medical transcription business is estimated to be worth US$10 to $25 billion annually and growing 15 percent each year. The main reason for outsourcing is stated to be the cost advantage due to cheap labor in developing countries and their currency rates as compared to the U.S. dollar.

There is a volatile controversy on whether medical transcription work should be outsourced, mainly due to three reasons:

1. The greater majority of MTs presently work from home offices rather than actually in hospitals, working off-site for "national" transcription services. It is predominantly those nationals located in the United States who are striving to outsource work to other-than-US-based transcribers. In outsourcing work to sometimes lesser-qualified and lower-paid non-US MTs, the nationals unfortunately can force US transcribers to accept lower rates, at the risk of losing business altogether to the cheaper outsourcing providers. In addition to the low line rates forced on US transcribers, US MTs are often paid as ICs (independent contractors); thus, the nationals save on employee insurance and benefits offered, etc. Unfortunately for the state of healthcare-related administrative costs in the United States, in outsourcing, the nationals still charge the hospitals the same rate as they did in the past for highly qualified US transcribers, but subcontract the work to non-US MTs, keeping the difference as profit.
2. There are concerns about patient privacy, with confidential reports going from the country where the patient is located (i.e. the US) to a country where the laws about privacy and patient confidentiality may not even exist, which was overcome as HIPAA (Healthcare information portability and accountability act) became mandatory for all the providers from the outsourced countries. Some of the countries that now outsource transcription work are the United States, Britain, and Australia, with work outsourced to Philippines, India, Pakistan, Canada and Barbados.
3. The quality of the finished transcriptions is not a concern. Many outsourced transcribers simply do have the requisite basic education to do the job with reasonable accuracy, additional, occupation-specific training in medical transcription. Many foreign MTs who can speak English are much familiar with American expressions and/or the slang doctors often use, are apparently familiar with medical reference books, and are familiar with American names and places. An MT editor, certainly, is then responsible for all work transcribed from these countries and under these conditions. These outsourced transcribers often work for a fraction of what transcribers are paid in the United States, even with the US MTs daily accepting lower and lower rates.

Among outsourcing countries, the Philippines has recently attracted increased amounts of MT outsourcing from the United States due to the fact that aside from the Filipino language, English is one of the official languages used in almost all government transactions in the country and the high literacy in the English language and perhaps, the capability of average Filipino to understand American idioms, colloquialism, and slang used in medical transcription. This is very concerning to the US MTs. The Health Insurance Portability and

Accountability Act (HIPAA) governs outsourcing of MT work. Stricter policies in compliance with HIPAA are implemented in such companies to enable security and confidentiality of work involved in such practices.

One of the main advantages of outsourcing Medical transcription services to offshore locations is that comparable services are offered in these countries at highly competitive rates as compared to the industry standards prevalent in the U.S. Besides the built-in cost benefits are many:

- Lower per line rate.
- Lower direct labor costs.
- Lower costs in HR, administrative and training areas.
- Lower annual maintenance costs for maintenance of digital and transcription equipment.

India also has a strong market share in medical transcription outsourcing because of its large resource of young, college-educated and productive workforce. The dominant use of English as the main medium of communication is another cause for India's traditional edge in medical transcription outsourcing. Exposure to English language and the influence of western media such as movies, TV channels and books makes the average Indian familiar with the American usage and accent. Best-in-class medical transcription training methodologies shore up the inherent advantage that India offers in medical transcription outsourcing.

The time zone differential between the U.S. and India works to the advantage of clients as medical records are downloaded, transcribed and transmitted back overnight for access by health practitioners in the U.S., the following working day. This ensures the fastest turnaround time in the industry.

The medical transcription outsourcing industry in India can loosely be organized into the following:

- Indian subsidiaries of the large U.S.-based players: The majority of medical transcription service providers in India are subsidiaries of U.S.-based medical transcription companies. They are aligned with the U.S. parent company in training processes, systems, technology, billing and client relationship management.
- Medium sized Indian medical transcription firms: These are medium-to-small Indian companies with a limited marketing presence in the U.S. These sometimes function as franchisees or vendors to the larger players. But they have growing clout in the market and are increasingly seen as strong contenders for delivering quality medical transcription services.
- Small independent firms: These employ fewer transcriptionists and rely largely on work outsourced from the first two groups. (en.wikipedia.org/wiki/Medical_transcription, 2009; www.outsource2india.com, 2009)

Medical Transcription in India

MT Services are a strategic and imperative fit for India as it offers immense job opportunities and ability to earn foreign exchange. A majority of the State Governments in India are offering incentives and infrastructure for setting up these services. The Central Government has provided Income Tax exemption to profits from export of these services. Moreover, setting up of these services is not capital intensive and is entrepreneur driven. India has emerged as the preferred global destination and the hub for MT Services. Major advantages offered by India for MT Services:

- A virtual 12-hour time zone difference between India and USA offers cost and time savings.
- A huge pool of English speaking and computer literate graduate workforce who can

continue to cater to the growing demand of professionals for MT Services.
- India enjoys very strong brand equity in global markets in the IT sector, thanks to its growing and globally competitive software industry.
- A special thrust has been given by the Department of Telecommunications, Government of India with reduction in prices of high speed data communication lease circuits.
- Government of India has provided Income Tax exemption to profits from export earnings of MT Services.

Central and state governments as well as the private sector are setting up state-of-the-art infrastructure for MT Services including IT Habitats.

Nasscom has constituted a Vision Group for IT Enabled Services (MT is classified as an IT Enabled service in India). This is a special forum mandated with the task of identifying opportunity segments in the areas of IT Enabled Services. This Nasscom group would also devise segment specific strategies for market development, encourage entrepreneurship and position India as a global hub for IT Enabled Services.

The following table amply projects the potential for employment and earnings from MT Services.

Medical Transcription: Major Foreign Exchange Earner

- Medical Transcription is likely to become one of the major foreign exchange earners for India.
- The entire American MT industry is currently worth $ 6.6 billion.
- MT faces no major problems from WTO restrictions, competition, governmental roadblocks, shortages, power cuts or import restrictions. (www.indianmarkets.com, 2008)

Table 2. Medical transcription/ medical coding & billing

Year	1999/2000	2007/2008 (Projected)
Workforce Employed	5,000	50,000
Rs. Crore	120	4,000
(Source: Nasscom)		

ISSUES, CONTRAVERSIES, PROBLEMS

There are several issues, contraversies, and problems involved in medical transcription process, which are being researched upon. The following report is an initial attempt at formulating some of the primary issues identified through the **Bentley College Medical Transcription research project**. They are:

1. Capturing and describing the "professional sense" required to perform transcription.
2. Examining the performance metrics used in the industry to gauge accuracy, productivity, profitability, customer service, and technological impact.
3. Determining the effect of speech recognition technologies and other healthcare documentation technologies on work and the industry.
4. Describing the medical transcriptionist profession in terms of its demographics, background, experience, and challenges.
5. Identifying challenges and opportunities for the medical transcription workers and industry.

Controversies regarding technological impact involves the implementation of speech-recognition technology (SRT). The goal of SRTs is to accomplish a relatively complete draft of the dictated voice file as the dictator speaks with editing being done either on the "front-end" (by the dictator) or the "back-end" (by another person who may or may not be an MT). While the allure of SRTs lies in their promise of a quicker TAT and cheaper process (by assuming a reduced role of the MTs), there is no complete understanding of the impact of this technology on healthcare documentation production. **R.M. Issenman** and Jaffer (2004) found that there was increased frustration with "training" the SRT system (with 1 in 4 physicians actually completing the trial), a loss of efficiency (with the SRT being 66% less effective than MTs) and an increase in cost. This uncertainty regarding the impact of SRTs has led for calls for "a return on investement analysis" that includes "assessments of time spent by both the MTs and the physicians." (van Terheyden 2005:45). (David, 2008)

The key problems faced in transcribing are:

- Unfamiliar medication names or terminology.
- Unclear enunciation/dictation by doctors.
- Speedy dictations by doctors in departments such as ER(emergency room), which are severely time-challenged.
- Poor voice quality due to technical snags in the recording device.

SOLUTIONS AND RECOMMENDATIONS

Like everything, medical transcription has also been through phases of evolution. Medical transcription is a rather dynamic industry with new experiments and additions going on everyday. It provides unlimited intellectual challenge and the opportunity to make a unique contribution to quality health care and service.

To improve the medical transcription process and make it completely error free, firstly, the transcriptionists are encouraged to:

- Research intensively on the internet, when in doubt.
- Access printed and online resources and medical dictionaries.
- Flag off any file that is incomplete, unclear or inconsistent.

Apart from the above, technology vendors and the health information management (HIM) directors and Chief Information Officers (CIOs) that buy production technologies have predicted for over a decade that in a "few years" speech recognition and transcription technologies will render MTs obsolete resulting in significant savings to off-set the growing cost of healthcare.

Also, technological change involves the use of electronic medical record systems and platforms. The implementation of these enterprise-wide solutions is predicated on the belief that through a technologically-based re-engineering, healthcare organizations can gain a greater efficiency and reduce the turnaround time. An error analysis chart for each document categorizing and tracking the undetected errors by noting the occurrence of repeated types of mistakes (differentiating between medical language errors and English language errors), should be developed so that the MTs/SRT could identify problem areas and improve performance.

FUTURE RESEARCH DIRECTIONS

The medical transcription industry will continue to undergo metamorphosis based on many contributing factors like advancement in technology, practice workflow, regulations etc. The evolution toward the electronic patient record demonstrates that, over time, documentation habits will change either through standards and regulations or through personal preferences Any attention given to medical transcription typically revolves around three themes: the potentially lucrative nature of the industry, the off-shoring of medical records, and the "promise" of MT elimination through technology.

With this aspect in mind, voice recognition is one technology area that is being actively researched upon and one can expect a near perfect voice recognition software in the future that will make the transcriptionist's job much easier. Speech/voice recognition and internet technologies automate and reduces time required to transform medical dictation into medical transcription. This process is significantly faster and less expensive than typed transcription. The result is accurate and timely medical transcriptions that do not require healthcare providers to change the way they work. The transcription companies benefit by using new Internet communication and improved editing software.

It appears that physician adoption of EMR technology and speech recognition technology will have a significant impact over time on how reports are created by providers; however, in many provider organizations, adoption of these technologies is still a few years out. Many of the larger MTSOs are starting to use speech recognition technology to enhance their services, at least in the short term. However, it is unknown what the adoption will be further into the future.

Home-based transcription (HBT) is also emerging as a new technology for which various softwares have been made and are being researched upon to ease the process of HBT.

CONCLUSION

Medical transcription professionals play a critical role in the evolving future, a new breed of professional will be required. This new hybrid medical transcription professional will need to step up to the documentation management table with a broader portfolio of value-added skills. This will require not only retooling medical transcription professionals to be proficient in new technologies (speech recognition, electronic medical records, data tagging, etc), but also pushing them toward a deeper and more fundamental knowledge of clinical medicine to position themselves as documentation auditors to ensure the quality and accuracy of the document. At the point of provider entry, whether the data is input via **point-and-click template software**, speech-recognition software, or traditional dictation, this new medical transcription professionals will need to be positioned to funnel that information, verify its accuracy, and ensure its formatting for database upload and reimbursement.

Medical transcription can be a lifelong, satisfying career providing the constant challenge of an expanding and advancing technology. The changes occurring in the healthcare industry promise to provide even more challenges to the forward-looking medical transcription professionals. It is a portable skill that allows for professional and geographic mobility.

REFRENCES

AHDI. (2009). *Approved Medical Transcription Education Programs*. Modesto, CA: Association for Healthcare Documentation Integrity.

Caribbean (2009). *Barbados Looks to Become Medical Transcription Capital*". Caribbean Press Releases. Retrieved from http://www.caribbeanpressreleases.com/articles/4520/1/Barbados-Looks-to-Become-Medical-Transcription-Capitl/Page1.html

David, G. C. (2008). *Finding the Place of Technology in Medical Transcription.* Paper presented at the annual meeting of the American Sociological Association Annual Meeting, Sheraton Boston, Boston, MA. Retrieved from http://www.allacademic.com/meta/p242233_index.html

Em-t. (2009). *Em-t.* Retrieved from www.em-t.com.

Escubes (2009). *Escubes Technologies*. Retrieved from www.escubestechnologies.com/facilities.htm

Exchange, M. T. (2008). *The MT school wars*, MT Exchange. Retrieved from http://mtexchange.com/mtx/school_wars

HIPAA (1996). *The Health Insurance Portability and Accountability Act*. Retrieved from HIPAA.org

Indian Market. (2008). *Indian Market* Retrieved from www.indianmarket.com

Outsource2india (2009). *Outsource2india*. Retrieved from www.outsource2india.com

Outsource Strategies International. (2008). *Medical Transcription Tools and Equipment*. Retrieved from http://www.outsourcestrategies.com/blog/medical-transcription/2008/02/ medical-transcription-tools-and.html

Webraydian (2009). *Webraydian*. Retrieved from www.webraydian.com/content/view/1009/32/

Wise Geek. (2009). *Wise Geek*. Retrieved from http://www.wisegeek.com/ what-is-home-based-medical-transcription.htm

KEYTERMS AND DEFINITIONS

Medical Transcriptionist: An individual who performs medical transcription is known as a medical transcriptionist or an MT.

EMR: An electronic medical record (EMR) is a medical record in digital format.

HIPAA: Health Insurance Portability & Accountability Act (HIPAA) of 1996, Public Law 104-191, also known as the "Kennedy-Kassebaum Act." This U.S. law protects employees' health insurance coverage when they change or lose their jobs and provides standards for patient health, administrative, and financial data interchange.

HBT: Home-based transcription

SRT: Speech-recognition technology (SRT) is the ability of a machine or program to identify words and phrases in spoken language and convert them to a machine-readable format.

CSR: Continuous speech recognition (CSR) understands natural speech without pauses and is the most process intensive.

CAMT: The Computer Aided Medical Transcription (CAMT) software change spoken words to texts.

Hybrid: It is a combination of two or more different things, aimed at achieving a particular objective or goal.

Retooling: To revise and reorganize, especially for the purpose of updating or improving.

Metamorphosis: Any complete change in appearance, character, circumstances, etc.

Obsolete: No longer in use or practice.

Vendor: A vendor, or a supplier, is a supply chain management term meaning anyone who provides goods or services to a company.

Foot Pedal: Foot pedal means the foot operated lever designed to operate the mechanical linkage that trips a full revolution clutch.

Blue Cross/ Blue Shield: A nonprofit organization that offers its members health insurance covering hospitalization, surgical, and medical expenses.

Chapter 14
Artificial Intelligence in Medical Field

Satyanarayana Rentala
Jawaharlal Nehru Technological University, India

Uma Maheswara Rao Ganguru
Jawaharlal Nehru Technological University, India

Prameela Devi Yalavarthy
Jawaharlal Nehru Technological University, India

Lakshmi Narasu Mangamoori
Jawaharlal Nehru Technological University, India

ABSTRACT

Making the knowledge and expertise of human experts more widely available through computer consultation systems has been recognized as an important tool for improving the access to high quality health care. The software development exploits the potential of human intelligence such as reasoning, making decision, learning (by experiencing) and many others. Artificial intelligence is not a new concept, yet it has been accepted as a new technology in computer science. It has been applied in many areas such as education, business, medical and manufacturing. This chapter explores the potential of artificial intelligence techniques in medical applications.

INTRODUCTION

Intelligence is the computational part of the ability to achieve goals in the world. Varying kinds and degrees of intelligence occur in people, many animals and some machines. R. Jensen[1], a leading researcher in human intelligence, suggests 'as a heuristic hypothesis' that "all normal humans have the same intellectual mechanisms and that differences in intelligence are related to 'quantitative biochemical and physiological conditions'. I see them as speed, short term memory, and the ability to form accurate and retrievable long term memories." Whether or not Jensen is right about human intelligence, the situation in Artificial Intelligence (AI) today is the reverse. After World War II, a number of people independently started to work on intelligent machines. The English mathematician Alan Turing may have been the

DOI: 10.4018/978-1-61692-004-3.ch014

first to start AI research. He also may have been the first to decide that AI was best researched by programming computers rather than by building machines. By the late 1950s, there were many researchers on AI, and most of them were basing their work on programming computers. So, what is artificial intelligence? The answer is simple, "It is the science and engineering of making intelligent machines, especially intelligent computer programs". It is related to the similar task of using computers to understand human intelligence, but AI does not have to confine itself to methods that are biologically observable. The ultimate effort is to make computer programs that can solve problems and achieve goals in the world as well as humans. However, many people involved in particular research areas are much less ambitious. Medical informatics is "a developing body of knowledge and a set of techniques concerning the organizational management of information in support of medical research, education, and patient care". Medical informatics combines medical science with several technologies and disciplines in the information and computer sciences and provides methodologies by which these can contribute to better use of the medical knowledge base and ultimately to better medical care. In most developing countries insufficient of medical specialist has increase the mortality of patients suffered from various diseases. Current practice for medical treatment required patients to consult specialist for further diagnosis and treatment. However, the waiting time for treatments normally takes a few days, weeks or even months. Computer technology could be used to reduce the number of mortality and reduce the waiting time to see the specialist. Initially AI was applied to medicine, later to biostatistics, economics, cognitive psychology etc.

There are two kinds of AI

- factual AI - eg, anatomy of the heart
- problem solving AI - eg, diagnosis

Employing the technology especially Artificial Intelligence (AI) techniques in medical applications could reduce the cost, time, human expertise and medical error.

The **objectives** of this chapter are, to:

- Establish relationship between AI and medical field
- Study analytical perspectives in the applications of artificial intelligence in medical field
- Study the Novel issues in artificial intelligence in medical field
- Study the Novel perspectives in the field of artificial intelligence in Medicine
- Model expert systems in medical field
- Solve controversies and problems of Artificial Intelligence in medicine (AIM)
- Future of AI in medical diagnosis

ARTIFICIAL INTELLIGENCE IN MEDICINE (AIM)

The main goals of AI in medicine (AIM) are[1]

- To assist but not to replace the physician- do what computer does the best: memory, processing
- To focus attention
- To provide diagnosis
- To facilitate management

The potential of AI in medicine has been expressed by a number of researchers. Hoong[2] (1988) summarized the advantages of AI techniques in medicine as follows:

- Provides a laboratory for the examination, organization, representation and cataloguing of medical knowledge.
- Produces new tools to support medical decision-making, training and research.

- Integrates activities in medical, computer, cognitive and other sciences.
- Offers a content-rich discipline for future scientific medical specialty.
- Focuses on diagnosis and therapy rather than on facts
- Encourages experimentation and exploration
- It gives better measure of competency than multiple choice test

AI in Medicine (AIM) is AI specialized to medical applications. Researchers in AIM need not engage in the controversy introduced above. Although we employ human- like reasoning methods in the programs we write, we may justify that choice either as a commitment to a human/ computer equivalence sought by some or as a good engineering technique for capturing the best-understood source of existing expertise on medicine—the practice of human experts. Most researchers adopt the latter view.

Before embarking on an investigation of the tools and methods available for expert system design and implementation, it is important to identify the distinct phases in their development. The problem is one in which knowledge from a human expert (or a set of experts) must be transferred to a knowledge-acquisition methods. The output of this phase of expert system design is a "paper-based" system. To be of any use, this system must be represented in a form that can be implemented as a computer program.

The choice to model the behavior of a computer expert in medicine on the expertise of human consultants is by no means logically necessary. If we could understand the functioning in health and in disease of the human body in sufficient depth to model the detailed disease processes which disturb health, then, at least. In principle, we could perform diagnosis by fitting our model to the actually observable characteristics of the patient at hand. Further, we could try out possible therapies on the model to select the optimum one to use on the patient. Unfortunately, although biomedical research strives for such a depth of understanding, it has not been achieved in virtually any area of medical practice. The AIM methodology does not dogmatically reject the use of non-human modes of expertise in the computer. Indeed, accurate computations of probabilities and solutions of simple differential equations—tasks at which human experts are rather poor without special training--play a role in some of our programs. Nevertheless, most of what we know about the practice of medicine we know from interrogating the best human practitioners; therefore, the techniques we tend to build into our programs mimic those used by our clinician informants.

ANALYTICAL PERSPECTIVES IN THE APPLICATIONS OF ARTIFICIAL INTELLIGENCE IN MEDICAL FIELD

Artificial intelligence in medicine possesses the unique skills in combining knowledge management techniques with information technology within a healthcare setting. Artificial intelligence in medicine offers its clients specialist advice in the following areas[17-20]:

- IT-Enabled Evidence-Based Clinical Practices
- Medical Decision Support Systems
- Diagnostics Decision Making Systems
- Multimedia Healthcare solutions
- Healthcare Content Management
- Clinical Knowledge Architectures
- Sharing of Healthcare Knowledge between different healthcare groups using currently available information technologies
- Healthcare context-dependent knowledge supply

Evidence-Based Clinical Practices

Evidence-based practice is an approach that has gained recognition for facilitating the transfer of evidence into quality clinical practice. While occupational therapy clinicians have a professional responsibility to ensure that their practice is effective, managers also have a responsibility to implement structures and systems that will support therapists in doing so. It demonstrated limited evidence of specific organizational models of practice to facilitate the transfer of knowledge into occupational therapy practice. This paper outlines the steps undertaken by occupational therapists in a large tertiary teaching hospital to develop and implement a model of research utilization. The resulting Research and Evidence in Practice model and the enabling strategies for its implementation are presented. A challenge for the future is to conduct a formal evaluation of the model.

Medical Decision Support Systems

A Decision Support System (DSS) is a class of information systems (including but not limited to computerized systems) that support business and organizational decision-making activities. A properly designed DSS is an interactive software-based system intended to help decision makers compile useful information from a combination of raw data, documents, personal knowledge, or business models to identify and solve problems and make decisions.

Typical information that a decision support application might gather and present are:

- An inventory of all of your current information assets (including legacy and relational data sources, cubes, data warehouses, and data marts),
- Comparative sales figures between one week and the next, projected revenue figures based on new product sales assumptions.

Medical Decision Support Systems are "active knowledge systems which use two or more items of patient data to generate case-specific advice" Medical DSSs are typically designed to integrate a medical knowledge base, patient data and an inference engine to generate case specific advice. Four key functions of electronic medical decision support systems are outlined in

Administrative: Supporting clinical coding and documentation, authorization of procedures, and referrals.
Managing clinical complexity and details: Keeping patients on research and chemotherapy protocols; tracking orders, referrals follow-up and preventive care.
Cost control: Monitoring medication orders; avoiding duplicate or unnecessary tests.
Decision support: Supporting clinical diagnosis and treatment plan processes; and promoting use of best practices, condition-specific guidelines, and population-based management."

Diagnostics Decision Making Systems

Viewing diagnosis as a process of decision making under uncertainty, analogous to other decision processes studied in psychological decision theory. We have to address questions such as: How do diagnostic decision makers represent and use their knowledge, how do they create mental models, what cognitive heuristics do they use, how does mood influence decision making processes? We have to study the correctness of these diagnostic processes, and how and where computerized decision support is suitable.

Multimedia Healthcare Solutions

Increasingly mobile doctors, nurses and technicians require easy access to each other and to medical devices, databases and e-mail. To support this mobility, solutions stretch across technologies, from wireless connectivity to advanced Voice over IP (VoIP) systems that deliver new cost- and timesaving, real-time communications.

Healthcare Content Management

Healthcare information growth is unrelenting. Much of this information - up to 80 percent - is unstructured and often inaccessible to existing systems. Retention policies, legal discovery requests, and regulatory requirements add to the challenge. Successfully managing healthcare information is a critical part of providing quality care, increasing clinician satisfaction, and improving operational efficiencies - all while complying with regulatory mandates. To meet these requirements, more healthcare providers and payers are turning to Enterprise Content Management (ECM) solutions. The attendee of this web-cast will find out how enterprise content management can differentiate the healthcare organization from the competition. The attendee will also learn how solutions from EMC help healthcare providers and payers manage clinical, financial, and operational healthcare information - and ensure regulatory compliance.

Clinical Knowledge Architectures

A common implementation strategy for expert systems is to separate the delivery of knowledge from the knowledge itself. That is useful for several reasons. First, knowledge engineers and software developers can implement the system in parallel. Deployment and ongoing maintenance can occur in parallel, as well. Second, the knowledge can be decoupled from a particular implementation language or framework, thus making it portable, interoperable, and resilient to change. Software developed without this decoupling is often referred to as *conventional software*.

Sharing of Healthcare Knowledge

The representation of medical knowledge is not a trivial task, as it is necessary to use a highly expressive, platform-independent formalism that would allow several scattered and poorly coordinated peers to communicate and exchange knowledge. There is also need for a powerful query language able to make complex queries over complex data. Trying to address a similar problem, i.e., integrate heterogeneous information available in the Web, the Semantic Web initiative created in the last years standards that aim at universal forms of knowledge representation.

Healthcare Context-Dependent Knowledge Supply

The transformation in health related research can be traced to new scientific domains such as Bioinformatics and Cybernetics which have evolved due to trans-disciplinary research. Due to this research, healthcare systems have an increased interest in recycling knowledge acquired from previous best practices. Professionals from the Knowledge Management (KM) and Knowledge Engineering (KE) domains had attempted to bring together different methodologies for knowledge recycling. The focus of KE practitioners has been to put emphasis on codified knowledge (i.e. to discover new ways of effectively representing healthcare related information). Practitioners from KM have concentrated on macro/policy aspects on how healthcare-related information can best be disseminated to support knowledge recycling and creation of new knowledge. This contrasting approach by practitioners from these two domains is leading to the emergence of the knowledge age in healthcare.

NOVEL ISSUES IN ARTIFICIAL INTELLIGENCE IN MEDICAL FIELD[9-12, 21]

Recent developments in medical informatics research have afforded possibilities for great advances in health care delivery. These exciting opportunities also present a number of challenges to the implementation and integration of technologies in the workplace. As in most domains, there is a gulf between technologic artifacts and end users, which compromises the culture of safety in the workplace. Because clinical practice is a human endeavor, there is a need for bridging disciplines to enable clinicians to benefit from rapid technologic advances. This, in turn, necessitates a broadening of disciplinary boundaries to consider cognitive and social factors related to the design and use of technology. The authors argue for a place of prominence for cognitive science in understanding nursing factors associated with patient safety. Cognitive science provides a framework for the analysis and modeling of complex human performance. Studies of clinical cognition can meaningfully inform and shape design, development and assessment of information systems. Furthermore, they have a decisive impact on whether information technology has a positive influence on human performance and are especially important in understanding and promoting safe practices. The below issues have been discussed in the context of artificial intelligence in medical field.

- The emergence of "dot coms," new information technology companies fueled by readily available venture capital that have attracted several prominent researchers from academe to the private sector
- An increased interest in information resources directly serving the needs of health care consumers
- The rapid development of the field of bioinformatics, applying information technology to computational problems in modern molecular biology
- The evolution of mega-systems of health care, and the corresponding emergence of the technologic challenge of integrating information systems across multi-billion-dollar businesses
- The appearance of a new generation of vendor products, including sophisticated electronic health record systems with intelligent features that had previously been available only to a small number of medical centers that had developed such systems locally
- The gradual emergence of new business procedures and policies governing health care, requiring care providing organizations to acquire sophisticated information systems to support administrative and financial aspects of their operations
- The increasing interest in information systems addressing the health of identified populations, directing the development of information systems to monitor the health states of intact regions, and allowing early intervention in the event of disease outbreaks

NOVEL PERSPECTIVES IN THE FIELD OF ARTIFICIAL INTELLIGENCE IN MEDICINE

Genome-Enabled Science and Health Care[7]

Genomic science can be seen in two ways—as a structural component to map the genome and thus understand nature's blueprint for biological action, and, as we increasingly understand how these molecular signatures affect living systems in action, as a functional component. With the structural map of many organisms now complete, we are moving beyond a primary focus on molecular sequence and well into the era of functional genomics, which now makes it possible to identify molecular signatures of specific diseases. Microarray technology to measure gene expression, the primary scientific apparatus of functional genomics, generates data that are multi-dimensional and noisy. Current analytic methodology, using statistical clustering algorithms and manual identification of gene loci, is crude but nonetheless has identified some important linkages between the approximately 10,000 known human genes, with 20,000 known expression patterns, and a small number of diseases such as large cell lymphoma for which gene expression is strongly predictive of prognosis. A next generation of analytic tools for functional genomics envisions the simultaneous measurement of the expression patterns of all the approximately 35,000 genes that the human genome is expected to comprise. These tools would automatically find correlations between gene expression patterns and normal metabolic homeostasis, nonspecific reactions to disease stimuli, and specific disease states. These correlations, in turn, will enable a next phase of genomics, "personal genomics," whereby the gene maps of individuals can be used to diagnose risks and states of illness and to plan therapy. With a few exceptions, the community of scientists traditionally associated with medical informatics has not played a significant role in the work of structural genomics. This can and should change as we proceed into the eras of functional and personal genomics, because these eras require linkage of molecular data with "person data," the traditional purview of our field. Moreover, the challenges to create ontologies that promote understanding of the problems to be solved, to build systems that are scalable to the magnitude of the computational challenges that the functional genomics problem creates, to identify new algorithms that offer efficient and creative solutions to the computational problems at hand, and to reconcile the various vocabularies used to represent information are challenges that medical informatics has successfully addressed in the past. The question facing the field of medical informatics, the group historically identified with AMIA and ACMI, is whether to remain firmly planted on traditional turf or take aggressive steps to build collaborations with the communities of biologists who are extending their own expertise to include computational methods. The cost of not acting at all is to be left behind regarding many of the most exciting future developments in informatics and health care.

Education to Reduce Reliance on Memory and Opinion

Cognitive psychologists distinguish between the internal "knowledge in the head" of an individual completing a task and the external knowledge available to that individual "in the world." How an individual— for example, a health care practitioner or biomedical researcher—completes a task will invariably be directed by knowledge in the head, but it can be amplified by appropriate integration of knowledge in the world. Whereas knowledge in the head is automatically available to practitioners, knowledge in the world must often be sought, understood, and integrated before it can play a helpful role. Too much reliance on either kind of knowledge inhibits effective professional practice. A practitioner too reliant on knowledge in the world will be overburdened by the relatively slow process of accessing external information sources; a practitioner too reliant on knowledge in the head can be misled by faulty recollection or guided by knowledge that is not valid. In health care, the current problem is excessive dependency on knowledge in the head, leading to excessive reliance by practitioners on flawed memory and learned opinions that have become, for these persons, pseudo-facts. By no means is the only cause of medical errors, acting in the belief that one's personal knowledge is correct, when in fact it is wrong, certainly one of the major causes of suboptimal professional performance in health care. A grand goal of medical informatics has always been the creation of knowledge resources that facilitate the incorporation of "knowledge in the world" into professional practice. Such tools would make the search for and integration of this knowledge sufficiently fluid that practitioners can be supported by external knowledge without bogging themselves down to the point of hopeless inefficiency. Making this vision into reality, however, poses numerous challenges. Although easily searchable sources of validated biomedical knowledge are now widely available at the bedside and in the examination room, this addresses only one piece of the problem. How to integrate this external knowledge into the practitioner's "thought flow" and work flow remains largely unsolved. An external knowledge resource addressing the thought-flow problem would provide an answer matching the practitioner's question, since the practitioner framed the question. The external knowledge must be not only correct and relevant but also appropriately granular and specific. If the practitioner has to *think* too hard to recognize that the external resource is indeed providing potentially useful knowledge, the external resource will not be used. Similarly, an external knowledge resource addressing work flow should not add additional discrete tasks to the process of caring for patients. If the practitioner has to *work* too hard to recognize that the external resource is indeed providing potentially useful knowledge, the external resource will not be used. Tools that solve the work flow and thought flow problem are still sparse, but they are becoming palpably more prevalent. The technical side of this problem will be solved first, as ongoing research produces better information retrieval tools, and as dissemination of electronic health record systems provides a basis for integrating these resources into work flow and thought flow. Culture and tradition—and, notably, the "guild mentality" addressed later in this report—pose addition- al, and even more substantial, challenges to the integration of external knowledge into professional practice. The culture and tradition of the health professions value knowledge in the head. Traditional models of clinical teaching reward students, who can, when asked, instantly recall pertinent facts about a patient or quote the classic differential diagnosis or treatment of choice. Attending physicians who "know a lot" are revered in the culture. Experienced nurses who accurately and almost instantaneously assess a patient's changing condition are respected by other nurses and physicians alike. While the biomedical literature is valued as the source of authoritative knowledge, the legitimate model for using this external knowledge resource is to read and remember rather than to integrate it continuously. Continuing education programs that bombard a passive audience with facts, with the implied expectation that these facts will be remembered, both reflect and reinforce these values. These values, instilled into the work habits of trainees in the teaching hospital and clinic, become enshrined in practice and perpetuated by the next generation of teachers. Although it is a relatively slow solution, changing the educational process is the most effective way of promoting the integration of external knowledge into practice. Attending physicians and expert nurses should be revered for their ability to find and integrate external information with their personal knowledge. This is the primary challenge facing medical informatics. A field that has largely ignored health professions education now has the opportunity to revolutionize it.

System Mindedness and Error Reduction[8]

William Richardson wrote, "Human beings, in all lines of work, make errors. Errors can be prevented by designing systems that make it hard for people to do the wrong thing and easy for people to do the right thing." Estimating that errors in U.S. hospitals cause from 44,000 to 98,000 deaths per year, this report put medical errors, even at the more conservative estimate, above the eighth leading cause of death. Hundreds of thousands more

Americans experience non-fatal medical errors each year. Resources consumed in treating the injuries caused by medical errors add to the cost of health care without improving the benefits. In its second report, *Crossing the Quality Chasm: A New Health System for the 21st Century*[9], the Committee on Quality of Health Care in America noted that "What is perhaps most disturbing is the absence of real progress toward restructuring health care systems to address both quality and cost concerns, or toward applying advances in information technology to improve administrative and clinical processes." Most medical errors are not reckless. They occur because information that could prevent the error, information that exists somewhere, is not available when and where it is needed. The challenge to Artificial intelligence in medical and the whole field of biomedical informatics is clear: We must integrate the delivery and use of knowledge and information into new and better systems of health care delivery. As we strive to meet this challenge, problems of technology and information collide with problems of professional culture and tradition. Health care continues to depend on the decision-making capacity and reliability of autonomous individual practitioners to resolve problems that routinely exceed the bounds of human cognition. If we are to reduce errors, we must transform our culture to one in which caregivers exercise their unique human capacities within supportive systems that compensate for their inevitable human limitations. Achieving that vision, however, requires that we first build the systems and demonstrate their utility. Only then can we expect clinicians to integrate these new tools into their practices and to adopt system-oriented values. How can the field of medical informatics promote rapid development of appropriate tools to transform the culture and systems of health care? In a few academic medical centers, informaticians have already developed and successfully implemented systems for order entry, care management, and quality improvement that provide both real-time decision support and long-term learning from clinical data for quality improvement. These sites should conduct systematic evaluations and demonstrations to show – the effects on error reduction of order sets and care plans based on current scientific knowledge and customized to the individual patient. The additional effects on error reduction of quality improvement systems that reference patient data to produce knowledge for changing care and that provide specific decision support. The responses of clinicians to the changes in cognitive, psychomotor, and interpersonal processes of care that the information systems entail- The changes in organizational processes that occur when health care systems become cybernetic—that is, when clinicians and managers use information derived from patient care data and current knowledge to adjust and improve care processes and outcomes. The ethical values and issues that arise when responsibility for patient welfare is viewed not as the sole province of the individual clinician but as a shared responsibility in a system of care A multi-site study using common research methods and data definitions would facilitate the aggregation of data across sites, where appropriate, and comparisons among sites and systems. Unique aspects of particular sites and systems would, of course, have to be evaluated in ways suited to their own objectives and impact. Results of these evaluations and demonstrations should be the subject of meta-analyses to differentiate generalizable from particularized knowledge. From such findings could come detailed recommendations for using information systems to reduce medical errors? Review and critique at each stage, from design to conclusions, by an independent advisory panel—perhaps even the Committee on Quality of Health Care in America itself—would ensure the rigor of the investigation and the validity of the findings. Undertaking such a comprehensive evaluation of the most successful information systems designed to reduce medical errors will require a significant commitment of resources. Informatics leaders, institutions, and funding

Figure 1. Knowledge based human-computer architecture

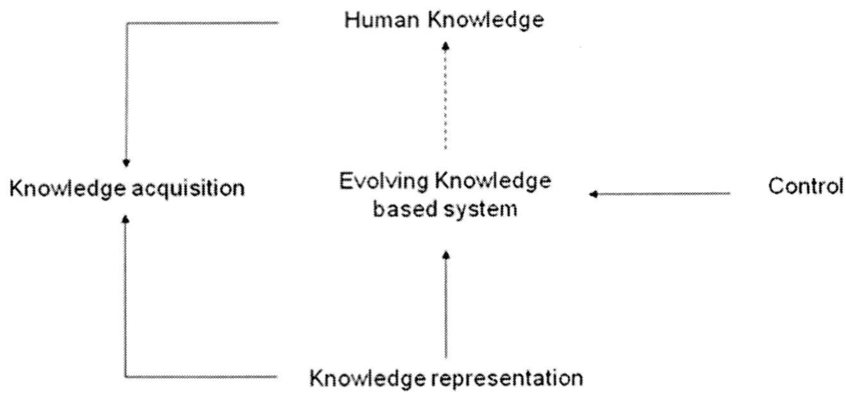

agencies would have to make this assessment of the state of the science a top priority. Not acting, however, would provide the archetypal example of allowing relevant knowledge to lie unused while (uninformed) humans decide how to respond to the crisis.

MODELING OF EXPERT SYSTEMS IN MEDICAL FIELD[13-16]

Before embarking on an investigation of the tools and methods available for expert system design and implementation, it is important to identify the distinct phases in their development (see Figure 1). The problem is one in which knowledge from a human expert (or a set of experts) must be transferred to a computer program for dissemination. Domain-specific knowledge is elicited from the human expert by knowledge-acquisition methods. The output of this phase of expert system design is a "paper-based" system. To be of any use, this system must be represented in a form that can be implemented as a computer program. A number of methods and tools are available to perform such tasks; these are detailed below. A different type of knowledge is required for the control strategy, i.e., decisions on when to use or "fire," specific rules in the knowledge base. In practice, these procedures are equated with different types of search strategies, such as depth-first, breadth-first, or various implementations of optimized search strategies.

What are not captured in (Figure 1) are issues dealing with evaluation of the system of human-computer interactions. These are interesting topics worthy of investigation but are outside the scope of this chapter.

Relying on the knowledge of human experts to build expert computer programs is actually helpful for several additional reasons: First, the decisions and recommendations of a program can be explained to its users and evaluators in terms which are familiar to the experts. Second, because we hope to duplicate the expertise of human specialists, we can measure the extent to which our goal is achieved by a direct comparison of the program's behavior to that of the experts. The flow of information through artificial intelligence in medical field has been viewed in (Figure 2).

Finally, within the collaborative group of computer scientists and physicians engaged in AIM research, basing the logic of the programs on human models supports each of the three somewhat disparate goals that the researchers may hold:

- To develop expert computer programs for clinical use, making possible the inexpensive dissemination of the best medical ex-

Figure 2. Flow of information though artificial intelligence in medical field

```
                        Artificial Intelligence System
                                 |
                                 V
 +--> data input -------> inference engine
 |                           |     | | |
 |                           V     | | |
 |      +------------ diagnosis    | | |
 |      |                         V | |
 |      +------------  explanation | |
user <--+                           V |
 ^      +---------------- questions   |
 |                                    V
 +------  patient <-------------  therapy
```

pertise to geographical regions where that expertise is lacking, and making consultation help available to non-specialists who are not within easy reach of expert human consultants.

- To formalize medical expertise, to enable physicians to understand better what they know and td give them a systematic structure for teaching their expertise to medical students.
- To test AI theories in a "real world" domain and to use that domain to suggest novel problems for further AI research.

Many intelligent systems have been developed for the purpose of enhancing health-care and provide better health care facilities, reduce cost and etc. Early studies in intelligent medical system such as MYCIN, CASNET, PIP and Internist-I have shown to out performs manual practice of diagnosis in several disease domain[3]. MYCIN was developed in the early 1970s to diagnose certain antimicrobial infections and recommends drug treatment. It has several facilities such as explanation facilities, knowledge acquisition facilities, teaching facilities and system building facilities. MYCIN uses production rules with certainty factors and these certainty factors allows fuzzy statements.

```
For eg,
IF
   infection is meningitis
   type of infection is bacte-
rial
   ...
THEN (certainty = 0.80)
   cause may be pnuemoccus or
neisseria
```

It also interprets user's "why?" question. CASNET (Causal ASsociational NETworks) was developed in early 1960s is a general tool for building expert system for the diagnosis and treatment of diseases. CASNET major application was the diagnosis and recommendation of treatment for glaucoma. PIP an abbreviation for Present Illness Program was developed in 1970s to simulate the behavior of an expert nephrologist in taking the history of the present illness of a patient with underlying renal disease.

In 1990s, the studies in intelligent system were enhanced to utilize the system based on current needs. In several studies two or more techniques were combined and utilized the function of the system to ensure system performance. ICHT (An

Intelligent Referral System for Primary Child Health Care) developed to reduce children mortality especially in rural areas[4]. The success of the system is mainly considered in catering common pediatric complaints, monitoring factors such as weight, immunization, development milestones and nutrition. ICHT utilized expert system in the process of taking the history data from patients. Other expert system have been developed such as HERMES (HEpathology Rule-based Medical Expert System) an expert system for prognosis of chronic liver diseases[5], Neo-Dat an expert system for clinical trials, SETH an expert system for the management on acute drug poisoning, PROVANES a hybrid expert system for critical patients in Anesthesiology and ISS (Interactive Sexually transmitted diseases Station) for diagnosis of sexually transmitted diseases. AI in Medicine (AIM) is AI specialized to medical applications. Researchers in AIM need not engage in the controversy introduced above. Although we employ human- like reasoning methods in the programs we write, we may justify that choice either as a commitment to a human/computer equivalence sought by some or as a good engineering technique for capturing the best-understood source of existing expertise on medicine--the practice of human experts. Most researchers adopt the latter view.

There are a number of methods for software development: iterative, agile, extreme programming, and waterfall. Each has a particular role that is contingent upon the size and complexity of the project and the organizational setting. We can use the *agile* method. Its basic approach is iterative: it incrementally delivers increasing portions of a software project, one step at a time. Agile development methods promote development iterations, teamwork, collaboration and process adaptability throughout the life cycle. All of them, however, follow the same pattern: requirements gathering, specifications, architecture, design, implementation and testing, deployment and maintenance. The agile method employs steps that are completed in "time-boxes." Teamwork is vital to this method. The team's size and membership can either increase or reduce the chance of success. Too large a consensus is a challenge; too small, and the required expertise leaves the development vacuous. Ideally, a team is made of five to nine members, with one domain expert representative. In our case, using a single domain expert would have eliminated the multi-domain expertise needed to capture specialized medical knowledge.

SOLUTIONS TO CONTROVERSIES AND PROBLEMS OF ARTIFICIAL INTELLIGENCE IN MEDICINE (AIM)

Just how good are AIM programs now? Each existing program has, in some trials, been judged comparable to expert physicians in their competence--this is indeed an outstanding result. Some have been shown statistically indistinguishable from experts in the field, others were judged as giving expert advice by true experts. Although the trials have ranged in rigor from well-controlled experiments to almost anecdotal testimonials, an objective examination of their performance clearly demonstrates that they have captured an important aspect of what it means to be an expert in a particular field of medicine and provided a good demonstration of their capabilities on some significant medical cases.

However, the programs' performance can also be non-uniform, exhibiting the "plateau and cliff effect" well known to all program developers: the program is outstanding on the core set of anticipated applications, but degrades rather ungracefully for problems just outside its domain of coverage. On very difficult cases, which are not typical of the ones used in formal evaluations, the programs may even be misled in cases that fall within their central domain by complex interactions or multiple disorders that are they are unable to untangle successfully.

We cannot ask, naturally, that an AIM program

be flawless before it can be acceptable, when the domain of its expertise is subject to uncertainties of knowledge and lack of data that can equally trip up a human expert. Nevertheless, for programs to function effectively in a typically human role, advising on decisions where life may hang in the balance, very high degrees of competence and reliability will be demanded. Can they be achieved?

The answer depends on two considerations: Is the AIM methodology sound enough to base the work on, or is it profoundly flawed by our lack of understanding of common sense human reasoning? Is the depth of knowledge which is expressible with the techniques we now have adequate to yield highly competent and reliable programs? To the first question, we will suggest "yes" as the answer, based on the observation that medical expertise is already rather formal (as argued above). To deal with the second, we point to some currently-developing ideas which suggest that richer representations are probably needed and probably achievable. First, however, we touch briefly on another aspect of AIM programs acceptability in clinical use.

We must realize that although current AIM programs already give quite impressive demonstrations of the success of the techniques used and of the dedication of the investigators, none of the programs reported on here or developed by other, similar efforts is in current clinical use. Perhaps, as it has been argued, programs will only be clinically accepted once their indispensability is established only when successful demonstrations exist that physicians or other medical personnel working with such programs are more successful than those without. Alternatively, social and administrative mechanisms may be more responsible for the ultimate utilization or abandonment of these tools. In any case, improved competence and reliability will surely be necessary and perhaps sufficient to help propel the programs into use.

As we approach the end of the 1990s, methodological developments in both the representation of knowledge and inference methods in medicine, however impressive in terms of their improvements over those of 20 or 30 years ago, still have not resulted in systems that are routinely used in the clinic. Reasons given for this usually include limitations in scope or ability to customize advice, lack of trust in automated advising systems, inadequate timeliness in critical situations, perception of the computer as a competitor, and most importantly, that decision support systems have yet to become indispensable adjuncts in medical practice situations. Problems and opportunities for medical AI in the 1990s have been identified and discussed with varying degrees of optimism or pessimism, depending on the author It has been suggested that the emphasis on decision support is misguided, and should be redirected towards medical education which would empower health care workers. This would tap into the developing theories

of clinical cognition and the use of clinical simulations to train and enhance learning at various levels of expertise. However, the systems reviewed were general diagnostic aids, which most physicians find less than indispensible given their own training and expertise. Another comparative study reported positive contributions to health care in three out of ten decision support systems reviewed. Most of the shortcomings came in systems that did not have to perform complex modeling or numerical computations, where computer-based assistance is often indispensable. Fields such as specialized laboratory test interpretation, treatment dosage planning and review, instrumentation monitoring and control, and multimodality imaging all suggest more essential domains for the application of AI methods.

The great computing success story of the 1990s has been the World Wide Web, and the proliferation of

web-based information services. The ease of designing good graphical user interfaces (GUIs) has resulted in a concomitant ease of interaction with our networked machines. E-mail has become ubiquitous, and various standard data interchange formats across platforms have been developed in medicine as in other fields. This presents AI in medical decision-making with a number of challenges and opportunities. The first is to characterize and build the knowledge-bases that can help improve medical decision-making; the second is to integrate them into useful, working, indispensable clinical systems; the third is to validate, standardize, and share medical knowledge as widely and economically as is possible. Development of standard medical vocabularies and nomenclatures; coding schemes, and the Unified Medical Language System (UMLS), are all essential to the standardization of medical knowledge representation. The availability of large digital image datasets has resulted in the creation of systems and knowledge bases for handling spatial information in anatomy, and has been accelerated by the widely disseminated multimodality image data from the Visible Human Project. The reusability of software is greatly facilitated by the development of ontologies for different types of knowledge and problem solving—a classical type of AI research which has received considerable new impetus from the needs of rapid knowledge transfer and scalability of web-based systems. In medicine, the PROTEGE system has become a model for such software re-use experiments, while other systems based on ontologies have also been developed. Software integration for multiple uses is increasingly spurred by initiatives such as IAIMS, and inclusion of useful decision support modules may evolve naturally as productive computing environments become more commonplace. One method for connecting clinical databases to knowledge bases used in decision support that is gaining acceptance is the Arden syntax. Automatic extraction of clinical data from narrative reports is also progressing due to a combination of statistical and linguistic methods. Meanwhile, AI systems are being designed to provide patients with intelligent access to medical information. The present situation, then, can be characterized as one of consolidation in integrating a variety of methods and techniques for different types of medical decision tasks while at the same time involving considerable reassessment and change in terms of expectations about the imminent application of decision-making systems within health care environments. On the one hand, the forthcoming increase in networking of various knowledge sources, digital libraries, and multimedia information opens up a whole new set of opportunities for filtering knowledge to the overwhelmed practitioner, whether in medicine, law, engineering, or other professions. On the other hand, the hard issues of understanding the role of human judgment and responsibility for clinical decisions and actions when using increasingly complex computerized instrumentation and systems presents an ongoing challenge to researchers in medicine, biomedical engineering and computer science, medical informatics, and all other fields essential to the solution of these problems.

ARTIFICIAL INTELLIGENCE IN FUTURE MEDICAL DIAGNOSIS

Networks are usually defined as a set of *layers*, each layer providing service to the layer above it. The networking infrastructure suitable in a campus environment today is called a *local area network* (LAN). In contrast, when communication is required over long distances (e.g., and organization which has offices all over the world), services from a long distance carrier company are required to establish what is called a *wide area network* (WAN). The protocols at higher layers work transparently over LANs and WANs, thus providing transparency to applications. Currently, software solutions are appearing that use distributed programs in order to achieve total network transparency and data integration from the end-user viewpoint. These are popularly termed *middleware*. Finally, there are specific solutions and standards pertinent to the health care environment which addresses medical domain problems which may be called *medical domain middleware*. In the following, we elaborate further on each of these concepts.

Middleware

At higher layers of networking, the client-server computing paradigm is becoming an alternative to central host-based computing. By distributing the work over several nodes on the network, more efficient and flexible solutions are created. These solutions integrate data for the end-users at the front end while hiding the multiplicity of origins of the data at the back end. A reliable, distributed file system, distributed printing services, consolidated directory services, network-based security service, and transparent invocation of applications residing elsewhere are examples of middleware. In the medical center context, it is extremely important to establish standards at this level to effectively tame the heterogeneity. Specific examples of middleware include Open Software Foundation's Distributed Computing Environment (DCE), SUN's Open Network Computing (ONC), OSI X.500 directory services, MIT kerberos security service, and OMG Common Object Request Broker Architecture (CORBA).

The **World Wide Web** (commonly abbreviated as "**the Web**") is a system of interlinked hypertext documents accessed via the Internet. With a Web browser, one can view Web pages that may contain text, images, videos, and other multimedia and navigate between them using hyperlinks. Using concepts from earlier hypertext systems, the World Wide Web was started in 1989 by the English physicist Sir Tim Berners-Lee[6], who is now the Director of the World Wide Web Consortium. The web-based collaborative system for Medical diagnosis uses the Computer and network technologies, the Internet to provide and support healthcare when distance separates the participants. Multi-threaded Server and client model is used in web-based medical diagnosis system that a client sends information to server and server echoes back to all clients and participants. Multiple clients are connected to single server. TCP/IP and Internet protocol is used to make server and clients communicate. The server application is generally set up in Linux machine, which runs Apache web server as this system is based on World Wide Web. The link with Linux operating system and current Apache web server allow this system to have all the benefit of Linux and Apache such as security. The client application is loaded when user accesses to the web site providing applet connecting back to server. A model for Web-Based Medical Diagnosis and Prediction is given in (Figure 3).

The Internet supports two-ways communications between users around the world at minimum cost. In medical, communication is very important as new information or new discovery is the key for the future survival. In addition, communications helps doctors sharing their knowledge or expertise. As an example, a specialist from Sydney can provide on-line medical assistance to doctor at Kuala Lumpur who is treating a patient that suffers from serious cancer problem. Another doctor from other country such as United Kingdom can share his experience dealing with the same cases. Communications between doctors or specialist from other region helps doctor at Kuala Lumpur diagnosing his patient and provides appropriate treatment. In telemedicine, Multimedia and Internet (or computer network) are two of the main tools that support the collaboration and distribution of information. Multimedia is a combination of media such as text, audio, visual and graphics can be used in medical application such as in image transmission (X-Ray images, pictures and etc.).

Clinicians, not machines, are responsible for clinical decisions. Advanced clinical decision support systems are designed to support those decisions. This is no small task. The simple example offered herein has shown that with, as little as, two factors, over 120 decision points must be considered. In the not too distant future maintaining these data will be challenging enough

Figure 3. A model for web-based medical diagnosis and prediction

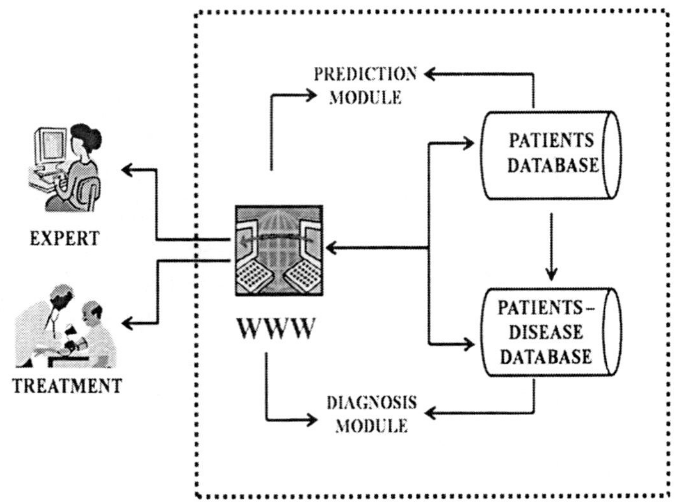

to require a semi-automated method for scanning scientific literature and selecting those factors that are germane to the decision. We call this tool an *artificial expert.* Completing the expert module questions is labor intensive. Full completion required about 20 hours. In our case we relied on the goodwill of colleagues. This method, however noble, extended the timeline to what would be unacceptable in a production environment. Future efforts should include some form of incentive. It is important to construct a modular system as a framework. The rapid change in emerging clinical knowledge will require regular updates to length, width, and depth of the knowledge base. Using this approach we have been able to add clinical modules, adolescent suicide linguistic analysis and other well-known analytical tools.

The use of networks at health care practice centers has provided value by increasing data availability, flexibility, and efficiency of operations. The graphical-user-interface-based applications, along with client- server paradigm of computing have begun to appear on these networks. The next generation of multimedia applications will require higher bandwidth networks, which have already begun to appear. In addition, the national efforts to link health care industries and providers in order to improve efficiency will now be possible due to the networks that have become the fourth utility—after electricity, water, and heat—in many medical centers. Individual doctor's offices, clinics, and practice settings are connecting to computer networks that accomplish the communication functions of the larger health care business networks.

CONCLUSION

The main features in medical diagnosis and prediction using artificial intelligence techniques will make the consultation to be more interactive. As clinical decision making inherently requires reasoning under uncertainty, expert systems and fuzzy logic will be suitable techniques for dealing with partial evidence and with uncertainty regarding the effects of proposed interventions. For the prediction tasks, Neural Networks have been proven to produce better results compared to other techniques (such as statistics). Such techniques are worth to explore and integrate in the system for medical diagnosis and prediction. The present situation, then, can be characterized as one of consolidation in integrating a variety of methods and techniques for different types of medical decision tasks while at the same time involving considerable reassessment and change in terms of expectations about the imminent application of decision-making systems within health care environments. On the one hand, the forthcoming increase in networking of various knowledge sources, digital libraries, and multimedia information opens up a whole new set of opportunities for filtering knowledge to the overwhelmed practitioner, whether in medicine, law, engineering, or other professions. On the other hand, the hard issues of understanding the role of human judgment and responsibility for clinical decisions and actions when using increasingly complex computerized instrumentation and systems presents an ongoing challenge to researchers in medicine, biomedical engineering and computer science, medical informatics, and all other fields essential to the solution of these problems. The Internet will be used as the medium to provide the tele-healthcare to the clinician or to the public. In addition, researchers in medical applications could use the data in their investigation of a new medical solution, patient's management and treatment.

REFERENCES

Berners-Lee, T., & Cailliau, R. (1990, November 12). *WorldWideWeb: Proposal for a HyperText Project* (Technical report), Genève, Switzerland: CERN.

Boehm, B., & Turner, R. (2004). Balancing Agility and Discipline: A Guide for the Perplexed. Reading, MA: Addison-Wesley publishers.

Bonfa, I., Maioli, C., Sarti, F., Milandri, G. L., & Monte, P. R. D. (1993). *HERMES: An Expert System for the Prognosis of Hepatic Diseases* (Technical Report UBLCS-93- 19), Universiti of Bologna.

Coiera, E. (2003). Guide to Health Informatics, 2 Ed. Oxford, UK: A Hodder Arnold Publication.

Duch, W., Matykiewicz, P., & Pestian, J. (2008). Neurolinguistic approach to natural language processing with applications to medical text analysis. *Neural Networks*, *21*(10), 1500–1510. doi:10.1016/j.neunet.2008.05.008

Giarratano, J., & Riley, G. (2004). Expert Systems: Principles and Programming, Fourth Edition. Florence, KY: Course Technology publishers.

Greenes, R. (2007). *Clinical Decision Support: The road ahead.* Burlington, MA: Elsevier publishers.

Guttmache, A. E., Porteous, M. E., & Mclnerney, J. D. (2007). Educating health-care professionals about genetics and genomics. *Nature Reviews. Genetics*, *8*(2), 151–157. doi:10.1038/nrg2007

Harrison, J. P., & McDowell, G. M. (2008). The role of laboratory information systems in healthcare quality improvement. *International Journal of Health Care Quality Assurance*, *21*(7), 679–691. doi:10.1108/09526860810910159

Hoong, N. K. (1988). Medical Information Science - Framework and Potential. In *Proceedings of the International Seminar and Exhibition Computerization for Development-the Research Challenge*, (pages 191-198). Kuala Lumpur: Universiti Pertanian Malaysia.

Jensen, A. R. (1998, November). Does IQ matter? *Commentary Magazine,* 20-21.

Kirchheiner, J., Nickchen, K., & Bauer, M. (2004). Pharmacogenetics of antidepressants and antipsychotics: the contribution of allelic variations to the phenotype of drug response. *Molecular Psychiatry*, *9*(5), 442–473. doi:10.1038/sj.mp.4001494

Larman, C., & Basili, V. (2003). Iterative and Incremental Development: A Brief History. *Computer*, *36*(6), 47–56. doi:10.1109/MC.2003.1204375

Lipton, J., & Hazelzet, J. A. (2009). Clinical decision support systems: Important tools when appropriately used. *Pediatric Critical Care Medicine*, *10*(1), 128–129. doi:10.1097/PCC.0b013e31819838f9

Mack, E. H., Wheeler, D. S., & Embi, P. J. (2009). Clinical decision support systems in the pediatric intensive care unit. *Pediatric Critical Care Medicine*, *10*(1), 23–28. doi:10.1097/PCC.0b013e3181936b23

Mahabala, H. N., Chandrasekhara, M. K., Baskar, S., Ramesh, S., & Somasundaram, M. S. (1992). ICHT: *An Intelligent Referral System for Primary Child Health Care*. In [*Conference of the South East Asia Regional Computer Confederation*. Kuala Lumpur.]. *Proceedings of SEARCC*, *92*, XI.

Quinlan, R. M. (1966). *Semantic Memory*. Cambridge, MA: Bolt Beranek and Newman.

Roots, I., Gerloff, T., & Meisel, C. (2004). Pharmacogenetics-based new therapeutic concepts. *Drug Metabolism Reviews*, *36*(3–4), 617–638. doi:10.1081/DMR-200033458

Rugg, M. D., & Curran, T. (2007). Event-related potentials and recognition memory. *Trends in Cognitive Sciences*, *11*(6), 251–257. doi:10.1016/j.tics.2007.04.004

Shortliffe, E. H. (1988). Computer Programs to Support Clinical Decision Making. *Journal of the American Medical Association*, *258*(1), 61–66. doi:10.1001/jama.258.1.61

Taffel, B. (2008). From data interoperability to value-driven healthcare. *Tennessee Medicine*, *101*(12), 31.

KEY TERMS AND DEFINITIONS

Medical Diagnosis: A label given for a medical condition or disease identified by its signs, symptoms, and from the results of various diagnostic procedures. The term "diagnostic criteria" designates the combination of signs, symptoms, and test results that allows the doctor to ascertain the diagnosis of the respective disease.

Artificial Intelligence: John McCarthy, who coined the term in 1956, defines it as "the science and engineering of making intelligent machines".

Expert System: Software that attempts to provide an answer to a problem, or clarify uncertainties where normally one or more human experts would need to be consulted.

Medical Informatics: Deals with the resources, devices, and methods required to optimize the acquisition, storage, retrieval, and use of information in health and biomedicine.

Diagnostics Decision Making Systems: Link health observations with health knowledge to influence health choices by clinicians for improved health care". This definition has the advantage of simplifying Clinical Decision Support to a functional concept.

World Wide Web: A system of interlinked hypertext documents accessed via the Internet. With a web browser, one can view web pages that may contain text, images, videos, and other multimedia and navigate between them using hyperlinks.

Cognitive Psychology: A discipline within psychology that investigates the internal mental processes of thought such as visual processing, memory, problem solving, and language.

Chapter 15
Cryopreservation of Spermatozoa:
Recent Biotechnological Advancement in Gamete Preservation Technology

Chanakya Nath Kundu
KIIT University, India

Gopal C Majumder
Jadavpur University, India & Indian Institute of Chemical Biology, India

Ranjan Preet
KIIT University, India

ABSTRACT

Cryopreservation of sperm has many applications in agriculture, biotechnology, and clinical medicine. The spermatozoon is a very specialized cell that loses the ability of biosynthesis, repair, growth and cell division during the final phase of spermatogenesis. Cryopreservation of sperm generally requires a reduction or arrest of the metabolism of cells, thereby prolonging their life. Semen samples of mammalian species are diluted with a suitable diluent [containing a complex extender (e.g., egg-yolk, milk, milk-whey), cryoprotectant (e.g., glycerol)] and processed through different freezing protocol prior to storage in liquid nitrogen (-196°C). Despite the use of complex media and cryoprotectants, a substantial portion of the cells die during freezing and thawing (recovery rate do not exceeds more than 50%). As the complex media contain large numbers of undefined biomolecules (proteins, lipids, carbohydrates), it is difficult to analyze the beneficial/detrimental effects of a particular compound on sperm cryopreservation. In the present book chapter we have briefly discussed the knowledge and limitations of the current semen cryopreservation technology and mainly focused on the development of a simple cryopreservation model using chemically-defined medium and goat cauda-epididymal sperm. Using this model system, several novel cryoprotectants have been identified and biochemical basis of sperm membrane damage during cryopreservation has been investigated.

DOI: 10.4018/978-1-61692-004-3.ch015

INTRODUCTION

Reproductive medicine is now drastically transforming our lives. Couples with impaired reproductive abilities are increasingly availing its benefits to conceive and realize their dreams of having a family. A major force in making this widely available is the ability to preserve fertility (sperms, eggs and embryos) using cryopreservation (storing cells in liquid nitrogen) (Bagchi *et al.,* 2008). Many cancer patients are also electing to preserve their fertility prior to undergoing chemotherapy or radiation (which can destroy reproductive abilities) to have the option of conceiving post-treatment. Cryopreservation of sperm has been highly successful in establishing pregnancies through artificial insemination (AI) and in vitro fertilization (IVF). Semen preservation is a subject of paramount interest because of the extensive use of frozen semen for artificial AI in cattle breeding to improve the production of milk, wool and meat. It is also a useful way of banking cells until needed for experimentation or other applications.

Research on semen preservation has had a long history over two centuries but till date the problem is that even with the best preservation techniques to date post-thaw survival is restricted to about 40-50% of the sperm population. Mammalian spermatozoa have been frozen stored by various methods based on systematic manipulation of cryopreservation protocol (e.g. dilution, cooling, freezing and thawing). Semen samples are generally diluted with a suitable diluent containing a complex extender (*e.g.,* egg-yolk, milk, milk-whey) and a cryoprotectant (*e.g.,* glycerol) prior to storage in liquid nitrogen (-196°C) (Hu *et al.*, 2009; Purdy 2006; Witte *et al.,* 2009). During cryopreservation a substantial portion of sperm cells undergo damage there-by reducing greatly motility/fertility potential of spermatozoa (Watson, 2000). But the biochemical basis of cryodamage is largely unknown. Complex media (egg yolk, milk, milk whey *etc.*) have been used as an extender **(cryopreservation medium and cryoprotectant)** for preservation of ejaculated spermatozoa by most of the investigators. Such media were also used for investigating the effect of multiple cryoprotectants (*e.g.* glycerol, sucrose, trehalose *etc.*). As this media contain a large number of undefined biomolecules (proteins, carbohydrate, lipids *etc.*), it is rather difficult to assess the biochemical basis of cryodamage and beneficial or detrimental effects of a particular compound on sperm cryopreservation.

For such an investigation it will be ideal to develop a simple sperm model for cryopreservation in a chemically-defined medium. Mature cauda epididymal sperm is a better model than the ejaculated sperm because the latter cells in view of their exposure to a variety of undefined constituents from the secretions of seminal vesicles, prostate that may complicate the interpretation of the data. An important advantage of the cauda-sperm model is that spermatozoa can be extracted from the epididymides that can be procured rather easily from the slaughter houses. Studies on cryoprotection mechanism using a cell model will require large amount of spermatozoa that will be rather difficult to procure from the ejaculated mammalian semen samples. Recently, we have developed a simple cryopreservation technique using a chemically-defined medium and goat cauda-epididymal sperm as the model system. (Kundu *et al.,* 2000)

In the present chapter we have discussed the existing knowledge and limitations of cryopreservation techniques including extenders, cryoprotectants and freeze-thaw protocol. Emphasis has been given on the development of a novel cauda-epididymal sperm cryopreservation model (using a chemically-defined medium) for screening the better cryoprotectant. Using that model system we have already screened cryoprotecting potentiality of several compounds. Finally, we have provided a novel hypothesis for cryoprotection mechanism offered by cryoprotectant.

CRYOBIOLOGY IN PRESERVATION

Cryobiology has an important application in preservation of biological materials leading to development of "organ", "tissue bank", "blood bank", "semen bank" etc. for maintaining viability *in vitro* at subzero temperature. The preserved organ has immense utility values in the modern surgical grafting techniques. Cryobiology thus confronts with the necessity of finding out the methods of keeping cells dormant but potentially alive by cooling or freezing at subzero temperature. This is obviously a challenging programme because water, the essential constituent of living cells, crystallises to ice which is fatal in most of the living systems. Dehydration due to the freezing brings about the following changes: [a] increase in the electrolyte concentration; [b] increase the ionic strength of the suspending medium; [c] precipitation of protein from solution; and [d] changes in pH values and concentration of certain solute to toxic levels (*e.g.* urea, gases *etc.*) *etc.* Addition of cryoprotective agents may overcome some of the above effects of cryo-injury but the knowledge about the mechanism of damage as well as protective action is still not adequate. Despite of this problem, the application of cryobiology for the preservation and maintenance of some important biological materials such as blood, protozoa, bacteria *etc.* has long been performed (Gluckman, 2009; Krenek & Berendonk, 2009; Kawahara, *et al.,* 2009).

BIOPHYSICS OF FREEZING

Under isotonic conditions, water in biological systems has an equilibrium melting point of approximately -0.6°C (Karlsson & Toner, 1996). The water is thermodynamically unstable below this temperature and increasingly favors its crystalline state, ice. There is certainly a degree of supercooling, before the first ice nucleus is formed during which the water remains in an unstable state. Although this degree of supercooling varies, the temperature at which nucleation first takes place is usually approximately -5°C (Woods *et al.,* 2004). Between -5 and -15°C, ice begins to form preferentially in the extracellular medium due to a spontaneous breakdown of the metastable state. The nucleation at high temperature can also be induced by the deliberate external seeding of ice. At these temperatures, water inside the cells remains unfrozen. The actual cause for this is not known but it is believed that the cell membrane prevents extracellular ice crystals from penetrating into the cell and seeding ice formation. The lack of efficient ice nucleators within the cell has also been cited as a possible reason (Mazur, 1970). The formation of ice in the external medium greatly influences the freezing response of cells. As the ice phase grows with decreasing temperature, solutes are rejected from the ice lattice into the unfrozen fraction of the extracellular medium, which becomes increasingly concentrated. This creates a chemical potential imbalance between the cytosol and the extracellular medium and sets up driving forces for the diffusion of solutes into the cell and for a water flux out of the cell. Due to the semi-permeable nature of the plasma membrane, a net osmotic gradient for the efflux of water from the cells is created. On the other hand, decreasing temperature increases the degree of intracellular supercooling, thus increasing the tendency for water inside the cell to freeze. There are, thus, two distinct, competing processes that tend to restore the thermodynamic equilibrium that is disrupted by the formation of extracellular ice. The cell can attain equilibrium either by losing water, thereby concentrating the cytosol and restoring the chemical potential, or by freezing intracellularly (Karlsson & Toner, 1996). The actual route to equilibrium depends on the velocity of cooling. If the cooling is sufficiently slow, the cell water has sufficient time to leave before it supercools significantly and, hence, the dominant mechanism of equilibration at low cooling rates is dehydration. The kinetics of water transport during freezing was elegantly first described in a mathematical model by Mazur (Mazur, 1963). Mazur's original model, and its subsequent variations (Toner, 1993; Pitt, 1992), have assumed that the rate of water efflux from the cells is directly proportional to the osmotic pressure difference across the plasma membrane and the permeability of the plasma membrane to water and is given by (Mazur, 1963): i)

$$\frac{dV}{dt} = \frac{L_P ART}{v_w} In \frac{p_e}{p_i}$$

where V is the volume of cell water, t is the time, L_p is the permeability coefficient for water, A is the cell surface area, R is the gas constant, T is the temperature, v_w is the molar volume of water, and p_e and p_i are the external and internal vapor pressures of water (Bagchi, *et al.,* 2008). The permeability coefficient is strongly temperature dependent and is given by:

$$L_p = L_{pg} \exp\left[-\frac{E_{L_P}}{R}\left(\frac{1}{T_{ref}} - \frac{1}{T}\right)\right]$$

where L_{pg} is the permeability at the reference temperature T_{ref} and E_{Lp} is the activation energy for water transport. It can thus be seen that the rate of water efflux from the cell is dependent on a variety of parameters, and since the values of these can vary significantly among various cell types, there will be a corresponding variability in the response of various cells to the same freezing protocol. At higher cooling rates, however, the probability of intra cellular ice formation (IIF) is greater. In this case, the rate of temperature decrease is much more rapid that the rate of water efflux from the cells causing the cell water to supercool significantly, thus favoring IIF. The actual mechanism of IIF, however, is not clearly understood and there are several hypotheses which have been proposed to explain it. Experimental evidence suggests that ice formation in cells frozen in the presence of extracellular ice occurs at significantly higher temperatures than in cells frozen without it, indicating that the external ice induces or catalyzes IIF (Bagchi *et al.,* 2008).

Based on this, Mazur proposed a mechanism of IIF in which ice crystals growing through pores in the plasma membrane nucleate ice formation inside cells (Mazur, 1965). An opposing theory is the membrane failure hypothesis, which posits that IIF is seeded by the extracellular ice following the rupture of the plasma membrane and the subsequent exposure of the cytoplasm to extracellular ice (Muldrew & McGann, 1990). A third mechanism of IIF has been proposed by Toner, *et al.*, in which IIF takes place by nucleation on intracellular catalytic sites (Toner *et al.,* 1990). The cooling velocity can affect the freezing response of cells in another very different way. With decreasing temperature, the viscosities of the extracellular and intracellular solutions keep increasing. This, in turn, decreases the diffusivity of water and low s the rate of ice formation. At the so-called glass-transition temperature, the viscosity of the solution is high enough to preclude any molecular diffusion, thereby stopping all phase transitions and creating a metastable, amorphous glassy state (Uhlmann, 1973). Although ice formation can occur at any temperature above the glass transition temperature, the amount of ice formed is dictated by the rate of cooling. If the cooling to this temperature is extremely rapid, the amount of ice formed will be negligible and the entire cell suspension will vitrify. This process is known as vitrification. Vitrification is an alternative to the freeze–thaw method of cryopreservation and is often preferred due to its avoidance of ice formation.

SPERMATOZOA

The spermatozoon is the last descendent of the male germ cell. It is synthesized in testis by spermatogenesis process and finally stored in epididymides. A mature mammalian spermatozoon (Figure 1) measures about 60 µm in length and can be commonly divided into the head, and the tail. The proportions between them can vary from 1:5 to 1:12.

The head is oval in shape and measures approximately 4.6 µ in length, 2.6 µ in width and 1.5 µ in thickness. The components of the sperm head are plasma membrane, acrosome and nucleus. The plasma membrane is a stable membrane that envelops the nucleus and acrosome of sperm head. The acrosome is a membrane-limited vesicle applied over a variable portion of the rostral surface of the sperm head in the form of a cap. It is essential for fertilization.

Sperm tail generates the propulsive force considered essential for penetration of the egg vestments. The main components of sperm tail are outer dense fiber, mitochondria, fibrous sheath and axoneme. The tail is divided into mid piece, principal or main piece and end or terminal piece. Anterior portion of the tail (midpiece) is the engine room of spermatozoa. The midpiece is a long cylinder, about 1 µm in diameter and 7 µm long. The main component of midpiece mitochondria, are the main site for synthesis of ATP, which is essential for providing energy for bending of tail flagellar motility.

CRYOPRESERVATION OF SPERMATOZOA

The spermatozoon has lost the ability of biosynthesis, repair, growth and cell division during the final phase of spermatogenesis. Conservation of sperm generally requires a reduction or arrest of metabolism of sperm cells, thereby prolonging their life.

Two major systems (liquid and frozen) of storage technologies have been developed for sperm conservation until the 20th century. For short and long term preservation, semen samples of various species are stored in refrigerated (4-5°C) or ambient temperature (18-24°C) and liquid nitrogen (-196°C), respectively.

Figure 1. Mature spermatozoon [Odell, W.D. and Moyer, D.L. (1971) In 'Physiology of Reproduction', Mosby, St. Louis, p. 56].

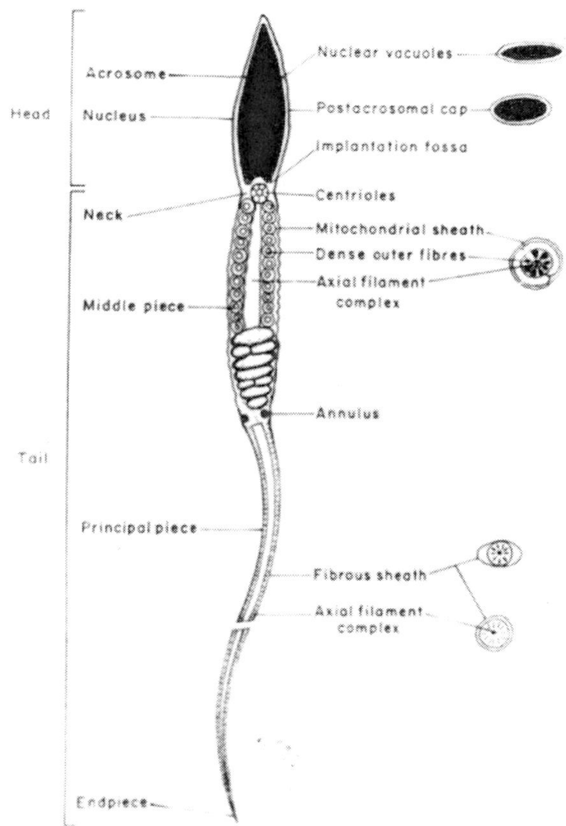

Liquid Storage

For short-term preservation, semen samples of mammalian species are stored in refrigerated or ambient temperature in liquid condition. Liquid preservation of semen has been done at refrigerated temperature in presence of a zwitterionic buffer (*e.g.* Tris, HEPES, TES, Citrate *etc.*) and a complex diluent (egg-yolk, skimmed milk, coconut oil *etc.*) (Farstad, 2009; Scherzer *et al.*, 2009). The life span of spermatozoa varies from species to species. The maximum life span are 2, 4-6 and 8-12 days for bull, goat, and boar, respectively

(Watson, 1990, 2000). In order to store semen at temperature above 5⁰C and achieve satisfactory results, alternative methods of metabolic inhibition were attempted. Thus, Van Denmark & Sharma (1957), proposed CO_2 narcosis, Norman *et al.,* (1958) suggested lowering the pH and Shannon (1965) proposed N_2 gassing as methods to inhibit the metabolic activity of spermatozoa. It was then postulated that storage at ambient temperature may be superior to at 5⁰C, provided the medium in which the spermatozoa are suspended, inhibits those pathways that are detrimental to their survival at higher temperature (Shannon and Curson, 1984). Egg-yolk, glucose, amino acids, several antioxidant, catalase, caproic acids are generally used for ambient temperature preservation of semen (5-20 ⁰C. 10-15 day may be the optimum survival period for ambient preservation (Sone *et al.,* 1992). Although liquid storage of semen has several advantages like low cost of preservation, greater insemination rate etc, but the major limitation of this process is limited shelf life of sperm cells.

Frozen Storage

To extend the life span of spermatozoa beyond a few days, the temperature must be reduced still further, introducing the additional stresses of freezing and thawing. At temperature of liquid nitrogen, -196°C, the thermodynamic processes are virtually halted, and theoretically the only deterioration of cells arising from background cosmic radiation. The observation of Mantegazza in 1866, that human spermatozoa survived freezing in semen frozen to -17°C must be ranked as one of the earliest reports of the recovery of mammalian cells after exposure to a temperature below freezing point (Mantegazza, 1866). It was a long time, however, before Jahnel in 1938 showed that a proportion of human spermatozoa survived after storage for a comparatively longer period in semen frozen to the temperature of solid carbon dioxide (-79°C) or liquid gases (Jahnel, 1938). Further experiments by Parkes (1945) revived the interest in this subject and a few years latter in 1949, one of the most important advantages was made by the discovery of protective effect of glycerol on the spermatozoa of several species (Polge *et al.,* 1949). This opened up the field tremendously, not only to work further on spermatozoa but also to carry out experiments on a wide variety of other cells and tissues.

Spermatozoa of more than 50 species have been cryopreserved (Watson, 1990; 95; Yang & Tiersch, 2009). It is important to recognize that cryopreservation cycle includes the entire process from sperm preparation, dilution, freezing and the post-thaw maintenance of functional over an extended period. At each of the stages, spermatozoa can loose their ability to function normally. Although some of the stages can relatively be innocuous, others (*e. g.* cooling and thawing) are very stressful. So, all the stages starting from ejaculation, freezing and return to body temperature should be considered carefully for successful cryopreservation of semen.

Dilution

After ejaculation from healthy donor, semen samples are diluted with a suitable diluent (e.g. Egg-yolk-citrate, egg-yolk-tris, egg-yolk-lactose, egg-yolk-HEPES, etc) for preservation of semen of almost all species (Farstad, 2009). Phillps (1939) made a crucial discovery when he found that egg-yolk added to the semen diluent had a beneficial effect on fertility. Phillips & Lardy (1940) recommended the use of diluent containing equal parts of phosphate buffer and egg-yolk a protective agent against cold shock. Salisbary *et al.,* (1941) presented conception results from field trials with bovine semen diluted in an egg-yolk sodium citrate diluent (EYC). The amount of egg-yolk commonly used in freezing media is between 15% and 30% on a volume to volume basis. Milk and its components (*e. g.* whole milk, milk whey, skimmed milk) are other commonly used diluents for the storage of mammalian spermatozoa (Scherzer *et al.*, 2009). A 10% whole milk or skimmed milk diluent in combination with 7% glycerol and antibiotics has very successfully been used as a diluent for freezing semen for many years. The main disadvantage with the milk extenders is the poor viability of spermatozoa under microscope, which makes the post-thaw evaluations difficult for this reason egg-yolk diluents in combination with Tris and citrate are preferred.

Cryoprotactants

For survival, most of the cell types require an optimum concentration of cryoprotective agent, which confers protection specifically during freezing and thawing. Cryoprotectants are generally classified into two main groups - penetrating which penetrate into the cells (*viz.* methanol, dimethyl sulfoxide, ethylene glycol, glycerol *etc.*) and non-penetrating which can not permeate into the cell (*viz.* polyvinylpyrrolidone, various sugars, protein *etc.*) (Watson, 1990; 1995; 2000; Varisli *et al.*, 2009). For spermatozoa of most mammalian species no cryoprotectant has been found as satisfactory as glycerol, although DMSO has been used alone or in combination with glycerol (Farshad *et al.*, 2009). For rabbit spermatozoa, however, DMSO is the cryoprotectant of choice (Makarevich *et al.*, 2008). Generally, glycerol concentrations of the order of 4-9% (v/v) are used depending on the cooling rate and species. Some sugar and polyols have been shown to give satisfactory results with rapidly frozen bull semen (Hu *et al.*, 2009).

Apart from the major cryoprotectants, other agents like amino acid and amino acid related compounds, butylated hydroxytoluene (BHT), hydrophobic aromatic compounds have cryoprotecting properties on ram, boar stallion, and human spermatozoa (Bamba & Miyagawa, 1992; Sanchez-Partida, 1998; Trimeche *et al.*, 1999; Ehmcke & Schlatt, 2008). Some anti-freeze peptide (Type 1 found in winter flounder) and anti-freeze glycoprotein (from Antarctic cod) have positive cryoprotection of ram spermatozoa when used at 1-10 μg/ ml in a standard diluent containing egg-yolk and glycerol (Payne *et al.*, 1994).

Processing Before Freezing (Equilibration)

Spermatozoa from some species require a pause (above 0°C) of several hours before freezing in order to develop maximal resistance to freezing (Gilbert & Almquist, 1978; Watson, 1990). This was allowed time for membrane changes or ionic fluxes to occur which rendered membranes more rigorous to cooling. This view is supported by the fact that when the spermatozoa are cooled slowly they have less need to holding period before freezing (Ennen *et al.*, 1976). Boar spermatozoa developed considerable resistance to cold shock on incubation for several hours prior to cooling (Pursel *et al.*, 1972) and ram spermatozoa show some evidence of similar effect (Robertson & Watson, 1986). Apparently, acquired resistance to cooling above 0°C may confer an additional resistance to freezing and thawing.

Freezing and Thawing

Generally, after dilution and equilibration the semen sample are packaged into 0.25 ml or 0.5 ml plastic straws. Then the straws are cooled and freezed at different rates (by simple holding the straws on the liquid nitrogen vapour or by computer controlled programmable bio-freezer) prior to storage in liquid nitrogen (-196°C). But several researchers showed that a major portion of cells die during cooling as well as freezing. Although the optimum rate of cooling and freezing not only depends on species but also on optimum concentration of cryoprotectants used (Mortimer *et al.*, 1976; Purdy, 2006).

Cryo-injury to a variety of cell organelles is regarded as being due the two major stresses of cryopreservation, *i.e.*, temperature decrease (cooling) and increase (thawing). Optimum cooling rate for semen of the domestic mammals are generally considered to be in the range of 10-100°C per minute (Watson, 1990). Sudden cooling of ram and bovine spermatozoa from body temperatures to the above freezing temperature affects their motility, (Watson & Martin, 1972) carbohydrate metabolism (Blackshaw, 1958), release of intracellular enzymes (Harrison & White, 1972), lipids (Darin-Bennett *et al.,* 1973) and redistribution of ions (Quinn & White, 1966). Cooling from 37°C to 5°C causes a specific alteration that is related to membrane lipid phase transition, loss of the selective permeability characteristic of biological membranes (Gilmore *et al.,* 2000). These changes are accompanied by morphological changes evident particularly in the acrosome (Watson, 1981b). This injury is the direct result of sudden cooling or "cold shock" depends on the rate of cooling [Morris & Watson, 1984] and on the final temperature to which semen is cooled. This detrimental effect of rapid cooling on spermatozoa may be minimised by introducing exogenous compounds (Watson, 1981a) and changing cooling rate.

Straws are generally thawed by immersion in a water bath at 37°C. Re-warming in hot water (upto 75°C for a few seconds) has generally been shown to improve the motility and acrosomal integrity of ram, bull and stallion spermatozoa (Watson & Martin, 1972; Muiño-Blanco, 2008). Some investigators have found that relatively lower temperature (36 to 45°C) is better for acrosomal maintenance (Chandler *et al.,* 1984). A recent observation that rapid dilution and warming in the temperature range of 5-37°C caused acrosomal damage to boar spermatozoa (Bamba & Cran, 1985) is consistent with these findings. The benefits of fast thawing were not reflected in fertility status (Rugg *et al.,* 1977).

THE CHALLENGE AND RESPONSE

Although current cryopreservation technology is useful, some limitations exist because the post-thaw motility of spermatozoa is too low for some application (restricted to 40- 50%). During cryopreservation a substantial portion of sperm cells undergo damage from thermal, mechanical, chemical and osmotic stresses there-by reducing greatly motility/fertility potential of spermatozoa (Watson, 1990, 1995, 2000). Cell damage during freezing and thawing is believed to be due to extensive dehydration and cellular ice crystallization (Bagchi *et al.,* 2008). Ice crystal mediated damage of plasma membrane is believed to be a major cause of cell death during cryopreservation. A high proportion of cell death has been documented when the transition period from the liquid to solid phase or *vice versa* is prolonged. Cooling from 37 to 5°C causes a specific type of alteration that is related to membrane lipid phase transitions and is very different from those caused by freezing and thawing e.g., osmotic, mechanical stresses (Watson, 1981a, Hammerstedt *et al.,* 1990).The optimum cryopreservation of semen depends not only on the species but also on cryopreservation medium, cryoprotectants, and freeze-thaw protocol.

Media containing the complex extenders such as egg yolk, milk, skim milk, and milk whey are routinely used for cryopreservation of sperm of different species (Farstad, 2009; Scherzer *et al.,* 2009). Despite the use of complex media and cryoprotectants, a substantial portion of the cells die during freezing and thawing. As the complex media contain large numbers of undefined biomolecules (proteins, lipids, carbohydrates), it is rather difficult to analyze the beneficial effects of a particular compound on sperm cryopreservation. Due to occasional outbreaks of avian influenza is a matter of growing concern throughout the world as transportation of frozen or chilled semen exposed to egg yolk could be extremely hazardous. Several countries have in fact, prohibited export and import of frozen animal semen samples containing egg yolk. Animal derived products (such as milk, milk whey, etc,) used as extenders for semen cryopreservation, may also contain hazardous viruses and microbes.

A synthetic medium will be most appropriate for investigating the biochemical basis of sperm cryodamage as well as cryoprotection offered by the cryoprotectants. Mature cauda-epididymal sperm is a better model than the ejaculated sperm because the latter cells are exposed to variety of undefined constituents from the secretions of seminal vesicles, prostrate that may complicate the interpretation of the data. Studies from our laboratory during the last two decades have shown that goat cauda-sperm is a suitable model for investigating the biochemical regulation of sperm motility (Majumder *et al.,* 1990, 1999). Methodologies have been developed for measuring intactness and forward motility of these cells (Majumder *et al.,* 1990, 1999). A method has also been evolved for isolation of highly purified sperm plasma membranes (Rana & Majumder, 1987). It has been investigated the functional characteristics of the cell membrane with special reference to cell adhesion, cell-surface antigens, protein phosphorylation/dephosphorylation mechanisms (Dey & Majumder, 1990; Nath & Majumder, 1999, Jaiswal *et al.,* 2009), lipid phase fluidity, lipid constituents, phospholipid asymmetry (Rana & Majumder, 1990; Chakrabarty *et al.,* 2007). An important advantage of the cauda-sperm model is that spermatozoa can be extracted from the epididymides that can be procured rather easily from the slaughter houses. Studies on cryoprotection mechanism using a cell model will require large amount of spermatozoa that will be rather difficult to procure from the ejaculated mammalian semen samples. Therefore goat cauda sperm is the ideal model for developing a simple sperm cryopreservation technology and to analyze the biochemical mechanism of cryopreservation of these cells.

EPIDIDYMAL SPERM CRYOPRESERVATION

The epididymis is closely apposed tubule to the testicles that fuse with the vasa efferentia at their testicular end and the vas deferens at its distal end (Figure 2). It can be roughly divided into three parts; the enlarged proximal end known as the head - caput, the slender middle region or the corpus, and the pointed tail end or cauda (Figure 2). During the transit the spermatozoa from caput to cauda, it undergo a number of maturational changes, in the course of which they develop the capacity for forward motility and the ability to fertilise the eggs.

The ability to carry a male genetic contribution beyond its natural life span is remarkably important. Cryopreservation of epididymal sperm is one of the methods to conserve genetic resources in mammals. In many cases, due to the lack of technicians and instrument, it is very difficult to collect and freeze epididymal-sperm from extinct and pedigreed animal in the field after their sudden death. If their epididymides are transported to a laboratory and the sperm were collected and frozen there, it would be useful method for conserving mammalian genetic resources. Cryopreserved epididymal spermatozoa would be also useful for the transgenic production of animal, for the conservation of endangered species, and for solving some of the problems of human male infertility- a global social problem.

Limited studies have been carried out for the preservation of epididymal sperm of mammalian species (Luvoni, 2006). Cryopreserved epididymal sperm have been used for rectifying some of the problems of male infertility using intra-cytoplasmic sperm injection (ICSI) (Patrizio, 2000). The investigators used complex media (egg-yolk, milk) and a cryoprotectant (glycerol) for the preservation of epididymal spermatozoa of various species (e.g cat (Hermansson & Axner, 2007), red deer (Fernandez-Santos *et al.,* 2006), spanish ibex (Santiogo-Moreno *et al.,* 2007),

Figure 2. Diagram showing the parts of the testis and epididymis [Redrawn from Odell, W.D. and Moyer, D.L. (1971) In 'Physiology of Reproduction', Mosby, St. Louis, p. 44].

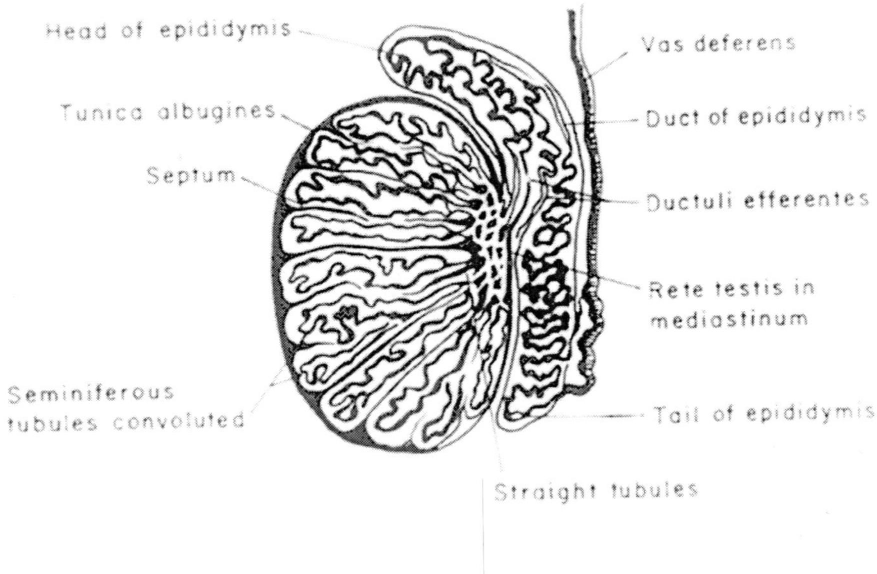

mice (Yamashiro *et al.,* 2007) and rhesus monkey (Dong & Vandevoort, 2009) in liquid nitrogen. Thuwanut et al., 2008 reported that cysteine and vitamin E has cryoprotectant potentiality for cat epididymal spermatozoa (Thuwanut *et al.,* 2008).

DEVELOPMENT OF NOVEL CRYOPRESERVATION TECHNOLOGY

A novel cryopreservation methodology has been developed for the first time using a chemically-defined medium (modified Ringer's solution) and goat cauda-epididymal sperm as the model (Kundu *et al.,* 2000). The cryopreservation model has been developed by careful manipulation of rates of cooling with the help of a computer-controlled bio-freezer by following way.

Preparation of Spermatozoa and Epididymal Plasma

Goat epididymides were collected from theslaughterhouses. Spermatozoa were extracted from the epididymides within 2–3 h of slaughtering (Mandal *et al.,* 1989).

Mature goat epididymal spermatozoa were isolated at room temperature (30 ± 2°C) from the cauda segments of the epididymis by the procedure described by Mandal *et al.,* 1989. Cauda epididymides were cut into four to five pieces with a sharp razor blade and were suspended in modified Ringer's solution (RPS medium -119 mM NaCl, 5 mM KCl, 1.2 mM MgSO4, 10 mM glucose, penicillin G (50 unit/ml), and 16.3 mM potassium phosphate, pH 6.9.) to get the sperm for experimentation. After 5 min, the sperm suspension was filtered through four layers of cotton cheese cloth. Spermatozoa were sedimented by centrifugation at 800*g* for 5 min at room temperature and the pellet was washed twice with RPS medium. The spermatozoal pellet was dispersed in RPS medium, and this spermatozoa preparation was used for the studies. The sperm preparation was highly purified as judged by phase contrast microscopy, and it contained less than 2% broken or damaged cells. The number of spermatozoa in the sample was determined with a hemocytometer and the spermatozoa preparation was left at room temperature for subsequent use. Goat cauda epididymal plasma (EP) was prepared by the procedure described earlier (Mandal *et al.,* 1989). Freshly extracted sperm preparations were centrifuged at 800*g* for 5 min when most of the spermatozoa were removed as a pellet. The resulting supernatant, which appeared to be slightly turbid, were again spun at 14,000*g* for 10 min yielding the cell free EP.. The concentration of EP was expressed as its protein content.

Motility Assay Method

The percentages of forward motility (FM) and total motility (TM) were assayed pre-freeze (initial sperm motility in RPS medium prior to the addition of cryoprotectant) and post-thaw (i.e., after thawing and removing cryoprotectant) by the conventional microscopic method using the hemocytometer as the counter chamber. The motility assay was carried out in the presence of EP (1.2 mg protein/ml) to prevent the adhesion of sperm to glass (Roy & Majumder, 1989). Spermatozoa (0.5 X10^6 cells) were incubated with EP (0.6 mg protein) at room temperature (30 ±2°C) for 1 min in a total volume of 0.5 ml of RPS medium. A portion of the cell suspension was then injected into the hemocytometer. Immediately spermatozoa that showed well-defined FM (FM cells) (cells that moved in small or large circles were excluded) and TM (including all types of motile cells) and total cell numbers were counted under a phase contrast microscope at 400 magnification. The percentages of FM and TM cells were then calculated.

Cryopreservation Procedure

Freezing

The sperm freezing procedure is carried out as described by Kundu *et.al,* 2000. Specified concentrations of reagents were prepared by dissolving them in RPS medium. Sperm preparations were then added to the cryopreservation media in such a way that the concentration of sperm cells was 60-80×10^6 cells per ml. In each experiment the sperm preparation contained about 30-40% forward motility and 50-60% total motility. Aliquots of the sperm suspension were loaded with and without cryoprotectant (i.e. control) into the plastic straws having capacity of 0.5 ml and the open ends of the straws were sealed by polyvinyl chloride powder, which was then dipped in double distilled water for complete sealing. Then the straws were put into the teflon made straw holder and placed inside the computer controlled programmable biofreezer (PTC-1000 C, Apex Instruments, Calcutta, India) for freezing.

The processed sperm preparations were frozen by following protocol from room temperature (30 ± 2^0 C) to 5^0 C at the rate of 0.25^0 C min^{-1}, then from 5^0 C to -20^0 C at the rate of 5^0 C min^{-1}, again from -20^0 C to -100^0 C at the rate of 20^0 C min^{-1}. When the run was completed, the straws were removed from the freezing chamber and immediately plunged into liquid nitrogen (-196^0 C) for storage.

Thawing

After 24 hours, the straws were removed from storage cryocan and rapidly thawed in a 37^0 C water bath for 2-3 minutes. Both ends of the sealed straws were cut by sharp razor blade and the spermatozoa were suspended in RPS medium. The cryoprotectants were removed from the sperm suspension by gentle centrifugation at 800 × g for five minutes at room temperature using a table top centrifuge and pellet was washed twice with RPS medium. Finally, the pellet was suspended in the same medium. Then the motility was determined by the methods described above.

Calculation of Motility Recovery (%)

The motility recovery was calculated by comparing the pre-freeze and post-thaw motilities. If M_b and M_f be the percentage of motility of spermatozoa before and after freezing, then recovery (%) would be $(M_f / M_b) \times 100$.

STATISTICAL ANALYSIS

Results were expressed as means (±) standard deviation. Significant test was carried out by Student's "t" test and compared with standard table. P value of $P<0.02$ was considered statistically significant.

STANDARDIZATION OF FREEZING PROTOCOL USING GLYCEROL (0.87 M) AS CRYOPROTECTANT

Standardization of freezing protocol for cryopreservation of sperm cells has been done by Kundu *et al.,* (2000). In brief, cooling process consisted of four stages of cooling: [a] from room temperature (30 ± 2)°C to 5°C, [b] 5°C to -20°C, [c] -20°C to -100°C (or -50°C), and [d] immersion in liquid nitrogen (-196°C). The cooling rates of individual steps were optimized by a computer controlled programmable biofreezer using 0.87 M glycerol in modified Ringer's solution as cryopreservation medium. When the chamber was cooled at the rate of 5°C per min and 1°C per min from room temperature (30 ± 2°C) to 5°C, all the spermatozoa lost their motility (Figure 3). With the lowering of the rate, the motility recovery first increased up to 0.25°C per min. On further lowering of the rate, the recovery of FM decreased but TM remained same ($p<0.01$). The percent motility recovered was 15 ± 1.2% (FM) and 23 ± 2% (TM) when the cooling rate was 0.5°C per min (Figure 3). The optimum recovery was found to be 32 ± 3% (FM) and 35 ± 2% (TM) at the rate of 0.25°C per min ($p<0.01$) (Figure 3). But motility recovery was 18 ± 1.5% (FM) and 35 ± 2.5% (TM) at the cooling rate 0.2°C per min. So, initial cooling rate 0.25°C per min was better than 0.2°C per min.

The optimum recovery of motility was not only dependent on initial cooling rate but also on initial freezing rate (5°C to -20°C). Freezing at 5°C per min was better than 10°C per min. When the straws were cooled at 10°C per min, all the sperm cells lost their motility. But at 5°C per min the motility recovery was 15 ± 1.2% (FM) and 23 ± 2% (TM) (Figure 3).

In the third step, the cooling and freezing rates were kept constant but different maximum freezing temperatures were used to assess the motility recovery. When the straws were frozen to -50°C prior to transfer into liquid nitrogen, the optimum motility recovery was 16 ± 2% (FM), 34 ± 2% (TM). But when they were cooled to -100°C before transfer into liquid nitrogen, the recovery was 18 ± 1.5% (FM) and 35 ± 2.5% (TM) (Figure 3). This result suggests that cooling to -100°C appeared to be superior to that of -50°C.

An experiment was designed to elucidate the importance of the various stages of cooling on the sperm cryopreservation (Figure 4). Spermatozoa lost their motility completely when the straws were plunged directly into liquid nitrogen either from room temperature or 5°C. But the recovery of FM and TM was 15± 2% and 18 ± 3% when the straws were transferred to liquid nitrogen from -20°C. However, maximal recovery (FM – 32 ± 2%; TM – 35 ± 3%) was obtained when the straws were plunged into liquid nitrogen from -100°C. The data shows that all the three stages of cooling are important for optimal cryopreservation of the cells.

*Figure 3. Effect of different cooling rate on motility recovery of goat-epididymal sperm using glycerol (0.87M) as cryoprotectant. Values indicate the mean ± S.D. of five experiments. *The prefreeze motility (control) was 35±5% for FM and 60 ± 5% for TM, respectively. ** RT represents room temperature (30 ± 2)°C. (Reproduced from Kundu et al., 2000, Cryobiology 40, 117-125)*

Protocol	Motility Recovery* (%)	
	FM	TM
RT** $\xrightarrow{5^\circ C/min}$ 5°C $\xrightarrow{5^\circ C/min}$ -20°C $\xrightarrow{20^\circ C/min}$ -100°C	0	0
RT $\xrightarrow{1^\circ C/min}$ 5°C $\xrightarrow{5^\circ C/min}$ -20°C $\xrightarrow{20^\circ C/min}$ -100°C	0	0
RT $\xrightarrow{0.5^\circ C/min}$ 5°C $\xrightarrow{10^\circ C/min}$ -20°C $\xrightarrow{20^\circ C/min}$ -100°C	0	0
RT $\xrightarrow{0.5^\circ C/min}$ 5°C $\xrightarrow{5^\circ C/min}$ -20°C $\xrightarrow{20^\circ C/min}$ -100°C	15 ± 1.2	23 ± 2
RT $\xrightarrow{0.2^\circ C/min}$ 5°C $\xrightarrow{5^\circ C/min}$ -20°C $\xrightarrow{20^\circ C/min}$ -100°C	18 ± 1.5	35 ± 2.5
RT $\xrightarrow{0.2^\circ C/min}$ 5°C $\xrightarrow{5^\circ C/min}$ -20°C $\xrightarrow{20^\circ C/min}$ -50°C	16 ± 2	34 ± 2
RT $\xrightarrow{0.25^\circ C/min}$ 5°C $\xrightarrow{5^\circ C/min}$ -20°C $\xrightarrow{20^\circ C/min}$ -100°C	32 ± 3	35 ± 2

EFFECTS OF CRYOPROTECTANTS ON MOTILITY RECOVERY

Penetrating Agents

Highly motile spermatozoa dispersed in Ringer's solution, were subjected to the freezing protocol: cooling 0.25°C per min to 5°C, 5°C per min to -20°C, 20°C per min to –100°C, prior to plunging into liquid nitrogen (Kundu *et al.*, 2000). In absence of any cryoprotective agent, all of the spermatozoa lost their motility. Addition of glycerol (0.22 to 0.87 M) caused a dose-dependent increase of sperm motility recovery. The highest recovery of forward and total motility was (32 and 35% respectively) at 0.87 M (Figure 5).Like glycerol, DMSO and ethylene glycol also showed dose-dependent increase of motility recovery. At optimal concentrations, DMSO (1.00 M) and ethylene glycol (1.29 M) were effective to recover sperm motility to the extent of 20% and 13% respectively (Figure 5).Thus these reagents have markedly lower cryoprotection potential than glycerol. The motility recovery of sperm cells was significantly increased in presence of the combination of glycerol and DMSO. The highest motility recovery was found (FM 45 ± 2% and TM 48 ± 2%) at 0.76 M DMSO in presence of glycerol (Figure 5).

Non-Penetrating Agents

Amino Acids (AAs)

In Absence of Other Cryoprotectants

Studies were carried out to investigate the cryoprotecting efficacy of amino acids (e.g., L-proline, L-glutamine, L-histidine, L-arginine, L-lysine, L-alanine and glycine) at a wide range of concentrations (0.02 - 0.2 M) in presence of RPS medium, using the above model system (Kundu *et al.*, 2001). Motility recoveries were relatively higher in presence of alanine, proline (FM 10-15% and TM 15-20%) as compared to glutamine and glycine (FM 5 - 10% and TM 10 - 15%). Little (0 - 5%) motility recovery was found in the presence of histidine. Alanine offered the best cryoprotection (recovery FM 12 ± 1 and TM 19 ± 2%) at

*Figure 4. Cryorecovery of goat epididymal spermmotility after each stage of cooling using glycerol (0.87M) as cryoprotectant Values indicate the mean ± S.D. of five experiments. *The prefreeze motility (control) was 37 ± 3% for FM and 62 ± 2% for TM, respectively. ** RT represents room temperature (30 ± 2)°C. (Reproduced from Kundu et al., 2000, Cryobiology 40, 117-125)*

Protocol	Motility Recovery* (%)	
	FM	TM
RT** → LN_2	0	0
RT $\xrightarrow{0.25°C/min}$ 5°C → LN_2	0	0
RT $\xrightarrow{0.25°C/min}$ 5°C $\xrightarrow{5°C/min}$ -20°C → LN_2	15 ± 2	18 ± 3
RT $\xrightarrow{0.25°C/min}$ 5°C $\xrightarrow{5°C/min}$ -20°C $\xrightarrow{20°C/min}$ -100°C → LN_2	32 ± 2	35 ± 3

*Figure 5. Effect of penetrating cryoprotectants on goat–cauda sperm motility recovery after freezing and thawing. Values indicate the mean ± S.D. of five experiments *The prefreeze motility (control) was 37 ± 3% for FM and 62 ± 2% for TM, respectively.*

SL No	Cryoprotectant (concentration)	Motility recovery* %	
		FM	TM
1	Glycerol (0.87M)	32 ± 3	35 ± 2
2	DMSO (1.0M)	16 ± 3	20 ± 3
3	Ethylene Glycol (1.29M)	10 ± 1	13 ± 1
4	Glycerol (0.87M)+DMSO (0.76M)	45 ± 2	48 ± 2

0.135 M ($p < 0.02$). The highest recoveries were observed in the presence of proline, glutamine, glycine, and histidine at 0.13 M (FM 12 ± 1 and TM 17 ± 2%), 0.1 M (FM 8 ± 1 and TM 11 ± 2%), 0.15 M (FM 8 ± 1 and TM 10 ± 2%) and 0.12 M (FM 4 ± 2 and TM 6 ± 1%), respectively (Kundu *et al.*, 2001) (Figure 6).

In Presence of Other Cryoprotectants

Studies were carried out to investigate the combined action of amino acids with glycerol and glycerol *plus* DMSO (Kundu *et al.*, 2001). In presence of AAs, the cryoprotecting potentiality of glycerol increased (approx. 8-12%). Proline showed concentration dependent- increase (0.01 – 0.02 M) in motility recovery of sperm cells offering maximum cryoprotection (recovery FM 43 ± 2 and TM 46 ± 2%, respectively) at 0.02 M concentration ($p < 0.02$) (Figure 6). The cryoprotection profiles of other amino acids were similar to that of proline. The highest motility recoveries obtained in presence of alanine, glycine, glutamine, and histidine were at 0.04 M (FM 40 ± 3 and TM 42 ± 2%), 0.04 M (FM 38 ± 2 and

*Figure 6. Effects of amino acids on cryopreservation of goat-cauda sperm motility after freezing and thawing. Values indicate the mean ± S.D. of five experiments *The prefreeze motility (control) was 37 ± 3% for FM and 62 ± 2% for TM, respectively.*

Sl No	Cryoprotectant (concentration)	Motility Recovery* %	
		FM	TM
1	L-Lysine	0	0
2	L-Arginine	0	0
3	L-alanine (0.135)	12 ± 1	19 ± 2
4	L-proline (0.13M)	12 ± 1	17 ± 2
5	Glycine (0.15M)	8 ± 1	10 ± 2
6	L-glutamine (0.1M)	8 ± 1	11 ± 2
7	L-Histidine (0.12M)	4 ± 2	6 ± 1
8	Glycerol (0.87M) + L-proline (0.02M)	43 ± 2	46 ± 2
9	Glycerol (0.87M) + DMSO (0.76M) + L-proline (0.02M)	55 ± 3	58 ± 2
10	Glycerol (0.87M) + L-alanine (0.04M)	40 ± 3	42 ± 2
11	Glycerol (0.87M) + DMSO (0.76M) + L-alanine (0.04M)	52 ± 3	54 ± 3
12	Glycerol (0.87M) + Glycine (0.04M)	38 ± 2	42 ± 2
13	Glycerol (0.87M) + DMSO (0.76M) + Glycine (0.04M)	51 ± 2	56 ± 1
14	Glycerol (0.87M) + L-glutamine (0.07M)	40 ± 3	43 ± 2
15	Glycerol (0.87M) + DMSO (0.76M) + L-glutamine (0.06M)	52 ± 2	56 ± 2
16	Glycerol (0.87M) + L-Histidine (0.06M)	38 ± 2	41 ± 2
17	Glycerol (0.87M) + DMSO (0.76M) + L-Histidine (0.04M)	50 ± 2	53 ± 2

TM 42 ± 2%), 0.07 M (FM 40 ± 3 and TM 43 ± 2%) and 0.06 M (FM 38 ± 2 and TM 41 ± 2%), respectively (Figure 6). Thus, the results show that in presence of glycerol, AAs were more effective as cryoprotectants at lower concentrations than those required in the absence of glycerol.

Cryoprotecting potentiality of glycerol was further increased (5-10%) when different concentration of AAs was added to the optimal formulation of glycerol (0.87 M) and DMSO (0.76 M) (Figure 6). The optimal formulation of glycerol (0.87 M) and DMSO (0.76M) showed approx. 48% motility recovery (Figure 5). The best cryoprotection potential (recovery FM 55 ± 3 and TM 58 ± 2%) was observed in the presence of 0.02 M proline ($p < 0.02$) and the motility recoveries in the presence of other AAs (glutamine, alanine, glycine, and histidine) were nearly the same as with proline. The highest motility recoveries were observed at 0.04 M (FM 52 ± 3 and TM 54 ± 3%), 0.04 M (FM 51 ± 2 and TM 56 ± 1%), 0.06 M (FM 52 ± 2 and TM 56 ± 2%), and 0.04 M (FM 50 ± 2 and TM 53 ± 2%) in presence of alanine, glycine, glutamine, and histidine, respectively (Figure 6).

*Figure 7. Effects of carbohydrates on goat –cauda-sperm cryopreservation in terms of motility recovery. Values indicate the mean ± S.D. of five experiments *The prefreeze motility (control) was 37 ± 3% for FM and 62 ± 2% for TM, respectively.*

l 'o	Cryoprotectant (concentration)	Motility Recovery* % FM	TM
	Maltose (0.175M)	17 ±2	20 ± 2
	Trehalose (0.234M)	16 ± 1	18 ± 2
	Raffinose (0.1M)	19 ± 2	22 ± 2
	Dextran 10 kDa (8.42mM)	23 ± 1.5	25 ± 1.5
	Glycerol (0.87M) + Maltose (0.175M)	44 ± 2	47 ± 2
	Glycerol (0.87M) + Trehalose (0.234M)	42 ± 2	46 ± 2
	Glycerol (0.87M) + Raffinose (0.1M)	46 ± 2	50 ± 3
	Glycerol (0.87M) + Dextran 10 kDa (6.27mM)	50 ± 3	53 ± 3
	Glycerol (0.87M) + DMSO (0.76M) + Dextran 10 kDa (6.27mM)	60 ± 3	65 ± 2

Carbohydrates

In The Absence of Other Cryoprotectants

Studies were also carried out to investigate the cryoprotecting efficacy of several low molecular weight carbohydrates (*e.g.* monosaccharide, disaccharide, and trisaccharide) using the goat-epididymal cryopreservation model (Figure 7). After freezing and thawing, all the sperm cells lost their flagellar motility in absence of carbohydrate. Glucose, a monosaccharide has no appreciable cryoprotecting potentiality at a wide range of concentrations (0.01 to 0.65 M), but disaccharides like maltose and trehalose have significant cryoprotective ability to sperm cells. They showed characteristic cryoprotecting potentiality of sperm cells. The cryoprotecting efficacy of disaccharide was biphasic in nature. Maltose caused a dose -dependent (0.058 - 0.175 M) increase of motility recovery of sperm cells. The maximum motility recovery (FM 17 ± 2 and TM 20 ± 2%, respectively) was obtained at 0.175 M. The cryoprotecting efficacy of trehalose was similar to that of maltose. The highest motility recovery (FM-16 ± 1 and TM 18 ± 2%, respectively) was found at 0.234 M (Figure 7). The profile of cryo-recovery in presence of trisaccharide was same as disaccharide. Raffinose (a trisaccharide) showed a dose- dependent (0.33 - 0.1 M) increase in the motility recovery of sperm cells having the highest motility recovery of FM 19 ± 2 and TM 22 ± 2%, respectively, at 0.1 M (Figure 7).

In Presence of Other Cryoprotectants

To increase the percentage of motility recovery of sperm cells, we have added carbohydrates (*e.g.* trehalose, maltose and raffinose) in a fixed concentration of glycerol (0.87 M). All the carbohydrates showed a characteristic cryoprotecting potentiality of sperm cells in presence of glycerol. Cryoprotective efficacy of glycerol significantly increased (15 - 20%) in presence of carbohydrates. Maltose caused a dose dependent (0.058 - 0.175 M) increase in motility recovery of sperm cells and it offered maximum cryoprotection at 0.175

M (recovery FM 44 ± 2% and TM 47 ± 2%, respectively) (Figure 7).The cryoprotection profile of trehalose was similar to that of maltose, but trehalose offered highest motility recovery of 42 ± 2% for FM and 46 ± 2% for TM, respectively, at 0.234 M ($p < 0.02$) (Figure 7).The cryoprotecting efficacy of trisaccharide was slightly higher than disaccharide in presence of glycerol. Raffinose caused a dose dependent (0.33 - 0.1M) increase in motility recovery of frozen spermatozoa and the highest cryoprotection was observed (recovery FM 46 ± 2% and TM 50 ± 3%, respectively) at 0.1 M. Thus it appears that carbohydrates caused a partially additive effect for cryoprotection of sperm cells in presence of glycerol.

Biopolymer

In Absence of Other Cryoprotectants

Studied have been carried out to check the cryoprotecting potentiality of biopolymer dextran (polymer of carbohydrate) using the above mentioned goat-epididymal sperm model (Kundu *et al.,* 2000). All the compounds have significant cryoprotecting potentiality on the sperm cells. Cryoprotecting efficacy of dextrans was biphasic in nature. Initially, with increasing concentration of dextran, the motility recovery increased and at a particular concentration showed maximum cryoprotection (Kundu *et al.,* 2002). With further increase of the dose of dextran, the sperm motility recovery fell slowly. The highest recovery of sperm motility (FM 23 ± 1.5% and TM 25 ± 1.5%) was found with 8.42 mM of 10 kDa dextran (Figure 7).

In Presence of Other Cryoprotectants

To increase the motility recovery and to investigate the cryoprotection property of dextran, different concentrations of dextran have been added (10 kDa) to the fixed concentration of glycerol (0.87 M). There was a concentration-dependent (2.0 - 6.27 mM) increase in motility recovery (approx. 20%) of sperm cells Kundu *et al.,* 2002). The highest motility recovery (FM 50 ± 3 and TM 53 ± 3%, respectively) was found at 6.27 mM dextran (Figure 7).

OPTIMUM FORMULATION

Studies have shown that among the membrane-penetrating cryoprotectants, glycerol, at a concentration of 0.87 M, provides the most effective cryoprotection (recovery of total motility approximately 35%) (Kundu *et al.,* 2000). Addition of amino acids enhanced (approx. 7–10%) the cryoprotection efficacy glycerol and a combination of glycerol and dimethyl sulfoxide. The combined cryoprotecting action of glycerol, dimethyl sulfoxide, and amino acids provided motility recovery as high as 52% (Figure 6). For the formulation of an optimum cryoprotection medium, we have tried different combination of cryoprotectant (e.g. glycerol, DMSO, amino acid, biopolymer etc). The best motility recovery was obtained in combination with dextran and a mixture of two membrane-penetrating compounds, glycerol and DMSO. The percentage recovery of motility increased when different concentrations of 10 kDa dextran were used with the optimum concentrations of glycerol plus DMSO. Maximum recovery of motility (forward motility 60 ± 3% and total motility 65 ± 2%) was observed at a concentration of 10 kDa dextran of 6.27 mM (Figure 7).

MECHANISM OF CRYOPROTECTION ACTION OF CRYOPROTECTANT

It is well known that elevated levels of extracellular reagents will increase osmotic pressure of the media thereby inflicting greater damage to the cells (Liu & Foote, 1998). Consequently each cryoprotectant is expected to have a characteristic optimal concentration for cryosurvival of the cells. Further increase of the level of cryoprotectant

Figure 8. A schematic diagram showing the formation of protective coats due to the interaction of glycerol with phospholipids of the membrane by H-bonding. The H-bond is formed between oxygen atom of the phospholipid head group and OH-group of glycerol. '……… ' lines represents H-bond

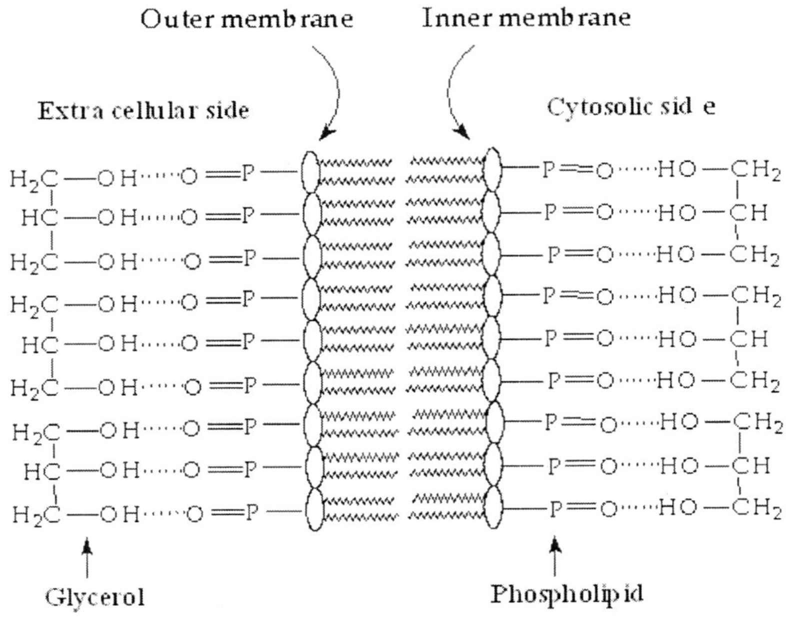

will damage the cells primarily due to elevated osmotic pressure of the media and as a result there will be lower cryosurvival of the cells. The biphasic curves on the action of the cryoprotectants can thus be explained. Although glycerol is widely used as a cryoprotectant for a variety of mammalian cells, its mechanism of action is still not clear. The main cause of cell damage is the formation of intra- and extra-cellular ice-crystals during freezing. Glycerol is believed to protect the cells by minimizing the ice-crystal formation (Bagchi *et al.*, 2008). Glycerol (CH_2OH-CHOH-CH_2OH) has three OH groups and hydrogen atoms of these OH groups are likely to form H-bonding with the oxygen atoms of the phosphate groups of the membrane phospholipids. Ethylene glycol (CH_2OH-CH_2OH) by virtue of having two -OH groups may as well bind to the sperm membrane by H-bonding. In aqueous solution DMSO occurs as a charged molecule [$(CH_3)_2S^+$-O^-] that may interact electrostatically with phosphate head groups of the sperm inner/outer membranes. Based on this postulated mechanism, cryoprotectants will form a coating on the inner as well as the outer cell membranes that may serve as a protective cushion against the ice crystals (Figure 8)

The data shows that the membrane penetrating reagent, glycerol at 0.87 M level offers optimal cryoprotection (motility recovery 35%) of the goat cauda-epididymal spermatozoa (Figure 5).This study also shows that biopolymer dextran, the membrane non-penetrating reagents can serve as efficient cryoprotectant (Figure 7). It is interesting to note that a mixture of biopolymer and glycerol has much better cryoprotecting efficacy than either of the cryoprotectants when used in optimal concentrations (Figure 7). The observed nearly additive cryoprotecting efficacy of these reagents (Figure 7) shows that the mechanisms of action of these cryoprotectants are clearly different. It is generally believed that the major cause of cell damage during cryopreservation is the formation of ice crystals (Bagchi *et al.*, 2008). Several investigators have speculated that the cryoprotectants (*e.g.* glycerol) protect the cells by the formation of H-bond between their –OH groups (Figure 3) and the oxygen atoms of the phospholipid head groups of the membrane thereby forming a protective layer over the cell membrane that serves as a cushion for cryoprotection against the ice-crystals (Liu *et al.*, 1998, Aboagla & Terada, 2003, Bagchi *et al.*, 2008). Biopolymer, by virtue of having innumerable numbers of OH-groups, may as well form a layer on the sperm surface by forming H-bond with the phosphate head groups of the membrane phospholipids. If H-bonding is the mechanism for cryoprotection of cells, glycerol alone at optimal level (0.87 M) will offer full cryoprotection by forming H-bonds with the inner as well as outer cell surfaces. Addition of biopolymer (*e.g.* 6.27 mM, 10 kDa dextran) is not expected to offer additional cryoprotection in presence of optimum glycerol concentration because through H-bonding glycerol will occupy all the free phosphate head groups of the sperm membrane. Furthermore, glycerol, by virtue of its lower molecular size as well as higher optimal concentration as compared to biopolymer, will have an edge for its interaction with the phosphate head groups of the cell membrane. It thus appears that the earlier postulated mechanism of action of cryoprotectants through the H-bonding is not correct. A synthetic polymer, polyvinylpyrrolidone has cryoprotecting potentiality for a variety of cell types including spermatozoa (De-Leeuw *et al.*, 1990). Bamba & Miyagawa (1992) showed that the hydrophobic aromatic compounds (*e.g.* napthalene) serve as cryoprotectants for boar spermatozoa. These compounds are serving as cryoprotectants despite the fact that they are incapable of forming H-bonds with phospholipid head groups as they do not have –OH groups. These observations are consistent with the above view. On the other hand, polyethylene glycol (MW 600 - 1000 kDa), having innumerable –OH groups has no cryoprotecting potentiality on goat sperm cells [Kundu & Majumder, unpublished observation]. These data strengthen further the above contention.

As indicated above glycerol and biopolymer (dextran) cryoprotect the sperm cells by two different mechanisms whose biochemical basis is not clear. During freezing ice-crystals are formed and these crystals formed in the cytoplasmic part of spermatozoa are believed to damage of the plasma membrane thereby causing the death of the cells (Bagchi *et al.*, 2008). Ice-crystal formation process is believed to be associated with the major steps: unit ice-crystals are first formed that finally unite to give rise to a large crystal (Dupuy *et al.*, 1982). For the formation of a unit ice-crystal lattice structure five water molecules are essential in tetrahedral arrangement (Dupuy *et al.*, 1982) and the water molecules are attached to each other with H-bonds. The unit ice-crystals join together through H-bonds to form large ice-crystals. Cryoprotectants may interfere with the formation of ice-crystals and thereby may protect the cells from the ice-crystal-mediated cell damage. Glycerol (0.87 M) that offers optimal cryoprotection of the cells (Figure 5) may interfere with the formation of unit ice-crystal by competing with some of the water molecules of the tetrahedral structure resulting in the formation of distorted rather than well-defined unit ice-crystals. Glycerol may also offer mechanical obstruction for the formation of the tetrahedral arrangement of the water molecules during cooling. Because of the huge excess of the water molecules as compared to glycerol in the cryoprotecting medium, glycerol-mediated blockage of the unit ice-crystal formation will only be partial. As the unit crystals are essential for the formation of large ice-crystals, glycerol will cause partial inhibition of large ice-crystal formation. As glycerol is a non-ionic low molecular weight substance, it enters into the cells. Glycerol thus cryoprotect the cells by inhibiting ice-crystal formation within the cell as well as in the extracellular medium. The observation that glycerol despite its presence in the inner and outer environments of the cells protects only about 32% cells (Figure 5) can be explained based on the proposed limited inhibitory action of the cryoprotectant on ice-crystal formation. It is possible that dextrans, by virtue of their remarkably high molecular size, cause mechanical obstruction for the second phase of ice-crystal formation, *i.e.,* the formation of large ice-crystals from the unit ice-crystals. Because of the large molecular size, the biopolymers will not enter the sperm cells. Thus, the dextrans will cryoprotect the cells from the damaging action of ice-crystals formed in the extracellular medium. Dextran-mediated cryoprotection is only partial (motility recovery approx. 25%) as it cannot protect the cells from the ice-crystals formed intra-cellularly. The data implicate that the intracellular ice-crystal and the ice-crystals formed in the extracellular medium as well damage the cells, and the cryoprotectants protect the cells from the harmful effects of these crystals.

CONCLUSION

The present study has developed for the first time a chemically-defined model system for the cryopreservation of spermatozoa. This model is likely to be highly useful to identify the novel cryoprotectants and to delineate the mechanism of actions of the cryoprotectants. Using the goat cauda-epididymal sperm model, we have already identified cryoprotecting potentiality of different compounds and developed a synthetic medium that permits cryorecovery of about 65% of the motile sperm cells. The novel diluent is thus likely to be highly beneficial for improving the cryopreservation of ejaculated sperm delivered from various species. This improved cryopreservation technology may be useful for solving some of the problems of cattle breeding, conservation of endangered species, sperm banking and human male infertility - a social global problem. The body of research documents that there are many acceptable methods for cryopreserving semen. The focus of research should now be on maximizing fertility with a minimum number of sperm following cryopreservation. To accomplish this goal, alternative

semen cryopreservation media, which is described here will be more beneficial. Exploitation of methodologies such as these will require minimum processing where no centrifugation to remove seminal plasma will be necessary. This should result in greater numbers of viable cells following cryopreservation, due to less physical damage being inflicted on the sperm due to processing. If fewer sperm are used for insemination, then this will result in increased economic advantage to producers by more insemination doses being produced per ejaculate. In addition, less time will be spent in processing semen and will also results in greater efficiency for the producer and consequently greater profits.

FUTURE RESEARCH DIRECTIONS

In common practice, cryopreserved ejaculated semen is extensively used for the AI and other purposes. Our results as demonstrated above are based on epididymal spermatozoa. So question arises whether our exciting observation is applicable for ejaculated sperm. Therefore future direction will be to apply above formulation directly to the ejaculated semen of mammalian species. It is also well recognized that sperm motility is only one of several parameters that define post-thaw sperm quality, but our data consists entirely of motility assessments. Further investigation will be needed in terms of viability, acrosomal integrity, DNA fragmentation status and mitochondrial activity, which would provide a more comprehensive indication of outcomes.

REFERENCES

Aboagla, E. M. E., & Terada, T. (2003). Trehalose-enhanced fluidity of the goat sperm membrane and its protection during freezing. *Biology of Reproduction*, *69*, 1245–1250. doi:10.1095/biolreprod.103.017889

Bagchi, A., Woods, E. J., & Crister, J. K. (2008). Cryopreservation and vitrification: recent advances in fertility preservation technologies. *Expert Review of Medical Devices*, *5*, 359–370. doi:10.1586/17434440.5.3.359

Bamba, K., & Cran, D. G. (1985). Effect of rapid warming of boar semen on sperm morphology and physiology. *Journal of Reproduction and Fertility*, *75*, 133–138. doi:10.1530/jrf.0.0750133

Bamba, K., & Miyagawa, N. (1992). Protective action of aromatic compounds against cold-shock injuries in boar spermatozoa. *Cryobiology*, *29*, 533–536. doi:10.1016/0011-2240(92)90057-9

Blackshaw, A. W. (1958). The effects of incubation temperature and cold shock on the metabolism of ram spermatozoa. *Australian Journal of Biological Sciences*, *11*, 581–588.

Chakrabarty, J., Banerjee, D., Pal, D., De, J., Ghosh, A., & Majumder, G. C. (2007). Shedding off specific lipid constituent from sperm cell membrane during cryopreservation. *Cryobiology*, *54*, 27–35. doi:10.1016/j.cryobiol.2006.10.191

Chandler, J. E., Adkinson, R. W., & Nebel, R. L. (1984). Thawing optimums for bovine spermatozoa processed by three methods and packaged in continental and french straws. *Journal of Dairy Science*, *67*, 398–404. doi:10.3168/jds.S0022-0302(84)81315-6

Darin-Bennett, A., Poulos, A., & White, I. G. (1973). The effect of cold-shock and freeze thawing on the release of phospholipids by ram, bull, and boar spermatozoa. *Australian Journal of Biological Sciences*, *26*, 1409–1420.

De-Leeuw, E. F., De-Leeuw, A. M., Den-Dass, J. H. G., Colenbrander, B., & Verkleij, A. J. (1990). Cold-induced ultrastructural changes in bull and boar sperm plasma membranes. *Cryobiology*, *30*, 32–44.

Dey, C. S., & Majumder, G. C. (1990). Maturation specific type II cyclic AMP- dependent protein kinase in goat sperm plasma membrane. *Biochemistry International*, *21*, 659–665.

Dong, Q., & Vandevoort, C. A. (2009). Effect of egg yolk on cryopreservation of Rhesus monkey ejaculated and epididymal sperm. *Journal of Andrology*, *30*, 309–316. doi:10.2164/jandrol.108.006395

Dupuy, J., Jal, J. F., Ferradou, C., Chieux, P., Wright, A. F., Calemczuk, R., & Angel, C. A. (1982). Controlled nucleation and quasi-ordered growth of ice-crystals from low temperature electrolyte solution. *Nature*, *296*, 138–140. doi:10.1038/296138a0

Ehmcke, J., & Schlatt, S. (2008). Animal models for fertility preservation in the male. *Reproduction (Cambridge, England)*, *136*, 717–723. doi:10.1530/REP-08-0093

Ennen, B. D., Berndtson, W. E., Mortimer, R. G., & Pickett, B. W. (1976). Effect of processing procedures on motility of bovine spermatozoa frozen in 0.25ml straws. *Journal of Animal Science*, *43*, 651–656.

Farshad, A., Khalili, B., & Fazeli, P. (2009). The effect of different concentrations of glycerol and DMSO on viability of Markhoz goat spermatozoa during different freezing temperatures steps. *Pakistan Journal of Biological Sciences*, *12*, 239–245. doi:10.3923/pjbs.2009.239.245

Farstad, W. (2009). Cryopreservation of canine semen – new challenges. *Reproduction in Domestic Animals*, *44*, 336–341. doi:10.1111/j.1439-0531.2009.01418.x

Fernández-Santos, M. R., Esteso, M. C., Soler, A. J., Montoro, V., & Garde, J. J. (2006). Effects of egg yolk and cooling rate on the survival of refrigerated red deer (*Cervus elaphus hispanicus*) epididymal spermatozoa. *Reproduction in Domestic Animals*, *41*, 114–118. doi:10.1111/j.1439-0531.2006.00649.x

Gilbert, G. R., & Almquist, J. O. (1978). Effects of processing procedures on post-thaw acrosomal retention and motility of bovine spermatozoa packaged in 3ml straws at room temperature. *Journal of Animal Science*, *46*, 225–231.

Gilmore, J. A., Liu, J., Woods, E. J., Peter, A. T., & Critser, J. K. (2000). Cryoprotective agent and temperature effects on human sperm membrane permeabilities: Convergence of theoretical and empirical approaches for optimal cryopreservation methods. *Human Reproduction (Oxford, England)*, *15*, 335–343. doi:10.1093/humrep/15.2.335

Gluckman, E. (2009). Ten years of cord blood transplantation: from bench to bedside. *British Journal of Haematology*, *147*, 192–199. doi:10.1111/j.1365-2141.2009.07780.x

Hammerstedt, R. H., Graham, J. K., & Nolan, J. P. (1990). Cryopreservation of mammalian sperm: what we ask them to survive. *Journal of Andrology*, *11*, 73–88.

Harrison, R. A. P., & White, I. G. (1972). Glycolytic enzymes in the spermatozoa and cytoplasmic droplets of bull, boar and ram, their leakage after shock. *Journal of Reproduction and Fertility*, *30*, 105–115. doi:10.1530/jrf.0.0300105

Hermansson, U., & Axner, E. (2007). Epididymal and ejaculated cat spermatozoa are resistant to cold shock but egg yolk promotes sperm longevity during cold storage at 4°C. *Theriogenology*, *67*, 1239–1248. doi:10.1016/j.theriogenology.2007.01.008

Hu, J. H., Li, Q. W., Jiang, Z. L., Yang, H., Zhang, S. S., & Zhao, H. W. (2009). The cryoprotective effect of trehalose supplementation on boar spermatozoa quality. *Reproduction in Domestic Animals*, *44*, 571–575. doi:10.1111/j.1439-0531.2007.00975.x

Jahnel, F. (1938). Resistance of human spermatozoa to deep cold. *Klinische Wochenschrift*, *17*, 1273–1274. doi:10.1007/BF01775125

Jaiswal, B. S., Das, K., Saha, S., Dungdung, S. R., & Majumder, G. C. (2009, September 30). Purification and characterization of a motility initiating protein from caprine epididymal plasma. *Journal of Cellular Physiology*; Epub ahead of print.

Karlsson, J. O. M., & Toner, M. (1996). Long-term storage of tissues by cryopreservation: critical issues. *Biomaterials*, *17*, 243–256. doi:10.1016/0142-9612(96)85562-1

Kawahara, H., Higa, S., Tatsukawa, H., & Obata, H. (2009). Cryoprotection and cryosterilization effects of type I antifreeze protein on E. coli cells. *Biocontrol Science*, *14*, 49–54. doi:10.4265/bio.14.49

Krenek, S., & Berendonk, T. U. (2009). A long-term conservation tool for cell characteristics: cryopreservation of Paramecium caudatum. *Protist*, *160*, 355–363. doi:10.1016/j.protis.2009.03.002

Kundu, C. N., Chakrabarty, J., Dutta, P., Battacharyya, D., Ghosh, A., & Majumdar, G. C. (2002). Effect of dextrans on cryopreservation of goat cauda epididymal spermatozoa using a chemically defined medium. *Reproduction (Cambridge, England)*, *123*, 907–913. doi:10.1530/rep.0.1230907

Kundu, C. N., Chakrabarty, J., Dutta, P., Bhattacharyya, D., Ghosh, A., & Majumder, G. C. (2000). Development of a simple sperm cryopreservation model using a chemically defined medium and goat cauda epididymal spermatozoa. *Cryobiology*, *40*, 117–125. doi:10.1006/cryo.2000.2230

Kundu, C. N., Das, K., & Majumder, G. C. (2001). Effect of amino acids on goat cauda-epididymal sperm cryopreservation using a chemically defined model system. *Cryobiology*, *41*, 21–27. doi:10.1006/cryo.2001.2296

Liu, Z., & Foote, R. H. (1998). Osmotic effects on volume and motility of bull sperm exposed to membrane permeable and nonpermeable agents. *Cryobiology*, *37*, 207–218. doi:10.1006/cryo.1998.2116

Liu, Z., Foote, R. H., & Brockett, C. C. (1998). Survival of bull sperm frozen at different rates in media varying in osmolarity. *Cryobiology*, *37*, 219–230. doi:10.1006/cryo.1998.2117

Luvoni, G. C. (2006). Gamete cryopreservation in the domestic cat. *Theriogenology*, *66*, 101–111. doi:10.1016/j.theriogenology.2006.03.012

Majumder, G. C., Dey, C. S., Haldar, S., & Barua, M. (1990). Biochemical parameters of initiation and regulation of sperm motility. *Archives of Andrology*, *24*, 287–303. doi:10.3109/01485019008987585

Majumder, G. C., Jaiswal, B. S., Nath, D., Banerjee, S., Barua, M., & Sarkar, M. (1999). Biochemistry of sperm motility initiation during epididymal maturation. In Ray, K. P., Krishna, A., & Halder, C. (Eds.), *Comparative Endocrinology and Reproduction*. New Delhi, India: Narosa.

Makarevich, A. V., Chrenek, P., Olexikova, L., Popelkova, M., Turanova, Z., Ostro, A., & Pivko, J. (2008). Post-thaw survival, cell death and actin cytoskeleton in gene-microinjected rabbit embryos after vitrification. *Theriogenology*, *70*, 675–681. doi:10.1016/j.theriogenology.2008.04.043

Mandal, M., Banerjee, S., & Majumder, G. C. (1989). Stimulation of forward motility of goat cauda epididymal spermatozoa by a sperm glycoprotein factor. *Biology of Reproduction*, *41*, 983–989. doi:10.1095/biolreprod41.6.983

Mantegazza, P. (1866)... *R.C. Ist. Lombardo*, *3*, 183–196.

Mazur, P. (1963). Kinetics of water loss from cells at subzero temperatures and the likelihood of intracellular freezing. *The Journal of General Physiology*, *47*, 347–369. doi:10.1085/jgp.47.2.347

Mazur, P. (1965). The role of cell membranes in the freezing of yeast and other signal cells. *Annals of the New York Academy of Sciences*, *125*, 658–676. doi:10.1111/j.1749-6632.1965.tb45420.x

Mazur, P. (1970). Cryobiology: the freezing of living systems. *Science*, *168*, 939–949. doi:10.1126/science.168.3934.939

Morris, G. J., & Watson, P. F. (1984). Cold shock-a widespread cellular reaction. *Cryo Letters*, *5*, 352–372.

Mortimer, R. G., Berndtson, W. E., Ennen, B. D., & Pickett, B. W. (1976). Influence of glycerol concentration and freezing rate on post-thaw motility of bovine spermatozoa in continental Straws. *Journal of Dairy Science*, *59*, 2134–2137. doi:10.3168/jds.S0022-0302(76)84499-2

Muiño-Blanco, T., Pérez-Pé, R., & Cebrián-Pérez, J. A. (2008). Seminal plasma proteins and sperm resistance to stress. *Reproduction in Domestic Animals*, *43*, 18–31. doi:10.1111/j.1439-0531.2008.01228.x

Muldrew, K., & McGann, L. E. (1990). Mechanisms of intracellular ice formation. *Biophysical Journal*, *57*, 525–533. doi:10.1016/S0006-3495(90)82568-6

Nath, D., & Majumder, G. C. (1999). Maturation dependent modification of protein phosphorylation profile of isolated goat sperm plasma membrane. *Journal of Reproduction and Fertility*, *115*, 29–37. doi:10.1530/jrf.0.1150029

Norman, C., Johnson, C. E., Porterfield, I. D., & Dunbar, R. S. (1958). Effect of pH on the Life-Span and Metabolism of Bovine Sperm Kept at Room Temperatures. *Journal of Dairy Science*, *41*, 1803–1812. doi:10.3168/jds.S0022-0302(58)91167-6

Parkes, A. S. (1945). Preservation of human Spermatozoa at Low Temperatures. *British Medical Journal*, *2*, 212. doi:10.1136/bmj.2.4415.212

Patrizio, P. (2000). Cryopreservation of epididymal sperm. *Mol. Cell. Endrol.*, *169*, 11–14. doi:10.1016/S0303-7207(00)00344-0

Payne, S. R., Oliver, J. E., & Upreti, G. C. (1994). Effect of antifreeze proteins on the motility of ram spermatozoa. *Cryobiology*, *31*, 180–184. doi:10.1006/cryo.1994.1021

Phillips, P. H. (1939). Preservation of bull semen. *The Journal of Biological Chemistry*, *130*, 415.

Phillips, P. H., & Lardy, H. A. (1940). A yolk-buffer pabulum for the preservation of bull semen. *Journal of Dairy Science*, *23*, 399–404.

Pitt, R. E. (1992). Thermodynamics and intracellular ice formation. In Steponkus, P. (Ed.), *Advances in Low-Temperature Biology* (*Vol. 1*, pp. 63–99). London: JAI press.

Polge, C., Smith, A. U., & Parkes, A. S. (1949). Revival of spermatozoa after vitrification and dehydration at low temperature. *Nature*, *164*, 666–668. doi:10.1038/164666a0

Purdy, P. H. (2006). A review on goat sperm cryopreservation. *Small Ruminant Research*, *63*, 215–225. doi:10.1016/j.smallrumres.2005.02.015

Pursel, V. G., Johnson, L. A., & Schulman, L. L. (1972). Interaction of extender composition and incubation period on cold shock susceptibility of boar spermatozoa. *Journal of Animal Science*, *35*, 580–584.

Quinn, P. J., & White, I. G. (1966). The effect of cold shock and deep freezing on the concentration of major cations in spermatozoa. *Journal of Reproduction and Fertility*, *12*, 263–270. doi:10.1530/jrf.0.0120263

Rana, A. P. S., & Majumder, G. C. (1987). Factors influencing the yield and purity of goat sperm plasma membranes isolated by means of an aqueous two- phase polymer system. *Preparative Biochemistry*, *17*, 261–281. doi:10.1080/00327488708062493

Rana, A. P. S., & Majumder, G. C. (1990). Changes in the fluidity of the goat sperm plasma membrane in the transit from caput to cauda epididymis. *Biochemistry International*, *21*, 797–803.

Robertson, L., & Watson, P. F. (1986). Calcium transport in diluted or cooled ram semen. *Journal of Reproduction and Fertility*, *77*, 177–185. doi:10.1530/jrf.0.0770177

Roy, N., & Majumder, G. C. (1989). Purification and characterization of an antisticking factor from goat epididymal plasma that inhibits sperm–glass and sperm–sperm adhesion. *Biochimica et Biophysica Acta*, *991*, 114–122.

Rugg, C. D., Berndtson, W. E., Mortimer, R. G., & Pickett, B. W. (1977). Effect of Thawing Procedures on Fertility of Bovine Spermatozoa Frozen in. 25-ml Straws. *Journal of Animal Science*, *44*, 266–270.

Salisbury, G. W., Fuller, H. K., & Willett, E. L. (1941). Preservation of Bovine Spermatozoa in Yolk-Citrate Diluent and Field Results from its Use. *Journal of Dairy Science*, *24*, 905–910.

Sanchez-Partida, L. G., Setchell, B. P., & Maxwell, W. M. C. (1998). Effect of compatible solutes and diluent composition on the post thaw motility of ram sperm. *Reproduction, Fertility, and Development*, *10*, 347–357. doi:10.1071/R98053

Santiago-Moreno, J., Toledano-Díaz, A., Dorado, J., Pulido-Pastor, A., Coloma, M. A., & López-Sebastián, A. (2007). Recovery and cryopreservation of Spanish ibex epididymal spermatozoa. *Archives of Andrology*, *53*, 309–316. doi:10.1080/01485010701730674

Scherzer, J., Fayrer-Hosken, R. A., Aceves, M., Hurley, D. J., Ray, L. E., Jones, L., & Heusner, G. L. (2009). Freezing equine semen: the effect of combinations of semen extenders and glycerol on post-thaw motility. *Australian Veterinary Journal*, *87*, 275–279. doi:10.1111/j.1751-0813.2009.00452.x

Shannon, P. (1965). Contribution of seminal plasma, sperm numbers, and gas phase to dilution effects of bovine spermatozoa. *Journal of Dairy Science*, *48*, 1357–1361. doi:10.3168/jds.S0022-0302(65)88463-6

Shannon, P., & Curson, B. (1984). Effect of storage temperature on the viability and fertility of bovine sperm diluted and stored in Caprogen. *New Zealand Journal of Agricultural Research*, *27*, 173–177.

Sone, M., Chikyu, M., Yoshida, M., Bamba, K., & Ogasa, A. (1992). Prolonged storage of boar semen in liquid form. *Jpn. J. Swine Sci.*, *29*, 41–50.

Thuwanut, P., Chatdarong, K., Techakumphu, M., & Axner, E. (2008). The effect of antioxidants on motility, viability, acrosome integrity and DNA integrity of frozen thawed epididymal cat spermatozoa. *Theriogenology*, *70*, 233–740. doi:10.1016/j.theriogenology.2008.04.005

Toner, M. (1993). Nucleation of ice crystals inside biological cells. In Steponkus, P. (Ed.), *Advances in Low-Temperature Biology* (*Vol. 2*, pp. 1–51). London: JAI press.

Toner, M., Cravalho, E. G., & Karel, M. (1990). Thermodynamics and kinetics of intracellular ice formation. *Journal of Applied Physics*, *67*, 1582–1592. doi:10.1063/1.345670

Trimeche, A., Yvon, J. M., Vidament, M., Palmer, E., & Magistrini, M. (1999). Effects of glutamine, proline, histidine and betaine on post-thaw motility of stallion spermatozoa. *Theriogenology*, *52*, 181–191. doi:10.1016/S0093-691X(99)00120-X

Uhlmann, D. R. (1973). A kinetic treatment of glass formation. *Journal of Non-Crystalline Solids*, *7*, 337–348. doi:10.1016/0022-3093(72)90269-4

Van Denmark, N. L., & Sharma, U. D. (1957). Preliminary Fertility Results from the Preservation of Bovine Semen at Room Temperatures. *Journal of Dairy Science*, *40*, 438–439.

Varisli, O., Uguz, C., Agca, C., & Agca, Y. (2009). Effect of chilling on the motility and acrosomal integrity of rat sperm in the presence of various extenders. *Journal of the American Association for Laboratory Animal Science; JAALAS*, *48*, 499–505.

Watson, P. F. (1981a). The effects of cold shock on sperm cell membranes. In Morris, G. J., & Clarke, A. (Eds.), *Effect of Low Temperature on Biological Membranes* (pp. 189–218). London: Academic Press.

Watson, P. F. (1981b). The roles of lipid and protein in the protection of ram spermatozoa at 5°C by egg-yolk lipoprotein. *Journal of Reproduction and Fertility*, *62*, 483–492. doi:10.1530/jrf.0.0620483

Watson, P. F. (1990). Arficial insemination and the preservation of semen. In Lamming, G. M. (Ed.), *Marshall's Physiology of Reproduction* (*Vol. 2*, pp. 747–869). New York: Churchill Livingstone.

Watson, P. F. (1995). Recent development and concepts in the cryopreservation of spermatozoa, the assessment of their post thawing function. *Reproduction, Fertility, and Development*, *7*, 871–891. doi:10.1071/RD9950871

Watson, P. F. (2000). The causes of reduced fertility with cryopreserved semen. *Animal Reproduction Science*, *60-61*, 481–492. doi:10.1016/S0378-4320(00)00099-3

Watson, P. F., & Martin, I. C. A. (1972). A comparison of changes in the acrosomes of deep-frozen ram and bull spermatozoa. *Journal of Reproduction and Fertility*, *28*, 99–101. doi:10.1530/jrf.0.0280099

Witte, T. S., Schafer-Somi, S., Kuchar, A., Mostl, E., Iben, C., & Aurich, C. (2009). Effect of hen's egg yolk on capacitation and acrosome reaction of diluted canine spermatozoa. *Animal Reproduction Science*, *110*, 293–305. doi:10.1016/j.anireprosci.2008.01.022

Woods, E. J., Benson, J. D., Agca, Y., & Critser, J. K. (2004). Fundamental cryobiology of reproductive cells and tissues. *Cryobiology*, *48*, 146–156. doi:10.1016/j.cryobiol.2004.03.002

Yamashiro, H., Han, Y. j., Sugawara, A., Tomioka, I., Hoshino, Y., & Sato, E. (2007). Freezability of rat epididymal sperm induced by raffinose in modified Krebs-Ringer bicarbonate (mKRB) based extender solution. *Cryobiology*, *55*, 285–294. doi:10.1016/j.cryobiol.2007.08.011

Yang, H., & Tiersch, T. R. (2009). Current status of sperm cryopreservation in biomedical research Fish models: Zebrafish, medaka, and Xiphophorus. *Comparative Biochemistry and Physiology*, *149*(Part C), 224–232.

KEY TERMS AND DEFINITIONS

Cryopreservation: Preservation of biological material at low temperature (generally -196 ^{0} C for long time.

Spermatozoa: The mature fertilizing gamete of a male organism, usually consisting of a round or cylindrical nucleated cell, a short neck, and a thin long tail by which it moves to fertilize the female ovum.

Biopolymer: A macromolecule in a living organism that is formed by linking together several smaller molecules, as a protein from amino acids, DNA from nucleotides, Dextran from carbohydrates etc.

Cryoprotectant: A special type of compounds which protect the cell from cold shock during freeing and thawing. e.g. Glycerol, DMSO etc

Synthetic medium: A solution composed of different synthetic compounds.

Goat: A hollow-horned, bearded ruminant mammals of the genus *Capra*, originally of mountainous areas of the Old World, especially any of the domesticated forms of *C. hircus*, raised for wool, milk, and meat.

Epididymis: The epididymis is closely apposed tubule to the testicles that fuse with the vasa efferentia at their testicular end and the vas deferens at its distal end. It can be roughly divided into three parts; the enlarge proximal end known as the head - caput, the slender middle region or the corpus, and the pointed tail end or cauda. During the transit the spermatozoa from caput to cauda, it undergo a number of maturational changes, in the course of which they develop the capacity for forward motility and the ability to fertilise the eggs.

Chapter 16

Analysis and Prediction of DNA-Recognition by Zinc Finger Proteins: Applications in Genome Modification

Anita Sarkar
Indian Institute of Technology (IIT), India

Sonu Kumar
Indian Institute of Technology (IIT), India

Ankita Punetha
Indian Institute of Technology (IIT), India

Abhinav Grover
Indian Institute of Technology (IIT), India

Durai Sundar
Indian Institute of Technology (IIT), India

ABSTRACT

Zinc fingers are the most abundant class of DNA-binding proteins encoded in the eukaryotic genomes. Custom-designed zinc finger proteins attached to various DNA-modifying domains can be used to achieve highly specific genome modification, which has tremendous applications in molecular therapeutics. Analysis of sequence and structure of the zinc finger proteins provides clues for understanding protein-DNA interactions and aid in custom-design of zinc finger proteins with tailor-made specificity. Computational methods for prediction of recognition helices for C2H2 zinc fingers that bind to specific target DNA sites could provide valuable insights for researchers interested in designing specific zinc finger proteins for biological and biomedical applications. In this chapter, we describe the zinc finger protein-DNA interaction patterns, challenges in engineering the recognition-specificity of zinc finger proteins, the computational methods of prediction of proteins that recognize specific target DNA sequence and their applications in molecular therapeutics.

DOI: 10.4018/978-1-61692-004-3.ch016

INTRODUCTION

The Human Genome Project (HGP) was a landmark achievement for science in more ways than one. The immense data generated by this effort, and thereafter, has given us a holistic view of our genetic make-up. The pool of refined data that we obtain as a result of this endeavor will be the reference source for all future biomedical research. Although the human genome is almost 99.9% similar in everybody, individuality stems from the millions of single-base DNA mutations that vary from person to person. These are also the reason for every individual's varying susceptibility towards cardiovascular disease, diabetes, arthritis, cancers etc. and a determinant of how that person reacts to environmental factors. Deft mining of the biological data generated by the HGP to obtain useful information is essential for researchers who are working in the areas of Genomics and Proteomics. As a result, a new field of science called Computational Genomics and Bioinformatics has emerged, in which the focus is on developing efficient algorithms and computational tools to obtain valuable information which is of interest to the user. The design of such tools and databases is such that the user is readily able to extract useful information from the ever-rising pool of biological sequence and structure data.

The human genome has gene-rich (G≡C rich) and gene-poor (A=T rich) centers. The G≡C rich regions frequently appear adjacent to the gene-rich areas, acting as barriers between genes and junk DNA and aiding gene regulation. This is thus, taken as an indicative in certain computational tools, like those designed for gene identification to detect the presence of genes.

Gene expression in all organisms is controlled by DNA-protein complexes. Every person carries, approximately, half a dozen defective genes, but remains ignorant about their susceptibility till a close relation suffers from a genetic disease. The easy availability of complete genomes has provided a new platform for developing new therapeutic strategies by modulating the transcription of the gene(s) of interest.

Protein-nucleic acid interaction remains the central theme in the area of molecular recognition and transcription factors have been given a priority for many reasons for research in this area. Transcription factors are proteins that regulate gene expression by binding to the promoter elements lying upstream of genes and either facilitate or inhibit transcription. Transcription factors are composed of two essential functional regions: a DNA-binding domain and an activator domain. The DNA-binding domain consists of amino acids that recognize specific DNA bases at the beginning of transcription. Transcription factors are typically classified according to the structure of its DNA-binding domain, which are of one of the following types: zinc fingers, helix-turn-helix, leucine zipper, helix-loop-helix, and high mobility groups (Sauer, 1990; Schwabe & Rhodes, 1991). The class of zinc finger proteins (ZFPs) is especially fascinating due to its ability to recognize DNA, RNA as well as other proteins. Though there are pointers to predict DNA-protein interactions, changing binding specificities of existing transcription factors and probably even devising a rational way to design proteins that would recognize and bind to a particular target DNA sequence, there is no simple formula (or code) for DNA recognition by transcription factors. Advancements in design and engineering of DNA-binding proteins have led to the use of zinc fingers in gene targeting for therapeutic purposes. In this chapter, we discuss the progress towards computational prediction of DNA recognition of zinc finger proteins, the different approaches developed to design them and its potential applications in biomedicine in areas such as cancer, monogenic diseases and detecting infectious disease-causing pathogens. Several important leads have been obtained in such applications for the treatment of Severe Combined Immunodeficiency Disease (SCID) and infectious diseases such as hepatitis B and HIV,

Alzheimer's disease, peripheral artery disease, diabetic neuropathy, heart disease etc.

Zinc Finger Proteins

Zinc finger are those proteins which contain a finger-shaped fold, that coordinate zinc ions with a combination of cysteine and histidine residues for their fold stabilization, to achieve (mostly regulatory) functions in eukaryotic cells by binding to DNA, RNA or other proteins. Zinc fingers are naturally present in the nucleus of each organism, where their function is to regulate gene activity by binding to the latter and turning them on or off. They are also commonly used by the cell's machinery for gene splicing.

The modular structure of zinc finger (ZF) motifs and modular recognition by ZF domains make them the most versatile of the DNA recognition motifs for designing artificial DNA binding proteins (Beerli & Barbas, 2002; Pabo, Peisach, & Grant, 2001). Each ZF motif consists of about 30 amino acids and folds into ββα structure, which is stabilized by chelation of a zinc ion by the conserved Cys2His2 residues. The ZF motifs bind DNA by inserting the α-helix into the major groove of the DNA double helix (Pavletich & Pabo, 1991). The ZF motifs bind DNA by inserting the α-helix into the major groove of the DNA double helix (Kandavelou, Mani, Durai, & Chandrasegaran, 2005).

Each finger primarily binds to a triplet within the DNA substrate (Figure 1A). Key amino acid residues at positions –1, +1, +2, +3, +4, +5 and +6 relative to the start of the α-helix of each ZF motifs contribute to most of the sequence specific interactions with the DNA site (Elrod-Erickson & Pabo, 1999; Pavletich & Pabo, 1991; Shi & Berg, 1995). These amino acids can be changed while maintaining the remaining amino acids as a consensus backbone to generate ZF motifs with different triplet sequence specificities (Desjarlais & Berg, 1993; Wolfe, Greisman, Ramm, & Pabo, 1999). Binding to longer DNA sequences is achieved by linking several of these ZF motifs in tandem to form zinc finger proteins (Figure 1B) (Alwin et al., 2005; Beerli, Segal, Dreier, & Barbas, 1998; J. S. Kim & Pabo, 1998; Q. Liu, Segal, Ghiara, & Barbas, 1997). The designed ZFPs provide a powerful platform technology since other functionalities like non-specific FokI cleavage domain (N), transcription activator domains (A), transcription repressor domains (R) and methylases (M) can be fused to a ZFPs to form respectively zinc finger nucleases (ZFN) (Alwin et al., 2005; Y. G. Kim, Cha, & Chandrasegaran, 1996; Mani, Kandavelou, Dy, Durai, & Chandrasegaran, 2005; Smith et al., 2000) zinc finger transcription activators (ZFA) (Bartsevich, Miller, Case, & Pabo, 2003; Dai et al., 2004; P. Q. Liu et al., 2001; Rebar, 2004; Rebar et al., 2002; Zhang et al., 2000), zinc finger transcription repressors (ZFR) (Bartsevich & Juliano, 2000; Ren, Collingwood, Rebar, Wolffe, & Camp, 2002; Snowden et al., 2003) and zinc finger methylases (ZFM) (McNamara, Hurd, Smith, & Ford, 2002; Xu & Bestor, 1997). The binding of DNA and protein is mainly dependent upon chemical and stereochemical factors.

Chemical Factors

The intrinsic ability of a given residue and a base to produce non-covalent interaction determines the chemical rules of binding. On studying the chemical features of amino acid residues and DNA bases, the possible partners can be determined. Binding specificity stems from the chemical contacts made between the amino acid side chains and the nucleotide bases in the major groove. Some amino acids have stronger binding specificity than others due to their ability to form strong hydrogen bonds and hydrophobic interactions. Others have weak interactions and hence are not very important for determining binding specificity. Serine is a special case as its side chain can act as both hydrogen bond acceptor as well as hydrogen bond donor and consequently,

Figure 1. A schematic representation of zinc finger protein and its target double-stranded DNA site. (A) The ββα–structure of a single zinc finger protein domain (ZFP) bound to three base DNA target site (B) Diagram of a three zinc finger domain protein (Zif268) wrapping around the target DNA; the zinc finger amino acid side chains at the alpha helical positions -1, 3 and 6 makes sequence-specific hydrogen bond interactions with the nucleotides on the top DNA strand; a cross-strand interaction to the complementary DNA strand is also depicted (amino acid side chain at position 2 makes the cross-strand interaction)

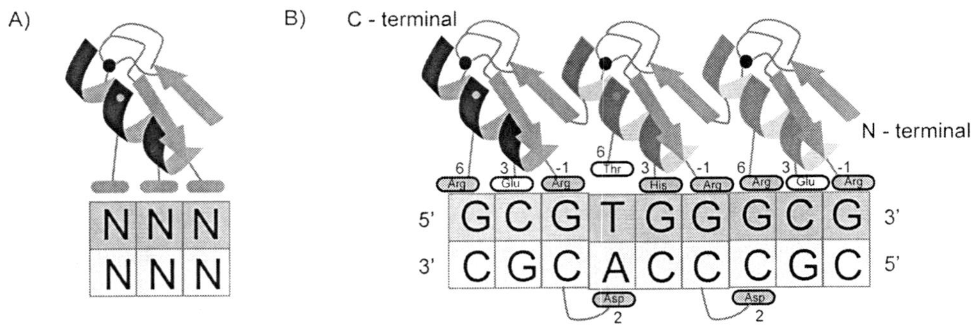

bind to any base. Some residues form bridges between two nucleotides either on the same strand or on different DNA strands, depending upon the distances between the two interacting chemical groups. Besides these considerations, the size and chemical nature of the amino acid residues also play a decisive role in bond formation with DNA bases (Suzuki, 1994).

Stereochemical Factors

Members of the same family of proteins have a specific binding geometry and consequently they make contact with the amino acid and base positions following a similar pattern. Binding geometries are determined by two major structural factors- tight fitting of the DNA-protein surfaces and the position-matching of the DNA-protein residues. Further, binding geometry is limited by the requirement of at least three contacts between the recognition helix and the DNA base for confirming sequence specificity. Thus, to determine binding geometry both the specific (comprising of the direct protein –DNA residue interactions) and non-specific (interactions between protein-sugar and protein-phosphate) interactions have to be taken into account. The pattern of binding can be derived using information from NMR and crystal structures and refined further using data from biochemical and genetic experiments (Suzuki, Brenner, Gerstein, & Yagi, 1995).

The stereochemical pattern defines the binding of the recognition helix to the DNA major groove. Further, to specify the stereochemical interactions, the sizes of the residues that interact with the DNA bases must be known. With this information, the positions in the transcription factors that specifically target the nucleotides become evident and show the compatibility of the amino acid residue sizes at these positions (Suzuki, Gerstein, & Yagi, 1994).

Recognition Helix

Alpha helices are the predominant secondary structures in transcription factors that form the interaction surface, aiding in the recognition of their DNA counterparts in the major groove. The recognition helices are between 7-12 residues long and cover the important interaction sites. All DNA recognition helices of eukaryotic transcription factors, excluding ZFPs, share common features

Figure 2. Custom-designed zinc finger protein can be fused to different DNA modification domains that have applications in functional genomics and molecular therapeutics. (A) Highly specific custom-designed zinc finger proteins can be fused to nuclease domain to achieve targeted chromosomal cleavage, recombination and site-specific gene correction. (B) Zinc finger domains attached to methyltransferase can find applications in turning-off gene expression. (C) Activator domains fused to custom-designed zinc finger domains can be employed for activation (turn-on) of specific genes. (D) Zinc finger domains fused to repressor domains can find applications to repress (turn-off) specific genes.

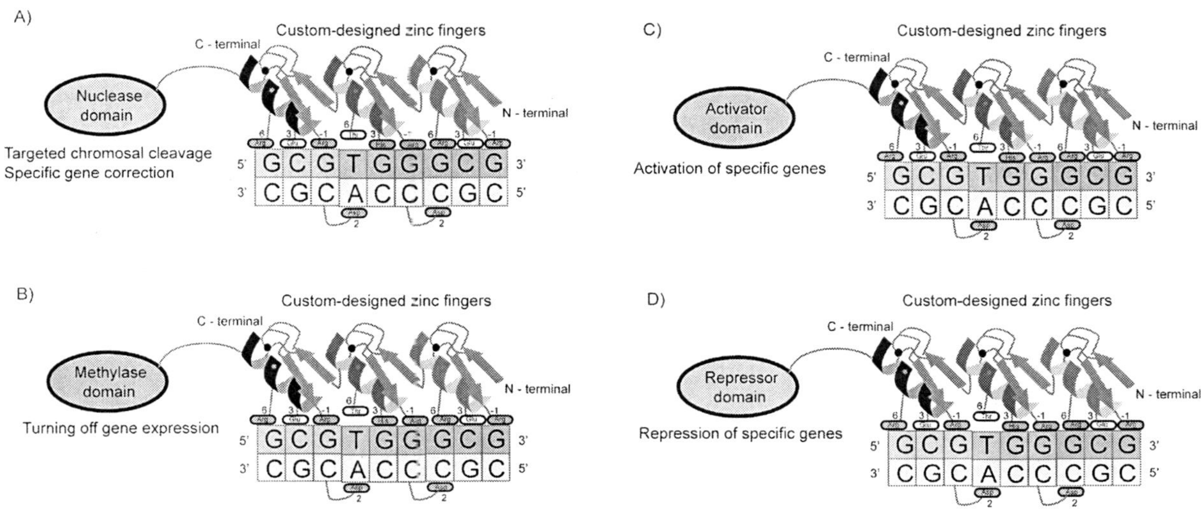

in their amino acid primary structures (Suzuki, 1993). This makes dealing with ZFPs challenging.

Applications (of Engineered Zinc Finger Protein Technology)

The capability of fusing zinc finger proteins with effector domains has led to the technology of engineering chimeric DNA-modifying enzymes (Figure 2). A variety of catalytic domains that act directly on DNA, namely DNA methyltransferase, integrase (W. Tan, Zhu, Segal, Barbas, & Chow, 2004), resolvase and nuclease (Carroll, 2004; Urnov et al., 2005), combined with designer zinc fingers can be employed to modify DNA in a site-specific manner at a desired chromosomal locus. By fusing zinc finger peptides to activator or repressor domains, genes can be selectively switched on and off.

Zinc fingers find their major applications in gene regulation using transcription factors (Figure 2C). The designer transcription factors (an activator domain fused to custom-designed zinc finger protein) can be used for validating genes as drug targets and can also be used for human therapeutics (Jamieson, Miller, & Pabo, 2003). Several studies on how artificial transcription factors based on zinc fingers can target the promoter region in order to control endogenous gene expression have been reported in literature (Papworth, Kolasinska, & Minczuk, 2006). These include up-regulation of the human erythropoietin gene (EPO1) (Zhang et al., 2000), the vascular endothelial growth factor A (VEGF-A) (P. Q. Liu et al., 2001), the erbB-3 protoncogene (Beerli, Dreier, & Barbas, 2000) as well as silencing of the multidrug resistance 1 gene (MDR1) (also known as ABCB1), the erbB-2 protooncogene (Beerli et al., 2000) the peroxisome proliferator activated receptor-γ gene (PPARγ) (Ren et al., 2002) and checkpoint kinase 2 (CHK2) (S. Tan et al., 2003). Regulation of expression of specific genes using zinc finger artificial transcription factors in mammalian cell cultures were the first reported successful experiments (Beerli & Barbas, 2002; Segal & Barbas, 2001). Studies are underway to utilize vascular zinc finger proteins, that activate endothelial growth factor (VEGF), to treat human peripheral arterial disease by stimulating vascular growth (Klug, 2005; Papworth et al., 2006).

Zinc finger proteins have also been fused to independent repressor domains Kruppel associated box (KRAB), ERF repressor domain (ERD), Mad SID or even parts of TATA-box binding protein (TBP) to generate transcription factors (Figure 2D) (Bartsevich et al., 2003; Beerli et al., 1998; Li et al., 2008; Stege, Guan, Ho, Beachy, & Barbas, 2002; Thiesen, Bellefroid, Revelant, & Martial, 1991; C. Tian et al., 2009; C. Y. Tian, Zhang, & He, 2006).

Gene silencing by targeted DNA methylation has potential applications in basic research and therapy (Figure 2B). Though progress in this area has been little slow because of the toxicity of the methylase domains, there have been reports where zinc finger domain-methylase fusion protein was selected to bind the p53 site from the p21WAF1/CIP1 gene to achieve targeted methylation of the oligonucleotides that contained specific binding sites *in vitro* (Xu & Bestor, 1997). Additionally, methylation has also be shown to target *in vivo* to a potentially broad range of sequences using specifically engineered zinc-finger proteins (Carvin, Parr, & Kladde, 2003).

Another application of zinc fingers is the application of zinc finger-nuclease domain fusions (ZFN) to create a DNA double strand break at specific genomic location (Durai et al., 2005; Moehle et al., 2007). These can be used in targeted gene therapy strategies and in targeted engineering of plant and mammalian genomes (Figure 2A). Double-stranded breaks stimulate natural DNA-repair mechanism of the cell at the specific locus. ZFNs has been reported in manipulation of genomes of many higher organisms including Drosophila melanogaster, Caenorhabditis elegans, tobacco, various types of mammalian cells (Carroll, 2008) and zebra fish (Doyon et al., 2008). Clinical trials are underway to evaluate the disruption of CCR5 gene in CD4+ human T-cells using ZFNs and look at a potential treatment for HIV/AIDS. Monogenic disorders such as X-linked severe combined immune deficiency (SCID) (Urnov et al., 2005), sickle-cell anemia (SCA), haemophilia etc. are currently being studied to replace the gene copy with an extra chromosomal DNA donor by means of homologous recombination using ZFNs. This gene correction would be possible by employing a ZFN at or near the location of the mutation.

PREDICTING THE RECOGNITION OF DNA BY ZINC FINGER PROTEINS COMPUTATIONALLY

Background and Challenges

A protein domain can be designed to bind to a particular sequence with high specificity (Pavletich & Pabo, 1991). This is convenient from a technical stand-point because DNA-binding module fused to a functional domain is relevant to the specific experimental goal encoded by a single chimeric cDNA which the cell eventually transcribes and translates. Evolution has favored the degeneracy of transcription factor binding sequences to confer different levels of activity to different promoters. But out of the predicted 1850 transcription factors in the human genome, very few have well-characterized binding specificities. The challenge lies in characterizing these specificities for identifying their target genes and their probable mode of transcriptional regulatory control. High throughput techniques simplify and accelerate the understanding of the locations and combinatorial interaction mode of transcription factors. This dearth of experimental data poses major challenges to computational prediction of ZFPs and even if the predicted ZFPs bind well *in vitro* this may not be the case observed *in vivo*.

The versatility of ZFs stems from their modular structure and recognition (Pabo et al., 2001). No simple DNA-protein recognition rules exist, unlike the genetic code. Even the binding patterns that are observed are subject to degeneracy and the docking arrangement of the protein with its target DNA site. The currently available computational techniques for prediction of zinc fingers focus on the modular prediction of these fingers, (i.e. they do not take in to account the effect of the binding of other zinc fingers in the vicinity). *In vivo* studies indicate that the attachment of a zinc finger to its target DNA is the major groove of DNA influences the binding of subsequent fingers near it. Thus, alongside the modular approach, a synergistic view also needs to be taken to more effectively tackle the complexity of zinc fingers from a robust application point of view.

Presently, no such tool for zinc finger prediction is available. Towards this end, the authors of this chapter have developed a zinc finger prediction tool (available at http://web.iitd.ac.in/~sundar/zifpredict) that is capable of predicting zinc fingers in both modular and synergistic fashion, according to the user's requirements. The tool also predicts zinc finger nucleases which are widely manipulated to engineer custom chimeric zinc finger proteins that can be used for targeted genome editing.

1. **Computational Algorithms for ZFP prediction:** ZFPs can play a pivotal role in several biological processes like replication, cell defense etc., which rely upon very specific sequence recognition. The recognition of DNA binding sites and the identification of ZFPs have primarily followed an approach dependent upon the sequence and structural data that has been generated through experiments or past predictions till date. DNA-recognition prediction is an active part of Computational Genomics. The interest is because of the high pace of discovery of new protein sequences in genome sequencing experiments. However, there are still many challenges in this area and newer prediction protocols can help in better understanding of DNA-protein interactions as well as design of newer zinc finger proteins. In the following section, we have presented the different algorithms that are currently available, which are based on different properties of the protein.

a. *Algorithm based on chemical and stereo-chemical binding properties:* As described earlier in the chapter, the protein-DNA binding is dependent upon its chemical, stereochemical interactions and binding geometry that is deciphered from the structural information generated from X-ray crystallography and NMR experiments (Suzuki et al., 1995; Suzuki et al., 1994). This data is eventually utilized in analyzing any protein-DNA interface by feeding them in to a computer program that has been designed to score all the contacts (indicative of the binding energy) between the zinc fingers proteins and DNA in the major groove. The numerical values of the compatibility between amino acid residues of the zinc finger proteins and the nucleotide residue are used for the computational evaluation of the binding scores, depending upon the respective canonical models of the individual zinc finger proteins.

b. *Algorithm based on hydrogen bonding:* This algorithm utilizes the bonding patterns (hydrogen and hydrophobic) recorded in 53 co-crystal structures of a variety of proteins extracted from Protein data Bank (PDB) and Nucleic Acid Database (NDB) that have atomic interactions in the DNA major groove (Mandel-Gutfreund & Margalit, 1998). It is an application representing the general trends in protein-DNA interactions that scores protein-DNA interactions considering the individual pairs to be independent of one another.

c. *Probabilistic algorithms*

Based on SELEX and Phage Experiment Data

This is a probabilistic model based on different types of interactions derived from SELEX data (where specific proteins extract oligonucleotide target sequences from a randomized pool that is specific to them), phage experiment data (where the protein is randomized keeping the DNA target sequence fixed). It uses a position-specific energy matrix for scoring the maximum specificity of a protein to its target DNA site (Benos, Lapedes, & Stormo, 2002).

Based on Three and Four Finger Zinc Finger Proteins in the TRANSFAC Database

This probabilistic method is trained on binding site data of three and four finger zinc finger proteins derived from the TRANSFAC database. The model is trained using expectation maximization of the probabilities associated to the location of the binding DNA sites as well as the contacts in the canonical model of the zinc finger protein, and the scoring of potential binding sites is predicted based on the number of position-specific interactions in the canonical model (Kaplan, Friedman, & Margalit, 2005).

2. **Databases:** Efforts made towards the assimilation of zinc finger proteins have been compiled as web-accessible resources for both natural and engineered zinc finger proteins. Here is a brief description of a few such databases available presently.
   a. *Database 1: Zinc Finger Database (ZiFDB):* ZiFDB is a C2H2 zinc finger repository that stores information regarding 716 individual zinc finger modules as well as engineered zinc fingers (Fu et al., 2009). They have worked on the idea that selection methods are more reliable than modular assembly in the case of zinc finger proteins which they have based upon a selection-based technique called OPEN (Oligomerized Pool Engineering) developed by the same group (Maeder et al., 2008).
   b. *Database 2: Structural Classification of Zinc Fingers:* This database enables a comprehensive classification of the spatial structures of zinc finger proteins in one of the eight groups depending upon the type of folding observed. The categorization is based on the structural properties observed in the vicinity of the zinc finger binding site (Krishna, Majumdar, & Grishin, 2003). This classification database helps in the understanding of the structure-function relationships and the evolutionary patterns observed in zinc fingers.
   c. *Database 3: SysZNF:* SysZNF is a systematic repository of the human and mouse C2H2-ZNF genes, with each entry having a physical location, gene model (including the various transcripts), affymetrix gene expression probes, protein domain structures, homologs (and synteny) between the human and mouse genes and PubMed references and links to other relevant public databases (Ding, Lorenz, Kreutzer, Li, & Thiesen, 2009). Searching is made simple through text search and sequence search.
   d. *Database 4: ZifBASE:* ZiFBase is an elaborate zinc finger protein collection (both natural and engineered constructs included). It provides information on the sequence, including class, type, framework, number of fingers,

residues, position, recognition site and physio-chemical properties of 50 natural and 89 engineered zinc finger proteins (http://web.iitd.ac.in/~sundar/zifbase) (Jayakanthan et al., 2009).

3. **Prediction tools:** The above database information is not sufficient as not much binding site information has been collected for zinc finger proteins experimentally. To overcome this hurdle and to give a better insight for understanding DNA- zinc finger interactions, a few tools for zinc finger prediction have been developed and posted on the web. Some of these are as mentioned below:
   a. *Tool 1: ZIFIBI:* This is a Hidden Markov Model based tool that utilizes publically available data to detect possible patterns of interaction between nucleotides of DNA in the major groove and amino acids of zinc fingers. The user's query is "fit" into the target DNA sites available with the database and the best corresponding amino acid stretch is provided as output (Cho, Chung, Park, Park, & Lee, 2008).
   b. *Tool 2: Predicting DNA Recognition by C2H2 Zinc finger Proteins:* This is a Support Vector Machine (SVM) approach for C2H2 zinc finger binding prediction. This additionally incorporates weak protein-DNA interactions as well as information where there is no binding found at all. It includes both linear and polynomial kernels for prediction that is indicative of the binding dependency based on canonical binding model (Persikov, Osada, & Singh, 2009).
   c. *Tool 3: Zinc finger Tools:* Zinc finger Tools is a utility that detects appropriate DNA target sites in the input DNA sequence that is especially sensitive to target sites involved in gene regulation or in detecting zinc finger nucleases. It can also predict the target binding sites for a known zinc finger protein sequence (Mandell & Barbas, 2006).
   d. *Tool 4: ZiF-Predict:* ZiF-Predict is a web-server for the prediction of C2H2 zinc fingers that bind to specific DNA targets on the major groove using artificial neural network (ANN). It allows the user the freedom to choose between modular and synergistic prediction approaches. Further, it also predicts zinc finger nucleases that are very important in targeted genome editing. The web-server also provides the user with information on the already published zinc fingers on selecting this specific option. (http://web.iitd.ac.in/~sundar/zifpredict) (Molparia et al., 2010).

CONCLUSION

The current methods for prediction of zinc finger proteins are based on protein structure and amino acid sequence. The structure based prediction methods work pretty well only for those proteins whose structures are available. In this chapter, we have described the methods of prediction that looks into various properties of proteins including positively charged electrostatic patches, DNA-binding structural motifs, protein sequence composition, solvent accessibility and secondary structure, net charge, dipole and quadrapole moments, and size of largest positive surface patch and amino acid composition, etc. Many of the protein-DNA interactions are flexible and redundant and hence many of the interactions are poorly understood. Moreover, the structures of many of the proteins are also not available and this leads to difficulties in accurate prediction. All these need to be unraveled and completely addressed to evolve an accurate prediction protocol, which could be routinely used by genome scientists before they proceed with designing proteins to target a specific site on any genome.

FUTURE SCOPE

In the post-genomic era, custom-designed zinc finger proteins are becoming very valuable tools for "gene-editing" and "directed mutagenesis" of plant and mammalian genomes including the human genome. The specificity of the chimeric proteins (custom-designed zinc finger proteins fused to DNA-modifying domains) for their targets is driven by the specificity of designed zinc finger proteins. Identification of zinc finger proteins binding to specific DNA-target site can only been accomplished through laborious and time consuming experiments. Therefore, computational identification may provide a good alternative that focuses on identifying the target (binding) sites of the C2H2 fingers and predicting the protein recognition helices that bind to them. The determination of DNA-binding specificity in zinc fingers is functionally relevant. Design of specific zinc finger proteins to target a particular chromosomal locus, requires highly sensitive prediction protocol. An ideal prediction should incorporate sequence data, structural data and genome-specific information and all possible knowledge of biological function. Many of the difficulties associated with prediction are likely to be overcome if one comes up with all the features that could be incorporated for precise prediction of DNA-binding specificity in zinc fingers. Recent developments in this area could vastly increase and improve the accuracy of prediction protocols, thereby, enabling the wet laboratory researchers to design these predicted proteins for novel therapeutic applications. Advances in the development of prediction protocols may lead to creation of highly specific custom-designed ZFPs that will have tremendous applicability in genome editing and molecular therapeutics.

REFERENCES

Alwin, S., Gere, M. B., Guhl, E., Effertz, K., Barbas, C. F. III, & Segal, D. J. (2005). Custom zinc-finger nucleases for use in human cells. *Molecular Therapy*, *12*(4), 610–617. doi:10.1016/j.ymthe.2005.06.094

Bartsevich, V. V., & Juliano, R. L. (2000). Regulation of the MDR1 gene by transcriptional repressors selected using peptide combinatorial libraries. *Molecular Pharmacology*, *58*(1), 1–10.

Bartsevich, V. V., Miller, J. C., Case, C. C., & Pabo, C. O. (2003). Engineered zinc finger proteins for controlling stem cell fate. *Stem Cells (Dayton, Ohio)*, *21*(6), 632–637. doi:10.1634/stemcells.21-6-632

Beerli, R. R., & Barbas, C. F. III. (2002). Engineering polydactyl zinc-finger transcription factors. *Nature Biotechnology*, *20*(2), 135–141. doi:10.1038/nbt0202-135

Beerli, R. R., Dreier, B., & Barbas, C. F. III. (2000). Positive and negative regulation of endogenous genes by designed transcription factors. *Natl. Acad. Sci.*, *97*(4), 1495–1500. doi:10.1073/pnas.040552697

Beerli, R. R., Segal, D. J., Dreier, B., & Barbas, C. F. III. (1998). Toward controlling gene expression at will: specific regulation of the erbB-2/HER-2 promoter by using polydactyl zinc finger proteins constructed from modular building blocks. *Natl. Acad. Sci.*, *95*(25), 14628–14633. doi:10.1073/pnas.95.25.14628

Benos, P. V., Lapedes, A. S., & Stormo, G. D. (2002). Probabilistic code for DNA recognition by proteins of the EGR family. *Journal of Molecular Biology*, *323*(4), 701–727. doi:10.1016/S0022-2836(02)00917-8

Carroll, D. (2004). Using nucleases to stimulate homologous recombination. *Methods in Molecular Biology (Clifton, N.J.)*, *262*, 195–207.

Carroll, D. (2008). Progress and prospects: zinc-finger nucleases as gene therapy agents. *Gene Therapy*, *15*(22), 1463–1468. doi:10.1038/gt.2008.145

Carvin, C. D., Parr, R. D., & Kladde, M. P. (2003). Site-selective in vivo targeting of cytosine-5 DNA methylation by zinc-finger proteins. *Nucleic Acids Research*, *31*(22), 6493–6501. doi:10.1093/nar/gkg853

Cho, S. Y., Chung, M., Park, M., Park, S., & Lee, Y. S. (2008). ZIFIBI: Prediction of DNA binding sites for zinc finger proteins. *Biochemical and Biophysical Research Communications*, *369*(3), 845–848. doi:10.1016/j.bbrc.2008.02.106

Dai, Q., Huang, J., Klitzman, B., Dong, C., Goldschmidt-Clermont, P. J., & March, K. L. (2004). Engineered zinc finger-activating vascular endothelial growth factor transcription factor plasmid DNA induces therapeutic angiogenesis in rabbits with hindlimb ischemia. *Circulation*, *110*(16), 2467–2475. doi:10.1161/01.CIR.0000145139.53840.49

Desjarlais, J. R., & Berg, J. M. (1993). Use of a zinc-finger consensus sequence framework and specificity rules to design specific DNA binding proteins. *Natl. Acad. Sci.*, *90*(6), 2256–2260. doi:10.1073/pnas.90.6.2256

Ding, G., Lorenz, P., Kreutzer, M., Li, Y., & Thiesen, H. J. (2009). SysZNF: the C2H2 zinc finger gene database. *Nucleic Acids Research*, *37*(Database issue), 267–273. doi:10.1093/nar/gkn782

Doyon, Y., McCammon, J. M., Miller, J. C., Faraji, F., Ngo, C., & Katibah, G. E. (2008). Heritable targeted gene disruption in zebrafish using designed zinc-finger nucleases. *Nature Biotechnology*, *26*(6), 702–708. doi:10.1038/nbt1409

Durai, S., Mani, M., Kandavelou, K., Wu, J., Porteus, M. H., & Chandrasegaran, S. (2005). Zinc finger nucleases: custom-designed molecular scissors for genome engineering of plant and mammalian cells. *Nucleic Acids Research*, *33*(18), 5978–5990. doi:10.1093/nar/gki912

Elrod-Erickson, M., & Pabo, C. O. (1999). Binding studies with mutants of Zif268. Contribution of individual side chains to binding affinity and specificity in the Zif268 zinc finger-DNA complex. *The Journal of Biological Chemistry*, *274*(27), 19281–19285. doi:10.1074/jbc.274.27.19281

Fu, F., Sander, J. D., Maeder, M., Thibodeau-Beganny, S., Joung, J. K., & Dobbs, D. (2009). Zinc Finger Database (ZiFDB): a repository for information on C2H2 zinc fingers and engineered zinc-finger arrays. *Nucleic Acids Research*, *37*(Database issue), 279–283. doi:10.1093/nar/gkn606

Jamieson, A. C., Miller, J. C., & Pabo, C. O. (2003). Drug discovery with engineered zinc-finger proteins. *Nature Reviews. Drug Discovery*, *2*(5), 361–368. doi:10.1038/nrd1087

Jayakanthan, M., Muthukumaran, J., Chandrasekar, S., Chawla, K., Punetha, A., & Sundar, D. (2009). ZifBASE: a database of zinc finger proteins and associated resources. *BMC Genomics*, *10*, 421. doi:10.1186/1471-2164-10-421

Kandavelou, K., Mani, M., Durai, S., & Chandrasegaran, S. (2005). "Magic" scissors for genome surgery. *Nature Biotechnology*, *23*(6), 686–687. doi:10.1038/nbt0605-686

Kaplan, T., Friedman, N., & Margalit, H. (2005). Ab initio prediction of transcription factor targets using structural knowledge. *PLoS Computational Biology*, *1*(1). doi:10.1371/journal.pcbi.0010001

Kim, J. S., & Pabo, C. O. (1998). Getting a handhold on DNA: design of poly-zinc finger proteins with femtomolar dissociation constants. *Natl. Acad. Sci.*, *95*(6), 2812–2817. doi:10.1073/pnas.95.6.2812

Kim, Y. G., Cha, J., & Chandrasegaran, S. (1996). Hybrid restriction enzymes: zinc finger fusions to Fok I cleavage domain. *Natl. Acad. Sci.*, *93*(3), 1156–1160. doi:10.1073/pnas.93.3.1156

Klug, A. (2005). Towards therapeutic applications of engineered zinc finger proteins. *FEBS Letters*, *579*(4), 892–894. doi:10.1016/j.febslet.2004.10.104

Krishna, S. S., Majumdar, I., & Grishin, N. V. (2003). Structural classification of zinc fingers: survey and summary. *Nucleic Acids Research*, *31*(2), 532–550. doi:10.1093/nar/gkg161

Li, Y., Yang, D., Bai, Y., Mo, X., Huang, W., & Yuan, W. (2008). ZNF418, a novel human KRAB/C2H2 zinc finger protein, suppresses MAPK signaling pathway. *Molecular and Cellular Biochemistry*, *310*(1-2), 141–151. doi:10.1007/s11010-007-9674-4

Liu, P. Q., Rebar, E. J., Zhang, L., Liu, Q., Jamieson, A. C., & Liang, Y. (2001). Regulation of an endogenous locus using a panel of designed zinc finger proteins targeted to accessible chromatin regions. Activation of vascular endothelial growth factor A. *The Journal of Biological Chemistry*, *276*(14), 11323–11334. doi:10.1074/jbc.M011172200

Liu, Q., Segal, D. J., Ghiara, J. B., & Barbas, C. F. III. (1997). Design of polydactyl zinc-finger proteins for unique addressing within complex genomes. *Natl. Acad. Sci.*, *94*(11), 5525–5530. doi:10.1073/pnas.94.11.5525

Maeder, M. L., Thibodeau-Beganny, S., Osiak, A., Wright, D. A., Anthony, R. M., & Eichtinger, M. (2008). Rapid "open-source" engineering of customized zinc-finger nucleases for highly efficient gene modification. *Molecular Cell*, *31*(2), 294–301. doi:10.1016/j.molcel.2008.06.016

Mandel-Gutfreund, Y., & Margalit, H. (1998). Quantitative parameters for amino acid-base interaction: implications for prediction of protein-DNA binding sites. *Nucleic Acids Research*, *26*(10), 2306–2312. doi:10.1093/nar/26.10.2306

Mandell, J. G., & Barbas, C. F., 3rd. (2006). Zinc Finger Tools: custom DNA-binding domains for transcription factors and nucleases. *Nucleic Acids Res, 34*(Web Server issue), 516-523.

Mani, M., Kandavelou, K., Dy, F. J., Durai, S., & Chandrasegaran, S. (2005). Design, engineering, and characterization of zinc finger nucleases. *Biochemical and Biophysical Research Communications*, *335*(2), 447–457. doi:10.1016/j.bbrc.2005.07.089

McNamara, A. R., Hurd, P. J., Smith, A. E. F., & Ford, K. G. (2002). Characterisation of site-biased DNA methyltransferases: specificity, affinity and subsite relationships. *Nucleic Acids Research*, *30*(17), 3818–3830. doi:10.1093/nar/gkf501

Moehle, E. A., Rock, J. M., Lee, Y. L., Jouvenot, Y., DeKelver, R. C., & Gregory, P. D. (2007). Targeted gene addition into a specified location in the human genome using designed zinc finger nucleases. *Natl. Acad. Sci.*, *104*(9), 3055–3060. doi:10.1073/pnas.0611478104

Molparia, B., Goyal, K., Sarkar, A., Kumar, S., & Sundar, D. (2010). (in press). Zif-Predict: a web tool for predicing DNA-binding specificity in C2H2 zinc finger proteins. *Genomics, Proteomics & Bioinformatics*.

Pabo, C. O., Peisach, E., & Grant, R. A. (2001). Design and selection of novel Cys2His2 zinc finger proteins. *Annual Review of Biochemistry*, *70*, 313–340. doi:10.1146/annurev.biochem.70.1.313

Papworth, M., Kolasinska, P., & Minczuk, M. (2006). Designer zinc-finger proteins and their applications. *Gene*, *366*(1), 27–38. doi:10.1016/j.gene.2005.09.011

Pavletich, N. P., & Pabo, C. O. (1991). Zinc finger-DNA recognition: crystal structure of a Zif268-DNA complex at 2.1 A. *Science*, *252*(5007), 809–817. doi:10.1126/science.2028256

Persikov, A. V., Osada, R., & Singh, M. (2009). Predicting DNA recognition by Cys2His2 zinc finger proteins. *Bioinformatics (Oxford, England)*, *25*(1), 22–29. doi:10.1093/bioinformatics/btn580

Rebar, E. J. (2004). Development of pro-angiogenic engineered transcription factors for the treatment of cardiovascular disease. *Expert Opinion on Investigational Drugs*, *13*(7), 829–839. doi:10.1517/13543784.13.7.829

Rebar, E. J., Huang, Y., Hickey, R., Nath, A. K., Meoli, D., & Nath, S. (2002). Induction of angiogenesis in a mouse model using engineered transcription factors. *Nature Medicine*, *8*(12), 1427–1432. doi:10.1038/nm795

Ren, D., Collingwood, T. N., Rebar, E. J., Wolffe, A. P., & Camp, H. S. (2002) PPARgamma knockdown by engineered transcription factors: exogenous PPARgamma2 but not PPARgamma1 reactivates adipogenesis. *Genes & Development*, *16*(1), 27–32. doi:10.1101/gad.953802

Sauer, R. T. (1990). Transcriptional control. Scissors and helical forks. *Nature*, *347*(6293), 514–515. doi:10.1038/347514b0

Schwabe, J. W., & Rhodes, D. (1991). Beyond zinc fingers: steroid hormone receptors have a novel structural motif for DNA recognition. *Trends in Biochemical Sciences*, *16*(8), 291–296. doi:10.1016/0968-0004(91)90121-B

Segal, D. J., & Barbas, C. F. III. (2001). Custom DNA-binding proteins come of age: polydactyl zinc-finger proteins. *Current Opinion in Biotechnology*, *12*(6), 632–637. doi:10.1016/S0958-1669(01)00272-5

Shi, Y., & Berg, J. M. (1995). A direct comparison of the properties of natural and designed zinc-finger proteins. *Chemistry & Biology*, *2*(2), 83–89. doi:10.1016/1074-5521(95)90280-5

Smith, J., Bibikova, M., Whitby, F. G., Reddy, A. R., Chandrasegaran, S., & Carroll, D. (2000). Requirements for double-strand cleavage by chimeric restriction enzymes with zinc finger DNA-recognition domains. *Nucleic Acids Research*, *28*(17), 3361–3369. doi:10.1093/nar/28.17.3361

Snowden, A. W., Zhang, L., Urnov, F., Dent, C., Jouvenot, Y., & Zhong, X. H. (2003). Repression of vascular endothelial growth factor A in glioblastoma cells using engineered zinc finger transcription factors. *Cancer Research*, *63*(24), 8968–8976.

Stege, J. T., Guan, X., Ho, T., Beachy, R. N., & Barbas, C. F. III. (2002). Controlling gene expression in plants using synthetic zinc finger transcription factors. *The Plant Journal*, *32*(6), 1077–1086. doi:10.1046/j.1365-313X.2002.01492.x

Suzuki, M. (1993). Common features in DNA recognition helices of eukaryotic transcription factors. *The EMBO Journal*, *12*(8), 3221–3226.

Suzuki, M. (1994). A framework for the DNA-protein recognition code of the probe helix in transcription factors: the chemical and stereochemical rules. *Structure (London, England)*, *2*(4), 317–326. doi:10.1016/S0969-2126(00)00033-2

Suzuki, M., Brenner, S. E., Gerstein, M., & Yagi, N. (1995). DNA recognition code of transcription factors. *Protein Engineering*, *8*(4), 319–328. doi:10.1093/protein/8.4.319

Suzuki, M., Gerstein, M., & Yagi, N. (1994). Stereochemical basis of DNA recognition by Zn fingers. *Nucleic Acids Research*, *22*(16), 3397–3405. doi:10.1093/nar/22.16.3397

Tan, S., Guschin, D., Davalos, A., Lee, Y. L., Snowden, A. W., & Jouvenot, Y. (2003). Zinc-finger protein-targeted gene regulation: genomewide single-gene specificity. *Natl. Acad. Sci.*, *100*(21), 11997–12002. doi:10.1073/pnas.2035056100

Tan, W., Zhu, K., Segal, D. J., Barbas, C. F. III, & Chow, S. A. (2004). Fusion proteins consisting of human immunodeficiency virus type 1 integrase and the designed polydactyl zinc finger protein E2C direct integration of viral DNA into specific sites. *Journal of Virology*, *78*(3), 1301–1313. doi:10.1128/JVI.78.3.1301-1313.2004

Thiesen, H. J., Bellefroid, E., Revelant, O., & Martial, J. A. (1991). Conserved KRAB protein domain identified upstream from the zinc finger region of Kox 8. *Nucleic Acids Research*, *19*(14), 3996. doi:10.1093/nar/19.14.3996

Tian, C., Xing, G., Xie, P., Lu, K., Nie, J., & Wang, J. (2009). KRAB-type zinc-finger protein Apak specifically regulates p53-dependent apoptosis. *Nature Cell Biology*, *11*(5), 580–591. doi:10.1038/ncb1864

Tian, C. Y., Zhang, L. Q., & He, F. C. (2006). Progress in the study of KRAB zinc finger protein. *Yi Chuan*, *28*(11), 1451–1456. doi:10.1360/yc-006-1451

Urnov, F. D., Miller, J. C., Lee, Y. L., Beausejour, C. M., Rock, J. M., & Augustus, S. (2005). Highly efficient endogenous human gene correction using designed zinc-finger nucleases. *Nature*, *435*(7042), 646–651. doi:10.1038/nature03556

Wolfe, S. A., Greisman, H. A., Ramm, E. I., & Pabo, C. O. (1999). Analysis of zinc fingers optimized via phage display: evaluating the utility of a recognition code. *Journal of Molecular Biology*, *285*(5), 1917–1934. doi:10.1006/jmbi.1998.2421

Xu, G. L., & Bestor, T. H. (1997). Cytosine methylation targetted to pre-determined sequences. *Nature Genetics*, *17*(4), 376–378. doi:10.1038/ng1297-376

Zhang, L., Spratt, S. K., Liu, Q., Johnstone, B., Qi, H., & Raschke, E. E. (2000). Synthetic zinc finger transcription factor action at an endogenous chromosomal site. Activation of the human erythropoietin gene. *The Journal of Biological Chemistry*, *275*(43), 33850–33860. doi:10.1074/jbc.M005341200

KEY TERMS AND DEFINITIONS

Zinc Finger Protein: A DNA-binding protein domain consisting of zinc fingers ranging from to nine. They occur in nature as the part of transcription factors conferring DNA sequence specificity as the DNA-binding domain.

Zinc-Finger Nucleases: Synthetic proteins consisting of an engineered zinc finger DNA-binding domain fused to the cleavage domain of the FokI restriction endonuclease and can be used to induce double-stranded breaks (DSBs) in specific DNA sequences. Zinc finger domains can be engineered to target desired DNA sequences which enable zinc-finger nucleases to target unique sequence within a complex genome. By taking advantage of endogenous DNA repair machinery, these reagents can be used to precisely alter the genomes of higher organisms.

Recognition Helix: DNA recognition by zinc finger protein occurs through its alpha-helical region called recognition helix, which is made up of seven amino acids (positions -1 to +7 relative the start of the alpha helix in the finger).

Backbone Sequence: The backbone sequence consists of the zinc finger backbone which does not interact with the DNA. Interactions with DNA are mediated by the zinc finger helix, which is variable depending upon the triplet recognized. The backbone sequences provided include the 2 N-term ß-strands (in the N-term backbone), the C-terminal portion of the alpha-helix (in the C-term backbone), and a linker between proximal fingers.

Genome: The genome is the entirety of an organism's hereditary information. It is encoded either in DNA or, for many types of virus, in RNA. The genome includes both the genes and the non-coding sequences of the DNA.

Algorithm: A specific set of instructions for carrying out a procedure or solving a problem which results in a predictable end-state from a known beginning. Specific algorithms sometimes also go by the name method, procedure, or technique. The process of applying an algorithm to an input to obtain an output is called a computation.

Support Vector Machines (SVMs): A set of related supervised learning methods used for classification and regression. In simple words, given a set of training data belonging to two distinct subsets, this method automatically assigns further data to one of the subsets. A support vector machine constructs a hyperplane or set of hyperplanes in a high or infinite dimensional space, which can be used for classification, regression or other tasks. Intuitively, a good separation is achieved by the hyperplane that has the largest distance to the nearest training datapoints of any class (so-called functional margin), since in general the larger the margin the lower the generalization error of the classifier.

Hidden Markov Model: A HMM is a statistical model in which the system being modeled is assumed to be a Markov process with unobserved state. In a regular Markov model, the state is directly visible to the observer, and therefore the state transition probabilities are the only parameters. In a hidden Markov model, the state is not directly visible, but output dependent on the state is visible. Each state has a probability distribution over the possible output tokens. Therefore the sequence of tokens generated by a HMM gives some information about the sequence of states.

Artificial Neural Network: An ANN is a mathematical model or computational model that tries to simulate the structure and/or functional aspects of biological neural networks. It consists of an interconnected group of artificial neurons and processes information using a connectionist approach to computation. Neural networks are non-linear statistical data modeling tools. They can be used to model complex relationships between inputs and outputs or to find patterns in data.

Protein Data Bank (PDB): The PDB is a repository for the 3-D structural data of experimentally-determined s large biological molecules such as proteins, nucleic acids, and complex assemblies. The Protein Data Bank (PDB) format provides a standard representation for macromolecular structure data derived from X-ray diffraction and NMR studies. This representation was created in the 1970's and a large amount of software using it has been written. The PDB is overseen by an organization called the Worldwide Protein Data Bank, wwPDB.

Nucleic Acid Database (NDB): NDB is a repository of three-dimensional structural information about nucleic acids and serves as a resource for research and education. The NDB's goal is to provide access to nucleic acid structure. The services include an atlas that provides multiple X-ray and NMR images, areas where data can be deposited and downloaded, and a search function. The NDB is supported by funds from the National Science Foundation and the Department of Energy.

Compilation of References

Abbasi, K. (2006). Journals join the podcast revolution. *Journal of the Royal Society of Medicine*, *99*, 329. doi:10.1258/jrsm.99.7.329

Abdelgawad, M., Watson, M. W. L., Young, E. W. K., Mudrik, J. M., Ungrin, M. D., & Wheeler, A. R. (2008). Soft lithography: masters on demand. *Lab on a Chip*, *8*(8), 1379–1385. doi:10.1039/b804050h

Aboagla, E. M. E., & Terada, T. (2003). Trehalose-enhanced fluidity of the goat sperm membrane and its protection during freezing. *Biology of Reproduction*, *69*, 1245–1250. doi:10.1095/biolreprod.103.017889

Abraham, & Nath, B. (2001). A Neuro-fuzzy approach for modelling electricity demand in Victoria, *Appl. Soft Comput. 1*, 127–138.

Abramowitz, M., & Stegun, I. A. (1970). *Handbook of Mathematical Functions*. New York: Dover Publications.

Adair, R. K. (1991). Constraints on biological effects of weak extremely-low-frequency electromagnetic-fields. *Physical Review A.*, *43*(2), 1039–1048. doi:10.1103/PhysRevA.43.1039

Adair, R. K. (1992). Criticism of lednev mechanism for the influence of weak magnetic-fields on biological-systems. *Bioelectromagnetics*, *13*(3), 231–235. doi:10.1002/bem.2250130307

Adair, R. K. (1998). A physical analysis of the ion parametric resonance model. *Bioelectromagnetics*, *19*(3), 181–191. doi:10.1002/(SICI)1521-186X(1998)19:3<181::AID-BEM6>3.0.CO;2-Y

Adams, A. A., Okagbare, P. I., Feng, J., Hupert, M. L., Patterson, D., & Gottert, J.. (2208). Highly efficient circulating tumor cell isolation from whole blood and label-free enumeration using polymer-based microfluidics with an integrated conductivity sensor. *Journal of the American Chemical Society*, *130*, 8633–8641. doi:10.1021/ja8015022

Adams, R., Calcraft, L., & Davey, N. (2009). Using a genetic algorithm to investigate efficient connectivity in associative memories . *Neurocomputing*, *72*(4-6), 732–742. doi:10.1016/j.neucom.2008.05.017

Adamson, D. N., Mustafi, D., Zhang, J. X. J., Zheng, B., & Ismagilov, R. F. (2006). Production of arrays of chemically distinct nanolitre plugs via repeated splitting in microfluidic devices. *Lab on a Chip*, *6*(9), 1178–1186. doi:10.1039/b604993a

Adler-Milstein, J., & Bates, D. W. (2009). U.S. Regional health information organizations: progress and challenges. *Health Affairs (Project Hope)*, *28*(2), 483–492. doi:10.1377/hlthaff.28.2.483

Adler-Milstein, J., & McAfee, A. P. (2008). The state of regional health information organizations: current activities and financing. *Health Affairs (Project Hope)*, *27*(1), 60–69. doi:10.1377/hlthaff.27.1.w60

Aharoni, A., Griffiths, A. D., & Tawfik, D. S. (2005). High-throughput screens and selections of enzyme-encoding genes. *Current Opinion in Chemical Biology*, *9*(2), 210–216. doi:10.1016/j.cbpa.2005.02.002

AHDI. (2009). *Approved Medical Transcription Education Programs*. Modesto, CA: Association for Healthcare Documentation Integrity.

Albanese, M., & Mitchell, S. (1993). Problem-based learning: A review of the literature on its outcomes and implementation issues. *Academic Medicine*, *68*, 52–81. doi:10.1097/00001888-199301000-00012

Alexander, H. R. Jr. (2008). Isolation Perfusion . In De-Vita, V. T., Lawrence, T. S., & Rosenberg, S. A. (Eds.),

Cancer Principles and Practice of Oncology (8th ed., pp. 701–710). Philadelphia: Lippincott, Williams, & Wilkins.

Alexe, G. (2006). Breast cancer prognosis by combinatorial analysis of gene expression data. *Breast Cancer Research*, *8*(4). doi:10.1186/bcr1512

Alizadeh, A. A. (2000). Distinct types of diffuse large B-cell lymphoma identified by gene expression profiling. *Nature*, *403*(6769), 503–511. doi:10.1038/35000501

Alwin, S., Gere, M. B., Guhl, E., Effertz, K., Barbas, C. F. III, & Segal, D. J. (2005). Custom zinc-finger nucleases for use in human cells. *Molecular Therapy*, *12*(4), 610–617. doi:10.1016/j.ymthe.2005.06.094

American Association of Family Physicians. (2009). *Patient-Centered Medical Home*. Retrieved from http://www.aafp.org/online/en/home/membership/initiatives/pcmh.html.

Amin, M. F., & Murase, K. (2009). Single-layered complex-valued neural network for real-valued classification problems . *Neurocomputing*, *72*(4-6), 945–955. doi:10.1016/j.neucom.2008.04.006

Anand, D., & Niranjan, U. (1988). *Watermarking Medical Images with Patient Information*. In *Proceedings of the IEEE/EMBS Conference*, (pp. 703-706).

Ang, J. H., Tan, K. C., & Al-Mamun, A. (2008). Training neural networks for classification using growth probability-based evolution . *Neurocomputing*, *71*(16-18), 3493–3508. doi:10.1016/j.neucom.2007.10.011

Anon., (1968). A definition of irreversible coma. Report of the ad hoc committee of the Harvard Medical School to examine the definition of brain death. *Journal of the American Medical Association*, *205*(6), 337–340. doi:10.1001/jama.205.6.337

Anon., (1979). *National Commission for the Protection of Human Subjects of Biomedical and Behavioral Research (National Commission). Belmont Report: Ethical Principles and Guidelines for the Protection of Human Subjects of Research*. Washington, DC: US Government Printing Office.

Antezana, E., Kuiper, M., & Mironov, V. (2009). Biological knowledge management: the emerging role of the Semantic Web technologies. *Briefings in Bioinformatics*, *10*, 392–407. doi:10.1093/bib/bbp024

Antia, M., Herricks, T., & Rathod, P. K. (2007). Microfluidic modeling of cell-cell interactions in malaria pathogenesis. *PLoS Pathogens*, *3*(7), e99. doi:10.1371/journal.ppat.0030099

Appleby, C. (1995). The trouble with CHINS (community health information networks). *Hospitals & Health Networks*, *69*(9), 42–44.

Assenheimer, M., Laver-Moskovitz, O., Malonek, D., Manor, D., Nahaliel, I., Nitzan, R., & Saad, A. (2001). The T-SCAN™ technology: electrical impedance as a diagnostic tool for brest cancer detection . *Physiological Measurement*, *22*(1), 1–8. doi:10.1088/0967-3334/22/1/301

Atreja, A., Messinger-Rapport, B., Jain, A., & Mehta, N. (2006). Using Web 2.0 technologies to develop a resource for evidence based medicine. In *Proceedings of the AMIA Annu. Symp.,* (pg. 847).

Ayala, D. E., Hermida, R. C., Mojon, A., & Iglesias, M. (2002). Circadian blood pressure variability in healthy human pregnancy. Comparison with gestational hypertension. In *Proceedings of Engineering in Medicine and Biology Society, IEEE Annual Conference,* (vol. 1., pp. 639 – 640).

Ayala, D. E., Hermida, R. C., Mojon, A., Fernandez, J. R., Alonso, I., Silva, I., et al. (2002). Blood pressure and heart rate variability during gestation in healthy and hypertensive pregnant women, In *Proceedings of the Engineering in Medicine and Biology Society, Ann. Int. Conf. IEEE,*(vol.1., pp 367 – 370).

Babaeizadeh, S., Brooks, D. H., & Isaacson, D. (2007). 3-D Electrical Impedance Tomography for Piecewise Constant Domains With Known Internal Boundaries. *IEEE Transactions on Bio-Medical Engineering*, *54*(1), 2–10. doi:10.1109/TBME.2006.886839

Bagchi, A., Woods, E. J., & Crister, J. K. (2008). Cryopreservation and vitrification: recent advances in fertility preservation technologies. *Expert Review of Medical Devices*, *5*, 359–370. doi:10.1586/17434440.5.3.359

Ball, M. J., & Gold, J. (2006). Banking on health: Personal records and information exchange. *Journal of Healthcare Information Management*, *20*(2), 71–83.

Bamba, K., & Cran, D. G. (1985). Effect of rapid warming of boar semen on sperm morphology and physiology.

Journal of Reproduction and Fertility, *75*, 133–138. doi:10.1530/jrf.0.0750133

Bamba, K., & Miyagawa, N. (1992). Protective action of aromatic compounds against cold-shock injuries in boar spermatozoa. *Cryobiology*, *29*, 533–536. doi:10.1016/0011-2240(92)90057-9

Bange, A., Halsall, H. B., & Heineman, W. R. (2005). Microfluidic immunosensor systems. [Review]. *Biosensors & Bioelectronics*, *20*(12), 2488–2503. doi:10.1016/j.bios.2004.10.016

Barber, D. C., & Brown, B. H. (1984). Applied Potential Tomography. *Journal of Physics. E, Scientific Instruments*, *17*, 723–733. doi:10.1088/0022-3735/17/9/002

Barber, D. C., Brown, B. H., & Avis, N. J. (1992). Image Reconstruction in Electrical Impedance Tomography Using Filtered Back-Projection. *Proceedings of the Annual International Conference IEEE EMBS* (Paris, France), *14*, 1691 -1692.

Barnes, F. S. (2006). *Bioengineering and biophysical aspects of Electromagnetic fields*. Boca Raton, FL: CRC.

Barone, F. C., & Feuerstein, G. Z. (1999). Inflammatory mediators and stroke: New opportunities for novel therapeutics. [Review]. *Journal of Cerebral Blood Flow and Metabolism*, *19*(8), 819–834. doi:10.1097/00004647-199908000-00001

Barrows, H. S. (1983). Problem-based, self-directed learning. *Journal of the American Medical Association*, *250*, 3077–3080. doi:10.1001/jama.250.22.3077

Barrows, H. S., & Bennett, K. (1982). Experimental studies on the diagnostic (problem-solving) skill of the neurologist, their implications for neurological training. *Archives of Neurology*, *26*, 273–277.

Bartsevich, V. V., & Juliano, R. L. (2000). Regulation of the MDR1 gene by transcriptional repressors selected using peptide combinatorial libraries. *Molecular Pharmacology*, *58*(1), 1–10.

Bartsevich, V. V., Miller, J. C., Case, C. C., & Pabo, C. O. (2003). Engineered zinc finger proteins for controlling stem cell fate. *Stem Cells (Dayton, Ohio)*, *21*(6), 632–637. doi:10.1634/stemcells.21-6-632

Baten, C. T. M., Moerkerk, H. V., Kingma, I., Dien, J. V., Dolan, T., Veltink, P. H., & Hermens, H. J. (2000). Ambulatory low back load exposure estimation. In *Proceedings of the IEA 2000/44th Annual Meeting HFES 2000*, (4, pp. 609–612).

Baten, C. T. M., Oosterhoff, P., Kingma, I., Veltink, P. H., & Hermens, H. J. (1996). Inertial sensing in ambulatory back load estimation. In *Proceedings of the 18th Annual International Conference of the IEEE Engineering in Medicine and Biology Society*, (2, pp. 497–498).

Becker, H., & Gärtner, C. (2008). Polymer microfabrication technologies for microfluidic systems. *Analytical and Bioanalytical Chemistry*, *390*(1), 89–111. doi:10.1007/s00216-007-1692-2

Beerli, R. R., & Barbas, C. F. III. (2002). Engineering polydactyl zinc-finger transcription factors. *Nature Biotechnology*, *20*(2), 135–141. doi:10.1038/nbt0202-135

Beerli, R. R., Dreier, B., & Barbas, C. F. III. (2000). Positive and negative regulation of endogenous genes by designed transcription factors. *Natl. Acad. Sci.*, *97*(4), 1495–1500. doi:10.1073/pnas.040552697

Beerli, R. R., Segal, D. J., Dreier, B., & Barbas, C. F. III. (1998). Toward controlling gene expression at will: specific regulation of the erbB-2/HER-2 promoter by using polydactyl zinc finger proteins constructed from modular building blocks. *Natl. Acad. Sci.*, *95*(25), 14628–14633. doi:10.1073/pnas.95.25.14628

Begg, R., Lai, D. T. H., & Palaniswami, M. (2007). *Computational Intelligence in Biomedical Engineering*. Boca Raton, FL: Taylor & Francis Books Inc.

Begg, R. K., Palaniswami, M., & Owen, B. (2005). Support vector machines for automated gait classification. *IEEE Transactions on Bio-Medical Engineering*, *52*(5), 828–838. doi:10.1109/TBME.2005.845241

Benos, P. V., Lapedes, A. S., & Stormo, G. D. (2002). Probabilistic code for DNA recognition by proteins of the EGR family. *Journal of Molecular Biology*, *323*(4), 701–727. doi:10.1016/S0022-2836(02)00917-8

Berger, M., Castelino, J., Huang, R., Shah, M., & Austin, R. H. (2001). Design of a microfabricated magnetic cell separator. *Electrophoresis*, *22*(18), 3883–3892.

doi:10.1002/1522-2683(200110)22:18<3883::AID-ELPS3883>3.0.CO;2-4

Berners-Lee, T., & Fischetti, M. (1999). *Weaving the Web: the original design and ultimate destiny of the world wide web by its inventor*. San Francisco: Harper San Francisco.

Berners-Lee, T., & Hendler, J. (2001). Publishing on the semantic web. *Nature*, *26*, 1023–1024. doi:10.1038/35074206

Berners-Lee, T., & Cailliau, R. (1990, November 12). *WorldWideWeb: Proposal for a HyperText Project* (Technical report), Genève, Switzerland: CERN.

Berryman, J. G., & Kohn, R. V. (1990). Variational Constraints for Electrical Impedance Tomography. *Physical Review Letters*, *65*(3). doi:10.1103/PhysRevLett.65.325

Beyor, N., Seo, T. S., Liu, P., & Mathies, R. A. (2008). Immunomagnetic bead-based cell concentration microdevice for dilute pathogen detection. *Biomedical Microdevices*, *10*(6), 909–917. doi:10.1007/s10544-008-9206-3

Bier, M. (2006). How to evaluate the electric noise in a cell membrane? *Acta Physica Polonica B*, *37*(5), 1409.

Binhi, V. N. (2000). Amplitude and frequency dissociation spectra of ion-protein complexes rotating in magnetic fields. *Bioelectromagnetics*, *21*(1), 34–45. doi:10.1002/(SICI)1521-186X(200001)21:1<34::AID-BEM6>3.0.CO;2-8

Binhi, V. N., Alipov, Y. D., & Belyaev, Y. I. (2001). Effect of static magnetic field on E. coli cells and individual rotations of ion - protein complexes. *Bioelectromagnetics*, *22*, 79–86. doi:10.1002/1521-186X(200102)22:2<79::AID-BEM1009>3.0.CO;2-7

Bird, R. B., Stewart, W. E., & Lightfoot, E. N. (1960). *Transport Phenomena*. New York: John Wiley and Sons.

Bittner, M. (2000). Molecular classification of cutaneous malignant melanoma by gene expression profiling. *Nature*, *406*(6795), 536–540. doi:10.1038/35020115

Blackman, C. F., Benane, S. G., Rabinowitz, J. R., House, D. E., & Joines, W. T. (1985). A role for the magnetic-field in the radiation-induced efflux of calcium-ions from brain-tissue invitro. *Bioelectromagnetics*, *6*(4), 327–337. doi:10.1002/bem.2250060402

Blackman, C. F., Blanchard, J. P., Benane, S. G., & House, D. E. (1994). Empirical-test of an ion parametric resonance model for magnetic-field interactions with pc-12 cells. *Bioelectromagnetics*, *15*(3), 239–260. doi:10.1002/bem.2250150307

Blackman, C. F., Blanchard, J. P., Benane, S. G., & House, D. E. (1995). The ion parametric resonance model predicts magnetic-field parameters that affect nerve-cells. *The FASEB Journal*, *9*(7), 547–551.

Blackman, C. F., Blanchard, J. P., Benane, S. G., House, D. E., & Elder, J. A. (1998). Double blind test of magnetic field effects on neurite outgrowth. *Bioelectromagnetics*, *19*(4), 204–209. doi:10.1002/(SICI)1521-186X(1998)19:4<204::AID-BEM2>3.0.CO;2-5

Blackman, C. F., Kinney, L. S., House, D. E., & Joines, W. T. (1989). Multiple power-density windows and their possible origin. *Bioelectromagnetics*, *10*(2), 115–128. doi:10.1002/bem.2250100202

Blackshaw, A. W. (1958). The effects of incubation temperature and cold shock on the metabolism of ram spermatozoa. *Australian Journal of Biological Sciences*, *11*, 581–588.

Blair, R. (2006). RHIO nation. *Health Management Technology*, *27*(2), 56–62.

Blanchard, J. P., & Blackman, C. F. (1994). Clarification and Application of an Ion Parametric Resonance Model for Magnetic Field Interactions with Biological Systems. *Bioelectromagnetics*, *15*, 217–238. doi:10.1002/bem.2250150306

Boehm, B., & Turner, R. (2004). *Balancing Agility and Discipline: A Guide for the Perplexed*. Reading, MA: Addison-Wesley publishers.

Bonfa, I., Maioli, C., Sarti, F., Milandri, G. L., & Monte, P. R. D. (1993). *HERMES: An Expert System for the Prognosis of Hepatic Diseases* (Technical Report UBLCS-93- 19), Universiti of Bologna.

Borcea, L. (2003). Nonlinear multigrid for electrical impedance tomography, In *Proceedings of the SPIE - The International Society for Optical Engineering*: *Vol. 5016*(1), (pp. 49-58). Santa Clara, CA.

Bouhaddou, O., & Warnekar, P. (2008). Exchange of computable patient data between the Department of

Veterans Affairs (VA) and the Department of Defense (DoD): Terminology Mediation Strategy. *Journal of the American Medical Informatics Association*, *15*(2), 174–183. doi:10.1197/jamia.M2498

Boulos, M. N., Maramba, I., & Wheeler, S. (2006). Wikis, blogs and podcasts: a new generation of Web-based tools for virtual collaborative clinical practice and education. *BMC Medical Education*, *15*, 41. doi:10.1186/1472-6920-6-41

Bourke, A. K., O'Donovan, K. J., & Olaighin, G. (2008). The identification of vertical velocity profiles using an inertial sensor to investigate pre-impact detection of falls. *Medical Engineering & Physics*, *30*(7), 937–946. doi:10.1016/j.medengphy.2007.12.003

Braz, J. (2004, May). Med Biol Res Fuzzy expert system in the prediction of neonatal resuscitation. *Brazilian Journal of Medical and Biological Research*, *37*(5), 755–764.

Brennan, C. P. (1995). Managed care and health information networks. *Journal of Health Care Finance*, *21*(4), 1–5.

Brennan, P. F. (1999). Health informatics and community health: support for patients as collaborators in care. *Methods of Information in Medicine*, *38*(4-5), 274–278.

Brennan, P. F., Ferris, M., et al. (2005). Modeling participation in the NHII: operations research approach. In *Proceedings of the AMIA Annu. Symp.* (pp. 76-80).

Brown, B. H. (2003). Electrical Impedance Tomography (EIT): a review. *Journal of Medical Engineering & Technology*, *27*(3), 97–108. doi:10.1080/0309190021000059687

Burns, M. A., Johnson, B. N., Brahmasandra, S. N., Handique, K., Webster, J. R., & Krishnan, M. (1998). An integrated nanoliter DNA analysis device. *Science*, *282*(5388), 484–487. doi:10.1126/science.282.5388.484

Caribbean (2009). *Barbados Looks to Become Medical Transcription Capital*". Caribbean Press Releases. Retrieved from http://www.caribbeanpressreleases.com/articles/4520/1/Barbados-Looks-to-Become-Medical-Transcription-Capitl/Page1.html

Carroll, D. (2004). Using nucleases to stimulate homologous recombination. *Methods in Molecular Biology (Clifton, N.J.)*, *262*, 195–207.

Carroll, D. (2008). Progress and prospects: zinc-finger nucleases as gene therapy agents. *Gene Therapy*, *15*(22), 1463–1468. doi:10.1038/gt.2008.145

Carter, P., & Lemery, C. (2006). Privacy and security in health information exchange. *Journal of American Health Information Management Association*, *77*(10), 64A–64C.

Carvin, C. D., Parr, R. D., & Kladde, M. P. (2003). Site-selective in vivo targeting of cytosine-5 DNA methylation by zinc-finger proteins. *Nucleic Acids Research*, *31*(22), 6493–6501. doi:10.1093/nar/gkg853

Celik, M., Sharma,U. G. Saber, E. Tekalp, A. M. (n.d.). Hierarchical Watermarking for Secure Image Authentication with Localization. *IEEE Trans. Image Processing, 11*(6), pp.585-594.

Chakrabarty, J., Banerjee, D., Pal, D., De, J., Ghosh, A., & Majumder, G. C. (2007). Shedding off specific lipid constituent from sperm cell membrane during cryopreservation. *Cryobiology*, *54*, 27–35. doi:10.1016/j.cryobiol.2006.10.191

Chanda, B., & Majumder, D. D. *Digital Image Processing.* (2002), Prentice-Hall of India, ISBN-81-203-1618-5, 2003.

Chandler, J. E., Adkinson, R. W., & Nebel, R. L. (1984). Thawing optimums for bovine spermatozoa processed by three methods and packaged in continental and french straws. *Journal of Dairy Science*, *67*, 398–404. doi:10.3168/jds.S0022-0302(84)81315-6

Chao, H. M., Hsu, C. M., & Miaou, S. G. (2002). A Data-Hiding Technique with Authentication, Integration, and Confidentiality for Electronic Patients Records. *IEEE Transactions on Information Technology in Biomedicine*, *6*(1), 46–53. doi:10.1109/4233.992161

Chaudhuri, B. B., & Bhattacharya, U. (2000). Efficient training and improved performance of multilayer perceptron in pattern classification . *Neurocomputing*, *34*, 11–27. doi:10.1016/S0925-2312(00)00305-2

Chauvet, E., Fokapu, O., Hogrel, J.-Y., Gamet, D., & Duchene, J. (2003, November). Automatic Identification of Motor Unit Action Potential Trains from Electromyographic signals Using Fuzzy Techniques. *Journal of Medical and Biological Engineering and Computing . SpringerLink*, *41*(6), 646–653.

Chen, X., Cui, D. F., Liu, C. C., & Li, H. (2008). Microfluidic chip for blood cell separation and collection based on crossflow filtration. *Sensors and Actuators. B, Chemical*, *13*, 216–221. doi:10.1016/j.snb.2007.07.126

Cheney, M., & Isaacson, D. (1995). Issues in Electrical Impedance Imaging . *IEEE Computational Science & Engineering*, *2*, 53–62. doi:10.1109/99.476369

Cheng, K. S., Isaacson, D., Newell, J. C., & Gisser, D. G. (1989). Electrode Models for Electric Current Computed Tomography. *IEEE Transactions on Biomedical Engineering*, *36*(9), 918–924. doi:10.1109/10.35300

Cherepin, V. A., Karpov, A. Y., Korjenevsky, A. V., Kornienko, V. N., Kultiasov, Y. S., & Oshapkin, M. B. (2002). Three-Dimensional EIT Imaging of Breast Tissues: System Design and Clinical Testing. *IEEE Transactions on Medical Imaging*, *21*(6), 662–667. doi:10.1109/TMI.2002.800602

Chiabrera, A. (1992). From the Langevin-Lorentz to the Zeeman model of electromagnetic effects on ligand-receptor binding. *Bioelectrochemistry and Bioenergetics*, *28*, 355–365. doi:10.1016/0302-4598(92)80025-C

Chiabrera, A. B. B., Kaufman J. J., & Pilla A. A. (1989). *Interaction Mechanisms of Low Level Electromagnetic Fields in Living Systems*. Genoa, Italy: University of Genoa.

Cho, Y. K., Lee, J. G., Park, J. M., Lee, B. S., Lee, Y., & Ko, C. (2007). One-step pathogen specific DNA extraction from whole blood on a centrifugal microfluidic device. *Lab on a Chip*, *7*(5), 565–573. doi:10.1039/b616115d

Cho, S. Y., Chung, M., Park, M., Park, S., & Lee, Y. S. (2008). ZIFIBI: Prediction of DNA binding sites for zinc finger proteins. *Biochemical and Biophysical Research Communications*, *369*(3), 845–848. doi:10.1016/j.bbrc.2008.02.106

Chou, H. P., Spence, C., Scherer, A., & Quake, S. (1999). A microfabricated device for sizing and sorting DNA molecules. *Proceedings of the National Academy of Sciences of the United States of America*, *96*(1), 11–13. doi:10.1073/pnas.96.1.11

Christodoulos, I., & Pattichis, C. S. (1999, February). Unsupervided pattern recognition for the classification of EMG signals. *IEEE Trans. on BME*, *46*(2), 169–178. doi:10.1109/10.740879

CIA. (2008) *World Factbook*. Retrieved July 21, 2009 from https://www.cia.gov/library/publications/the-world-factbook/fields/2102.html

Cisler, S. (1994). Community computer networks: building electronic greenbelts . In Bishop, A. P. (Ed.), *Emerging Communities: Integrating Networked Information into Library Services: Clinic on Library Applications of Data Processing* (pp. 16–31).

Coatrieux, G., Maître, H., Sankur, B., Rolland, Y., & Collorec, R. (2000) *Relevance of watermarking in medical imaging*. In *Proceedings of 22nd International Conference of IEEE EMBS*, (pp 250–255).

Coatrieux, G., Sankur, B., & Maitre, H. (2001). *Strict Integrity Control of Biomedical Images*. In Proceedings of SPIE Conf. 4314: Security and Watermarking of Multimedia Contents III.

Cohen, M. E., & Hudson, D. L. (2002). Meta neural networks as intelligent agents for diagnosis . *Neural Networks*, *1*, 233–238.

Coiera, E. (2003). Interaction design theory. *International Journal of Medical Informatics*, *69*, 205–222. doi:10.1016/S1386-5056(02)00106-5

Coiera, E. (2003). *Guide to Health Informatics*, 2 Ed. Oxford, UK: A Hodder Arnold Publication.

Cokelet, G. R., Soave, R., Pugh, G., & Rathbun, L. (1993). Fabrication of in vitro microvascular blood flow systems by photolithography. *Microvascular Research*, *46*, 394–400. doi:10.1006/mvre.1993.1062

Collins, J. (2006). Education techniques for lifelong learning: writing multiple-choice questions for continuing medical education activities and self-assessment modules. *Radiographics*, *26*, 543–551. doi:10.1148/rg.262055145

Conceição, S. C., & Taylor, L. D. (2007). Using a constructivist approach with online concept maps: relationship between theory and nursing education. *Nursing Education Perspectives*, *28*, 268–275.

Conn, J. (2005). Destination RHIO. As regional data networks continue to grow in number, some find financial strength. *Mod Healthc*, *35*(42), 28, 32.

Conor, R., Collins, J. J., & Neill, M. O. (n.d.). *Grammatical Evolution - Evolving Programs for an Arbitrary Language*

Cook, D. A., & Dupras, D. M. (2004). A practical guide to developing effective web-based learning. *Journal of General Internal Medicine*, *19*, 698–707. doi:10.1111/j.1525-1497.2004.30029.x

Cooper, P. J., Garny, A., & Kohl, P. (2003). *Cardiac electrophysiology: Theoretical considerations of a potential target for weak electromagnetic field effects*. Oxford, UK: Oxford University Press.

Coulton, LA, B. A., Van Lierop JE, and Walsh MP. (2000). The effect of static magnetic fields on the rate of calcium/calmodulin-dependent phosphorylation of myosin light chain. *Bioelectromagnetics*, *21*, 189–196. doi:10.1002/(SICI)1521-186X(200004)21:3<189::AID-BEM6>3.0.CO;2-L

Countouriotis, A., Moore, T. B., & Sakamoto, K. M. (2002). Cell surface antigen and molecular targeting in the treatment of hematologic malignancies. [Review]. *Stem Cells (Dayton, Ohio)*, *20*(3), 215–229. doi:10.1634/stemcells.20-3-215

Courant, R., & Hilbert, D. (1989). *Methods of mathematical physics*. New York: Wiley.

Cox, I., Miller, M., & Bloom, J. (2002). *Digital Watermarking*. San Francisco: Morgan Kaufmann Publishers.

Dai, Q., Huang, J., Klitzman, B., Dong, C., Goldschmidt-Clermont, P. J., & March, K. L. (2004). Engineered zinc finger-activating vascular endothelial growth factor transcription factor plasmid DNA induces therapeutic angiogenesis in rabbits with hindlimb ischemia. *Circulation*, *110*(16), 2467–2475. doi:10.1161/01.CIR.0000145139.53840.49

Dammer, U., Hegner, M., Ansemetti, D., Wagner, P., Dreier, M., & Huber, W. (1996). Specific antigen/antibody interactions measured by force microscopy. *Biophysical Journal*, *70*, 2437–2441. doi:10.1016/S0006-3495(96)79814-4

Danesh, J., Collins, R., Appleby, P., & Peto, R. (1998). Association of fibrinogen, C-reactive protein, albumin, or leukocyte count with coronary heart disease - Meta-analyses of prospective studies. [Review]. *Jama-Journal of the American Medical Association*, *279*(18), 1477–1482. doi:10.1001/jama.279.18.1477

Darin-Bennett, A., Poulos, A., & White, I. G. (1973). The effect of cold-shock and freeze thawing on the release of phospholipids by ram, bull, and boar spermatozoa. *Australian Journal of Biological Sciences*, *26*, 1409–1420.

Daubechis, I. (1988). Orthogonal bases for Compactly Supported Wavelets. *Communications on Pure and Applied Mathematics*, *41*, 909–996. doi:10.1002/cpa.3160410705

David, G. C. (2008). *Finding the Place of Technology in Medical Transcription*. Paper presented at the annual meeting of the American Sociological Association Annual Meeting, Sheraton Boston, Boston, MA. Retrieved from http://www.allacademic.com/meta/p242233_index.html

Davis, J. A., Inglis, D. W., Morton, K. J., Lawrence, D. A., Huang, L. R., & Chou, S. Y. (2006). Deterministic hydrodynamics: Taking blood apart. *Proceedings of the National Academy of Sciences of the United States of America*, *103*(40), 14779–14784. doi:10.1073/pnas.0605967103

Davis, D., O'Brien, M. A., Freemantle, N., Wolf, F. M., Mazmanian, P., & Taylor-Vaisey, A. (1999). Impact of formal continuing medical education: do conferences, workshops, rounds, and other traditional continuing education activities change physician behaviour or health outcomes? *Journal of the American Medical Association*, *282*, 867–874. doi:10.1001/jama.282.9.867

Dayhoff, R. E., & Maloney, D. L. (1992). Exchange of Veterans Affairs medical data using national and local networks. *Annals of the New York Academy of Sciences*, *670*, 50–66. doi:10.1111/j.1749-6632.1992.tb26074.x

De Luca, C. J., Alexander, A., Wotiz, R., Gilmore, L. D., & Nawab, S. H. (2006). Decomposition of Surface EMG Signal. *Journal of Neurophysiology*, *96*, 1646–1657. doi:10.1152/jn.00009.2006

Dejnabadi, H., Jolles, B. M., & Aminian, K. (2005). A new approach to accurate measurement of uniaxial joint angles based on a combination of accelerometers and gyroscopes. *IEEE Transactions on Bio-Medical Engineering*, *52*(8), 1478–1484. doi:10.1109/TBME.2005.851475

De-Leeuw, E. F., De-Leeuw, A. M., Den-Dass, J. H. G., Colenbrander, B., & Verkleij, A. J. (1990). Cold-induced ultrastructural changes in bull and boar sperm plasma membranes. *Cryobiology*, *30*, 32–44.

Desjarlais, J. R., & Berg, J. M. (1993). Use of a zinc-finger consensus sequence framework and specificity rules to design specific DNA binding proteins. *Natl. Acad. Sci.*, *90*(6), 2256–2260. doi:10.1073/pnas.90.6.2256

Despont-Gros, C., Mueller, H., & Lovis, C. (2005). Evaluating user interactions with clinical information systems: a model based on human-computer interaction models. *Journal of Biomedical Informatics*, *38*, 244–255. doi:10.1016/j.jbi.2004.12.004

DesRoches, C. M., & Campbell, E. G. (2008). Electronic health records in ambulatory care--a national survey of physicians. *The New England Journal of Medicine*, *359*(1), 50–60. doi:10.1056/NEJMsa0802005

Dey, C. S., & Majumder, G. C. (1990). Maturation specific type II cyclic AMP- dependent protein kinase in goat sperm plasma membrane. *Biochemistry International*, *21*, 659–665.

Diamond, S. L. (2001). Reaction complexity of flowing human blood. [News Item]. *Biophysical Journal*, *80*(3), 1031–1032. doi:10.1016/S0006-3495(01)76083-3

Diamond, C., & Ricciardi, L. (2006). Building consumer trust into health information exchange. *J. AHIMA*, *77*(10),36, 38.

Ding, G., Lorenz, P., Kreutzer, M., Li, Y., & Thiesen, H. J. (2009). SysZNF: the C2H2 zinc finger gene database. *Nucleic Acids Research*, *37*(Database issue), 267–273. doi:10.1093/nar/gkn782

Dittrich, P. S., Jahnz, M., & Schwille, P. (2005). A new embedded process for compartmentalized cell-free protein expression and on-line detection in microfluidic devices. *ChemBioChem*, *6*(5), 811–814. doi:10.1002/cbic.200400321

Dittrich, P. S., & Manz, A. (2006). Lab-on-a-chip: microfluidics in drug discovery. *Nature Drug Discov.*, *5*, 210–218. doi:10.1038/nrd1985

Dobson, D. C. (1992). Convergence of a reconstruction method for the inverse conductivity problem. *SIAM Journal on Applied Mathematics*, *52*(2), 442–458. doi:10.1137/0152025

Dolgin, M., & Einziger, P. D. (2006). Reconstruction of Layered Biological Tissues via Electrical Impedance Tomography. *IEEE Transactions on Bio-Medical Engineering*, *53*(12), 2464–2471. doi:10.1109/TBME.2006.884638

Dolgin, M., & Einziger, P. D. (2004). Image series expansion for electrical impedance tomography. *Phyical. Review Letters*, *93*(14), 148101/1-4.

Dong, Q., & Vandevoort, C. A. (2009). Effect of egg yolk on cryopreservation of Rhesus monkey ejaculated and epididymal sperm. *Journal of Andrology*, *30*, 309–316. doi:10.2164/jandrol.108.006395

Donnelly, J., & Mussi, J. (2006). Building an interoperable regional health information network today with IHE integration profiles. *Journal of Healthcare Information Management*, *20*(3), 29–38.

D'Orazio, P. (2003). Biosensors in clinical chemistry. [Review]. *Clinica Chimica Acta*, *334*(1-2), 41–69. doi:10.1016/S0009-8981(03)00241-9

Dorn, O., Berteta-Aguirre, H., Berryman, J. G., & Papanicolaou, G. (1999). A nonlinear inversion method for 3D-electromagnetic imaging using adjoint fields. *Inverse Problems*, *15*, 1523–1558. doi:10.1088/0266-5611/15/6/309

Doyle, D. J., Ruskin, K. J., & Engel, T. P. (1996). The Internet and medicine: past, present, and future. *The Yale Journal of Biology and Medicine*, *69*, 429–437.

Doyon, Y., McCammon, J. M., Miller, J. C., Faraji, F., Ngo, C., & Katibah, G. E. (2008). Heritable targeted gene disruption in zebrafish using designed zinc-finger nucleases. *Nature Biotechnology*, *26*(6), 702–708. doi:10.1038/nbt1409

Draghici, S. (1997). A neural network based artificial vision system for license plate recognition, International Journal of Network Security . *International Journal of Neural Systems*, *8*(1). doi:10.1142/S0129065797000148

Duch, W., Matykiewicz, P., & Pestian, J. (2008). Neurolinguistic approach to natural language processing with applications to medical text analysis. *Neural Networks*, *21*(10), 1500–1510. doi:10.1016/j.neunet.2008.05.008

Duffy, D. C., McDonald, J. C., Schueller, O. J. A., & Whitesides, G. M. (1998). Rapid prototyping of microfluidic systems in poly(dimethylsiloxane). *Analytical Chemistry*, *70*(23), 4974–4984. doi:10.1021/ac980656z

Dulinska, I., Targosz, M., Strojny, W., Lekka, M., Czuba, P., & Balwierz, W. (2006). Stiffness of normal and pathological erythrocytes studied by means of atomic force microscopy. *Journal of Biochemical and Biophysical Methods*, *66*(1-3), 1–11. doi:10.1016/j.jbbm.2005.11.003

Dupuy, J., Jal, J. F., Ferradou, C., Chieux, P., Wright, A. F., Calemczuk, R., & Angel, C. A. (1982). Controlled nucleation and quasi-ordered growth of ice-crystals from low temperature electrolyte solution. *Nature*, *296*, 138–140. doi:10.1038/296138a0

Durai, S., Mani, M., Kandavelou, K., Wu, J., Porteus, M. H., & Chandrasegaran, S. (2005). Zinc finger nucleases: custom-designed molecular scissors for genome engineering of plant and mammalian cells. *Nucleic Acids Research*, *33*(18), 5978–5990. doi:10.1093/nar/gki912

Durney, C. H., Rushforth, C. K., & Anderson, A. A. (1988). Resonant AC – DC magnetic fields: calculated response. *Bioelectromagnetics*, *9*, 315–336. doi:10.1002/bem.2250090402

Durney, C. H., Massoudi, H., & Iskander, M. F. (1986). *Radiofrequency radiation dosimetry handbook* (4 ed.). New York: Wiley.

Effenhauser, C. S., Bruin, G. J. M., Paulus, A., & Ehrat, M. (1997). Integrated capillary electrophoresis on flexible silicone microdevices: Analysis of DNA restriction fragments and detection of single DNA molecules on microchips. *Analytical Chemistry*, *69*(17), 3451–3457. doi:10.1021/ac9703919

eHealth Initiative. (2009). *HIE Directory*. Retrieved from http://www.ehealthinitiative.org/directory-health-information-exchange-initiatives.html

eHealth Initiative. (2009, October 1). *Migrating Toward Meaningful Use: The State of Health Information Exchange. Retrievedfrom*http://www.ehealthinitiative.org/sites/default/files/file/2009%20Survey%20Report%20FINAL.pdf

Ehmcke, J., & Schlatt, S. (2008). Animal models for fertility preservation in the male. *Reproduction (Cambridge, England)*, *136*, 717–723. doi:10.1530/REP-08-0093

Eichwald, C., & Walleczek, J. (1998). Magnetic field perturbations as a tool for controlling enzyme-regulated and oscillatory biochemical reactions. *Biophysical Chemistry*, *74*(3), 209–224. doi:10.1016/S0301-4622(98)00180-X

Einbinder, J. S., & Bates, D. W. (2007). Leveraging information technology to improve quality and safety. *Yearbook of Medical Informatics*, 22–29.

Einziger, P. D., Livshitz, L. M., & Mizrahi, J. (2002). Rigorous image-series expansions of quasi-static Green's functions for regions with planar stratification. *IEEE Transactions on Antennas and Propagation*, *50*(12), 1813–1823. doi:10.1109/TAP.2002.807365

Einziger, P. D., Livshitz, L. M., & Mizrahi, J. (2006). Image Theory and Applications in Bioelectromagnetics . In Misra, J. C. (Ed.), *Biomathematics: Modeling and Stimulation* (pp. 315–358). Singapore: World Scientific. doi:10.1142/9789812774859_0012

El-Ali, J., Gaudet, S., Gunther, A., Sorger, P. K., & Jensen, K. F. (2005). Cell stimulus and lysis in a microfluidic device with segmented gas-liquid flow. *Analytical Chemistry*, *77*(11), 3629–3636. doi:10.1021/ac050008x

Elrod-Erickson, M., & Pabo, C. O. (1999). Binding studies with mutants of Zif268. Contribution of individual side chains to binding affinity and specificity in the Zif268 zinc finger-DNA complex. *The Journal of Biological Chemistry*, *274*(27), 19281–19285. doi:10.1074/jbc.274.27.19281

Em-t. (2009). *Em-t*. Retrieved from www.em-t.com.

Enderle, J. D., Blanchard, S. M., & Bronzino, J. D. (Eds.). (2005). *Introduction to Biomedical Engineering* (2nd ed.). Oxford: Elsevier Academic Press.

Engstrom, S. (1996). Dynamic properties of Lednev's parametric resonance mechanism. *Bioelectromagnetics*, *17*(1), 58–70. doi:10.1002/(SICI)1521-186X(1996)17:1<58::AID-BEM8>3.0.CO;2-5

Engstrom, S. (1997). What is the time scale of magnetic field interaction in biological systems? *Bioelectromagnetics*, *18*(3), 244–249. doi:10.1002/(SICI)1521-186X(1997)18:3<244::AID-BEM7>3.0.CO;2-2

Engstrom, S., & Bowman, J. D. (2004). Magnetic resonances of ions in biological systems. *Bioelectromagnetics*, *25*(8), 620–630. doi:10.1002/bem.20028

Ennen, B. D., Berndtson, W. E., Mortimer, R. G., & Pickett, B. W. (1976). Effect of processing procedures on motility of bovine spermatozoa frozen in 0.25ml straws. *Journal of Animal Science*, *43*, 651–656.

Er, M. J., & Zhou, Y. (2008). A novel framework for automatic generation of fuzzy neural networks . *Neurocomputing*, *21*(4-6), 584–591. doi:10.1016/j.neucom.2007.03.015

Erdelyi, A. (1954). *Tables of integral transforms* (*Vol. II*). New York: McGraw-Hill.

Erer, K. S. (2007). Adaptive usage of the butterworth digital filter. *Journal of Biomechanics*, *40*(13), 2934–2943. doi:10.1016/j.jbiomech.2007.02.019

Escubes (2009). *Escubes Technologies*. Retrieved from www.escubestechnologies.com/facilities.htm

Estudillo, F. J., Martinez, C. H., Gutierrez, P. A., & Estudillo, A. C. (2008). Evolutionary product-unit neural networks classifiers . *Neurocomputing*, *72*(1-3), 548–561. doi:10.1016/j.neucom.2007.11.019

Exchange, M. T. (2008). *The MT school wars*, MT Exchange. Retrieved from http://mtexchange.com/mtx/school_wars

Farber, G. K. (1999). New approaches to rational drug design. *Pharmacology & Therapeutics*, *84*, 327–332. doi:10.1016/S0163-7258(99)00039-X

Farshad, A., Khalili, B., & Fazeli, P. (2009). The effect of different concentrations of glycerol and DMSO on viability of Markhoz goat spermatozoa during different freezing temperatures steps. *Pakistan Journal of Biological Sciences*, *12*, 239–245. doi:10.3923/pjbs.2009.239.245

Farstad, W. (2009). Cryopreservation of canine semen – new challenges. *Reproduction in Domestic Animals*, *44*, 336–341. doi:10.1111/j.1439-0531.2009.01418.x

Fernández-Santos, M. R., Esteso, M. C., Soler, A. J., Montoro, V., & Garde, J. J. (2006). Effects of egg yolk and cooling rate on the survival of refrigerated red deer (*Cervus elaphus hispanicus*) epididymal spermatozoa. *Reproduction in Domestic Animals*, *41*, 114–118. doi:10.1111/j.1439-0531.2006.00649.x

Ferrari, M. (2005). Cancer nanotechnology: Opportunities and challenges. *Nature Reviews. Cancer*, *5*(3), 161–171. doi:10.1038/nrc1566

Fever, R. S., & Luca, C. J. (1982, March). A procedure for decomposing the myoelectric signal into its constituent action potentials-part 1: Technique, Theory and Implementation. *IEEE Trans. on BME*, *29*(3), 149–157. doi:10.1109/TBME.1982.324881

Fever, R. S., Xenakis, A. P., & Luca, C. J. (1982, March). A procedure for decomposing the myoelectric signal into its constituent action potentials-part 2: Execution and Test for Accuracy. *IEEE Trans. on BME*, *29*(3), 158–164. doi:10.1109/TBME.1982.324882

Feynman, R. P. (1960). There's plenty of room at the bottom. *Engineering and Science*, 22–36.

Flexman, J. A., & Lazareck, L. (2007). Biomedical engineering and society: policy and ethics. In *Proceedings of IEEE Eng. Med. Biol. Soc., 6156-6158.*

Fogel, D. B., Wasson Iii, E. C., & Boughton, E. M. (1995). Evolving neural networks for detecting breast cancer. *Cancer Letters*, *96*(1), 49–53. doi:10.1016/0304-3835(95)03916-K

Frangi, A. R., Riu, P. J., Rosell, J., & Viergever, M. A. (2002). Propagation of measurement noise through backprojection reconstruction in electrical impedance tomography. *IEEE Transactions on Medical Imaging*, *21*(6), 566–578. doi:10.1109/TMI.2002.800612

Frisse, M. E., King, J. K., et al. (2008). A regional health information exchange: architecture and implementation. In *Proceedings of AMIA Annu. Symp.*, 212-216.

Frohlich, H. (1958). *Theory of dielectrics: dielectric constant and dielectric loss*. Oxford, UK: Clarendon Press.

Fu, A. Y., Spence, C., Scherer, A., Arnold, F. H., & Quake, S. R. (1999). A microfabricated fluorescence-activated cell sorter. *Nature Biotechnology*, *17*, 1109–1111. doi:10.1038/15095

Fu, F., Sander, J. D., Maeder, M., Thibodeau-Beganny, S., Joung, J. K., & Dobbs, D. (2009). Zinc Finger Database (ZiFDB): a repository for information on C2H2 zinc fingers and engineered zinc-finger arrays. *Nucleic Acids Research*, *37*(Database issue), 279–283. doi:10.1093/nar/gkn606

Fung, G., Mangasarian, O. L., & Shavlik, J. (2005). Knowledge-based support vector machine classifiers. In *Proceedings of NIPS 2002*.

Furie, B., & Furie, B. C. (2005). Thrombus formation in vivo. *The Journal of Clinical Investigation*, *115*, 3355–3362. doi:10.1172/JCI26987

Furukawa, M. (1997). Models for evolving community health information networks. *Topics in Health Information Management*, *17*(4), 11–29.

Gafurov, D., Helkala, K., & Soendrol, T. (2006). Gait recognition using acceleration from MEMS. In *Proceedings - First International Conference on Availability, Reliability and Security, ARES,* (pp. 432–439).

Gagnon, M. P., & Legare, F. (2009). Interventions for promoting information and communication technologies adoption in healthcare professionals. *Cochrane Database of Systematic Reviews*, (1): CD006093.

Gallagher, J. E., Dobrosielski-Vergona, K. A., Wingard, R. G., & Williams, T. M. (2005). Web-based vs. traditional classroom instruction in gerontology: a pilot study. *Journal of Dental Hygiene*, *79*, 7.

Gatti, R., Antonelli, G., Prearo, M., Spinella, P., Cappellin, E., & De Palo, E. F. (2009). Cortisol assays and diagnostic laboratory procedures in human biological fluids. [Review]. *Clinical Biochemistry*, *42*(12), 1205–1217. doi:10.1016/j.clinbiochem.2009.04.011

Gerber, A., Studer, R. M., Figueiredo, R. J. P., & Moschytz, G. S. (1984, December). A new framework and computer program for quantitative EMG signal analysis. *IEEE Trans. on BME*, *31*(12), 857–863. doi:10.1109/TBME.1984.325248

Gernot, A., & Fink, P. & Thomas (2006). Unsupervised Estimation of Writing Style Models for Improved Unconstrained Off-line Handwriting Recognition. In *Proceedings of the Tenth International Workshop on Frontiers in Handwriting Recognition*.

Ghosh, A., Biehl, M., & Hammer, B. (2005). Dynamical analysis of LVQ type learning rules. In *Proceedings of the Workshop on the Self-Organizing-Map WSOM'05*, Univ. de Paris (I).

Giakoumaki, A., Pavlopoulos, S., & Koutsouris, D. "*A Medical Image Watermarking Scheme Based on Wavelet Transform*", (Sept. 2003), In *Proceedings of the 25th Annual Int. Conf. of the IEEE-EMBS*, (pp. 856-859).

Giarratano, J., & Riley, G. (2004). *Expert Systems: Principles and Programming, Fourth Edition*. Florence, KY: Course Technology publishers.

Gilbert, G. R., & Almquist, J. O. (1978). Effects of processing procedures on post-thaw acrosomal retention and motility of bovine spermatozoa packaged in 3ml straws at room temperature. *Journal of Animal Science*, *46*, 225–231.

Gilden, D., Cohrs, R. J., Mahalingam, R., & Nagel, M. A. (2009). Varicella zoster virus vasculopathies: diverse clinical manifestations, laboratory features, pathogenesis, and treatment. [Review]. *The Lancet Neurology*, *8*(8), 731–740. doi:10.1016/S1474-4422(09)70134-6

Giles, J. (2005). Internet encyclopaedias go head to head. *Nature*, *15*, 900–901. doi:10.1038/438900a

Gill, K. C. M., Cummins, K. L., & Dorfman, L. J. (1985, July). Automatic decomposition of the clinical Electromyogram. *IEEE Trans. on BME*, *32*(7), 470–477. doi:10.1109/TBME.1985.325562

Gilleard, W., Lai, D. T. H., Levinger, P., & Begg, R. K. (2008, August 20-24). Detecting trunk motion changes due to pregnancy using pattern, recognition techniques. In *Proceedings of the 30th Annual International IEEE EMBS Conference*, British Columbia, Canada.

Gilmore, J. A., Liu, J., Woods, E. J., Peter, A. T., & Critser, J. K. (2000). Cryoprotective agent and temperature effects on human sperm membrane permeabilities: Convergence of theoretical and empirical approaches for optimal cryopreservation methods. *Human Reproduction (Oxford, England)*, *15*, 335–343. doi:10.1093/humrep/15.2.335

Glinkowski, W., & Ciszek, B. (2007). WWW-based e-teaching of normal anatomy as an introduction to telemedicine and e-health. *Telemedicine Journal and e-Health*, *13*, 535–544. doi:10.1089/tmj.2006.0077

Gluckman, E. (2009). Ten years of cord blood transplantation: from bench to bedside. *British Journal of Haematology, 147*, 192–199. doi:10.1111/j.1365-2141 2009.07780.x

Goedecke, N., McKenna, B., El-Difrawy, S., Carey, L., Matsudaira, P., & Ehrlich, D. (2004). A high-performance multilane microdevice system designed for the DNA forensics laboratory. *Electrophoresis, 25*(10-11), 1678–1686. doi:10.1002/elps.200305897

Goharian, M., Bruwer, M., Jegatheesan, A., & Moran, G.R., & MacGregor. (2007). A novel approach for EIT regularization via spatial and spectral principal component analysis. *Physiological Measurement, 28*(9), 1001–1016. doi:10.1088/0967-3334/28/9/003

Goldberg, M., Langer, R., & Jia, X. (2007). Nanostructured materials for applications in drug delivery and tissue engineering. *Journal of Biomaterials Science. Polymer Edition, 18*(3), 241–268. doi:10.1163/156856207779996931

Gonzalez, Woods. "Digital Image Processing", *Prentice-Hall of India*, ISBN-81-7808-629-8,.

Good, B. M., & Wilkinson, M. D. (2006). The Life Sciences Semantic Web is full of creeps! *Briefings in Bioinformatics, 7*, 275–286. doi:10.1093/bib/bbl025

Google. (2009). *Google Health*. Retrieved from https://www.google.com/health

Gotthardt, M., Siegert, M. J., Schlieck, A., Schneider, S., Kohnert, A., & Gross, M. W. (2006). How to successfully implement E-learning for both students and teachers. *Academic Radiology, 13*, 379–390. doi:10.1016/j.acra.2005.12.006

Grannis, S. J., Overhage, J. M., et al. (2002). Analysis of identifier performance using a deterministic linkage algorithm. In *Proceedings of AMIA Symp.*, (pp. 305-309).

Grannis, S. J., Overhage, J. M., et al. (2003). Analysis of a probabilistic record linkage technique without human review. In *Proceedings of AMIA Annu. Symp.*, (pp. 259-263).

Gravely, S. D., & Whaley, E. S. (2009). The next step in health data exchanges: trust and privacy in exchange networks. *Journal of Healthcare Information Management, 23*(2), 33–37.

Graves, A., Fernandez, S., Liwicki, M., Bunke, H., & Schmidhuber, J. (2008). Unconstrained Online Handwriting Recognition with Recurrent Neural Networks, In *Proceedings of Advances in Neural Information Processing Systems*.

Greenes, R. (2007). *Clinical Decision Support: The road ahead*. Burlington, MA: Elsevier publishers.

Grigore, O., & Gavat, I. (1998). Neuro-fuzzy Models for Speech Pattern Recognition in Romanian Language. In *Proceedings of European Symposium on Intelligent Techniques* (CONTI'98). Timisoara, Romania, (pp. 165–172).

Grossman, J. M., & Bodenheimer, T. S. (2006). Hospital-physician portals: the role of competition in driving clinical data exchange. *Health Affairs (Project Hope), 25*(6), 1629–1636. doi:10.1377/hlthaff.25.6.1629

Grossman, J. M., Kushner, K. L., et al. (2008). Creating sustainable local health information exchanges: can barriers to stakeholder participation be overcome? *Res Briefs*, (2), 1-12.

Gruvberger, S. (2001). Estrogen receptor status in breast cancer is associated with remarkably distinct gene expression patterns. *Cancer Research, 61*(16), 5979–5984.

Gutierrez, E., Petrich, B. G., Shattil, S. J., Ginsberg, M. H., Groisman, A., & Kasirer-Friede, A. (2008). Microfluidic devices for studies on shear-dependent platelet adhesion. *Lab on a Chip, 8*(9), 1486–1495. doi:10.1039/b804795b

Guttmache, A. E., Porteous, M. E., & Mclnerney, J. D. (2007). Educating health-care professionals about genetics and genomics. *Nature Reviews. Genetics, 8*(2), 151–157. doi:10.1038/nrg2007

Guyton, C., & Hall, J. E. (2006). *Textbook of medical physiology*. Philadelphia: Elsevier Inc.

Habash, R. (2004). *Biological Effects of Electromagnetic Fields, Handbook of Engineering Electromagnetic Fields*. Boca Raton, FL: CRC Press.

Haber, C. (2006). Microfluidics in commerical applications: an industry perspective. *Lab on a Chip, 6*, 1118–1121. doi:10.1039/b610250f

Hafezi-Moghadam, A., Thomas, K. L., & Cornelssen, C. (2004). A novel mouse-driven ex vivo flow chamber for the study of leukocyte and platelet function. *American*

Journal of Physiology. Cell Physiology, 286, C876–C892. doi:10.1152/ajpcell.00500.2003

Haga, J. H., & Beaudoin, A. J. W., J.G., & Strony, J. (1998). Quantification of the passive mechanical properties of the resting platelet. *Annals of Biomedical Engineering, 26*, 268–277. doi:10.1114/1.118

Halgamuge, M. N., Persson, B. R. R., Salford, L. G., Mendis, P., & Eberhardt, J. L. (2009). Comparison between Two Models for Interactions between Electric and Magnetic Fields and Proteins in Cell Membranes. *Environmental Engineering Science, 26*(10), 1473–1480. doi:10.1089/ees.2009.0014

Halgamuge, M. N., Abeyratne, C. D., & Mendis, P. (2009). *Effect of Cyclotron Resonance Frequencies in Particles Due to AC and DC ElectroMagnetic Fields.* Paper presented at the World Academy of Science, Rome, Italy.

Hammerstedt, R. H., Graham, J. K., & Nolan, J. P. (1990). Cryopreservation of mammalian sperm: what we ask them to survive. *Journal of Andrology, 11*, 73–88.

Hamming, R. W. (1986). *Numerical Methods for Scientists and Engineers.* New York: Dover.

Hammond, W. E. (2008). eHealth interoperability. *Studies in Health Technology and Informatics, 134*, 245–253.

Hara, N., & Kling, R. (1999). *Students' frustrations with a web-based distance education course: A taboo topic in the discourse.* Indiana University, Rob Kling Center for Social Informatics. Retrieved June 15, 2009, from http://rkcsi.indiana.edu/archive/CSI/WP/wp99_01-octoberB.html

Hara, N., & Kling, R. (2000). *Students' distress with a web-based distance education course: An ethnographic study of participants' experiences.* Indiana University, Rob Kling Center for Social Informatics. Retrieved June 15, 2009, from http://rkcsi.indiana.edu/archive/CSI/WP/wp00-01B.html

Harding, J. R., & Wright, A. M. (1996). Non-invasive imaging in the investigation of deep vein. In *Proceedings of the 18th Annual International Conference of the IEEE Engineering in Medicine and Biology Society.* Amsterdam: IR Imaging in Medicine I1 - Quantitative Clinical Applications.

Harnad, S. (1992). *Interactive Publication: Extending American Physical Society's Discipline-Specific Model for Electronic Publishing.* Serials Review, Special Issue on Economics Models for Electronic Publishing, pp. 58–61. Retrieved from http://users.ecs.soton.ac.uk/harnad/ Papers/Harnad/harnad92.interactivpub.html

Harris, C. E. Jr. (2008). The good engineer: giving virtue its due in engineering ethics. *Science and Engineering Ethics, 14*(2), 153–164. doi:10.1007/s11948-008-9068-3

Harrison, J. P., & McDowell, G. M. (2008). The role of laboratory information systems in healthcare quality improvement. *International Journal of Health Care Quality Assurance, 21*(7), 679–691. doi:10.1108/09526860810910159

Harrison, R. A. P., & White, I. G. (1972). Glycolytic enzymes in the spermatozoa and cytoplasmic droplets of bull, boar and ram, their leakage after shock. *Journal of Reproduction and Fertility, 30*, 105–115. doi:10.1530/jrf.0.0300105

Hashimoto, M., Chen, P. C., Mitchell, M. W., Nikitopoulos, D. E., Soper, S. A., & Murphy, M. C. (2004). Rapid PCR in a continuous flow device. *Lab on a Chip, 4*(6), 638–645. doi:10.1039/b406860b

Hassan, R., Hossain, M. M., Bailey, J., Macintyre, G., Ho, J., & Ramamohanarao, K. (2009). A voting approach to identify a small number of highly predictive genes using multiple classifiers . *BMC Bioinformatics, 10*(Suppl 1), S19. doi:10.1186/1471-2105-10-S1-S19

Hassan, R., Hossain, M. M., Begg, R. K., Ramamohanarao, K., & Morsi, Y. (2010). Breast-Cancer identification using HMM-fuzzy approach . *Computers in Biology and Medicine, 40*(Issue 3), 240–251. doi:10.1016/j.compbiomed.2009.11.003

Hassan, R. Begg,Y.Morsi,K.Lynch,HMM-fuzzy model forbreast cancer diagnosis, in: Proceedings of the 15th International Conference on Machines in Medicineand Biology,2006.

Hassan, R., Begg, R., & Taylor, S. (2006). Fuzzy logic-based recognition of gait changes due to trip-related falls. In *Proceedings of the 27th Annual International Conference of the IEEE Engineering in Medicine and Biology Society (IEEE Cat. No.05CH37611C)*, (pp. 4970–4973).

Haus, H. A., & Melcher, J. R. (1989). *Electromagnetic fields and energy*. Englewood Cliffs, NJ: Prentice-Hall.

Hayward, M. K., & Warren, R. D. (2007). Jackson Community Medical Record: a model for provider collaboration in a RHIO. *Journal of Healthcare Information Management*, *21*(3), 31–36.

He, M. Y., Edgar, J. S., Jeffries, G. D. M., Lorenz, R. M., Shelby, J. P., & Chiu, D. T. (2005). Selective encapsulation of single cells and subcellular organelles into picoliter- and femtoliter-volume droplets. *Analytical Chemistry*, *77*(6), 1539–1544. doi:10.1021/ac0480850

Hemker, H. C., Giesen, P., Al Dieri, R., Regnault, V., de Smedt, E., & Wagenvoord, R. (2003). Calibrated automated thrombin generation measurement in clotting plasma. *Pathophysiology of Haemostasis and Thrombosis*, *33*, 4–15. doi:10.1159/000071636

Hendee, S. P., Faour, F. A., Christensen, D. A., Patrick, B., Durney, C. H., & Blumenthal, D. K. (1996). The effects of weak extremely low frequency magnetic fields on calcium/calmodulin interactions. *Biophysical Journal*, *70*(6), 2915–2923. doi:10.1016/S0006-3495(96)79861-2

Henderson, R. P., & Webster, J. G. (1978). An Impedance Camera for Spatially Specific Measurements of the Thorax. *IEEE Transactions on Bio-Medical Engineering*, *25*, 250–254. doi:10.1109/TBME.1978.326329

Hermansson, U., & Axner, E. (2007). Epididymal and ejaculated cat spermatozoa are resistant to cold shock but egg yolk promotes sperm longevity during cold storage at 4°C. *Theriogenology*, *67*, 1239–1248. doi:10.1016/j.theriogenology.2007.01.008

Hessler, B. J., & Soper, P. (2009). Assessing the relationship between health information exchanges and public health agencies. *Journal of Public Health Management and Practice*, *15*(5), 416–424.

Hewavitharana, S., Fernando, H. C., & Kodikara, N. D. (2002). Off-line Sinhala Handwriting Recognition using Hidden Markov Models

Hinman, A. R., & Davidson, A. J. (2009). Linking children's health information systems: clinical care, public health, emergency medical systems, and schools. *Pediatrics*, *123*(2), S67–S73. doi:10.1542/peds.2008-1755D

HIPAA (1996). *The Health Insurance Portability and Accountability Act*. Retrieved from HIPAA.org

Holder, D. S. (Ed.). (2005). *Electrical Impedance Tomography, Methods, History and Applications*. Bristol, UK: IOP.

Holliman, M., & Memon, N. (2000). Counterfeiting Attacks on Oblivious Block-Wise Independent Invisible Watermarking Schemes. *IEEE Transactions on Image Processing*, *9*, 432–441. doi:10.1109/83.826780

Holmquest, D. L. (2007). Another lesson from Santa Barbara. *Health Affairs (Project Hope)*, *26*(5), 592–594. doi:10.1377/hlthaff.26.5.w592

Holobar, A., & Zazula, D. (2004). Correlation-based decomposition of surface electromyograms at low contraction forces. *Journal of Medical and Biological Engineering and Computing . SpringerLink*, *42*(4), 487–495.

Homola, J. (2008). Surface plasmon resonance sensors for detection of chemical and biological species. *Chemical Reviews*, *108*, 462–493. doi:10.1021/cr068107d

Honda, N., Lindberg, U., Andersson, P., Hoffman, S., & Takei, H. (2005). Simultaneous multiple immunoassays in a compact disc-shaped microfluidic device based on centrifugal force. *Clinical Chemistry*, *51*(10), 1955–1961. doi:10.1373/clinchem.2005.053348

Hoong, N. K. (1988). Medical Information Science - Framework and Potential. In *Proceedings of the International Seminar and Exhibition Computerization for Development-the Research Challenge*, (pages 191-198). Kuala Lumpur: Universiti Pertanian Malaysia.

Hu, Y.-C. (2008). Nonadditive grey single-layer perceptron with Choquet integral for pattern classification problems using genetic algorithms . *Neurocomputing*, *72*(1-3), 331–340. doi:10.1016/j.neucom.2008.01.008

Hu, J. H., Li, Q. W., Jiang, Z. L., Yang, H., Zhang, S. S., & Zhao, H. W. (2009). The cryoprotective effect of trehalose supplementation on boar spermatozoa quality. *Reproduction in Domestic Animals*, *44*, 571–575. doi:10.1111/j.1439-0531.2007.00975.x

Huang, B., Wu, H., Bhaya, D., Grossman, A., Granier, S., & Kobilka, B. K. (2007). Counting low-copy number proteins in a single cell. *Science*, *315*(5808), 81–84. doi:10.1126/science.1133992

Huang, R., Barber, T. A., Schmidt, M. A., Tompkins, R. G., Toner, M., & Bianchi, D. W. (2008). A microfluidics approach for the isolation of nucleated red blood cells (NRBCs) from the peripheral blood of pregnant women. *Prenatal Diagnosis*, *28*(10), 892–899. doi:10.1002/pd.2079

Huang, E. (2003). Gene expression predictors of breast cancer outcomes. *Lancet*, *361*(9369), 1590–1596. doi:10.1016/S0140-6736(03)13308-9

Huh, D., Gu, W., Kamotani, Y., Grotberg, J. B., & Takayama, S. (2005). Microfluidics for flow cytometric analysis of cells and particles. *Physiological Measurement*, *26*(3), R73–R98. doi:10.1088/0967-3334/26/3/R02

Hurd, A. (2008). The federated advantage. Data exchange between healthcare organizations in RHIOs is a hot topic. Can federated models end the debate? *Health Manag, Technol.*, *29*(4), 14, 16.

Hwang, G. H., Chen, J. M., Hwang, G. J., & Chu, J. C. (2006). A time scale-oriented approach for building medical expert systems. *Expert Systems with Applications*, 299–308. doi:10.1016/j.eswa.2005.09.050

Ibrahim, F., Taib, M. N., Saadiah, S., Abu Bakar, W., & Abas, W. (2001). Dengue fever and dengue haemorrhagic fever symptoms analysis from an expert system respective. In *Proceedings of the IEEE Int. Conf. 2001.*

Ikai, A., Smith, A., & Tsukada, M. (1999). Nanomechanics. *Current Nanoscience*, *3*(1), 1. doi:10.2174/157341307779940517

Iliescu, C., Xu, G., Barbarini, E., Avram, M., & Avram, A. (2009). Microfluidic device for continuous magnetophoretic separation of white blood cells. *Microsystem Technologies*, *15*, 1157–1162. doi:10.1007/s00542-008-0718-9

Ilter, N., Guvenir, H., & Altay (1998). *UCI Machine Learning Repository.* Rerieved from http://www.ics.uci.edu/~mlearn/MLRepository.html

Indian Market. (2008). *Indian Market* Retrieved from www.indianmarket.com

Ingerman, D. V. (2000). Discrete and continuous Dirichlet-to-Neumann maps in the layered case. *SIAM Journal on Mathematical Analysis*, *31*(6), 1214–1234. doi:10.1137/S0036141097326581

Intermountain Healthcare. (2009). Intermountain Healthcare. Retrieved from http://intermountainhealthcare.org/Pages/home.aspx

Isaacson, D., Mueller, J. L., Newell, J. C., & Siltanen, S. (2004). Reconstruction of Chest Phantoms by the D-Bar Method for Electrical Impedance Tomography. *IEEE Transactions on Medical Imaging*, *23*(7), 821–828. doi:10.1109/TMI.2004.827482

Isakov, V. (1998). *Inverse Problems for Partial Differential Equations.* Wichita, KA: Springer.

Ishii-Watabe, A., Uchida, E., Mizuguchi, H., & Hayakawa, T. (2000). On the mechanism of plasmin-induced platelet aggregation: implications of the dual role of granule ADP. *Biochemical Pharmacology*, *59*, 1345–1355. doi:10.1016/S0006-2952(00)00279-3

Israelachvili, J. (2006). *Intermolecular and surface forces.* New York: Academic Press.

Jagadish, N., Subbanna Bhat, P., Acharya, R., & Niranjan, U. C. (2004, June). Simultaneous storage of medical images in the spatial and frequency domain: a comparative study. *Biomedical Engineering Online*, *3*(1).

Jaggi, R. D., Sandoz, R., & Effenhauser, C. S. (2007). Microfluidic depletion of red blood cells from whole blood in high-aspect-ratio microchannels. *Microfluid. Nanofluid.*, *3*, 47–53. doi:10.1007/s10404-006-0104-9

Jahnel, F. (1938). Resistance of human spermatozoa to deep cold. *Klinische Wochenschrift*, *17*, 1273–1274. doi:10.1007/BF01775125

Jahnisch, K., Hessel, V., Lowe, H., & Baerns, M. (2004). Chemistry in microstructured reactors. *Angewandte Chemie International Edition*, *43*, 406–446. doi:10.1002/anie.200300577

Jaiswal, B. S., Das, K., Saha, S., Dungdung, S. R., & Majumder, G. C. (2009, September 30). Purification and characterization of a motility initiating protein from caprine epididymal plasma. *Journal of Cellular Physiology*; Epub ahead of print.

Jamieson, A. C., Miller, J. C., & Pabo, C. O. (2003). Drug discovery with engineered zinc-finger proteins. *Nature Reviews. Drug Discovery*, *2*(5), 361–368. doi:10.1038/nrd1087

Jang, J.-S. R. (1993). ANFIS: adaptive-network-based fuzzy inference system . *IEEE Transactions on Systems, Man, and Cybernetics*, *23*, 665–685. doi:10.1109/21.256541

Jang, K. S., Hwang, S. Y., Park, S. J., Kim, Y. M., & Kim, M. J. (2005). Effects of a Web-based teaching method on undergraduate nursing students' learning of electrocardiography. *The Journal of Nursing Education*, *44*, 35–39.

Jayakanthan, M., Muthukumaran, J., Chandrasekar, S., Chawla, K., Punetha, A., & Sundar, D. (2009). ZifBASE: a database of zinc finger proteins and associated resources. *BMC Genomics*, *10*, 421. doi:10.1186/1471-2164-10-421

Jensen, A. R. (1998, November). Does IQ matter? *Commentary Magazine,* 20-21.

Jerbi, K., Lionheart, W. R. B., Vauhkonen, P. J., & Vauhkonen, M. (2000). Sensitivity matrix and reconstruction algorithm for EIT assuming axial uniformity. *Physiological Measurement*, *21*, 61–66. doi:10.1088/0967-3334/21/1/308

Jha, A. K., & DesRoches, C. M. (2009). Use of electronic health records in U.S. hospitals. *The New England Journal of Medicine*, *360*(16), 1628–1638. doi:10.1056/NEJMsa0900592

Johnson, N. F., Duric, Z., & Jajodia, S. (2001). *Information Hiding: Steganography and Watermarking - Attacks and Countermeasures*. Amsterdam: Kluwer Academic Press.

Johnson, K. R., Freeman, S. R., & Dellavalle, R. P. (2007). Wikis: the application of Web 2.0. *Archives of Dermatology*, *143*, 1065–1066. doi:10.1001/archderm.143.8.1065

Kaelber, D. C., & Bates, D. W. (2007). Health information exchange and patient safety. *Journal of Biomedical Informatics*, *40*(6), 40–45. doi:10.1016/j.jbi.2007.08.011

Kaiser Permanente. (2009). *Kaiser Permanente*. Retrieved from https://www.kaiserpermanente.org/

Kak, S. C. (1998). On generalization by neural networks . *Information Sciences*, *111*, 293–302. doi:10.1016/S0020-0255(98)10009-9

Kala, R., Shukla, A., & Tiwari, R. (2009). Fuzzy Neuro Systems for Machine Learning for Large Data Sets. In *Proceedings of the IEEE International Advance Computing Conference*, (pp. 541-545) Patiala, India.

Kallman, J. S., & Berryman, J. G. (1992). Weighted least-squares criteria for electrical impedance tomography. *IEEE Transactions on Medical Imaging*, *11*(2), 284–292. doi:10.1109/42.141653

Kam, A., & Cohen, A. (April, 2000). Separation of twins fetal ECG by means of blind source separation (BSS). In *Proceedings of the 21st IEEE Electrical and Electronic Engineers in Israel.* (pp. 342 – 345).

Kamel Boulos, M. N., & Wheeler, S. (2007). The emerging Web 2.0 social software: an enabling suite of sociable technologies in health and health care education. *Health Information and Libraries Journal*, *24*, 2–23. doi:10.1111/j.1471-1842.2007.00701.x

Kamruzzaman, J., et al. (2005). Gene selection and classification of human lymphoma from microarray data, In *Lecture Notes in Computer Science (including subseries Lecture Notes in Artificial Intelligence and Lecture Notes in Bioinformatics* (pp. 379-390).

Kandavelou, K., Mani, M., Durai, S., & Chandrasegaran, S. (2005). "Magic" scissors for genome surgery. *Nature Biotechnology*, *23*(6), 686–687. doi:10.1038/nbt0605-686

Kang, L., Chung, B. G., Lang, R., & Khademhosseini, A. (2008). Microfluidics for drug discovery and development: From target selection to product lifecycle management. *Drug Discovery Today*, *13*(1), 1–13. doi:10.1016/j.drudis.2007.10.003

Kansky, J. (2008). Indiana Health Information Exchange: HIE success in the Heartland - Indiana Network for Patient Care. In *Proceedings of the 2008 HIMSS Conference.*

Kantak, A. S., Gale, B. K., Lvov, Y., & Jones, S. A. (2003). Platelet function analyzer: shear activation of platelets in microchannels. *Biomedical Microdevices*, *5*(3), 207–215. doi:10.1023/A:1025708225412

Kaplan, T., Friedman, N., & Margalit, H. (2005). Ab initio prediction of transcription factor targets using structural knowledge. *PLoS Computational Biology*, *1*(1). doi:10.1371/journal.pcbi.0010001

Karlsson, J. O. M., & Toner, M. (1996). Long-term storage of tissues by cryopreservation: critical issues. *Biomaterials*, *17*, 243–256. doi:10.1016/0142-9612(96)85562-1

Kastrup, C. J., Boedicker, J. Q., Pomerantsev, A. P., Moayeri, M., Bian, Y., & Pompano, R. R. (2008). Spatial localization of bacteria controls coagulation of human blood by 'quorum acting'. [Article]. *Nature Chemical Biology, 4*(12), 742–750. doi:10.1038/nchembio.124

Kastrup, C. J., Shen, F., Runyon, M. K., & Ismagilov, R. F. (2007). Characterization of the threshold response of initiation of blood clotting to stimulus patch size. [Article]. *Biophysical Journal, 93*(8), 2969–2977. doi:10.1529/biophysj.107.109009

Katzman, G. L. (2001). Adobe acrobat: an alternative electronic teaching file construction methodology independent of HTML restrictions. *Journal of Digital Imaging, 14*, 9–13. doi:10.1007/s10278-001-0018-8

Kawahara, H., Higa, S., Tatsukawa, H., & Obata, H. (2009). Cryoprotection and cryosterilization effects of type I antifreeze protein on E. coli cells. *Biocontrol Science, 14*, 49–54. doi:10.4265/bio.14.49

Keller, G. V., & Frischknecht, F. C. (1966). *Electrical Methods in Geophysical Prospecting.* Oxford, UK: Pergamon Press.

Khan, F. S., Maqbool, F., Razzaq, S., Irfan, K., & Zia, T. (2008, February). The Role of Medical Expert Systems in Pakistan. In *Proceedings of world academy of science, engineering and technology* (volume 27).

Khandpur, R. S. (1987). *Hand book of biomedical instrumentation.* New York: McGraw-Hill Publishing Company Limited.

Kim, J., Jang, S. H., Jia, G. Y., Zoval, J. V., Da Silva, N. A., & Madou, M. J. (2004). Cell lysis on a microfluidic CD (compact disc). *Lab on a Chip, 4*(5), 516–522. doi:10.1039/b401106f

Kim, T., Cheng, L.-J., Kao, M.-T., Hasselbrink, E. F., Guo, L. J., & Meyhofer, E. (2009). Biomolecular motor-driven molecular sorter. *Lab on a Chip, 9*, 1282–1285. doi:10.1039/b900753a

Kim, B. S., Boverman, G., Newell, J. C., Saulnier, G. J., & Isaacson, D. (2007). The complete electrode model for EIT in a mammography geometry. *Physiological Measurement, 8*(7), S57–S69. doi:10.1088/0967-3334/28/7/S05

Kim, J. S., & Pabo, C. O. (1998). Getting a handhold on DNA: design of poly-zinc finger proteins with femtomolar dissociation constants. *Natl. Acad. Sci., 95*(6), 2812–2817. doi:10.1073/pnas.95.6.2812

Kim, Y. G., Cha, J., & Chandrasegaran, S. (1996). Hybrid restriction enzymes: zinc finger fusions to Fok I cleavage domain. *Natl. Acad. Sci., 93*(3), 1156–1160. doi:10.1073/pnas.93.3.1156

Kirchheiner, J., Nickchen, K., & Bauer, M. (2004). Pharmacogenetics of antidepressants and antipsychotics: the contribution of allelic variations to the phenotype of drug response. *Molecular Psychiatry, 9*(5), 442–473. doi:10.1038/sj.mp.4001494

Kleine, B. J., vanDijk, B., Lapatki, M., & Zwarts, D., Stegeman. (2007). Using two-dimensional spatial information in decomposition of surface EMG signals. *Journal of Electromyography and Kinesiology, Elsevier, 17*(5), 535–548. doi:10.1016/j.jelekin.2006.05.003

Kline, T. R., Runyon, M. K., Pothiawala, M., & Ismagilov, R. F. (2008). ABO, D blood typing and subtyping using plug-based microfluidics. *Analytical Chemistry, 80*(16), 6190–6197. doi:10.1021/ac800485q

Klir, G. J., & Yuan, B. (1995). *Fuzzy Sets and Fuzzy Logic: Theory and Applications.* Englewood Cliffs, NJ: Prentice-Hall.

Klug, A. (2005). Towards therapeutic applications of engineered zinc finger proteins. *FEBS Letters, 579*(4), 892–894. doi:10.1016/j.febslet.2004.10.104

Koch, K., van Berkel, S. S., van de Wal, M. M. E. B., Nieuwland, P. J., van Hest, J. C. M., & Rutjes, F. P. J. T. (2009). Thrombin generation test in microfluidic systems. *Journal of Applied Physics, 105*, 102012–102017. doi:10.1063/1.3116634

Koch, C., Sommarin, M., Persson, B. R. R., Salford, L. G., & Eberhardt, J. L. (2003). Interaction between weak low frequency magnetic fields and cell membranes. *Bioelectromagnetics, 24*(6), 395–402. doi:10.1002/bem.10136

Kohn, R. V., & Vogelius, M. (1985). Determining conductivity by boundary measurements II. Interior results. *Communications on Pure and Applied Mathematics, 38*(5), 643–667. doi:10.1002/cpa.3160380513

Kolehmainen, V., Vauhkonen, M., Karjalainen, P. A., & Kaipio, J. P. (1997). Spatial inhomogeneity and regularization in EIT. *Proceedings of the 19th Annual International Conference of the IEEE Engineering in Medicine and Biology SocietY,* (1, pp. 449-452). Chicago.

Kong, X., & Feng, R. (2001, September). Watermarking Medical Signals for Telemedicine. *IEEE Transactions on Information Technology in Biomedicine*, *5*(3), 195–201. doi:10.1109/4233.945290

Korjenevsky, A., Cherepin, V., & Sapetsky, A. (2000). Magnetic Induction Tomography: experimental realisation. *Physiological Measurement*, *21*(1), 89–94. doi:10.1088/0967-3334/21/1/311

Koval, D. (2005). Real-world RHIO. A regional health information organization blazes a trail in Upstate New York. *Journal of American Health Information Management Association*, *76*(3), 44–48.

Kraemer, T., & Maurer, H. H. (1998). Determination of amphetamine, methamphetamine and amphetamine-derived designer drugs or medicaments in blood and urine. [Review]. *Journal of Chromatography. B, Analytical Technologies in the Biomedical and Life Sciences*, *713*(1), 163–187. doi:10.1016/S0378-4347(97)00515-X

Kralj, J. G., Sahoo, H. R., & Jensen, K. F. (2007). Integrated continuous microfluidic liquid-liquid extraction. *Lab on a Chip*, *7*(2), 256–263. doi:10.1039/b610888a

Krenek, S., & Berendonk, T. U. (2009). A long-term conservation tool for cell characteristics: cryopreservation of Paramecium caudatum. *Protist*, *160*, 355–363. doi:10.1016/j.protis.2009.03.002

Kribeche, A., Benderbous, S., Tranquart, F., Kouame, D., & Pourcelot, L. (2004). Detection and analysis of fetal movements by ultrasonic multi-sensor Doppler (ACTIFOETUS). In *Proceedings of the 2004 IEEE Ultrasonics Symposium*, (Vol. 2, pp. 1457 – 1460).

Krishna, S. S., Majumdar, I., & Grishin, N. V. (2003). Structural classification of zinc fingers: survey and summary. *Nucleic Acids Research*, *31*(2), 532–550. doi:10.1093/nar/gkg161

Kuhn, K. A., & Giuse, D. A. (2007). Expanding the scope of health information systems - from hospitals to regional networks, to national infrastructures, and beyond. *Methods of Information in Medicine*, *46*(4), 500–502.

Kukolj, D. (2002). Design of adaptive Takagi–Sugeno–Kang fuzzy models. *Applied Soft Computing*, *2*, 89–103. doi:10.1016/S1568-4946(02)00032-7

Kulp, M., Vaher, M., & Kaljurand, M. (2005). Miniaturization of sampling for chemical reaction monitoring by capillary electrophoresis. [Article]. *Journal of Chromatography. A*, *1100*(1), 126–129. doi:10.1016/j.chroma.2005.11.018

Kumar, R. A., & Clark, D. S. (2006). High-throughput screening of biocatalytic activity: application in drug discovery. *Current Opinion in Chemical Biology*, *10*(2), 162–168. doi:10.1016/j.cbpa.2006.02.033

Kumar, R. A., Dong, J. F., Thaggard, J. A., Cruz, M. A., Lopez, J. A., & McIntire, L. V. (2003). Kinetics of GPIb alpha-vWF-A1 tether bond under flow: Effect of GPIb alpha mutations on the association and dissociation rates. [Article]. *Biophysical Journal*, *85*(6), 4099–4109. doi:10.1016/S0006-3495(03)74822-X

Kundu, C. N., Chakrabarty, J., Dutta, P., Battacharyya, D., Ghosh, A., & Majumdar, G. C. (2002). Effect of dextrans on cryopreservation of goat cauda epididymal spermatozoa using a chemically defined medium. *Reproduction (Cambridge, England)*, *123*, 907–913. doi:10.1530/rep.0.1230907

Kundu, C. N., Chakrabarty, J., Dutta, P., Bhattacharyya, D., Ghosh, A., & Majumder, G. C. (2000). Development of a simple sperm cryopreservation model using a chemically defined medium and goat cauda epididymal spermatozoa. *Cryobiology*, *40*, 117–125. doi:10.1006/cryo.2000.2230

Kundu, C. N., Das, K., & Majumder, G. C. (2001). Effect of amino acids on goat cauda-epididymal sperm cryopreservation using a chemically defined model system. *Cryobiology*, *41*, 21–27. doi:10.1006/cryo.2001.2296

Kuo, R. J., Hong, S. M., Lin, Y., & Huang, Y. C. (2008). Continuous genetic algorithm-based fuzzy neural network for learning fuzzy IF–THEN rules. *Neurocomputing*, *71*(13-15), 2893–2907. doi:10.1016/j.neucom.2007.07.013

Kuznetsov, V. A. (1996). Syndrome approach for computer recognition of fuzzy systems and its application to immunological diagnostics and prognosis of human cancer. *Mathematical and Computer Modelling*, *23*(6), 95–119. doi:10.1016/0895-7177(96)00021-0

Lacroix, M. (2006). Significance, detection and markers of disseminated breast cancer cells. *Endocrine-Related Cancer, 13*(4), 1033–1067. doi:10.1677/ERC-06-0001

Lagally, E. T., Emrich, C. A., & Mathies, R. A. (2001). Fully integrated PCR-capillary electrophoresis microsystem for DNA analysis. *Lab on a Chip, 1*(2), 102–107. doi:10.1039/b109031n

Lai, D. T. H., Charry, E., Begg, R., & Palaniswami, M. (2008). Frequency analysis of inertial sensor data for measuring toe clearance. In *Proceedings of the International Conference on Intelligent Sensors, Sensor Networks and Information Processing - ISSNIP 2008*, (pp. 303–308).

Larman, C., & Basili, V. (2003). Iterative and Incremental Development: A Brief History. *Computer, 36*(6), 47–56. doi:10.1109/MC.2003.1204375

Lassila, K. S., & Pemble, K. R. (1997). Assessing the impact of community health information networks: a multisite field study of the Wisconsin Health Information Network. *Topics in Health Information Management, 18*(2), 64–76.

Lau, H. Y., & Tong, K. (2008). The reliability of using accelerometer and gyroscope for gait event identification on persons with dropped foot. *Gait & Posture, 27*(2), 248–257. doi:10.1016/j.gaitpost.2007.03.018

Lau, L. M., Banning, P. D., et al. (2005). Mapping Department of Defense laboratory results to Logical Observation Identifiers Names and Codes (LOINC). In *Proceedings of the AMIA Annu. Symp.*, (pp. 430-434).

Lawrence, D. (2007). "Doing it right. While the key to the perfect RHIO may still be a mystery, a number of them are off and running." Healthc Inform **24**(9): 38, 40.

Lednev, V. V. (1991). Possible mechanism for the influence of weak magnetic-fields on biological-systems. *Bioelectromagnetics, 12*(2), 71–75. doi:10.1002/bem.2250120202

Lednev, V. V., Srebnotskaya, L. K., & L'Yasova, I., Y. N., Rozhdestvenskaya., Z. Y., Klimov, A. A., Belova, N. A., et al. (1996). Magnetic parametric resonance in biosystems: experimental verification of the predictions of a theory using regenerating planarians Dugesia tigrina as a test system. *Biophysics, 41*, 825–835.

Lee, B. S., Lee, J. N., Park, J. M., Lee, J. G., Kim, S., & Cho, Y. K. (2009). A fully automated immunoassay from whole blood on a disc. *Lab on a Chip, 9*(11), 1548–1555. doi:10.1039/b820321k

Lee, W. C., Lien, K. Y., Lee, G. B., & Lei, H. Y. (2008). An integrated microfluidic system using magnetic beads for virus detection. *Diagnostic Microbiology and Infectious Disease, 60*(1), 51–58.

Lee, S. G., et al. (1999). A Neuro-Fuzzy Classifier for Land Cover Classification. In *Proceedings of the 1999 IEEE International Fuzzy Systems Conference Proceedings*, Seoul, Korea.

Levine, H. G., & Forman, P. B. (1973). A study of retention of knowledge of neurosciences information. *Journal of Medical Education, 48*, 867–869.

Levy, S., Adam, D., & Bresler, Y. (2002). Electromagnetic Impedance Tomography (EMIT): A New Method for Impedance Imaging. *IEEE Transactions on Medical Imaging, 21*(6), 676–687. doi:10.1109/TMI.2002.800573

Li, Y., Yang, D., Bai, Y., Mo, X., Huang, W., & Yuan, W. (2008). ZNF418, a novel human KRAB/C2H2 zinc finger protein, suppresses MAPK signaling pathway. *Molecular and Cellular Biochemistry, 310*(1-2), 141–151. doi:10.1007/s11010-007-9674-4

Liau, A., Karnik, R., Majumdar, A., & Cate, J. H. D. (2005). Mixing crowded biological solutions in milliseconds. *Analytical Chemistry, 77*(23), 7618–7625. doi:10.1021/ac050827h

Liboff, A. (1985). Cyclotron resonance in membrane transport . In *Interactions between Electromagnetic Fields and Cells*. New York: Wiley.

Liboff, A. R., Mc, S. S. D., & Leod, B. R. (1987). Mechanistic Approaches to Interactions of Electric and Electromagnetic Fields with Living Systems. *Bioelectrochemistry and Bioenergetics, 35*(1-2), 71–79.

Liboff, A. R., Rozek, R. J., Sherman, M. L., McLeod, B. R., & Smith, S. D. (1987). CA-2+-45 cyclotron-resonance in human-lymphocytes. *Journal of Bioelectricity, 6*(1), 13–22.

Liboff, A. R., Williams, T., Strong, D. M., & Wistar, R. (1984). Time-varying magnetic-fields - effect on DNA-synthesis. *Science, 223*(4638), 818–820. doi:10.1126/science.6695183

Lichtman, M. A., Beutler, E., Kipps, T. J., Seligsohn, U., Kaushanksy, K., & Prchal, J. T. (2006). *William's Hematology*. New York: McGraw-Hill.

Lin, C. J., Chung, I. F., & Chen, C. H. (2007). An entropy-based quantum neuro-fuzzy inference system for classification applications . *Neurocomputing, 70*(13-15), 2502–2516. doi:10.1016/j.neucom.2006.08.008

Lin, C. J., & Hong, S. J. (2007). The design of neuro-fuzzy networks using particle swarm optimization and recursive singular value decomposition . *Neurocomputing, 71*(1-3), 297–310. doi:10.1016/j.neucom.2006.12.016

Lin, T., Podilchuk, C. I., & Delp, E. J. (2000, January). Detection of image alterations using semi-fragile watermarks. In *Proceedings of the SPIE Int. Conf. on Security and Watermarking of Multimedia Contents II*, (vol. 3971, pp. 152-163).

Linderholm, P., Vannod, J., Barrandon, Y., & Renaud, P. (2007). Bipolar resistivity profiling of 3D tissue culture. *Biosensors & Bioelectronics, 22*, 789–796. doi:10.1016/j.bios.2006.02.016

Lionheart, W. R. (2004). EIT reconstruction algorithms: pitfalls, challenges and recent developments. *Physiological Measurement, 25*(1), 125–142. doi:10.1088/0967-3334/25/1/021

Lipton, J., & Hazelzet, J. A. (2009). Clinical decision support systems: Important tools when appropriately used. *Pediatric Critical Care Medicine, 10*(1), 128–129. doi:10.1097/PCC.0b013e31819838f9

Litovitz, T. A. K., D.; Mullins, J.M. (1991). Effect of coherence time of the applied magnetic field on ornithine decarboxylase activity. *Biochemical and Biophysical Research Communications, 178*, 862–865. doi:10.1016/0006-291X(91)90970-I

Liu, Z., & Foote, R. H. (1998). Osmotic effects on volume and motility of bull sperm exposed to membrane permeable and nonpermeable agents . *Cryobiology, 37*, 207–218. doi:10.1006/cryo.1998.2116

Liu, Z., Foote, R. H., & Brockett, C. C. (1998). Survival of bull sperm frozen at different rates in media varying in osmolarity. *Cryobiology, 37*, 219–230. doi:10.1006/cryo.1998.2117

Liu, P. Q., Rebar, E. J., Zhang, L., Liu, Q., Jamieson, A. C., & Liang, Y. (2001). Regulation of an endogenous locus using a panel of designed zinc finger proteins targeted to accessible chromatin regions. Activation of vascular endothelial growth factor A. *The Journal of Biological Chemistry, 276*(14), 11323–11334. doi:10.1074/jbc.M011172200

Liu, Q., Segal, D. J., Ghiara, J. B., & Barbas, C. F. III. (1997). Design of polydactyl zinc-finger proteins for unique addressing within complex genomes. *Natl. Acad. Sci., 94*(11), 5525–5530. doi:10.1073/pnas.94.11.5525

Livshitz, L. M., Einziger, P. D., & Mizrahi, J. (2001). A model of finite electrodes in layered media: a hybrid image series and moment method scheme. *Journal of the Applied Computational Electromagnetics, 16*(2), 145–154.

Lloyd, S. S. (1992). Automated information systems provide health information management support to veterans' healthcare. *Journal of American Health Information Management Association, 63*(6), 63–67.

Lo, K., & Diamond, S. L. (2004). Blood coagulation kinetics: high throughput method for real-time reaction monitoring. [Article]. *Thrombosis and Haemostasis, 92*(4), 874–882.

Lorenzi, N. (2003). *Strategies for Creating Successful Local Health Information Infrastructure Initiatives*. Nashville, TN: Vanderbilt University.

Loudon, G. H., Jone, N. B., & Sehmi, A. S. (1992, November). New signal processing techniques for the decomposition of EMG signals. *Medical & Biological Engineering & Computing, 30*(6), 591–599. doi:10.1007/BF02446790

Luvoni, G. C. (2006). Gamete cryopreservation in the domestic cat. *Theriogenology, 66*, 101–111. doi:10.1016/j.theriogenology.2006.03.012

Lynch, P. J., & Horton, S. (1998). Hypertext markup language as an authoring tool for CD-ROM production. *The Journal of Biocommunication, 25*, 20–25.

Mack, E. H., Wheeler, D. S., & Embi, P. J. (2009). Clinical decision support systems in the pediatric intensive care unit. *Pediatric Critical Care Medicine, 10*(1), 23–28. doi:10.1097/PCC.0b013e3181936b23

Macq, B., & Dewey, F. (1999, October). Trusted Headers for Medical Images. In *DFG VIII-D II Watermarking Workshop*.

Mader, S. S. (2008). *Human Biology* (10 ed.): McGraw Hill Higher Education.

Maeder, M. L., Thibodeau-Beganny, S., Osiak, A., Wright, D. A., Anthony, R. M., & Eichtinger, M. (2008). Rapid "open-source" engineering of customized zinc-finger nucleases for highly efficient gene modification. *Molecular Cell*, *31*(2), 294–301. doi:10.1016/j.molcel.2008.06.016

Maerkl, S. J., & Quake, S. R. (2007). A systems approach to measuring the binding energy landscapes to transcription factors. *Science*, *315*(5809), 233–237. doi:10.1126/science.1131007

Maffei, R. (2008). Determining Business Models for Financial Sustainability in Regional Health Information Organizations: A Literature Review. In *Proceedings of the AMIA Annu. Symp.*, (pg.1038).

Mahabala, H. N., Chandrasekhara, M. K., Baskar, S., Ramesh, S., & Somasundaram, M. S. (1992). ICHT: *An Intelligent Referral System for Primary Child Health Care*. In [*Conference of the South East Asia Regional Computer Confederation*. Kuala Lumpur.]. *Proceedings of SEARCC*, *92*, XI.

Majumder, G. C., Dey, C. S., Haldar, S., & Barua, M. (1990). Biochemical parameters of initiation and regulation of sperm motility. *Archives of Andrology*, *24*, 287–303. doi:10.3109/01485019008987585

Majumder, G. C., Jaiswal, B. S., Nath, D., Banerjee, S., Barua, M., & Sarkar, M. (1999). Biochemistry of sperm motility initiation during epididymal maturation . In Ray, K. P., Krishna, A., & Halder, C. (Eds.), *Comparative Endocrinology and Reproduction*. New Delhi, India: Narosa.

Makarevich, A. V., Chrenek, P., Olexikova, L., Popelkova, M., Turanova, Z., Ostro, A., & Pivko, J. (2008). Post-thaw survival, cell death and actin cytoskeleton in gene-microinjected rabbit embryos after vitrification. *Theriogenology*, *70*, 675–681. doi:10.1016/j.theriogenology.2008.04.043

Malepati, S., & Kushner, K. (2007). RHIOs and the value proposition. Value is in the eye of the beholder. *Journal of American Health Information Management Association*, *78*(3), 24–29, quiz 31–32.

Mallet, Y., Coomans, D., Kautsky, J., & Olivier, D. V. (1997, October). Classification using adaptive wavelets for feature extraction. *IEEE Trans. on PAMI*, *19*(10), 1058–1066.

Mandal, M., Banerjee, S., & Majumder, G. C. (1989). Stimulation of forward motility of goat cauda epididymal spermatozoa by a sperm glycoprotein factor. *Biology of Reproduction*, *41*, 983–989. doi:10.1095/biolreprod41.6.983

Mandel-Gutfreund, Y., & Margalit, H. (1998). Quantitative parameters for amino acid-base interaction: implications for prediction of protein-DNA binding sites. *Nucleic Acids Research*, *26*(10), 2306–2312. doi:10.1093/nar/26.10.2306

Mandell, J. G., & Barbas, C. F., 3rd. (2006). Zinc Finger Tools: custom DNA-binding domains for transcription factors and nucleases. *Nucleic Acids Res*, *34*(Web Server issue), 516-523.

Mandl, K. D., & Simons, W. W. (2007). Indivo: a personally controlled health record for health information exchange and communication. *BMC Medical Informatics and Decision Making*, *7*, 25. doi:10.1186/1472-6947-7-25

Mani, M., Kandavelou, K., Dy, F. J., Durai, S., & Chandrasegaran, S. (2005). Design, engineering, and characterization of zinc finger nucleases. *Biochemical and Biophysical Research Communications*, *335*(2), 447–457. doi:10.1016/j.bbrc.2005.07.089

Manion, F. J., & Robbins, R. J. (2009). Security and privacy requirements for a multi-institutional cancer research data grid: an interview-based study. *BMC Medical Informatics and Decision Making*, *9*, 31. doi:10.1186/1472-6947-9-31

Mantegazza, P. (1866)... *R.C. Ist. Lombardo*, *3*, 183–196.

Maravall, D., Lope, de, Martin, J., & Antonio, J. (2009). Hybridizing evolutionary computation and reinforcement learning for the design of almost universal controllers for autonomous robots . *Neurocomputing*, *72*(4-6), 887–894. doi:10.1016/j.neucom.2008.04.058

Marshall, G. F., & Gillespie, W. (2009). Privacy and security in Pennsylvania: ensuring privacy and security of health information exchange in Pennsylvania. *Journal of Healthcare Information Management*, *23*(2), 38–44.

Martin, M. W. (2002). Personal meaning and ethics in engineering. *Science and Engineering Ethics*, *8*(4), 545–560. doi:10.1007/s11948-002-0008-3

Martin, D. K. (1992). Making the connection: the VA-Regenstrief project. *M.D. Computing*, *9*(2), 91–96.

Martin, Z. (2007). Virginia RHIO taking baby steps. *Health Data Manag.*, *15*(2), 120, 122.

Martinez, A. W., Phillips, S. T., Butte, M. J., & Whitesides, G. M. (2007). Patterned paper as a platform for inexpensive, low-volume, portable bioassays. *Angewandte Chemie International Edition*, *46*, 1318–1320. doi:10.1002/anie.200603817

Martinez, A. W., Phillips, S. T., Carrilho, E., Thomas, S. W., Sindi, H., & Whitesides, G. M. (2008). Simple telemedicine for developing regions: Camera phones and paper-based microfluidic devices for real-time, off-site diagnosis. *Analytical Chemistry*, *80*(10), 3699–3707. doi:10.1021/ac800112r

Martinez, A. W., Phillips, S. T., & Whitesides, G. M. (2008). Three-dimensional microfluidic devices fabricated in layered paper and tape. *Proceedings of the National Academy of Sciences of the United States of America*, *105*, 19606–19611. doi:10.1073/pnas.0810903105

Mazur, P. (1963). Kinetics of water loss from cells at subzero temperatures and the likelihood of intracellular freezing. *The Journal of General Physiology*, *47*, 347–369. doi:10.1085/jgp.47.2.347

Mazur, P. (1965). The role of cell membranes in the freezing of yeast and other signal cells. *Annals of the New York Academy of Sciences*, *125*, 658–676. doi:10.1111/j.1749-6632.1965.tb45420.x

Mazur, P. (1970). Cryobiology: the freezing of living systems. *Science*, *168*, 939–949. doi:10.1126/science.168.3934.939

McClain, M. A., Culbertson, C. T., Jacobson, S. C., Allbritton, N. L., Sims, C. E., & Ramsey, J. M. (2003). Microfluidic devices for the high-throughput chemical analysis of cells. *Analytical Chemistry*, *75*(21), 5646–5655. doi:10.1021/ac0346510

McDonald, J. C., Duffy, D. C., Anderson, J. R., Chiu, D. T., Wu, H. K., & Schueller, O. J. A. (2000). Fabrication of microfluidic systems in poly(dimethylsiloxane). *Electrophoresis*, *21*(1), 27–40. doi:10.1002/(SICI)1522-2683(20000101)21:1<27::AID-ELPS27>3.0.CO;2-C

McDonald, C. J., & Overhage, J. M. (1999). The Regenstrief Medical Record System: a quarter century experience. *International Journal of Medical Informatics*, *54*(3), 225–253. doi:10.1016/S1386-5056(99)00009-X

McDonald, C. J., & Overhage, J. M. (2005). The Indiana network for patient care: a working local health information infrastructure. An example of a working infrastructure collaboration that links data from five health systems and hundreds of millions of entries. *Health Affairs (Project Hope)*, *24*(5), 1214–1220. doi:10.1377/hlthaff.24.5.1214

McGee, J. B., & Begg, M. (2008). What medical educators need to know about "Web 2.0". *Medical Teacher*, *30*, 164–169. doi:10.1080/01421590701881673

McGowan, J. J., Jordan, C., et al. (2007). Rural RHIOs: common issues in the development of two state-wide health information networks. In *Proceedings of the AMIA Annu. Symp.*, (pp. 528-532).

McGraw, D., & Dempsey, J. X. (2009). Privacy as an enabler, not an impediment: building trust into health information exchange. *Health Affairs (Project Hope)*, *28*(2), 416–427. doi:10.1377/hlthaff.28.2.416

McKimm, J., Jollie, C., & Cantillon, P. (2003). ABC of learning and teaching: Web based learning. *BMJ (Clinical Research Ed.)*, *19*, 870–873. doi:10.1136/bmj.326.7394.870

McLean, M. R. (2003). A framework for thinking ethically about human biotechnology. *BioProcess International*, *1*(6), 26–29.

McLean, R., Richards, B. H., & Wardman, J. I. (2007). The effect of Web 2.0 on the future of medical practice and education: Darwikinian evolution or folksonomic revolution? *The Medical Journal of Australia*, *6*, 174–177.

McLeod, B. R., & Liboff, A. R. (1986). Dynamic characteristics of membrane ions in multifield configurations of low-frequency electromagnetic-radiation. *Bioelectromagnetics*, *7*(2), 177–189. doi:10.1002/bem.2250070208

McLeod, B. R., Smith, S. D., Cooksey, K. E., & Liboff, A. R. (1987). Ion-cyclotron resonance frequencies enhance Ca++-dependent motility in diatoms. *Journal of Bioelectricity*, *6*(1), 1–12.

McNamara, A. R., Hurd, P. J., Smith, A. E. F., & Ford, K. G. (2002). Characterisation of site-biased DNA methyltransferases: specificity, affinity and subsite relationships. *Nucleic Acids Research*, *30*(17), 3818–3830. doi:10.1093/nar/gkf501

Medintz, I. L., Uyeda, H. T., Goldman, E. R., & Mattoussi, H. (2005). Quantum dot bioconjugates for imaging, labeling, and sensing. *Nature Materials*, *4*, 435–446. doi:10.1038/nmat1390

Meng, Q., Li, B., & Holstein, H. (2006). Recognition of human periodic movements from unstructured information using a motion-based frequency domain approach. *Image and Vision Computing*, *24*(8), 795–809. doi:10.1016/j.imavis.2006.01.033

Merck Manual Home Edition. (2007). *Introduction: Breast Disorders. Whitehouse Station.* NJ: Merck.

Metherall, P. (1998). *Three Dimensional Electrical Impedance Tomography of the Human Thorax*. (Ph.D. Thesis), University of Sheffield, UK.

Miaou, S., Hsu, C., Tsai, Y., & Chao, H. (2000, July, 23-28). A Secure Data Hiding Technique with Heterogeneous Data-Combining Capability for Electronic Patient Records. In *Proceedings of the 22nd Annual International Conference of the IEEE Engineering in Medicine and Biology Society*, (pp. 280-283).

Microsoft. (2009). *Microsoft HealthVault.* Retrieved from http://www.healthvault.com/

Miller, R. H., & Miller, B. S. (2007). The Santa Barbara County Care Data Exchange: what happened? *Health Affairs (Project Hope)*, *26*(5), 568–580. doi:10.1377/hlthaff.26.5.w568

Minerick, A. R. (2008). The rapidly growing field of micro and nanotechnology to measure living cells. *A.I.Ch.E.J.*, *54*(9), 2230–2237.

Mishra, S. (2007). Biotechnology: An Indian prospective. *Bioimpulse*, *1*(1), 12–15.

Miyazaki, S. (1997). Long-term unrestrained measurement of stride length and walking velocity utilizing a piezoelectric gyroscope. In . *Proceedings of the IEEE Transactions on Biomedical Engineering*, *44*(8), 753–759. doi:10.1109/10.605434

Moehle, E. A., Rock, J. M., Lee, Y. L., Jouvenot, Y., DeKelver, R. C., & Gregory, P. D. (2007). Targeted gene addition into a specified location in the human genome using designed zinc finger nucleases. *Natl. Acad. Sci.*, *104*(9), 3055–3060. doi:10.1073/pnas.0611478104

Molparia, B., Goyal, K., Sarkar, A., Kumar, S., & Sundar, D. (2010). (in press). Zif-Predict: a web tool for predicing DNA-binding specificity in C2H2 zinc finger proteins. *Genomics, Proteomics & Bioinformatics.*

Montelius, E., & Astrand, B. (2008). Individuals appreciate having their medication record on the web: a survey of attitudes to a national pharmacy register. *Journal of Medical Internet Research*, *10*(4), e35. doi:10.2196/jmir.1022

Monzon, J. E. (1999). Teaching ethical issues in biomedical engineering. *Int. J. Eng. Ed.*, *15*(4), 276–281.

Monzon, J. E., & Monzon-Wyngaard, A. (2008). Professional ethics in biomedical engineering practice and research. In *Proceedings of IEEE Eng. Med. Biol. Soc.* (pp. 2893-2896).

Moorthy, J., Mensing, G. A., Kim, D., Mohanty, S., Eddington, D. T., & Tepp, W. H. (2004). Microfluidic tectonics platform: A colorimetric, disposable botulinum toxin enzyme-linked immunosorbent assay system. *Electrophoresis*, *25*(10-11), 1705–1713. doi:10.1002/elps.200405888

Morris, S. J., & Paradiso, J. (2002). Shoe-integrated sensor system for wireless gait analysis and real-time feedback. In . *Proceedings of the Annual International Conference of the IEEE Engineering in Medicine and Biology*, *3*, 2468–2469.

Morris, G. J., & Watson, P. F. (1984). Cold shock-a widespread cellular reaction. *Cryo Letters*, *5*, 352–372.

Morse, P. M., & Feshbach, H. (1953). *Methods of Theoretical Physics.* New York: McGraw-Hill.

Morsy, A., & Flexman, J. (2008). Ethics in biomedical engineering. In *Proceedings of IEEE Eng. Med. Biol. Soc.* (p. 3823).

Mortimer, R. G., Berndtson, W. E., Ennen, B. D., & Pickett, B. W. (1976). Influence of glycerol concentration and freezing rate on post-thaw motility of bovine spermatozoa in continental Straws. *Journal of Dairy Science*, *59*, 2134–2137. doi:10.3168/jds.S0022-0302(76)84499-2

Moss, E. (2001). Multiple choice questions: their value as an assessment tool. *Current Opinion in Anaesthesiology*, *14*, 661–666. doi:10.1097/00001503-200112000-00011

Mu, C. S., Chien, H. C., Eugene, L., & Jonathan, L. (2006). A new approach to fuzzy classifier systems and its application in self-generating neuro-fuzzy systems . *Neurocomputing*, *69*(4-6), 586–614. doi:10.1016/j.neucom.2004.11.033

Muehsam, D. J., & Pilla, A. A. (1994). Weak magnetic-field modulation of ion dynamics in a potential well - mechanistic and thermal noise considerations. *Bioelectrochemistry and Bioenergetics*, *35*, 71–79. doi:10.1016/0302-4598(94)87014-4

Mueller, J. L., Siltanen, S., & Isaacson, D. (2002). A direct reconstruction algorithm for electrical impedance tomography. *IEEE Transactions on Medical Imaging*, *21*(6), 555–559. doi:10.1109/TMI.2002.800574

Muiño-Blanco, T., Pérez-Pé, R., & Cebrián-Pérez, J. A. (2008). Seminal plasma proteins and sperm resistance to stress. *Reproduction in Domestic Animals*, *43*, 18–31. doi:10.1111/j.1439-0531.2008.01228.x

Mukherjea, S. (2005). Information retrieval and knowledge discovery utilising a biomedical Semantic Web. *Briefings in Bioinformatics*, *6*, 252–262. doi:10.1093/bib/6.3.252

Muldrew, K., & McGann, L. E. (1990). Mechanisms of intracellular ice formation. *Biophysical Journal*, *57*, 525–533. doi:10.1016/S0006-3495(90)82568-6

Murthy, S. K., Sin, A., Tompkins, R. G., & Toner, M. (2004). Effect of flow and surface conditions on human lymphocyte isolation using microfluidic chambers. *Langmuir*, *20*, 11649–11655. doi:10.1021/la048047b

Nachman, A. I. (1996). Global Uniqueness for a Two-Dimensional Inverse Boundary Value Problem. *The Annals of Mathematics*, *143*(1), 71–96. doi:10.2307/2118653

Nagrath, S., Sequist, L. V., Maheswaran, S., Bell, D. W., Irimia, D., & Ulkus, L. (2007). Isolation of rate circulating tumor cells in cancer patients by microchip technology. *Nature*, *450*, 1235–1239. doi:10.1038/nature06385

Najafi, B., Aminian, K., Loew, F., Blanc, Y., & Robert, P. (2002). Measurement of stand-sit and sit-stand transitions using a miniature gyroscope and its application in fall risk evaluation in the elderly. *IEEE Transactions on Bio-Medical Engineering*, *49*(8), 843–851. doi:10.1109/TBME.2002.800763

Nandedkar, S. D., & Sanders, D. B. (1989, November). Median averaging of electromyographic motor unit action potentials: comparison with other techniques. *Medical & Biological Engineering & Computing*, *27*(6), 566–572. doi:10.1007/BF02441637

Nani, L., & Lumini, A. (2009). Particle swarm optimization for prototype reduction . *Neurocomputing*, *72*(4-6), 1092–1097. doi:10.1016/j.neucom.2008.03.008

Narasipura, S. D., & King, M. R. (2009). P-selectin-coated microtube for the purification of CD45+ hematopoietic cells directly from human peripheral blood. *Blood Cells, Molecules & Diseases*, *42*(2), 136–139. doi:10.1016/j.bcmd.2008.12.002

Narasipura, S. D., Wojciechowski, J. C., Duffy, B. M., Liesveld, L. J., & King, M. R. (2008). Purification of CD45+ hematopoietic cells directly from human bone marrow using a flow-based P-selectin-coated microtube. *American Journal of Hematology*, *83*(8), 627–629. doi:10.1002/ajh.21204

Nasir, M. S., & Jolley, M. E. (1999). Fluorescence polarization: An analytical tool for immunoassay and drug discovery. *Combinatorial Chemistry & High Throughput Screening*, *2*, 177–190.

Nath, D., & Majumder, G. C. (1999). Maturation dependent modification of protein phosphorylation profile of isolated goat sperm plasma membrane. *Journal of Reproduction and Fertility*, *115*, 29–37. doi:10.1530/jrf.0.1150029

NAUCK. D., NAUCK, U. AND KRUSE, R. (1996): 'Generating Classification rules with the Neuro Fuzzy system NEFCLASS', Proceedings of IEEE Conference, pp. 466-470.

Naurato, N., & Smith, T. J. (2003). Ethical considerations in bioengineering research. *Biomedical Sciences Instrumentation*, *39*, 573–578.

Neeves, K. B., Maloney, S. F., Fong, K. P., Schmaier, A. A., Kahn, M. L., & Brass, L. F. (2008). Microfluidic focal thrombosis model for measuring murine platelet deposition and stability: PAR4 signaling enhances shear-resistance of platelet aggregates. [Article]. *Journal of Thrombosis and Haemostasis*, *6*(12), 2193–2201. doi:10.1111/j.1538-7836.2008.03188.x

Nielsen, J. (1994). *Usability Engineering*. San Francisco: Morgan Kaufmann Publishers.

Noble, D., McKinlay, A., & Repacholi, M. (2005). Effects of static magnetic fields relevant to human health. *Progress in Biophysics and Molecular Biology*, *87*(2-3), 171–372.

Nocella, K. C., & Horowitz, K. J. (2008). Against all odds: designing and implementing a grassroots, community-designed RHIO in a rural region. *Journal of Healthcare Information Management*, *22*(2), 34–41.

Nolan, J. P., & Sklar, L. A. (1998). The emergence of flow cytometry for sensitive, real-time measurements of molecular interactions. *Nature Biotechnology*, *16*, 633–638. doi:10.1038/nbt0798-633

Norman, D. A. (1999). *The Invisible Computer: why good products can fail, the personal computer is so complex, and information appliances are the solution*. Cambridge, MA: MIT Press.

Norman, C., Johnson, C. E., Porterfield, I. D., & Dunbar, R. S. (1958). Effect of pH on the Life-Span and Metabolism of Bovine Sperm Kept at Room Temperatures. *Journal of Dairy Science*, *41*, 1803–1812. doi:10.3168/jds.S0022-0302(58)91167-6

Noss, B., & Zall, R. J. (2002). A review of CHIN initiatives: what works and why. *Journal of Healthcare Information Management*, *16*(2), 35–39.

O' Neill, M., & Ryan, C. (2001). Grammatical Evolution. *IEEE Transactions on Evolutionary Computation*, *5*(4).

O' Neill, M., & Brabazon, A. (2005). Recent Adventures in Grammatical Evolution. In *Proceedings of CMS 2005 Computer Methods and Systems*. (Vol. 1, pp. 245-253).

Open Source Health Records Exchange. (2009). *Open Source Health Records Exchange*. Retrieved from http://www.openhre.org/

Orlova, A. O., Dunnagan, M., et al. (2005). Electronic health record - public health (EHR-PH) system prototype for interoperability in 21st century healthcare systems. In Proceedings of the AMIA Annu. Symp., (pp, 575-579).

Orr, M. J. L. (1996). *Introduction to Radial Basis Function Networks (Technical report)*. Edinburgh, Scotland: Center for Cognitive Science, University of Edinburgh.

Osypka, M., & Gersing, E. (1995). Tissue impedance spectra and the appropriate frequencies for EIT. *Physiological Measurement*, *16*(3A), A49–A55. doi:10.1088/0967-3334/16/3A/005

Outsource Strategies International. (2008). *Medical Transcription Tools and Equipment*. Retrieved from http://www.outsourcestrategies.com/blog/medical-transcription/2008/02/ medical-transcription-tools-and.html

Outsource2india (2009). *Outsource2india*. Retrieved from www.outsource2india.com

Ozkaynak, M., Marquard, J., et al. (2007). Are lay people ready for health information exchange? In *Proceedings of the AMIA Annu. Symp.,* 1065.

Pabo, C. O., Peisach, E., & Grant, R. A. (2001). Design and selection of novel Cys2His2 zinc finger proteins. *Annual Review of Biochemistry*, *70*, 313–340. doi:10.1146/annurev.biochem.70.1.313

Packard, R. R. S., & Libby, P. (2008). Inflammation in atherosclerosis: From vascular biology to biomarker discovery and risk prediction. [Review]. *Clinical Chemistry*, *54*(1), 24–38. doi:10.1373/clinchem.2007.097360

Page, A. K. (2004). Ethical issues in international biomedical research: an overview. *Journal of Health Law*, *37*(4), 629–665.

Panagopoulos, D. J., Karabarbounis, A., & Margaritis, L. H. (2002). Mechanism for action of electromagnetic fields on cells. *Biochemical and Biophysical Research*

Communications, *298*(1), 95–102. doi:10.1016/S0006-291X(02)02393-8

Panagopoulos, D. J., Messini, N., Karabarbounis, A., Philippetis, A. L., & Margaritis, L. H. (2000). A mechanism for action of oscillating electric fields on cells. *Biochemical and Biophysical Research Communications*, *272*(3), 634–640. doi:10.1006/bbrc.2000.2746

Panaro, N. J., Lou, X. J., Fortina, P., Kricka, L. J., & Wilding, P. (2005). Micropillar array chip for integrated white blood cell isolation and PCR. *Biomolecular Engineering*, *21*, 157–162.

Pappas, I. P. I., Popovic, M., Keller, T., Dietz, V., & Morari, M. (2001). A reliable gait phase detection system. *IEEE Transactions on Neural Systems and Rehabilitation Engineering*, *9*(2), 113–125. doi:10.1109/7333.928571

Pappas, I., Keller, T., & Popovic, R. M. (1999). Experimental evaluation of the gyroscope sensor used in a new gait phase detection system. In *Proceedings of the 4th Annual Conference on the International Functional Electrical Stimulation Society, IFESS'99*, (pp. 23–27).

Papworth, M., Kolasinska, P., & Minczuk, M. (2006). Designer zinc-finger proteins and their applications. *Gene*, *366*(1), 27–38. doi:10.1016/j.gene.2005.09.011

Parkes, A. S. (1945). Preservation of human Spermatozoa at Low Temperatures. *British Medical Journal*, *2*, 212. doi:10.1136/bmj.2.4415.212

Patrizio, P. (2000). Cryopreservation of epididymal sperm . *Mol. Cell. Endrol.*, *169*, 11–14. doi:10.1016/S0303-7207(00)00344-0

Pavletich, N. P., & Pabo, C. O. (1991). Zinc finger-DNA recognition: crystal structure of a Zif268-DNA complex at 2.1 A. *Science*, *252*(5007), 809–817. doi:10.1126/science.2028256

Payne, S. R., Oliver, J. E., & Upreti, G. C. (1994). Effect of antifreeze proteins on the motility of ram spermatozoa. *Cryobiology*, *31*, 180–184. doi:10.1006/cryo.1994.1021

Payton, F. C., & Brennan, C. P. (1999). How a community health information network is really used. *Communications of the ACM*, *42*(12), 85–89. doi:10.1145/322796.322814

Payton, F. C., & Brennan, P. F. (1995). Cost justification of a community health information network: the ComputerLink for AD caregivers . In *Proceedings of Annu* (pp. 566–570). Symp. Comput. Appl. Med. Care.

Peng, C., Xiao, S., Nie, Z., & Wang, Z. (1996). Application of Bayes Theorem in medical expert system. In *Proceedings of the IEEE Engineering in medicine and Biology*.

Pereira, M. A., Schaefer, M. B., & Marques, J. L. B. (2004, Septmeber 1-5). Remote Expert System of Support the Prostate Cancer Diagnosis. In *Proceedings of the 26th Annual International Conference of the IEEE EMBS*. San Francisco, CA.

Persikov, A. V., Osada, R., & Singh, M. (2009). Predicting DNA recognition by Cys2His2 zinc finger proteins. *Bioinformatics (Oxford, England)*, *25*(1), 22–29. doi:10.1093/bioinformatics/btn580

Persson, A. (2006). Research ethics and the development of medical biotechnology. *Xenotransplantation*, *13*(6), 511–513. doi:10.1111/j.1399-3089.2006.00352_5.x

Pfau, T., Witte, T. H., & Wilson, A. M. (2005). A method for deriving displacement data during cyclical movement using an inertial sensor. *The Journal of Experimental Biology*, *208*(13), 2503–2514. doi:10.1242/jeb.01658

Philip, J. H. (•••). (No date.). 'Gasman' - Understanding Anesthesia Uptake & Distribution. [Computer software]. Chestnut Hill, MA: Med Man Simulations. *International Journal of Clinical Monitoring and Computing*, *3*, 165–173. doi:10.1007/BF01716358

Phillips, B. O., & Welch, E. E. (2007). Challenges for developing RHIOs in rural America: a study in Appalachian Ohio. *Journal of Healthcare Information Management*, *21*(3), 37–43.

Phillips, P. H. (1939). Preservation of bull semen. *The Journal of Biological Chemistry*, *130*, 415.

Phillips, P. H., & Lardy, H. A. (1940). A yolk-buffer pabulum for the preservation of bull semen. *Journal of Dairy Science*, *23*, 399–404.

Pinero, P. (2004). Sleep stage classification using fuzzy sets and machine learning techniques . *Neurocomputing*, *58–60*, 1137–1143. doi:10.1016/j.neucom.2004.01.178

Pitt, R. E. (1992). Thermodynamics and intracellular ice formation . In Steponkus, P. (Ed.), *Advances in Low-Temperature Biology* (*Vol. 1*, pp. 63–99). London: JAI press.

Polge, C., Smith, A. U., & Parkes, A. S. (1949). Revival of spermatozoa after vitrification and dehydration at low temperature. *Nature*, *164*, 666–668. doi:10.1038/164666a0

Popel, A. S., & Johnson, P. C. (2005). Microcirculation and hemorheology. *Annual Review of Fluid Mechanics*, *37*, 43–69. doi:10.1146/annurev.fluid.37.042604.133933

Public Health Informatics Institute. (2005). *Public Health Opportunities in Health Information Exchange*. Retrieved from http://www.phii.org/resources/doc/Opportunities_0605.pdf

Purdy, P. H. (2006). A review on goat sperm cryopreservation. *Small Ruminant Research*, *63*, 215–225. doi:10.1016/j.smallrumres.2005.02.015

Pursel, V. G., Johnson, L. A., & Schulman, L. L. (1972). Interaction of extender composition and incubation period on cold shock susceptibility of boar spermatozoa. *Journal of Animal Science*, *35*, 580–584.

Q A Pankhurst1, J Connolly2, S K Jones3 and J Dobson4 Applications of magnetic nanoparticles in biomedicine, J. Phys. D: Appl. Phys. **36** (2003) R167–R181 PII: S0022-3727(03)40035-1. topical review

Qu, B.-Y., Wu, Z.-Y., Fang, F., Bai, Z.-M., Yang, D.-Z., & Xu, S.-K. (2008). A glass microfluidic chip for continuous blood cell sorting by a magnetic gradient without labeling. *Analytical and Bioanalytical Chemistry*, *392*, 1317–1324. doi:10.1007/s00216-008-2382-4

Quake, S. R., & Scherer, A. (2000). From micro to nanofabrication with soft materials. *Science*, *290*(5496), 1536–1540. doi:10.1126/science.290.5496.1536

Quinlan, R. M. (1966). *Semantic Memory*. Cambridge, MA: Bolt Beranek and Newman.

Quinn, P. J., & White, I. G. (1966). The effect of cold shock and deep freezing on the concentration of major cations in spermatozoa. *Journal of Reproduction and Fertility*, *12*, 263–270. doi:10.1530/jrf.0.0120263

Rajagopal, P. (2003). *The Basic Kak Neural Network with Complex Inputs* (Master of Science in Electrical Engineering Thesis). Tamil Nadu, India: University of Madras

Ramsey, P. G., & Carline, J. D. (1991). Changes over time in the knowledge base of practicing internists. *Journal of the American Medical Association*, *266*, 1103–1107. doi:10.1001/jama.266.8.1103

Rana, A. P. S., & Majumder, G. C. (1987). Factors influencing the yield and purity of goat sperm plasma membranes isolated by means of an aqueous two- phase polymer system. *Preparative Biochemistry*, *17*, 261–281. doi:10.1080/00327488708062493

Rana, A. P. S., & Majumder, G. C. (1990). Changes in the fluidity of the goat sperm plasma membrane in the transit from caput to cauda epididymis. *Biochemistry International*, *21*, 797–803.

Raths, D. (2006). Real solutions for RHIO problems. Pioneering data exchange groups seek sustainability by solving business problems for members. *Healthcare Informatics*, *23*(8), 26–29.

Raths, D. (2008). Setting the standards stage. If health information exchange is to get to the next level, formulating standards will be an absolute key. *Healthcare Informatics*, *25*(3), 34–35.

Rebar, E. J. (2004). Development of pro-angiogenic engineered transcription factors for the treatment of cardiovascular disease. *Expert Opinion on Investigational Drugs*, *13*(7), 829–839. doi:10.1517/13543784.13.7.829

Rebar, E. J., Huang, Y., Hickey, R., Nath, A. K., Meoli, D., & Nath, S. (2002). Induction of angiogenesis in a mouse model using engineered transcription factors. *Nature Medicine*, *8*(12), 1427–1432. doi:10.1038/nm795

Reiss, J. (2001). *Bringing Your Medical Device to Market*. Washington, DC: FDLI Publ.

Ren, D., Collingwood, T. N., Rebar, E. J., Wolffe, A. P., & Camp, H. S. (2002). PPARgamma knockdown by engineered transcription factors: exogenous PPARgamma2 but not PPARgamma1 reactivates adipogenesis. *Genes & Development*, *16*(1), 27–32. doi:10.1101/gad.953802

Revzin, A., Sekine, K., Sin, A., Tompkins, R. G., & Toner, M. (2004). Development of a microfabricated cytometry platform for characterization and sorting of individual leukocytes. *Lab on a Chip*, *5*, 30–37. doi:10.1039/b405557h

Reynolds, P. A., Mason, R., & Harper, . (2008). The many faces of interaction. *British Dental Journal*, *24*, 565–570. doi:10.1038/sj.bdj.2008.409

Ridley, R. T. (2007). Interactive teaching: a concept analysis. *The Journal of Nursing Education*, *46*, 203–209.

Roach, L. S., Song, H., & Ismagilov, R. F. (2005). Controlling nonspecific protein adsorption in a plug-based microfluidic system by controlling interfacial chemistry using fluorous-phase surfactants. *Analytical Chemistry*, *77*(3), 785–796. doi:10.1021/ac049061w

Robertson, L., & Watson, P. F. (1986). Calcium transport in diluted or cooled ram semen. *Journal of Reproduction and Fertility*, *77*, 177–185. doi:10.1530/jrf.0.0770177

Rogoski, R. (2008). A lack of data standards & sets will hamper information exchange. Healthcare CIOs must pressure government bodies and industry organizations to make true data standards a reality. *Healthc. Inform.*, *25*(2), 58, 60.

Rollins, G. (2005). Finding RHIOs. HIM professionals seek, fill roles in emerging health data networks. *Journal of American Health Information Management Association*, *76*(8), 32–34, 36.

Rondelez, Y., Tresset, G., Tabata, K. V., Arata, H., Fujita, H., & Takeuchi, S. (2005). Microfabricated arrays of femtoliter chambers allow single molecule enzymology. *Nature Biotechnology*, *23*, 361–365. doi:10.1038/nbt1072

Rong, L., Zhiguo, D., Jianzhong, Z., & Ming, L. (2007). Identification of individual walking patterns using gait acceleration. In *Proceedings of the 1st International Conference on Bioinformatics and Biomedical Engineering, ICBBE*, (pp. 543–546).

Rong, L., Zhiguo, D., Jianzhong, Z., Ming, L , & Xiangfeng, H. (2007). A wearable acceleration sensor system for gait recognition. In *Proceedings of the Second IEEE Conference on Industrial Electronics and Applications*, (pp. 2654–2659).

Roots, I., Gerloff, T., & Meisel, C. (2004). Pharmacogenetics-based new therapeutic concepts. *Drug Metabolism Reviews*, *36*(3–4), 617–638. doi:10.1081/DMR-200033458

Rosenberg, R. D., & Aird, W. C. (1999). Vascular-bed - Specific hemostasis and hypercoagulable states. [Review]. *The New England Journal of Medicine*, *340*(20), 1555–1564. doi:10.1056/NEJM199905203402007

Ross, A. S., Saulnier, G. J., Newell, J. C., & Isaacson, D. (2003). Current Source Design for Electrical Impedance Tomography. *Physiological Measurement*, *24*(2), 509–516. doi:10.1088/0967-3334/24/2/361

Rosser, J. C., Lynch, P. J., Cuddihy, L., Gentile, D. A., Klonsky, J., & Merrell, R. (2007). The impact of video games on training surgeons in the 21st century. *Archives of Surgery (Chicago, Ill.)*, *142*, 181–186. doi:10.1001/archsurg.142.2.181

Roy, N., & Majumder, G. C. (1989). Purification and characterization of an antisticking factor from goat epididymal plasma that inhibits sperm–glass and sperm–sperm adhesion. *Biochimica et Biophysica Acta*, *991*, 114–122.

Rubin, R. (2003). The Community Health Information Movement: Where It's Been, Where It's Going . In O'Carroll, P. W., Yasnoff, W., Ward, M., Ripp, L., & Martin, E. (Eds.), *Public Health Informatics and Information Systems* (pp. 595–616). New York: Springer. doi:10.1007/0-387-22745-8_27

Rugg, M. D., & Curran, T. (2007). Event-related potentials and recognition memory. *Trends in Cognitive Sciences*, *11*(6), 251–257. doi:10.1016/j.tics.2007.04.004

Rugg, C. D., Berndtson, W. E., Mortimer, R. G., & Pickett, B. W. (1977). Effect of Thawing Procedures on Fertility of Bovine Spermatozoa Frozen in. 25-ml Straws. *Journal of Animal Science*, *44*, 266–270.

Runyon, M. K., Johnson-Kerner, B. L., & Ismagilov, R. F. (2004). Minimal functional model of hemostasis in a biomimetic microfluidic system. [Article]. *Angewandte Chemie International Edition*, *43*(12), 1531–1536. doi:10.1002/anie.200353428

Runyon, M. K., Johnson-Kerner, B. L., Kastrup, C. J., Van Ha, T. G., & Ismagilov, R. F. (2007). Propagation of blood clotting in the complex biochemical network of hemostasis is described by a simple mechanism. [Article]. *Journal of the American Chemical Society*, *129*(22), 7014–7015. doi:10.1021/ja072602p

Russon, A., Sethu, P., Irimia, D., Mindrinos, M. N., & Calvano, S. E. (2008). Microfluidic leukocyte isolation for gene expression analysis in critically ill hospitalized patients. *Clinical Chemistry*, *54*(5), 891–900. doi:10.1373/clinchem.2007.099150

Rutkowski, L. (2004). *Flexible Neuro-Fuzzy Systems, Structures, Learning and Performance Evaluation*. Amsterdam: Kluwer Academic Publishers.

Ryan, A. G., Louis, L. J., & Yee, W. C. (2005). Informatics in radiology (infoRAD): HTML and Web site design for the radiologist: a primer. *Radiographics*, *25*, 1101–1118. doi:10.1148/rg.254045119

Sabatini, A. M., Martelloni, C., Scapellato, S., & Cavallo, F. (2005). Assessment of walking features from foot inertial sensing . *IEEE Transactions on Bio-Medical Engineering*, *52*(3), 486–494. doi:10.1109/TBME.2004.840727

Saha, P., & Saha, S. (1986). Ethical responsibilities of the clinical engineer. *Journal of Clinical Engineering*, *11*(1), 17–25.

Saha, S., Misra, S., & Saha, P. (1985). Bioengineers, health-care technology and bioethics. *Journal of Medical Engineering & Technology*, *9*(2), 55–60. doi:10.3109/03091908509028765

Saha, S., & Saha, P. S. (1997). Biomedical ethics and the biomedical engineer: a review. *Critical Reviews in Biomedical Engineering*, *25*(2), 163–201.

Saha, S., & Saha, P. S. (2000). Ethical issues of animal and human experimentation in the development of medical devices . In Bronzino, J. D. (Ed.), *The Biomedical Engineering Handbook* (2nd ed.). Boca Raton: CRC Press LLC.

Sajeva, M. (2006). E-learning: Web-based education. *Current Opinion in Anaesthesiology*, *19*, 645–649. doi:10.1097/ACO.0b013e328010bec8

Salisbury, G. W., Fuller, H. K., & Willett, E. L. (1941). Preservation of Bovine Spermatozoa in Yolk-Citrate Diluent and Field Results from its Use. *Journal of Dairy Science*, *24*, 905–910.

Sanchez-Partida, L. G., Setchell, B. P., & Maxwell, W. M. C. (1998). Effect of compatible solutes and diluent composition on the post thaw motility of ram sperm. *Reproduction, Fertility, and Development*, *10*, 347–357. doi:10.1071/R98053

Sandhu, P. S., Salaria, D. S., & Singh, H. (2008). A Comparative Analysis of Fuzzy, Neuro-Fuzzy and Fuzzy-GA Based Approaches for Software Reusability Evaluation . In *Proceedings of Worlds Academy of Science* (*Vol. 29*). Engineering and Technology.

Santiago-Moreno, J., Toledano-Díaz, A., Dorado, J., Pulido-Pastor, A., Coloma, M. A., & López-Sebastián, A. (2007). Recovery and cryopreservation of Spanish ibex epididymal spermatozoa. *Archives of Andrology*, *53*, 309–316. doi:10.1080/01485010701730674

Sarvepalli, D. P., Schmidtke, D. W., & Nollert, M. U. (2009). Design considerations for a microfluidic device to quantify the platelet adhesion to collagen at physiological shear rates. *Annals of Biomedical Engineering*, *37*(7), 1331–1341. doi:10.1007/s10439-009-9708-z

Sauer, R. T. (1990). Transcriptional control. Scissors and helical forks. *Nature*, *347*(6293), 514–515. doi:10.1038/347514b0

Scalise, D. (2006). Technology. Which way RHIO? *Hosp. Health. Netw.*, *80*(6), 20, 22.

Schaff, U. Y., Xing, M. M., Lin, K. K., Pan, N., Jeon, N. L., & Simon, S. I. (2007). Vascular mimetics based on microfluidics for imaging the leukocyte - endothelial inflammatory response. *Lab on a Chip*, *7*(4), 448–456. doi:10.1039/b617915k

Scherzer, J., Fayrer-Hosken, R. A., Aceves, M., Hurley, D. J., Ray, L. E., Jones, L., & Heusner, G. L. (2009). Freezing equine semen: the effect of combinations of semen extenders and glycerol on post-thaw motility. *Australian Veterinary Journal*, *87*, 275–279. doi:10.1111/j.1751-0813.2009.00452.x

Schilling, K., Wiecha, J., Polineni, D., & Khalil, S. (2006). An interactive web-based curriculum on evidence-based medicine: design and effectiveness. *Family Medicine*, *38*, 126–132.

Schmid-Schonbein, G. W., Sung, K.-L. P., Tozeren, H., Skalak, R., & Chien, S. (1981). Passive mechanical properties of human leukocytes. *Biophysical Journal*, *36*, 243–256. doi:10.1016/S0006-3495(81)84726-1

Schmidt, H. G. (1993). Foundations of problem-based learning: some explanatory notes. *Medical Education, 27*, 422–432. doi:10.1111/j.1365-2923.1993.tb00296.x

Schwabe, J. W., & Rhodes, D. (1991). Beyond zinc fingers: steroid hormone receptors have a novel structural motif for DNA recognition. *Trends in Biochemical Sciences, 16*(8), 291–296. doi:10.1016/0968-0004(91)90121-B

Seebauer, E. G., & Barry, R. L. (2001). *Fundamentals of ethics for scientists and engineers*. New York: Oxford Press.

Seeman, N. C. (1999). DNA engineering and its application to nanotechnology. *Trends in Biotechnology, 17*(11), 437–443. doi:10.1016/S0167-7799(99)01360-8

Segal, D. J., & Barbas, C. F. III. (2001). Custom DNA-binding proteins come of age: polydactyl zinc-finger proteins. *Current Opinion in Biotechnology, 12*(6), 632–637. doi:10.1016/S0958-1669(01)00272-5

Sethi, S. K. (2007). Blog/web log - a new easy and interactive website building tool for a non-net savvy radiologist. *Journal of Thoracic Imaging, 22*, 115–119. doi:10.1097/01.rti.0000213578.47398.aa

Sethu, P., Moldawer, L. L., Mindrinos, M. N., Scrumpia, P. O., Tannahill, C. L., & Wilhelmy, J. (2006). Microfluidic isolation of leukocytes from whole blood for phenotype and gene expression analysis. *Analytical Chemistry, 78*, 5453–5461. doi:10.1021/ac060140c

Shadabi, F., Sharma, D., & Cox, R. (2006). Learning from Ensembles: Using Artificial Neural Network Ensemble for Medical Outcomes Prediction, *Innovations in Information Technology*, 1-5.

Shadbolt, N., & Berners-Lee, T. (2008). Web science emerges. *Scientific American, 299*, 76–81. doi:10.1038/scientificamerican1008-76

Shankar, G., & Simmons, A. (2009). Understanding ethics guidelines using an internet-based expert system. *Journal of Medical Ethics, 35*(1), 65–68. doi:10.1136/jme.2007.023358

Shannon, P. (1965). Contribution of seminal plasma, sperm numbers, and gas phase to dilution effects of bovine spermatozoa. *Journal of Dairy Science, 48*, 1357–1361. doi:10.3168/jds.S0022-0302(65)88463-6

Shannon, P., & Curson, B. (1984). Effect of storage temperature on the viability and fertility of bovine sperm diluted and stored in Caprogen. *New Zealand Journal of Agricultural Research, 27*, 173–177.

Shapiro, J. S. (2007). Evaluating public health uses of health information exchange. *Journal of Biomedical Informatics, 40*(6), 46–49. doi:10.1016/j.jbi.2007.08.003

Shevkoplyas, S. S., Gifford, S. C., Yoshida, T., & Bitensky, M. W. (2003). Prototype of an in vitro model of the microcirculation. *Microvascular Research, 65*, 132–136. doi:10.1016/S0026-2862(02)00034-1

Shevkoplyas, S. S., Yoshida, T., Munn, L. L., & Bitensky, M. W. (2005). Biomimetic autoseparation of leukocytes from whole blood in a microfluidic device. *Analytical Chemistry, 77*, 933–937. doi:10.1021/ac049037i

Shi, Y., & Berg, J. M. (1995). A direct comparison of the properties of natural and designed zinc-finger proteins. *Chemistry & Biology, 2*(2), 83–89. doi:10.1016/1074-5521(95)90280-5

Shi, D., Shu, W., & Liu, H. (1998). Feature Selection for Handwritten Chinese Character Recognition Based on Genetic Algorithms. In *Proceedings of the Intl' Conf. on Systems, man and Cybernetics*, (Vol. 5, No 5, pp. 4201-4206).

Shortliffe, E. H. (1988). Computer Programs to Support Clinical Decision Making. *Journal of the American Medical Association, 258*(1), 61–66. doi:10.1001/jama.258.1.61

Shui, L., Eijkel, J. C. T., & van den Berg, A. (2007). Multiphase flow in microfluidic systems - Control and applications of droplets and interfaces. *Advances in Colloid and Interface Science, 133*, 35–49. doi:10.1016/j.cis.2007.03.001

Shukla, S. S. (1985). Comparison of methods for numerical differentiation. *TrAC – . Trends in Analytical Chemistry, 4*(9), 229–233. doi:10.1016/0165-9936(85)85009-3

Shukla, A., Tiwari, R., & Kaur, P. (2009, March 6-7). Knowledge Based Approach for Diagnosis of Breast Cancer. In *Proceedings of the IEEE International Advance Computing Conference*. Patiala, India. (pp. 6-12).

Shukla, A., Tiwari, R., Janghel, R. R., & Kaur, P. (2009, March 6-7). Diagnosis of Thyroid Disorders using Artificial Neural Networks on (2009). IEEE International

Advance Computing Conference. Patiala, India, (pp. 2722-2726).

Shuvalova, L. A., Ostrovskaya, M. V., Sosunov, Y. A., & Lednev, V. V. (1991). Effect of parametric resonance magnetic-field on the rate of Ca2+-calmodulin dependent myosin phosphorylation. *Doklady Akademii Nauk SSSR*, *317*(1), 227–230.

Sievers, A. (1992). Free-Net in Cleveland and Case Western Reserve University Library: Linking Community and University. (pp. 187-203). *Clinic for Library Applications of Data Processing.* Urbana, IL: Graduate School of Library and Information Science.

Sin, A., Chin, K. C., Jamil, M. F., Kostov, Y., Rao, G., & Shuler, M. L. (2004). The design and fabrication of three-chamber microscale cell culture analog device with integrated dissolved oxygen sensors. *Biotechnology Progress*, *20*(1), 338–345. doi:10.1021/bp034077d

Smith, S. D., McLeod, B. R., Liboff, A. R., & Cooksey, K. (1987). Calcium cyclotron-resonance and diatom mobility. *Bioelectromagnetics*, *8*(3), 215–227. doi:10.1002/bem.2250080302

Smith, N. T., & Davidson, T. M. (1999). *'Body' simulation - Anesthesia, physiology and pharmacology simulation* [Computer software]. Point Roberts, WA: Advanced Simulation Corporation.

Smith, S. F., Roberts, N. J., & Partridge, M. R. (2007). Comparison of a web-based package with tutor-based methods of teaching respiratory medicine: subjective and objective evaluations. *BMC Medical Education*, *1*, 41. doi:10.1186/1472-6920-7-41

Smith, J., Bibikova, M., Whitby, F. G., Reddy, A. R., Chandrasegaran, S., & Carroll, D. (2000). Requirements for double-strand cleavage by chimeric restriction enzymes with zinc finger DNA-recognition domains. *Nucleic Acids Research*, *28*(17), 3361–3369. doi:10.1093/nar/28.17.3361

Snowden, A. W., Zhang, L., Urnov, F., Dent, C., Jouvenot, Y., & Zhong, X. H. (2003). Repression of vascular endothelial growth factor A in glioblastoma cells using engineered zinc finger transcription factors. *Cancer Research*, *63*(24), 8968–8976.

Soleimani, M., Powell, C. E., & Polydorides, N. (2005). Improving the Forward Solver for the Complete Electrode Model in EIT Using Algebraic Multigrid. *IEEE Transactions on Medical Imaging*, *24*(5), 577–583. doi:10.1109/TMI.2005.843741

Sollano, J. A., Kirsch, J. M., Bala, M. V., Chambers, M. G., & Harpole, L. H. (2008). The economics of drug discovery and the ultimate valuation of pharmacotherapies in the marketplace. *Clinical Pharmacology and Therapeutics*, *84*(2), 263–266. doi:10.1038/clpt.2008.117

Som, T., & Saha, S. (2008). Handwritten character recognition by using Neural-network and Euclidean distance metric. *Social Science Research Network.* Retrieved from http://ssrn.com/abstract=1118755

Somersalo, E., Cheney, M., Isaacson, D., & Isaacson, E. (1991). Layer stripping: a direct numerical method for impedance imaging. *Inverse Problems*, *7*, 899–926. doi:10.1088/0266-5611/7/6/011

Sone, M., Chikyu, M., Yoshida, M., Bamba, K., & Ogasa, A. (1992). Prolonged storage of boar semen in liquid form. *Jpn. J. Swine Sci.*, *29*, 41–50.

Song, H., Chen, D. L., & Ismagilov, R. F. (2006). Reactions in droplets in microfluidic channels. *Angewandte Chemie International Edition*, *45*, 7336–7356. doi:10.1002/anie.200601554

Song, H., Li, H. W., Munson, M. S., Van Ha, T. G., & Ismagilov, R. F. (2006). On-chip titration of an anticoagulant argatroban and determination of the clotting time within whole blood or plasma using a plug-based microfluidic system. *Analytical Chemistry*, *78*(14), 4839–4849. doi:10.1021/ac0601718

Soryani, M., & Rafat, N. (2006). Application of Genetic Algorithms to Feature Subset Selection in a Farsi OCR . In *Proceedings of World Academy of Science* (*Vol. 18*). Engineering and Technology.

Staes, C. J., & Xu, W. (2009). A case for using grid architecture for state public health informatics: the Utah perspective. *BMC Medical Informatics and Decision Making*, *9*, 32. doi:10.1186/1472-6947-9-32

Stashuk, D., & Bruin, H. D. (1988, January). Automatic decomposition of selective needle detected myoelectric signals. *IEEE Trans. on BME*, *35*(1), 1–10. doi:10.1109/10.1330

Stege, J. T., Guan, X., Ho, T., Beachy, R. N., & Barbas, C. F. III. (2002). Controlling gene expression in plants using synthetic zinc finger transcription factors. *The Plant Journal*, *32*(6), 1077–1086. doi:10.1046/j.1365-313X.2002.01492.x

Steigert, J., Grumann, M., Brenner, T., Riegger, L., Harter, J., & Zengerle, R. (2006). Fully integrated whole blood testing by real-time absorption measurement on a centrifugal platform. *Lab on a Chip*, *6*(8), 1040–1044. doi:10.1039/b607051p

Stein, T. (2006). Writing the RHIO fine print. Model policies and specifications speed data exchange start-ups. *Journal of American Health Information Management Association*, *77*(2), 38–40, 42.

Stone, H. A., Stroock, A. D., & Ajdari, A. (2004). Engineering flows in small devices: Microfluidics toward a lab-on-a-chip. *Annual Review of Fluid Mechanics*, *36*, 381–411. doi:10.1146/annurev.fluid.36.050802.122124

Stout, P. A., Villegas, J., & Kim, H. (2001). Enhancing learning through use of interactive tools on health-related websites. *Health Education Research*, *16*, 721–733. doi:10.1093/her/16.6.721

Summit Instruments (2005). Accelerometer offset drift reduction techniques, *Technical Note 404*.

Sundberg, S. A., Chow, A., Nikiforov, A., & Wada, H. G. (2000). Microchip-based systems for target validation and HTS. *Drug Discovery Today*, *5*, S92–S103. doi:10.1016/S1359-6446(00)80100-2

Suzuki, M. (1993). Common features in DNA recognition helices of eukaryotic transcription factors. *The EMBO Journal*, *12*(8), 3221–3226.

Suzuki, M. (1994). A framework for the DNA-protein recognition code of the probe helix in transcription factors: the chemical and stereochemical rules *Structure (London, England)*, *2*(4), 317–326. doi:10.1016/S0969-2126(00)00033-2

Suzuki, M., Brenner, S. E., Gerstein, M., & Yagi, N. (1995). DNA recognition code of transcription factors. *Protein Engineering*, *8*(4), 319–328. doi:10.1093/protein/8.4.319

Suzuki, M., Gerstein, M., & Yagi, N. (1994). Stereochemical basis of DNA recognition by Zn fingers. *Nucleic Acids Research*, *22*(16), 3397–3405. doi:10.1093/nar/22.16.3397

Sylvester, J. (1992). A convergent layer striping algorithm for the radially symmetric impedance tomography problem. *Communications in Partial Differential Equations*, *17*(11&12), 1955–1994.

Tachibana, H., Harauchi, H., Ikeda, T., Iwata, Y., Takemura, A., & Umeda, T. (2002, December). Practical Use of New Watermarking and VPN Techniques for Medical Image Communication and Archive. In *Proceedings of the RSNA 88th Scientific Assembly and Annual Meeting*.

Taffel, B. (2008). From data interoperability to value-driven healthcare. *Tennessee Medicine*, *101*(12), 31.

Tan, S., Guschin, D., Davalos, A., Lee, Y. L., Snowden, A. W., & Jouvenot, Y. (2003). Zinc-finger protein-targeted gene regulation: genomewide single-gene specificity. *Natl. Acad. Sci.*, *100*(21), 11997–12002. doi:10.1073/pnas.2035056100

Tan, W., Zhu, K., Segal, D. J., Barbas, C. F. III, & Chow, S. A. (2004). Fusion proteins consisting of human immunodeficiency virus type 1 integrase and the designed polydactyl zinc finger protein E2C direct integration of viral DNA into specific sites. *Journal of Virology*, *78*(3), 1301–1313. doi:10.1128/JVI.78.3.1301-1313.2004

Taur, J. S., & Tao, C. W. (2000). A New Neuro-Fuzzy Classifier with Application to On-Line Face Detection and Recognition. *The Journal of VLSI Signal Processing*, *26*, 397–409. doi:10.1023/A:1026515819538

Taylor-Mendes, C. (2007). Proceed with caution: using Wikipedia as a reference. *Neonatal Network*, *26*, 140–141.

Thiesen, H. J., Bellefroid, E., Revelant, O., & Martial, J. A. (1991). Conserved KRAB protein domain identified upstream from the zinc finger region of Kox 8. *Nucleic Acids Research*, *19*(14), 3996. doi:10.1093/nar/19.14.3996

Thompson, C. J., Briggs, K. M., Farrell, P., Fleming, A., Hocking, B., & Joyner, K. (1995). Nonlinear dynamics of charged-particles interacting with combined ac-dc electromagnetic-fields. *Physica A*, *220*(3-4), 471–484. doi:10.1016/0378-4371(95)00162-Z

Thuwanut, P., Chatdarong, K., Techakumphu, M., & Axner, E. (2008). The effect of antioxidants on motility, viability, acrosome integrity and DNA integrity of frozen thawed epididymal cat spermatozoa. *Theriogenology, 70*, 233–740. doi:10.1016/j.theriogenology.2008.04.005

Tian, C., Xing, G., Xie, P., Lu, K., Nie, J., & Wang, J. (2009). KRAB-type zinc-finger protein Apak specifically regulates p53-dependent apoptosis. *Nature Cell Biology, 11*(5), 580–591. doi:10.1038/ncb1864

Tian, C. Y., Zhang, L. Q., & He, F. C. (2006). Progress in the study of KRAB zinc finger protein. *Yi Chuan, 28*(11), 1451–1456. doi:10.1360/yc-006-1451

Toner, M., Cravalho, E. G., & Karel, M. (1990). Thermodynamics and kinetics of intracellular ice formation. *Journal of Applied Physics, 67*, 1582–1592. doi:10.1063/1.345670

Toner, M. (1993). Nucleation of ice crystals inside biological cells . In Steponkus, P. (Ed.), *Advances in Low-Temperature Biology* (*Vol. 2*, pp. 1–51). London: JAI press.

Tran, L., Farinas, J., Ruslim-Litrus, L., Conley, P. B., Muir, C., & Munnelly, K. (2005). Agonist-induced calcium response in single human platelets assayed in a microfluidic device. *Analytical Biochemistry, 341*, 361–368. doi:10.1016/j.ab.2005.02.024

Trigo, F. C., Gonzalez-Lima, R., & Amato, M. B. P. (2004). Electrical Impedance Tomography Using the Extended Kalman Filter. *IEEE Transactions on Medical Imaging, 51*(1), 72–81.

Trimeche, A., Yvon, J. M., Vidament, M., Palmer, E., & Magistrini, M. (1999). Effects of glutamine, proline, histidine and betaine on post-thaw motility of stallion spermatozoa. *Theriogenology, 52*, 181–191. doi:10.1016/S0093-691X(99)00120-X

Tripathi, M., & Delano, D. (2009). Engaging patients for health information exchange. *Health Affairs (Project Hope), 28*(2), 435–443. doi:10.1377/hlthaff.28.2.435

Tsoulos, I., Dimitris, G., & Glavas, E. (2008). Neural network construction and training using grammatical evolution . *Neurocomputing, 72*(1-3), 269–277. doi:10.1016/j.neucom.2008.01.017

Tsuchiya, K., Nakanishi, N., Uetsuji, Y., & Nakamachi, E. (2005). Development of blood extraction system for health monitoring system. *Biomedical Microdevices, 7*(4), 347–353. doi:10.1007/s10544-005-6077-8

Tsumoto, S. (2001). *Rule Induction System based on Characterization of Medical Diagnosis using Rough Sets*. Washington, DC: IEEE Press.

Turner, N. A., Moake, J. L., & McIntire, L. V. (2001). Blockade of adenosine diphosphate receptors P2Y(12) and P2Y(1) is required to inhibit platelet aggregation in whole blood under flow. [Article]. *Blood, 98*(12), 3340–3345. doi:10.1182/blood.V98.12.3340

Uhlmann, D. R. (1973). A kinetic treatment of glass formation. *Journal of Non-Crystalline Solids, 7*, 337–348. doi:10.1016/0022-3093(72)90269-4

Unger, M. A., Chou, H. P., Thorsen, T., Scherer, A., & Quake, S. R. (2000). Monolithic microfabricated valves and pumps by multilayer soft lithography. *Science, 288*(5463), 113–116. doi:10.1126/science.288.5463.113

Urnov, F. D., Miller, J. C., Lee, Y. L., Beausejour, C. M., Rock, J. M., & Augustus, S. (2005). Highly efficient endogenous human gene correction using designed zinc-finger nucleases. *Nature, 435*(7042), 646–651. doi:10.1038/nature03556

Valjus, J. (1996). Health risks of electric and magnetic fields caused by high-voltage systems in Finland. *Scandinavian Journal of Work, Environment & Health, 22*(2), 85–93.

Van Denmark, N. L., & Sharma, U. D. (1957). Preliminary Fertility Results from the Preservation of Bovine Semen at Room Temperatures. *Journal of Dairy Science, 40*, 438–439.

Van Ha, K. (1998). Hierarchical radial basis function networks. *Neural Networks Proceedings, 3*, 1893–1898.

VanWijk, M. J., VanBavel, E., Sturk, A., & Nieuwland, R. (2003). Microparticles in cardiovascular diseases. [Review]. *Cardiovascular Research, 59*(2), 277–287. doi:10.1016/S0008-6363(03)00367-5

Varisli, O., Uguz, C., Agca, C., & Agca, Y. (2009). Effect of chilling on the motility and acrosomal integrity of rat sperm in the presence of various extenders. *Journal of the American Association for Laboratory Animal Science; JAALAS, 48*, 499–505.

Veena Kumari, C., Sndara Rao, G., Madhusudhana Rao, G., & Reddy, K. V. V. S. (2002). *Expert system on neonatal birth injuries*, (vol. 6, pp. 1999 – 2000).

Vernon, D. T., & Blake, R. L. (1993). Does problem-based learning work? A meta-analysis of evaluative research. *Academic Medicine*, *68*, 550–563. doi:10.1097/00001888-199307000-00015

Verpoorte, E., & De Rooij, N. F. (2003). Microfluidics meets MEMS. [Review]. *Proceedings of the IEEE*, *91*(6), 930–953. doi:10.1109/JPROC.2003.813570

Vest, J. R. (2009). Health information exchange and healthcare utilization. *Journal of Medical Systems*, *33*(3), 223–231. doi:10.1007/s10916-008-9183-3

Vieira, A., & Barradas, N. (2003). A training algorithm for classification of high-dimensional data. *Neurocomputing*, *50*, 461–472. doi:10.1016/S0925-2312(02)00635-5

Vijver, Van De., He, M. J., et al. (2002). A gene-expression signature as a predictor of survival in breast cancer. *The New England Journal of Medicine*, *347*(25), 1999–2009. doi:10.1056/NEJMoa021967

Vogel, S. (1994). *Life in moving fluids* (2nd ed.). Princeton, NJ: Princeton University Press.

Voss, A. Baumert, M. Baier, V. Stepan, H. Walther, T. Faber, R., (2003). Analysis of interactions between heart rate and blood pressure in chronic hypertensive pregnancy, Engineering in Medicine and Biology. In *Proceedings of the Ann. Conf. of Biomedical Engineering Society*. (Vol. 2 pp. 1615-1616).

Vreeman, D. J. (2007). Keeping up with changing source system terms in a local health information infrastructure: running to stand still. *Studies in Health Technology and Informatics*, *129*(Pt 1), 775–779.

Wakatani, A. (2002, January). Digital Watermarking for ROI Medical Images by using Compressed Signature Image. In *Proceedings of the Annual Hawaii Int. Conf. on System Science*, (pp. 2043-2048).

Walker, J., & Pan, E. (2005). The value of health care information exchange and interoperability. *Health Affairs (Project Hope)*, (Suppl Web Exclusives), W5-10–W5-18.

Warnekar, P. P., Bouhaddou, O., et al. (2007). Use of RxNorm to exchange codified drug allergy information between Department of Veterans Affairs (VA) and Department of Defense (DoD). In Proceedings of AMIA Annu. Symp., (pp. 781-785).

Watson, S., Williams, R. J., Griffiths, H., Gough, W., & Morris, A. (2003). Magnetic induction tomography: phase versus vector-voltmeter measurement techniques. *Physiological Measurement*, *24*(2), 555–564. doi:10.1088/0967-3334/24/2/365

Watson, P. F. (1981b). The roles of lipid and protein in the protection of ram spermatozoa at 5°C by egg-yolk lipoprotein. *Journal of Reproduction and Fertility*, *62*, 483–492. doi:10.1530/jrf.0.0620483

Watson, P. F. (1995). Recent development and concepts in the cryopreservation of spermatozoa, the assessment of their post thawing function. *Reproduction, Fertility, and Development*, *7*, 871–891. doi:10.1071/RD9950871

Watson, P. F. (2000). The causes of reduced fertility with cryopreserved semen. *Animal Reproduction Science*, *60-61*, 481–492. doi:10.1016/S0378-4320(00)00099-3

Watson, P. F., & Martin, I. C. A. (1972). A comparison of changes in the acrosomes of deep-frozen ram and bull spermatozoa. *Journal of Reproduction and Fertility*, *28*, 99–101. doi:10.1530/jrf.0.0280099

Watson, P. F. (1990). Arficial insemination and the preservation of semen . In Lamming, G. M. (Ed.), *Marshall's Physiology of Reproduction* (*Vol. 2*, pp. 747–869). New York: Churchill Livingstone.

Watson, P. F. (1981a). The effects of cold shock on sperm cell membranes . In Morris, G. J., & Clarke, A. (Eds.), *Effect of Low Temperature on Biological Membranes* (pp. 189–218). London: Academic Press.

Webraydian (2009). *Webraydian*. Retrieved from www.webraydian.com/content/view/1009/32/

Weibel, D. B., DiLuzio, W. R., & Whitesides, G. M. (2007). Microfabrication meets microbiology. *Nature Reviews Microbiology*, *5*(3), 209–218. doi:10.1038/nrmicro1616

Weiner, S. J., & Barnet, B. (2005). Processes for effective communication in primary care. *Annals of Internal Medicine*, *142*(8), 709–714.

Whitesides, G. M. (2006). The origins and the future of microfluidics. *Nature*, *442*, 368–373. doi:10.1038/nature05058

Wiggins, R. H. III, Davidson, H. C., Harnsberger, H. R., Lauman, J. R., & Goede, P. A. (2001). Image file formats: past, present, and future. *Radiographics*, *21*, 789–798.

Wise Geek. (2009). *Wise Geek*. Retrieved from http://www.wisegeek.com/ what-is-home-based-medical-transcription.htm

Witte, T. S., Schafer-Somi, S., Kuchar, A., Mostl, E., Iben, C., & Aurich, C. (2009). Effect of hen's egg yolk on capacitation and acrosome reaction of diluted canine spermatozoa. *Animal Reproduction Science, 110*, 293–305. doi:10.1016/j.anireprosci.2008.01.022

WMA (World Medical Association). 2000. *Declaration of Helsinki Ethical Principles for Medical Research Involving Human Subjects*, Adopted by 18th WMA General Assembly, Helsinki, Finland, June 1964. Amended by the 29th WMA General Assembly, Tokyo, Japan, October 1975; 35th WMA General Assembly, Venice, Italy, October 1983; 41st WMA General Assembly, Hong Kong, September1989; 48th WMA General Assembly, Somerset West, Republic of South Africa, October 1996 and the 52nd WMA General Assembly, Edinburgh, Scotland, October 2000.

Wojciechowski, J. C., Narasipura, S. D., Charles, N., Mickelsen, D., Rana, K., & Blair, M. L. (2008). Capture and enrichment of CD34-positive haematopoietic stem and progenitor cells from blood circulation using P-selectin in an implantable device. *British Journal of Haematology, 140*(6), 673–681. doi:10.1111/j.1365-2141.2007.06967.x

Wolberg, W. H., & Mangasarian O. L., (1990). Multisurface method of pattern separation for medical diagnosis applied to breast cytology. *National Academy of Sciences, 87*(23), 9193-9196.

Wolberg, W. H., Mangasarian, O. L., & Aha, D. W. (1992). UCI Machine Learning Repository, University of Wisconsin Hospitals. Retrieved from http://www.ics.uci.edu/~mlearn/MLRepository.html

Wolfe, S. A., Greisman, H. A., Ramm, E. I., & Pabo, C. O. (1999). Analysis of zinc fingers optimized via phage display: evaluating the utility of a recognition code. *Journal of Molecular Biology, 285*(5), 1917–1934. doi:10.1006/jmbi.1998.2421

Wong, G., Greenhalgh, T., Russell, J., Boynton, P., & Toon, P. (2003). Putting your course on the Web: lessons from a case study and systematic literature review. *Medical Education, 37*, 1020–1023. doi:10.1046/j.1365-2923.2003.01673.x

Wong, P. W. (1998, October). *A Public Key Watermark for Image Verification and Authentication.* In *Proceedings of the IEEE International Conference on Image Processing*, (pp. 455-459).

Woods, E. J., Benson, J. D., Agca, Y., & Critser, J. K. (2004). Fundamental cryobiology of reproductive cells and tissues. *Cryobiology, 48*, 146–156. doi:10.1016/j.cryobiol.2004.03.002

Wootton, D. M., & Ku, D. N. (1999). Fluid mechanics of vascular systems, diseases, and thrombosis. [Review]. *Annual Review of Biomedical Engineering, 1*, 299–329. doi:10.1146/annurev.bioeng.1.1.299

Wright, A., & Sittig, D. F. (2008). SANDS: a service-oriented architecture for clinical decision support in a National Health Information Network. *Journal of Biomedical Informatics, 41*(6), 962–981. doi:10.1016/j.jbi.2008.03.001

Wu, J. D., Hsu, C.-C., & Chen, H.-C. (2009, May). An expert system of price forecasting for used cars using adaptive neuro-fuzzy inference. *Expert Systems with Applications, 36*(4), 7809–7817. doi:10.1016/j.eswa.2008.11.019

Wu, W. G., & Li, J. (2007). RSS made easy: a basic guide for librarians. *Medical Reference Services Quarterly, 26*, 37–50. doi:10.1300/J115v26n01_04

Xia, Y., & Whitesides, G. M. (1998). Soft lithography. *Angewandte Chemie International Edition, 37*, 550–575. doi:10.1002/(SICI)1521-3773(19980316)37:5<550::AID-ANIE550>3.0.CO;2-G

Xu, G. L., & Bestor, T. H. (1997). Cytosine methylation targetted to pre-determined sequences. *Nature Genetics, 17*(4), 376–378. doi:10.1038/ng1297-376

Yamashiro, H., Han, Y. j., Sugawara, A., Tomioka, I., Hoshino, Y., & Sato, E. (2007). Freezability of rat epididymal sperm induced by raffinose in modified Krebs-Ringer bicarbonate (mKRB) based extender solution. *Cryobiology, 55*, 285–294. doi:10.1016/j.cryobiol.2007.08.011

Yang, S. Y., Hsiung, S. K., Hung, Y. C., Chang, C. M., Liao, T. L., & Lee, G. B. (2006). A cell counting/sorting system incorporated with a microfabricated flow cytometer chip. *Measurement Science & Technology, 17*(7), 2001–2009. doi:10.1088/0957-0233/17/7/045

Yang, S. Y., Lien, K. Y., Huang, K. J., Lei, H. Y., & Lee, G. B. (2008). Micro flow cytometry utilizing a magnetic bead-based immunoassay for rapid virus detection. *Biosensors & Bioelectronics*, *24*(4), 855–862. doi:10.1016/j.bios.2008.07.019

Yang, H., & Tiersch, T. R. (2009). Current status of sperm cryopreservation in biomedical research Fish models: Zebrafish, medaka, and Xiphophorus. *Comparative Biochemistry and Physiology*, *149*(Part C), 224–232.

Yang, H., et al. (2003). A segmental nearest neighbor normalization and gene identification method gives superior results for DNA-array analysis. *National Academy of Sciences, 100*(3), 1122-1127.

Yegnanarayana, B. (2003). *Artificial Neural Networks*. New Delhi, India: Prentice Hall of India Pvt. Ltd.

Yorkey, T., Webster, J. G., & Tompkins, W. J. (1987). Comparing reconstruction algorithms for electrical impedance tomography. *IEEE Transactions on Bio-Medical Engineering*, *34*, 843–852. doi:10.1109/TBME.1987.326032

Yuen, P. K., Kricka, L. J., Fortina, P., Panaro, N. J., Sakazume, T., & Wilding, P. (2001). Microchip module for blood sample preparation and nucleic acid amplification reactions. *Genome Research*, *11*(3), 405–412. doi:10.1101/gr.155301

Zafar, A., & Dixon, B. E. (2007). Pulling back the covers: technical lessons of a real-world health information exchange. *Studies in Health Technology and Informatics*, *129*(Pt 1), 488–492.

Zaheeruddin, G. (2006, March). A neuro-fuzzy approach for prediction of human work efficiency in noisy environment. *Computing Volume, 283-294.*

Zain, J. M., & Clarke, M. (2007, September). Reversible Region of Non-Interest (RONI) Watermarking for Authentication of DICOM Images. *International Journal of Computer Science and Network Security*, *7*(9), 19–28.

Zary, N., Johnson, G., Boberg, J., & Fors, U. G. (2006). Development, implementation and pilot evaluation of a Web-based Virtual Patient Case Simulation environment--Web-SP. *BMC Medical Education*, *21*, 10. doi:10.1186/1472-6920-6-10

Zaytseva, N. V., Goral, V. N., Montagna, R. A., & Baeumner, A. J. (2005). Development of a microfluidic biosensor module for pathogen detection. *Lab on a Chip*, *5*(8), 805–811. doi:10.1039/b503856a

Zhang, L., Spratt, S. K., Liu, Q., Johnstone, B., Qi, H., & Raschke, E. E. (2000). Synthetic zinc finger transcription factor action at an endogenous chromosomal site. Activation of the human erythropoietin gene. *The Journal of Biological Chemistry*, *275*(43), 33850–33860. doi:10.1074/jbc.M005341200

Zheng, B., & Ismagilov, R. F. (2005). A microfluidic approach for screening submicroliter volumes against multiple reagents by using preformed arrays of nanoliter plugs in a three-phase liquid/liquid/gas flow. *Angewandte Chemie International Edition*, *44*(17), 2520–2523. doi:10.1002/anie.200462857

Zheng, B., Tice, J. D., & Ismagilov, R. F. (2004). Formation of arrayed droplets of soft lithography and two-phase fluid flow, and application in protein crystallization. *Advanced Materials (Deerfield Beach, Fla.)*, *16*(15), 1365–1368. doi:10.1002/adma.200400590

Zheng, B., Tice, J. D., Roach, L. S., & Ismagilov, R. F. (2004). A droplet-based, composite PDMS/glass capillary microfluidic system for evaluating protein crystallization conditions by microbatch and vapor-diffusion methods with on-chip X-ray diffraction. *Angewandte Chemie International Edition*, *43*(19), 2508–2511. doi:10.1002/anie.200453974

Zheng, S., Liu, J.-Q., & Tai, Y.-C. (2008). Streamline-based microfluidic devices for erythrocytes and leukocytes separation. *Journal of Microelectromechanical Systems*, *17*(4), 1029–1038. doi:10.1109/JMEMS.2008.924274

Zijlstra, W., & Hof, A. (2003). Assessment of spatio-temporal gait parameters from trunk accelerations during human walking. *Gait & Posture*, *18*(2), 1–10. doi:10.1016/S0966-6362(02)00190-X

Zlochiver, S., Freimark, D., Arad, M., Adunsky, A., & Abboud, S. (2006). Parametric EIT for monitoring cardiac stroke volume. *Physiological Measurement*, *27*, S139–S146. doi:10.1088/0967-3334/27/5/S12

Zlochiver, S., Rosenfeld, M., & Abboud, S. (2003). Induced-Current Electrical Impedance Tomography: A 2-D Theoretical Simulation. *IEEE Transactions on Medical Imaging*, *22*(12), 1550–1560. doi:10.1109/TMI.2003.820025

About the Contributors

Anupam Shukla is a Professor in the Information and Communication Technology Department of Indian Institute of Information Technology and Management, Gwalior, India. He has 21 years of teaching experience. His research interest includes Artificial Intelligence, Soft Computing, Biometrics, Bio-Medical Engineering, Bioinformatics Robotics, Animation and Signal processing. He has published around 100 papers in various national and international journals/conferences, authored nine book chapters and a book from CRC press. He is the editor and reviewer for reputed international journals/books/conferences; and also member of program and technical committees at international conferences. He received Young Scientist Award from Madhya Pradesh Government and Gold Medal from Jadavpur University in his post graduation.

Ritu Tiwari is an Assistant Professor in the Information and Communication Technology Department of Indian Institute of Information Technology and Management, Gwalior, India. She has 09 years of teaching experience. Her field of research includes Artificial Intelligence, Soft Computing, Biometrics, Bio-Medical Engineering, Robotics and Speech Signal processing. She has published around 40 papers in various national and international journals/conferences. She is the editor and reviewer for international journals/books/conferences and also members of program and technical committees at international conferences. She received Young Scientist Award from Chhattisgarh Council of Science & Technology and also received Gold Medal in her post graduation.

***

Charry Edgar received his B.Sc degree in Electrical Engineering from the University of São Paulo, São Paulo, Brazil in 2005. From 2006 until 2008, he worked at MEMS Ltda. in São Paulo with Instrumentation/Control Systems, specifically with MEMS sensors calibration and characterization. He has submitted his thesis towards the M.Sc degree from Melbourne University, Melbourne, Australia. Currently, he is working at Pro-Active Medical Pty Ltd in Melbourne, as an Electrical Engineer. His research interests include Digital Signal Processing, MEMS sensors in gait and low back pain analysis and Instrumentation/Control systems. He has over 10 peer-reviewed publications.

Chathurika D. Abeyrathne is a postgraduate student in the School of Engineering at the University of Melbourne, Australia. She received a Bachelor of Science degree in Electrical and Electronic Engineering from University of Peradeniya, Sri Lanka, in 2009. Her research interests include biological effects of weak, extremely low frequency electromagnetic fields.

Das Tirtha Sankar received his B. Tech degree in Electronics and Telecommunication Engineering from Vidyasagar University in 2002 and M.E. degree from Bengal Engineering & Science University, Shibpore in 2004 respectively and PhD degree in Digital Image Watermarking from Jadavpur University in 2009. At present he is an Assistant Professor in the department of Electronics and Communication Engineering at Future Institute of Engineering & Management, Kolkata. He has published around forty research papers in archive Journal and peer reviewed Conferences. His field of interest spans digital image processing, signal processing, communication and VLSI.

Dolgin Madlena received her B.Sc, M.Sc., and Ph.D. degrees in electrical engineering from the Technion - Israel Institute of Technology, Haifa, Israel, in 2000, 2002, and 2009 respectively. She is currently teaching at Sea of Galilee College. Her research interests includes: bioelectromagnetics, medical microwave imaging.

D. John Doyle is a Staff Anesthesiologist in the Department of General Anesthesiology at Cleveland Clinic, as well as Professor of Anesthesiology at the Cleveland Clinic Lerner College of Medicine of Case Western Reserve University. He received his MD degree in 1982 and his PhD degree in Biomedical Engineering in 1986, both from the University of Toronto. He has a long-standing interest in the use of educational technology in medical education.

Einziger Pinchas D. received the B.Sc. and M.Sc. degrees in electrical engineering from the Technion Israel Institute of Technology, Haifa, Israel, and the Ph.D. degree in electrophysics from the Polytechnic University, Brooklyn, NY, in 1976, 1978 and 1981, respectively.Since 1981 he has been on the Faculty of the Department of Electrical Engineering at the Technion. His main interests are electromagnetic wave theory, nonlinear wave phenomena, and bioelectromagnetics.

Ganguru Uma Maheswara Rao, research scholar, Centre for Biotechnology, Jawaharlal Nehru Technological University, Hyderabad, India finished his M.Sc. in Biotechnology form Bharathiar University, Coimbatore, India. He has more than 4 years of research experience and 4 years of teaching experience. At present he is working in Centre for Biotechnology, Jawaharlal Nehru Technological University-Hyderabad on Enzymatic methods for monitoring of toxic pollutants, Phytoremediation and Bioremediation.

Grover Abhinav,Abhinav Grover was born in the holy land of Kurukshetra, India. While pursuing schooling from a well disciplined school in his native place, he won accolades including National awards in Physics, Chemistry and Mathematics Olympiads. His academic proficiency paid him way to one of the India's best Engineering Institute - IIT Delhi, where his continued academic excellence rewarded him with internship offers from France and Australia funded by Embassy of France and Ian Wark Research Institute, Adelaide respectively. In Ian Wark, he worked on developing novel formulations for oral drug delivery. He stood in top twenty in GATE, a Masters' competitive qualifying exam in India. He also received a scholarship from Ministry of Human Resource & Development, Govt. of India and a Summer Undergraduate Research Award during his Masters degree. Throughout his graduation, he furnished himself with skills and expertise needed for a mature researcher and he is currently pursuing his Ph.D. in Science and Engineering from IIT Delhi.

Gundlapalli Adi, MD, PhD, MS is a tenure track Assistant Professor in Internal Medicine and Biomedical Informatics at the University of Utah School of Medicine. He is a practicing infectious diseases physician and active biomedical researcher. He is currently working on projects in public health, clinical and translational informatics. His specific research interests are in biosurveillance, biodefense, emerging infections, natural language processing, data exchange and data visualization. Adi received his medical degree from Madras Medical College, Chennai, India in 1990, PhD in immunology from the University of Connecticut in 1996 and MS in biomedical informatics from the University of Utah in 2007.

Halgamuge Malka N. is a Research Fellow of the Department of Civil and Environmental Engineering at the University of Melbourne. She completed her PhD in Department of Electrical & Electronic Engineering of The University of Melbourne, Australia, Masters of Engineering in Information Technology in School of Electrical & Computer Systems Engineering of RMIT University, Australia and BSc in Engineering, University of Peradeniya, SriLanka. She was awarded the Solander Fellowship for research collaboration with the Departments of Radiation Physics, Neurosurgery and Neuropathology at Lund University, Sweden, to conduct lab-based research using a rat model and cell model to investigate biological effects of non-thermal radio frequency electromagnetic fields of GSM mobile phones and extremely low frequency electromagnetic fields in 2007 & 2008. She is the Guest Editor of the Special Issue on Sensor Network for Building Monitoring on Electronic Journal of Structural Engineering, 2009.

Janghel R.R. is a PhD student in Department of Information Technology at Indian Institute of Information Technology and Management Gwalior. His areas of research are hybrid system design, artificial intelligence and soft computing and application of soft computing in biomedical field. He has published 5 papers in various international and national journals/conferences. He received secured first position in his post graduation from NIT, Raipur.

Jon Reid, MBA is an Informatics Portfolio Manager for the CDC-funded Rocky Mountain Center for Translational Research in Public Health Informatics at the University of Utah. He combines his business and information systems experience to successfully manage informatics project related to public health. Currently he is working with public and private health institutions in the state of Utah to successfully implement clinical health information exchange within those institutions. His main research focus is on electronic asynchronous communication to improve information sharing between clinical and public health workers. Jon received his MBA from the University of Utah in 2006 with a specialty in information systems.

Jose L. López-Ribot received his Pharm.D./Ph.D. in Pharmacy and Microbiology from University of Valencia in Spain in 1991, followed by a post-doctoral training at the Texas Tech University Health Science Center in Lubbock, TX, USA. He was an Assistant Professor and then an Associate Professor in the Department of Medicine/Infectious Diseases at the University of Texas Health Science Center at San Antonio, San Antonio, TX, USA from 1997 to 2005. He moved to the University of Texas at San Antonio in 2005, and is currently a Professor of Biology and South Texas Center for Emerging Infectious Diseases. He has published more than 100 peer-reviewed papers, and numerous conference proceedings. His research interests are in fungal biofilms, fungal pathogenesis, drug discovery, and high-throughput screening.

Kala Rahul, Rahul Kala is a student of final year of 5-year Integrated Post Graduate Course (BTech + MTech in IT) in Indian Institute of Information Technology and Management Gwalior. His areas of research are hybrid system design, robotic planning, design of algorithms, artificial intelligence and soft computing. He has published 18 papers in various international and national journals/conferences. He also takes a keen interest towards Free/Open Source Software.

Kumar Sonu ,With bachelors degree from Institute of Advanced Studies in Education (IASE) University, Rajasthan, India in Bioinformatics in 2006, Sonu started his biological career. After that he moved to New Delhi for his Master education, where he completed his masters in Bioinformatics from Jamia Millia Islamia in 2008. During his masters, he had worked on various small research project and developed one web-server entitled "Development of *in silico* Inhibitor Identification Tool, IS-IT?" in his master diploma. He was a Junior Research Fellow in Dr. Sundar's Lab at Indian Institute of Technology Delhi. There he had worked on Parkinson, GPCR, and web-server development and he got Schrodinger Best poster presentation and two publication (1 International and 1 National). Currently, he is a doctorate student at German Cancer Research Center, Heidelberg, Germany working on Glycoarray as a part of EuroGlycoArray consortium which is funded by Marie Curie Foundation.

Kundu Chanakya Nath is assistant professor at School of Biotechnology, KIIT University, Bhubaneswar, Orissa, India. He received PhD from Indian institute of Chemical Biology. Jadavpur, India in Biochemistry in specialization of reproductive technology. During his PhD he has developed a unique cryopreservation technology that will protect the sperm cell more than 80% after freezing and thawing. He did more than 7 years post doctoral training in various Universality and Institute in United States (Texas A &M University, Texas; University of Florida, Florida and Cleveland Clinic Foundation in, Ohio in signal transduction, cancer biology and DNA damage repair pathway. He has published more than 15 article in very high impact international journal like molecular cell, oncogene, etc.

Lai Daniel T.H. received his B.Eng degree in Electrical and Computer Systems from Monash University, Melbourne, Australia in 2002 and his PhD from Monash University in 2006. He is currently a Research Fellow within the Biomechanics Unit in Victoria University, Australia. His research interests include signal processing and intelligent modelling for gait analysis, and wireless sensor networks for healthcare engineering applications. He has over 40 peer-reviewed publications and is a current reviewer for several international journals. He has been actively involved in the organization of several conferences and workshops.

Majumder G. C. completed his Ph.D in Biochemistry from India in 1970 and went to USA for Post Doctoral studies on reproductive endocrinology. He came back to India in 1975 and joined the Indian Institute of Chemical Biology (IICB) in Scientist 'C' grade. Subsequently he retired in 2001 as Scientist 'G' (Director Grade) from the same Institute. Then he persuaded his scientific endeavor as an Emeritus Scientist of ICMR at IICB and completed his tenure in December 2006. Subsequently he has joined Center for Rural and Cryogenic Technologies, Jadavpur University as AICTE Emeritus Fellow in November 2007. Dr. Majumder's main research interest is male reproductive biology with special reference to sperm biochemistry. During this period he guided 16 Ph.D. students and published 130 research articles in different International and National Journals. He has served as reviewer for several International Journals. He has two Indian and seven foreign (USA, Japan) patents. Dr. Majumder is

Ph.D. thesis examiner and M.Sc. examiner of different Universities. He has visited USA, Canada, Germany, Japan, USSR for different scientific assignments. In 1976 he has received the prestigious Rafi Ahmed Kidwai Award of ICAR Along with several other honours he has also been elected as a Fellow of the West Bengal Academy of Science and Technology in 1994 Fellow of the National Academy of Sciences in 1998.

Mangamoori Lakshmi Narasu, Director, Institute of Science and Technology, Jawaharlal Nehru Technological University, Hyderabad, India, finished her Ph. D. in Microbiology from Indian Institute of Science (IISc) Bangalore in1987. She has 28 years of research experience and 19 years of teaching experience. She achieved All India Council for Technical Education career award for young teachers in the year 1996 for the proposed work on transformed root cultures of *Artemisia annua.* She has written 22 publications in international journals and more than 20 publications in National journals. Presently she is the coordinator for World Bank funded Program entitled Technical Education Quality Improvement Program (TEQIP) for the entire Institute (Budget involved is 128 Million Rupees) and also leading projects funded by Ministry of New and Renewable Energy. She is life time member, Indian Science Congress Association and holds many national and international fellowships.

Snehasish Mishra has a career spanning for more a decade and half, with experiences of more than eight years in research and extension, two years in industries, and about five years in academics and academic administration. He worked with some well-recognised international R&D agencies, such as the DFID, and NORAD. His two major current research areas of interest are Bioprocess Technology and Biotech Entrepreneurship with a strong outreach component. He has numerous national and international publications, both in peer-reviewed journals and science popularisation magazines. He headed the Entrepreneurship Development Cell (EDC) in one leading Engineering College in Delhi NCR region, and sensitised engineering graduates for entrepreneurship. He has received few awards and honours since his schooling days till date. He has successfully guided few MSc and MPhil students. Some of his students are now placed in various R&D assignments abroad. Currently, he is engaged as the Associate Dean.

Morsi Yos achieved his PhD from London University 1983 in the area of fluid modelling and diagnostics. He has held various academic positions in University College London, Loughborough University, University of New South Wales, Nottingham University. Currently he is the research director of the Bio-mechanics and tissue engineering laboratory. The majority of his research work, which he started in Imperial College London (ICL) and then University College London (UCL), is in the area of flow-field modelling and diagnostics. He has developed and used extensively various experimental laser diagnostics techniques and has gained substantial experience through his work as a consultant and R&D engineer in various engineering and industrial research establishments in UK and Australia. He has published over 150 journals and conference publication, one book and seven chapters and edited two proceedings in the area of tissue engineering, nanofabrications and fluid structure interaction of heart valves arteries and aorta.

Owida Amal obtained her PhD from Swinburne University of Technology in 2009. Her research interests cover, haemodynamic of Coronary Bypass Arteries, (CABG) nanofabrication and tissue engineering. She has more than 15 journals and conferences publications.

Preet Ranjan ,Ranjan Preet is Senior Research Fellow in KIIT Univ. Bhubaneswar. She is working in Cancer Biology in special reference to breast cancer. She has done her graduation from C. C. S. Univ., Meerut in Medical Laboratory Technology and Masters in Biochemistry from H.N.B. Garhwal Univ., Srinagar, India. She has also obtained Master of philosophy from C. D. L. Univ., Sirsa, India. She has also worked as Assistant Lecturer in Combined Institute of Medical Sciences and Research and also in SBS Post graduate Institute of Biomedical Sciences and Research, Dehradun, India. Her keen interest is in research to obtain the new findings for the goodwill of mankind.

Priyan Mendis is a Professor of Civil and Environmental Engineering at the University of Melbourne. He is leading the Advanced Protective Technology of Engineering Structures (APTES) research group at the University of Melbourne. He is also the Manager of the ARC Research Network for a Secure Australia (RNSA). RNSA involves 20 universities in Australia and facilitate collaboration on research areas related to security technology including bio security. He is also the Editor-in-chief of the Electronic Journal of Structural Engineering (EJSE). He has conducted research on human effects from extreme events in addition to other work on critical infrastructure protection. His peer-reviewed publications include 65 journal papers and 145 conference papers.

Pujing Shi is currently a PhD students working in the area of Lung Tissue Engineering.

Punetha Ankita ,Born in 1985, Ankita did her schooling from Gen. B. C. Joshi Army Public School and graduated from Kumaon University, securing the highest in her college. She did her Master's in Bioinformatics from Banasthali University. Her first project was on "Identification of Orthologous Proteins within Diatoms, Red Algae, Bryophytes and Pteridophytes using Chloroplast sequences and construction of Phylogenetic Tree based on their rRNA sequences". She got selected in the studentship of DBT at National Institute for Plant Genome Research and worked on building up of "Essential oil database for highly invasive weeds in India". In 2008, she joined in the laboratory of D. Sundar at IIT Delhi as Junior Research Fellows. Her work has been part of a couple of peer-reviewed international publications. Her research interests include understanding DNA-protein interactions and in molecular modeling studies.

Ramasubramanian Anand received his B.S. in Chemical Engineering from Annamalai University, India in 1994, an M.S. in Chemical Engineering from Indian Institute of Science, Bangalore, India in 1996, and a Ph.D. in Bioengineering from Rice University, Houston, TX, USA in 2004. He performed his post-doctoral training in Chemical Engineering at the University of California-Berkeley. He is currently an Assistant Professor in Biomedical Engineering and South Texas Center for Emerging Infectious Diseases. His research interests are in vascular bioengineering, microfluidics, and high-throughput screening.

Jan Root, Ph.D, is the President and CEO of the not-for-profit Utah Health Information Network (UHIN). Under Dr Root's leadership, Utah has actively moved into the development of a state-wide HIE. Dr Root has a long history working in health information exchange primarily in the area of administrative exchange: claims, remits, etc. She was the primary author of the 4010 HIPAA professional claim implementation guide, and a co-author of "The AMA's Field Guide to HIPAA". She received her PhD in health education from the University of Utah.

Rentala Satyanarayana, research scholar, Centre for Biotechnology, Jawaharlal Nehru Technological University, Hyderabad, India finished his M.Tech. in Biotechnology from Jawaharlal Nehru Technological University. He has more than 7 years of research experience and 8 years of teaching experience. He worked in National Institute of Immunology- New Delhi, Intas Pharma-Ahmedabad, Gujarat, and Justus-Liebig University-Giessen, Germany and at present in Centre for Biotechnology, Jawaharlal Nehru Technological University-Hyderabad on Stem Cells and Cancer Biology. He has trained many B.Tech. and M.Tech. students in Biomedical informatics.

Sarkar Anita ,She was born in Calcutta, the City of Joy, where she schooled and spent her formative years. She received the Jagriti Independence Scholarship from the Government of India, for excellence in academics [1998-1999]. She graduated from the University of Delhi in Zoology (Hons.) with a gold medal [2006]. She completed her Master's in Bioinformatics from Jamia Millia Islamia, New Delhi [2008]. Her Master's thesis was "Determination of Secondary Structure of ADF/Cofilin Protein from *Leishmania donovani* Using NMR Spectroscopy" at the Central Drug Research Institute, India. She was a Junior Research Fellow in the laboratory of D. Sundar at Indian Institute of Technology (IIT) Delhi [2008]. She worked on a few projects including Parkinson's disease, G-Protein Coupled receptors and Zinc Finger Proteins. She received the Schrödinger Best Poster Award for scientific poster presentation at the National Conference on Drug Discovery & Development [2009]. She received the Marie Curie Fellowship [2009] for Doctoral studies at CERMAV, CNRS in the EuroGlycoArrays Network. Her area of interests includes molecular modelling, protein-protein and protein-carbohydrate interactions, structure-functions relationships and structural biology.

Sarkar Subir Kumar received the B. Tech and M. Tech. Degree from the Institute of Radio Physics and Electronics, University of Calcutta in 1981 and 1983, respectively and PhD (Tech) degree in Micro-electronics from University of Calcutta. He joined as a faculty member in the Dept. of Electronics and Telecommunication Engineering, Bengal Engineering and Science University, Shibpur in 1992. Thereby he joined in Jadavpur University in the same dept. where he is presently a Professor. He has published three Engineering text books (from CRC, USA) and more than 300 technical research papers in archival journals and peer – reviewed conferences. Seventeen students have been awarded PhD (Engg) degree under his guidance and twelve more are presently perusing PhD under his guidance. He is on the TCP of several major international/ national conferences/ symposiums and was the organizing Secretary of International conferences on communications, devices and intelligent systems. As Principal Investigator he has successfully completed four R&D projects and two more are running. He has visited several countries like France, UK, Switzerland and Japan for Technical reasons like training, presenting papers or visiting sophisticated laboratories. He was invited as a post doctoral Research scholar in the Dept. of Electrical and Computer Engineering, Virginia Commonwealth University to work on quantum computing, spintronics, quantum dot memory and electronic transport in Nanostructures. His most recent research focus is in the areas of digital image processing, watermarking signal processing, low power VLSI design, ad hoc wireless networks, wireless mobile communication. He is a life Fellow of the Institution of Engineers and Institution of Electronics and Telecommunication Engineers, life member of Indian Association for the cultivation of Science.

Srinivasan Anand received his B.S. in Biotechnology from Anna University, Chennai, India in 2008. He is currently pursuing his M.S. in Biomedical Engineering at the University of Texas at San

Antonio, TX, USA. His research interests are in high-throughput screening, microfluidics, and anti-fungal drug discovery.

Srivastava Shilpi had born at Allahabad on September 29, 1975, and raised in Nagpur. Mrs. Srivastava had done her schooling from St. Joseph's Convent High School, Nagpur; graduation in BSc (Bio) from Nagpur University; and Masters in Industrial Relation and Personnel Management from Nagpur University. She had served as an editor in the medical transcription firm in Nagpur named DMC Management Consultants Ltd. and had worked as an home-based transcription editor with the same firm for 8 years. This is Mrs. Srivastava first publication as an author in the field of medical transcription, which provides a broader perspective on the impact of technology on the process of medical transcription and its academic interest.

Sundar Durai ,D. Sundar was born and raised in Pondicherry, India. He received his B.Sc., M.Sc. and M.Phil. degrees in Life Sciences from Pondicherry University, India. He also completed his Ph.D. from Pondicherry University, working with Prof. A.R. Reddy. After a Postdoctoral Fellowship with Srinivasan Chandrasegaran and Marc Ostermeier in the Department of Environmental Health Sciences and Department of Chemical and Biomolecular Engineering at the Johns Hopkins University, Baltimore, USA, he started his independent career in the Centre of Excellence in Bioinformatics at Pondicherry University in 2005. He moved to the Indian Institute of Technology (IIT) Delhi in 2008 as Assistant Professor in the Department of Biochemical Engineering and Biotechnology. His research interests are in understanding the molecular recognition processes and in Computational Genomics. He has been bestowed with prestigious national awards including the Young Scientist Awards from the Indian National Science Academy and Indian Science Congress, the Innovative Young Biotechnologist Award from the Department of Biotechnology, Govt. of India and the Outstanding Young Faculty Fellow recognition from the IIT Delhi.

Wadhwani A.K. obtained B.E. (Electrical) from Bhopal University in 1987 and M.E. Electrical (Measurement & Instrumentation) from University of Roorkee, Roorkee in 1993 and Ph. D. in Electrical from IIT Roorkee in 2003. At present he is working as Reader in Electrical Engineering at Madhav Institute of Technology & Science, Gwalior. He has guided 03 doctoral and more than 25 Master's thesis and has more than 50 research publications in National, International Journals and conferences. He has undertaken good number of sponsored research projects from government institutions.He holds membership of many professional bodies. He is life member of ISTE, fellow of The Institution of Engineers (I), Institution of Electronics and Telecommunications (IETE) etc. He has organized a number of staff development programme and national conferences for the benefit of student, faculty and field engineers. His areas of interest are application of neural network, fuzzy logic and wavelets in Electrical Engineering, digital signal processing.

Wadhwani Sulochana obtained her B.E. (Hons) in Electrical Engineering and ME degree (Hons) with specialization in Control Systems from Rani Durgavati University, Jabalpur in 1991 and 1994 respectively and Ph.D. from IIT Roorkeee in 2006. From 1994 to 1999, she was with Bhilai Institute of Technology, Drug as a lecturer in the Department of Electrical Engineering. She worked in a DST sponsored research project at UOR, Roorkee from Jan'2000-March'2001. From May 2001-Nov 2003, she was SRF (CSIR) in the Department of Electrical Engineering, IIT Roorkee. Since Dec'2003, she is with Madhav Institute of Technology & Science, Gwalior. She has guided 01 doctoral and more than 20 Master's thesis and has more than 40 research publications in National, International Journals and conferences. She has undertaken good number of sponsored research projects from government institutions. Her areas of interest are Condition Monitoring of Industrial Drives, Measurement and Instrumentation, and Application of Artificial Intelligence in Electrical Engineering.

Wu Xu, Ph.D. is the director for Office of Public Health Informatics in the Utah Department of Health. She also holds adjunct faculty status in the Department of Internal Medicine, University of Utah School of Medicine. Dr. Wu is a co-investigator for the CDC-funded Rocky Mountain Center for Translational Research in Public Health Informatics. She leads Utah Department of Health's participation in statewide clinical health information exchange (HIE) and coordinates statewide strategic planning to promote full participation in HIE from all interested parties. She has published in peer-reviewed journals and authored government reports on healthcare statistics and health informatics. She has also served on various national workgroups and advisory panels. To better connect informatics research to public health practice is one of her career goals. Dr. Xu received her Ph.D. from Utah State University in 1996 with a specialty in health demography.

Yalavarthy Prameela Devi, Professor, Centre for Biotechnology Institute of Science and Technology, Jawaharlal Nehru Technological University, Hyderabad, India, finished her Ph. D. in Zoology from Sri Venkateswara University, Tirupati in1984. She has 27 years of research experience and 24 years of teaching experience. She achieved University Grants Commission research awardee in the year 2006 for the proposed work on development of low cost field kits for monitoring of environmental toxic chemicals. She has written 31 publications in international journals and more than 22 publications in National journals. Presently she is working as visiting scientist and research officer in Centre for Biotechnology, JNTUH of Institute of Science and Technology.

Index

Breinigsville, PA USA
02 August 2010
242803BV00003B/1/P